DRUG RESISTANCE

CANCER TREATMENT AND RESEARCH

Emil J Freireich, M.D., D.Sc. (Hon.), *Series Editor*

Nathanson L. (ed): Malignant Melanoma: Biology, Diagnosis, and Therapy. 1988. ISBN 0-89838-384-6.

Pinedo H.M., Verweij J. (eds): Treatment of Soft Tissue Sarcomas. 1989. ISBN 0-89838-391-9.

Hansen H.H. (ed): Basic and Clinical Concepts of Lung Cancer. 1989. ISBN 0-7923-0153-6.

Lepor H., Ratliff T.L. (eds): Urologic Oncology. 1989. ISBN 0-7923-0161-7.

Benz C., Liu E. (eds): Oncogenes. 1989. ISBN 0-7923-0237-0.

Ozols R.F. (ed): Drug Resistance in Cancer Therapy. 1989. ISBN 0-7923-0244-3.

Surwit E.A., Alberts D.S. (eds): Endometrial Cancer. 1989. ISBN 0-7923-0286-9.

Champlin R. (ed): Bone Marrow Transplantation. 1990. ISBN 0-7923-0612-0.

Goldenberg D. (ed): Cancer Imaging with Radiolabeled Antibodies. 1990. ISBN 0-7923-0631-7.

Jacobs C. (ed): Carcinomas of the Head and Neck. 1990. ISBN 0-7923-0668-6.

Lippman M.E., Dickson R. (eds): Regulatory Mechanisms in Breast Cancer: Advances in Cellular and Molecular Biology of Breast Cancer. 1990. ISBN 0-7923-0868-9.

Nathanson, L. (ed): Malignant Melanoma: Genetics, Growth Factors, Metastases, and Antigens. 1991. ISBN 0-7923-0895-6.

Sugarbaker, P.H. (ed): Management of Gastric Cancer. 1991. ISBN 0-7923-1102-7.

Pinedo H.M., Verweij J., Suit, H.D. (eds): Soft Tissue Sarcomas: New Developments in the Multidisciplinary Approach to Treatment. 1991. ISBN 0-7923-1139-6.

Ozols, R.F. (ed): Molecular and Clinical Advances in Anticancer Drug Resistance. 1991. ISBN 0-7923-1212-0.

Muggia, F.M. (ed): New Drugs, Concepts and Results in Cancer Chemotherapy 1991. ISBN 0-7923-1253-8.

Dickson, R.B., Lippman, M.E. (eds): Genes, Oncogenes, and Hormones: Advances in Cellular and Molecular Biology of Breast Cancer. 1992. ISBN 0-7923-1748-3.

Humphrey, G. Bennett, Schraffordt Koops, H., Molenaar, W.M., Postma, A. (eds): Osteosarcoma in Adolescents and Young Adults: New Developments and Controversies. 1993. ISBN 0-7923-1905-2.

Benz, C.C., Liu, E.T. (eds): Oncogenes and Tumor Suppressor Genes in Human Malignancies. 1993. ISBN 0-7923-1960-5.

Freireich, E.J., Kantarjian, H. (eds): Leukemia: Advances in Research and Treatment. 1993. ISBN 0-7923-1967-2.

Dana, B.W. (ed): Malignant Lymphomas, Including Hodgkin's Disease: Diagnosis, Management, and Special Problems. 1993. ISBN 0-7923-2171-5.

Nathanson, L. (ed): Current Research and Clinical Management of Melanoma. 1993. ISBN 0-7923-2152-9.

Verweij, J., Pinedo, H.M., Suit, H.D. (eds): Multidisciplinary Treatment of Soft Tissue Sarcomas. 1993. ISBN 0-7923-2183-9.

Rosen, S.T., Kuzel, T.M. (eds): Immunoconjugate Therapy of Hematologic Malignancies. 1993. ISBN 0-7923-2270-3.

Sugarbaker, P.H. (ed): Hepatobiliary Cancer. 1994. ISBN 0-7923-2501-X.

Rothenberg, M.L. (ed): Gynecologic Oncology: Controversies and New Developments. 1994. ISBN 0-7923-2634-2.

Dickson, R.B., Kippman, M.E. (eds): Mammary Tumorigenesis and Malignant Progression. 1994. ISBN 0-7923-2647-4.

Hansen, H.H. (ed): Lung Cancer. Advances in Basic and Clinical Research. 1994. ISBN 0-7923-2835-3.

Goldstein, L.J., Ozols, R.F. (eds): Anticancer Drug Resistance. Advances in Molecular and Clinical Research. 1994. ISBN 0-7923-2836-1.

Hong, W.K., Weber, R.S. (eds): Head and Neck Cancer. Basic and Clinical Aspects. 1994. ISBN 0-7923-3015-3.

Thall, P.F. (ed): Recent Advances in Clinical Trial Design and Analysis. 1995. ISBN 0-7923-3235-0.

Buckner, C.D. (ed): Technical and Biological Components of Marrow Transplantation. 1995. ISBN 0-7923-3394-2.

Muggia, F.M. (ed): Concepts, Mechanisms, and New Targets for Chemotherapy. 1995. ISBN 0-7923-3525-2.

Klastersky, J. (ed): Infectious Complications of Cancer. 1995. ISBN 0-7923-3598-8.

Kurzrock, R., Talpaz, M. (eds): Cytokines: Interleukins and Their Receptors. 1995. ISBN 0-7923-3636-4.

Sugarbaker, P. (ed): Peritoneal Carcinomatosis: Drugs and Diseases. 1995. ISBN 0-7923-3726-3.

Sugarbaker, P. (ed): Peritoneal Carcinomatosis: Principles of Management. 1995. ISBN 0-7923-3727-1.

Dickson, R.B., Lippman, M.E. (eds): Mammary Tumor Cell Cycle, Differentiation, and Metastasis. 1995. ISBN 0-7923-3905-3.

Freireich, E.J., Kantarjian, H. (eds): Molecular Genetics and Therapy of Leukemia. 1995. ISBN 0-7923-3912-6.

Cabanillas, F., Rodriguez, M.A. (eds): Advances in Lymphoma Research. 1996. ISBN 0-7923-3929-0.

DRUG RESISTANCE

Edited by
WILLIAM N. HAIT, M.D., Ph.D.
The Cancer Institute of New Jersey
University of Medicine and Dentistry of New Jersey
Robert Wood Johnson Medical School
Piscataway, New Jersey

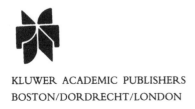

KLUWER ACADEMIC PUBLISHERS
BOSTON/DORDRECHT/LONDON

Distributors for North America:
Kluwer Academic Publishers
101 Philip Drive
Assinippi Park
Norwell, Massachusetts 02061 USA

Distributors for all other countries:
Kluwer Academic Publishers Group
Distribution Centre
Post Office Box 322
3300 AH Dordrecht, THE NETHERLANDS

Library of Congress Cataloging-in-Publication Data
Drug resistance / edited by William N. Halt.
    p. cm. — (Cancer treatment and research : CTAR 87)
    Includes bibliographical references and index.
    ISBN 0-7923-4022-1 (alk. paper)
    1. Drug resistance in cancer cells. I. Hait, William N.
II. Series: Cancer treatment and research ; v. 87,
    [DNLM: 1. Drug Resistance. 2. Antineoplastic Agents—
pharmacology. 3. Neoplasms—drug therapy. W1 CA693 v.87 1996 /
QV 267 D794 1996]
RC271.C3D78 1996
616.99'4061—dc20
DNLM/DLC
for Library of Congress   96-7538
                                       CIP

Printed on acid-free paper.

PRINTED IN THE UNITED STATES OF AMERICA

CONTENTS

CONTRIBUTING AUTHORS

James A. Allay, Ph.D.
Division of Hematology and Oncology
Department of Medicine and the CWRU/Ireland Cancer Center
Case Western Reserve University School of Medicine
University Hospitals of Cleveland
BRB-3
10900 Euclid Avenue
Cleveland, OH 44106-4937

Carmen J. Allegra, M.D.
Chief, NCI—Navy Medical Oncology Branch
National Cancer Institute
Division of Cancer Treatment
Naval Hospital Bethesda
8901 Wisconsin Avenue
Building 8, Room 5101
Bethesda, MD 20889-5105

Clay M. Anderson, M.D.
Fellow, Medical Oncology
Department of Medical Oncology
Melanoma/Sarcoma Section

Division of Medicine
The University of Texas
M.D. Anderson Cancer Center
Box 77
1515 Holcombe Blvd.
Houston, TX 77030

Brenda Brankin, Ph.D.
Vincent T. Lombardi Cancer Center
The Research Building, Room W405A
Georgetown University School of Medicine
3970 Reservoir Road NW
Washington, DC 20007-2197

Nils Brünner, M.D., Ph.D.
Finsen Laboratory
Strandboulevarden 49
Copenhagen, DK-2100
Denmark

Antonio C, Buzaid, M.D.
Assistant Professor of Medicine
Department of Medical Oncology
Melanoma/Sarcoma Section
Division of Medicine
The University of Texas
M.D. Anderson Cancer Center
Box 77
1515 Holcombe Blvd.
Houston, TX 77030

Anna M. Casazza, Ph.D.
Executive Director
Experimental Therapeutics
Oncology Drug Discovery
Bristol-Myers Squibb
Pharmaceutical Research Institute
P.O. Box 4000
Princeton, NJ 08543-4000

Yung-chi Cheng, Ph.D.
Yale Cancer Center
Yale University School of Medicine
Department of Pharmacology

333 Cedar St., NSB 287
New Haven, CT 06520

Edward Chu, M.D.
NCI—Navy Medical Oncology Branch
National Cancer Institute
National Institutes of Health
Bethesda, MD 20889

Robert Clarke, Ph.D.
Associate Professor
Department of Physiology & Biophysics
Director, Lombardi Cancer Center Animal Core Program
Georgetown University School of Medicine
The Research Building, Room W405A
Vincent T. Lombardi Cancer Center
3970 Reservoir Road NW
Washington, DC 20007-2197

Susan P.C. Cole, Ph.D.
Career Scientist of the Ontario Cancer Foundation
Professor of Oncology
Cancer Research Laboratories
Queen's University
Kingston, Ontario, Canada K7L 3N6

Roger G. Deeley, Ph.D.
Stauffer Research Professor
Cancer Research Laboratories
Queen's University
Kingston, Ontario, Canada K7L 3N6

Pu Duann, M.D., Ph.D.
Department of Pharmacology
University of Medicine and Dentistry of New Jersey
Robert Wood Johnson Medical School
Research Tower, Room 436
675 Hoes Lane
Piscataway, NJ 08854

Craig R. Fairchild
Oncology Drug Discovery & Exploratory Research
Bristol-Myers Squibb

Pharmaceutical Research Institute
P.O. Box 4000
Princeton, NJ 08543-4000

James M. Ford, M.D.
Departments of Biological Sciences and Internal Medicine (Oncology)
Herrin Biology Laboratories
Stanford University
Stanford, CA 94305-5020

Edward P. Gelmann, M.D.
Professor of Medicine and Cell Biology
Division of Hematology/Oncology
Department of Medicine
Lombardi Cancer Center
Georgetown University Medical Center
3800 Reservoir Road, NW
Washington, DC 20007

Stanton L. Gerson, M.D.
Division of Hematology and Oncology
Department of Medicine and the CWRU/Ireland Cancer Center
Case Western Reserve University School of Medicine
University Hospitals of Cleveland
BRB-3
10900 Euclid Avenue
Cleveland, OH 44106-4937

Elizabeth A. Grimm, Ph.D.
Professor of Biology
Department of Tumor Biology
Division of Research
The University of Texas
M.D. Anderson Cancer Center
Box 77
1515 Holcombe Blvd.
Houston, TX 77030

William N. Hait, M.D., Ph.D.
The Cancer Institute of New Jersey
Departments of Medicine and Pharmacology
University of Medicine and Dentistry of New Jersey
Robert Wood Johnson Medical School
679 Hoes Lane, Room 242

Piscataway, NJ 08854

Mattie James, M.S.
Vincent T. Lombardi Cancer Center
The Research Building, Room W405A
Georgetown University School of Medicine
3970 Reservoir Road NW
Washington, DC 20007-2197

Omer N. Koc, M.D.
Division of Hematology and Oncology
Department of Medicine and the CWRU/Ireland Cancer Center
Case Western Reserve University School of Medicine
University Hospitals of Cleveland
BRB-3
10900 Euclid Avenue
Cleveland, OH 44106-4937

Keunmyoung Lee, Ph.D.
Division of Hematology and Oncology
Department of Medicine and the CWRU/Ireland Cancer Center
Case Western Reserve University School of Medicine
University Hospitals of Cleveland
BRB-3
10900 Euclid Avenue
Cleveland, OH 44106-4937

Fabio Leonessa, M.D.
Vincent T. Lombardi Cancer Center and Department of Physiology & Biophysics
The Research Building, Room W405A
Georgetown University School of Medicine
3970 Reservoir Road NW
Washington, DC 20007-2197

Arnold J. Levine, Ph.D.
Department of Molecular Biology
Lewis Thomas Laboratory
Princeton University
Room 218
Princeton, NJ 08544

Tsai-Kun Li, Ph.D.
Department of Pharmacology
University of Medicine and Dentistry of New Jersey/

Robert Wood Johnson Medical School
Research Tower, Room 436
675 Hoes Lane
Piscataway, NJ 08854

Leroy Liu, Ph.D.
Professor and Chairman
Department of Pharmacology
University of Medicine and Dentistry of New Jersey
Robert Wood Johnson Medical School
Research Tower, Room 436
675 Hoes Lane
Piscataway, NJ 08854

Lili Liu, Ph.D.
Division of Hematology and Oncology
Department of Medicine and the CWRU/Ireland Cancer Center
Case Western Reserve University School of Medicine
University Hospitals of Cleveland
BRB-3
10900 Euclid Avenue
Cleveland, OH 44106-4937

Marc E. Lippman, M.D.
Vincent T. Lombardi Cancer Center
The Research Building, Room W405A
Georgetown University School of Medicine
3970 Reservoir Road NW
Washington, DC 20007-2197

Stuart Lutzker, M.D., Ph.D.
The Cancer Institute of New Jersey
University of Medicine and Dentistry of New Jersey/
Robert Wood Johnson Medical School
Department of Molecular Biology
Lewis Thomas Laboratory
Princeton University
Room 218
Princeton, NJ 08544

Daniel J. Medina, Ph.D.
Departments of Medicine and Molecular Biology
The Cancer Institute of New Jersey
University of Medicine and Dentistry of New Jersey

Robert Wood Johnson Medical School
679 Hoes Lane, Room 227
Piscataway, NJ 08854

Josephia R.F. Muindi, M.D., Ph.D.
Assistant Pharmacologist
Developmental Chemotherapy Service
Department of Medicine
Memorial Sloan-Kettering Cancer Center
1275 York Avenue
New York, NY 10021

John R. Murren, M.D.
Yale Cancer Center
Yale University School of Medicine
Department of Medicine
Section of Medical Oncology
333 Cedar Street NSB 287
New Haven, CT 06520

Philip G. Penketh, Associate Research Scientist
Department of Pharmacology
Yale Cancer Center
Yale University School of Medicine
Sterling Hall of Medicine
P.O. Box 208066
New Haven, CT 06520-8066

Weldon P. Phillips, Jr.
Division of Hematology and Oncology
Department of Medicine and the CWRU/Ireland Cancer Center
Case Western Reserve University School of Medicine
University Hospitals of Cleveland
BRB-3
10900 Euclid Avenue
Cleveland, OH 44106-4937

Giuseppe Pizzorno, Ph.D., Pharm.D.
Assistant Professor Internal Medicine
Pediatrics, and Pharmacology
Yale University School of Medicine
333 Cedar Street
P.O. Box 208032
New Haven, CT 06520-8032

Abhijit Raha, Ph.D.
Department of Pharmacology
Fox Chase Cancer Center
7701 Burholme Avenue
Philadelphia, PA 19111

Germana Rappa, M.D.
Yale Cancer Center
Yale University School of Medicine
Department of Pharmacology
Section of Medical Oncology
333 Cedar Street, NSB 287
New Haven, CT 06520

Elizabeth A. Rayl
Departments of Internal Medicine,
Pediatrics, and Pharmacology
Yale University School of Medicine
333 Cedar Street
P.O. Box 208032
New Haven, CT 06520-8032

Eric H. Rubin, M.D.
The Cancer Institute of New Jersey
University of Medicine and Dentistry of New Jersey/
Robert Wood Johnson Medical School
675 Hoes Lane, Room 526
Piscataway, NJ 08854

Alan C. Sartorelli
Alfred Gilman Professor of Pharmacology
Department of Pharmacology
Yale Cancer Center
Yale University School of Medicine
Sterling Hall of Medicine
P.O. Box 208066
New Haven, CT 06520-8066

Krishnamurthy Shyam
Associate Research Scientist
Department of Pharmacology
Yale Cancer Center
Yale University School of Medicine
Sterling Hall of Medicine

P.O. Box 208066
New Haven, CT 06520-8066

Todd Skaar, Ph.D.
Vincent T. Lombardi Cancer Center
The Research Building, Room W405A
Georgetown University School of Medicine
3970 Reservoir Road NW
Washington, DC 20007-2197

Roger K. Strair, M.D., Ph.D.
Departments of Medicine and Molecular Biology
The Cancer Institute of New Jersey
University of Medicine and Dentistry of New Jersey
Robert Wood Johnson Medical School
679 Hoes Lane, Room 102
Piscataway, NJ 08854

Kenneth D. Tew, Ph.D., D.Sc.
Department of Pharmacology
Fox Chase Cancer Center
7701 Burholme Avenue
Philadelphia, PA 19111

Jin-Ming Yang, Ph.D.
The Cancer Institute of New Jersey
University of Medicine and Dentistry of New Jersey/
Robert Wood Johnson Medical School
Department of Pharmacology
679 Hoes Lane, Room 239
Piscataway N J 08854

Nasir H. Zaidi, Ph.D.
Division of Hematology and Oncology
Department of Medicine and the CWRU/Ireland Cancer Center
Case Western Reserve University School of Medicine
University Hospitals of Cleveland
BRB-3
10900 Euclid Avenue
Cleveland, OH 44106-4937

INTRODUCTION

Resistance to treatment represents the final common outcome for far too many patients with cancer. Even our most promising new drugs fall victim to drug resistance. Hormones and newer biological therapies, though safe and active, also lose their activity over time.

In this volume of Drug Resistance, leading investigators in the field have reviewed the most basic mechanisms of drug resistance and have proposed ways to modulate resistance. These chapters cover a wide range of topics, including membrane transporters (*mdr* and *mrp*), resistance to microtubule agents such as Taxol, resistance to alkylating agents via glutathione S-transferase and O^6 alkyl transferase, and resistance to topoisomerase poisons. In addition, we have reviewed the mechanism of resistance to endocrine therapies, including agents that target the androgen and estrogen receptors, as well as resistance to differentiating agents, such as the retinoids. Lastly, Lutzker and Levine review the newly emerging role of P53 and apoptosis in chemosensitivity, Murren et al., review the development of multifunctional modulators of resistance, and Buzaid reviews the use of combination modalities to treat the most resistant of human malignancies, melanoma. This comprehensive volume should be of value for basic and clinical scientists who wish to delve more deeply into this intriguing problem in the laboratory and this devastating problem in the clinic.

W.N. Hait M.D., Ph.D.—
editor

I. MEMBRANE TRANSPORT MECHANISMS

1. P-GLYCOPROTEIN–MEDIATED MULTIDRUG RESISTANCE: EXPERIMENTAL AND CLINICAL STRATEGIES FOR ITS REVERSAL

JAMES M. FORD, JIN-MING YANG, AND WILLIAM N. HAIT

Clinical drug resistance to chemotherapeutic agents is a major obstacle for their curative potential in the treatment of human cancers. Multidrug resistance (MDR) is an important mechanism of cellular resistance to the cytotoxic activity of certain chemotherapeutic agents. Tumor cells selected for the MDR phenotype overexpress the *mdr*1 gene product, P-glycoprotein (P-gp), a membrane-bound drug efflux pump that confers resistance to a broad range of commonly used chemotherapeutic drugs and other agents. Numerous compounds have been identified that inhibit the efflux activity of P-gp, and reverse cellular resistance to cytotoxic agents in experimental systems [1]. This suggests that clinical drug resistance in human tumors, which often overexpress P-gp, may be potentially overcome through the concomitant administration to patients of a P-gp inhibitor with chemotherapeutic drugs.

P-glycoprotein–mediated MDR is only one of many cellular mechanisms by which tumor cells may evade the cytotoxic effects of anticancer agents, but remains one of the best understood and most intensively studied forms of mammalian drug resistance. Within two decades of the initial description of the MDR phenotype and its drug efflux characteristics [2,3,11], the cellular and biochemical pharmacologies of MDR have been carefully defined, the membrane protein responsible for drug efflux has been identified, its structure and function have been characterized, genes coding for P-gp and other related drug transport proteins have been cloned, P-gp has been shown to be functionally expressed in many human tumors as well as in normal tissues, a large number of drugs have been identified that inhibit the function of P-gp, and trials have been designed and executed to reverse clinical MDR in humans using these pharmacologic inhibitors. The scientific literature representative of the remarkable progess made in this field is now quite large, and many detailed reviews of these and other aspects of MDR have been published [1,4–8]. This chapter summarizes the biological mechanisms and clinical relevance of P-gp–mediated MDR and reviews the most exciting and important recent advances made in attempts to reverse MDR in both experimental and clinical settings.

CELLULAR PHARMACOLOGY AND MOLECULAR BIOLOGY OF MULTIDRUG RESISTANCE

The MDR phenotype was first described by Biedler and Riehm, who noted that following selection of mammalian tumor cells for resistance to a single cytotoxic drug, a broad crossresistance developed simultaneously to other structurally and functionally unrelated drugs [2]. Soon after, Dano noted that such drug-resistant cells displayed a decrease in accumulation of the anthracycline chemotherapeutic agent daunomycin due to its active outward transport [3]. Chemotherapeutic drugs now known to be affected by MDR include doxorubicin, mitoxantrone, vincristine, vinblastine, VP-16, taxol, and topotecan, but not drugs such as bleomycin, methotrexate, cisplatinum, or alkylating agents [6]. In addition, naturally occurring carcinogens, such as benzo(a)pyrene [9] and physiologic substances, such as hormonal steroids [10,80], also serve as substrates for the P-gp pump.

The most consistent alteration found in MDR cell lines is an increased expression of a high molecular weight cell surface glycoprotein (P-gp) not detectable in drug-sensitive cells, associated with an energy-dependent mechanism for the decreased accumulation and retention of cytotoxic drugs [11,12]. Ling and colleagues found that the presence of P-gp was correlated with both the degree of resistance and the relative decrease in drug accumulation [13]. Monoclonal antibodies to P-gp and nucleic acid probes for the mdr1 gene demonstrated that most MDR cell lines from rodent or human origin overexpress this gene [13,14].

Introduction of expression vectors containing cDNAs coding for P-gp confers the full MDR phenotype when transfected into drug-sensitive cells [15,16], and these stable transfectants overexpress P-gp and display enhanced efflux of cytotoxic drugs [17]. Furthermore, heterologous expression of mammalian mdr genes in bacteria [18] and yeast [19,20] confers drug resistance and ATP-dependent drug efflux of known P-gp substrates against a strong drug concentration gradient, independent of the membrane potential or transmembrane proton gradient [21]. Extensive studies of the biochemistry and molecular biology of the mdr1 gene product further support its role as an efflux pump of broad specificity that directly interacts with drug molecules to reduce their intracellular concentration. Structural analyses of P-gp accomplished by sequencing cDNA clones from P-gp encoding genes revealed it to consist of 2 homologous domains containing 12 predicted transmembrane segments, and 2 nucleotide binding domains [22,23], and to belong to a superfamily of ATPase proteins that behave as ion channels and transporters [24].

Rigorous proof of the drug efflux pump model for multidrug transport by functional reconstitution of P-gp in a highly defined system has long eluded

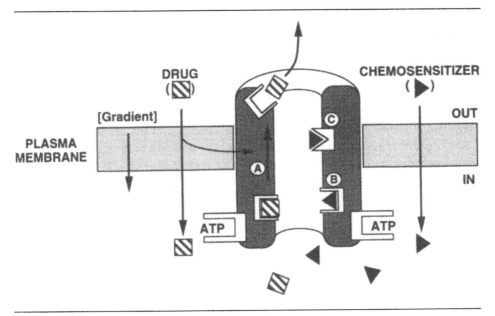

Figure 1–1. Functional representation of P-glycoprotein. The model depicts a translocating carrier protein, which utilizes ATP energy to actively transport drug substrate across the plasma membrane (A). Chemosensitizer may serve as a competitive inhibitor by occupying drug-binding sites (B) or as a noncompetitive inhibitor at chemosensitizer binding sites (C).

investigators due to difficulty in achieving efficient biochemical purification of the protein. However, several groups have now reported the purification and reconstitution of P-gp into phospholipid bilayers, which display constitutive ATP-dependent drug transport against a concentration gradient that is inhibited by chemosensitizers, and ATPase activity that is highly stimulated by chemosensitizers and MDR substrates [25,26].

Most models of P-gp suggest it functions to transport drugs across cell membranes in a manner analogous to that defined for active transport proteins (Figure 1–1). This model predicts that substrates (cytotoxic drugs) bind to specific domains of the protein, which subsequently undergoes an energy-dependent conformational change, allowing the substrate to be released on the exterior side of the membrane. Unlike other carrier molecules, P-gp is far less selective with regard to substrate. Identification and characterization of P-gp segments responsible for drug recognition and binding suggests that P-gp interacts directly with drug molecules. Efforts to map the drug-binding domains of P-gp by photoaffinity drug analogs and site-directed mutagenesis suggest that P-gp contains multiple nonoverlapping or partially overlapping drug-binding sites, each having different affinities for different drugs or classes of drugs [24,27–30].

In summary, P-gp functions as an energy-dependent multidrug transporter, and its expression forms the genetic basis for MDR. Furthermore, P-gp appears to function in a manner similar to that of active transport carrier proteins, although evidence remains insufficient to determine how closely it conforms to this model.

PHARMACOLOGIC REVERSAL OF P-GLYCOPROTEIN-MEDIATED MULTIDRUG RESISTANCE

A primary goal in the investigation of P-gp–mediated MDR is to discover specific means by which to reverse or circumvent it. Through the understanding of structural and functional features important for the inhibition of the MDR transporter, it is hoped that new agents for potential use in the clinic will be discovered. Tsuruo and coworkers first reported the pharmacologic reversal of MDR by showing that verapamil and trifluoperazine potentiated the antiproliferative activity of vincristine and produced an increased cellular accumulation of vincristine in an MDR murine leukemia cell line [31]. Since this original observation, numerous compounds have been shown to antagonize MDR in a variety of tissue culture assays and animal tumor models when coadministered with chemotherapeutic agents to which the cells are resistant. In general, agents used to antagonize MDR, termed *chemosensitizers* or *MDR modulators*, alter the drug accumulation defect present in MDR cells but exhibit little or no effect on drug-sensitive cells.

The majority of chemosensitizers described to date may be grouped into six broad categories, based on their primary pharmacologic activity: (1) calcium channel blockers, (2) calmodulin antagonists, (3) cyclosporines, (4) steroids and hormonal analogs, (5) dipyridamole, and (6) miscellaneous other compounds. Table 1–1 displays a partial list of the wide range of agents that have demonstrated ability to reverse MDR in preclinical models. Although these compounds share only broad structural similarities, all are lipophilic, and many are heterocyclic, positively charged substances.

Mechanism of multidrug resistance modulation

The primary mechanism by which most chemosensitizers are believed to antagonize MDR is through direct inhibition of drug efflux mediated by P-gp, resulting in restoration of cytotoxic drug concentrations in MDR cells. However, as is evident from Table 1–1, these compounds also possess a variety of other known cellular targets and pharmacologic effects. The broad and heterogeneous group of compounds that possess chemosensitizing activity and the multiple potential cellular targets for chemosensitizers suggest that a single, common target may not exist, but that a variety of interactions with different cellular targets may result in a similar effect on cytotoxic drug potentiation. Furthermore, there may be more than one receptor site on P-gp for anti-MDR drugs, which have unique structural requirements for efficient binding.

A simplified model of a potential mechanism of action for the ability of chemosensitizers to inhibit the MDR efflux pump is shown in Figure 1–1. In this scenario, P-gp functions as an active transport protein, which utilizes energy to transport cytotoxic substrates across the plasma membrane. Chemosensitizers may block cytotoxic drug efflux by acting as competitive or noncompetitive inhibitors,

Table 1–1. Selected pharmacologic agents with ability to reverse MDR

Calcium channel blockers[a]	*Immunosuppressive drugs*
Verapamil (5–10 μM)	Cyclosporin A (0.8–2 μM)
Nicardipine (3–10 μM)	SDZ PSC 833 (0.1 μM)
Niguldipine (10 μM)	SDZ 280-446 (0.1 μM)
Bepridil (2–4 μM)	FK506 (3 μM)
PAK-200 (5 μM)	Rapamycin (3 μM)
Ro11-2933 (2–6 μM)	
Calmodulin antagonists	*Vinca alkaloid analogs*
Trifluoperazine (3–5 μM)	Vindoline (20–50 μM)
Prochlorperazine (4 μM)	Thaliblastine (2 μM)
Fluphenazine (3 μM)	
trans-Flupenthixol (3 μM)	*Miscellaneous compounds*
	Dipyridamole (5–10 μM)
Protein kinase C inhibitors	BIBW 22 (1 μM)
Calphostin C (250 nM)	Quinidine (10 μM)
Staurosporine (200 nM)	Chloroquine (10–50 μM)
CGP 41251 (150 nM)	Terfenadine (3–6 μM)
NPC 15437 (60 μM)	Reserpine (5 μM)
	Amiodarone (4 μM)
	Methadone (75 μM)
Steroidal agents	S 9788 (1–3 μM)
Progesterone (2 μM)	GF120918 (0.02–0.1 μM)
Tamoxifen (2–10 μM)	Tolyporphin (0.1–0.5 μM)
Toremifene (5–10 μM)	
Megestrol acetate (5 μM)	
RU 486 (2–5 μM)	

[a] Concentrations in parentheses are those shown to have effect in reversing MDR in vitro.

perhaps by binding to similar drug/substrate binding sites, or to other chemosensitizer binding sites that cause allosteric changes resulting in inhibition of cytotoxic drug binding or transport. In support of this model, many studies have now demonstrated that certain chemosensitizers may directly bind to cellular membranes enriched for P-gp in a specific and saturable manner, and that this binding may be inhibited by other chemosensitizers and by chemotherapeutic drugs [27,32]. In addition, radiolabeled, photoactivatable chemosensitizer analogs irreversibly bind to P-gp, and this may be effectively inhibited by many other chemosensitizers [33–37].

An independent line of evidence that chemosensitizers interact with P-gp comes from the recent functional reconstitution of highly purified preparations of enzymatically active P-gp into phospholipid bilayers and the demonstration of an intrinsic ATPase activity that is stimulated by drug substrates and many chemosensitizers, but not by non-MDR chemotherapeutic agents [25,26]. However, conflicting evidence exists with regard to whether chemosensitizers of different classes function similar to inhibitors of drug efflux, how many binding sites exist for chemosensitizers on P-gp and where they are, and whether chemosensitizers share binding sites with cytotoxic substrates. Given the broad range of chemosensitizers, it is likely that several of these possibilites are relevant.

Recent studies utilizing P-gp molecules containing various mutations support the notion that more than one site of interaction for substrates and inhibitors exists. For example, substitution of a serine residue within the 11th predicted transmembrane domain of murine P-gp by any of six other amino acids resulted in both positive and negative effects on the modulatory abilities of different chemosensitizers [38]. Similarly, diverse effects were seen for the capacity of different chemosensitizers to inhibit drug efflux mediated by P-gp isoforms differing at a codon within the third transmembrane domain [39]. Also, photoactivatable binding of the chemosensitizer azidopine to P-gp has identified two distinct sites within the P-gp molecule, one between residues 198 and 440 of the amino half and the other within the carboxy portion of the protein [40].

Chemosensitizers may also serve as substrates themselves for the P-gp multidrug transporter, in support of their possible role as competitive ligands for drug-binding sites on P-gp. For example, verapamil , trans-flupenthixol, and cyclosporin A (CsA) are accumulated less in certain MDR cell lines [1,41,42]. Alternatively, certain chemosensitizers, such as the phenothiazines, might inhibit P-gp activity by interacting with physically separate sites on P-gp, such as the ATPase site or phosphorylation domains, or may act distantly, such as by inhibiting protein kinase C and altering the phosphorylation pattern of P-gp, thereby altering its activity. Indeed, phosphorylation of P-gp is associated with marked changes in drug transport [43], and many modulators of MDR are also inhibitors of protein kinase C [44]. The final delineation of P-gp drug-binding sites will be necessary to fully elucidate these mechanisms. Hopefully, a more sophisticated understanding of these processes will also lead to more powerful methods to manipulate P-gp function.

Classes of chemosensitizers

The variety of compounds identified as chemosensitizers (see Table 1–1) and their specific effect on MDR cell lines have been extensively reviewed elsewhere [1,6]. In the following section we discuss representative examples from each of the identified classes of chemosensitizers, and focus on those agents that hold potential for clinical use. The fact that many clinically used drugs are active chemosensitizers against MDR is a unique situation within the field of anticancer experimental therapeutics, since the clinical pharmacology of many of these drugs has been previously characterized. However, the necessity to achieve much higher than usual plasma and tissue levels presents considerable problems. Thus, knowledge of the dose-related toxicities and clinical pharmacokinetics for chemosensitizers is critical to the selection of optimal agents for successful use in humans.

Calcium channel blockers

The first identified compound with the ability to reverse MDR in vitro was verapamil [31,45,46], and it remains as an important standard agent for the comparison of potency and mechanism for all subsequently discovered chemosensitizers. This calcium channel blocker inhibits P-gp–associated, energy-dependent drug

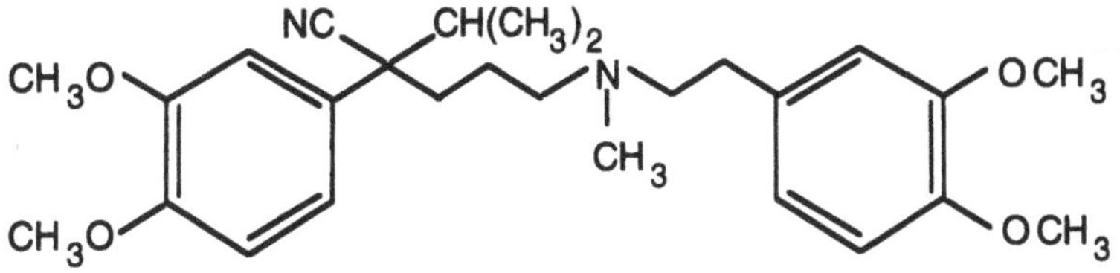

Verapamil

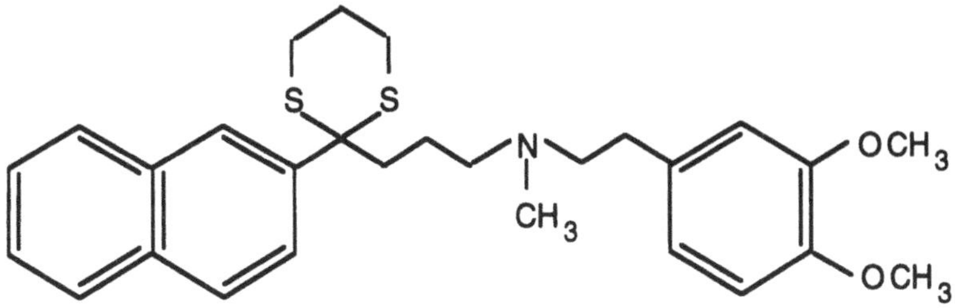

Ro11-2933

Figure 1–2. Structures of calcium channel blockers with chemosensitizing activity.

efflux in MDR cells, results in increased intracellular accumulation of chemotherapeutic agents, and is an effective antagonist of resistance to a number of drugs in most MDR cell lines in vitro [1]. Photoactivated verapamil analogs bind irreversibly to P-gp, and verapamil inhibits the binding of many chemotherapeutic drugs as well as other chemosensitizers to P-gp [27,34,47], suggesting that the mechanism of action of verapamil is through competitively blocking the binding of drugs to the transporter. Studies of many other MDR chemosensitizers demonstrate that most appear to function in a manner similar to that of verapamil, though with differing potencies, and perhaps with different sites of interaction on the P-gp molecule. Therefore, these critical studies of the effects of verapamil on the cellular pharmacology of MDR cell lines serve as a paradigm for the function of chemosensitizers in general.

In terms of clinical potential for MDR modulation, verapamil is limited by its cardiovascular effects in humans at plasma concentrations needed for antagonism of MDR in vitro [48]. Therefore, more potent and less toxic chemosensitizing agents than verapamil have been investigated. A structural analog of verapamil, Ro11-2933, was found to be up to 10-fold more potent than verapamil for increasing the cellular accumulation and sensitizing MDR cells to doxorubicin [49,50] (Figure 1–2). Plasma concentrations of Ro11-2933 effective for the reversal of MDR in cultured cells may be achieved, and this agent appears promising for clinical studies in humans.

A number of calcium channel blockers structurally dissimilar to verapamil have been studied for chemosensitizing activity and have been found to be active. While nifedipine is known to be a potent calcium channel blocker, it was a poor antagonist of MDR [51,52]. However, the dihydropyridine analogs, niludipine, nimodipine, and nicardapine, were found to be potent antagonists of MDR [51–53]. Recently, the chemosensitizing activity of 200 newly synthesized dihydropyridine analogs in human MDR cells was reported [54]. The lead compound, PAK-200, possessed the lowest calcium channel blocking activity, yet it fully reversed resistance to vincristine in a human MDR cell line. These studies confirmed the lack of correlation between pharmacologic calcium channel antagonism and anti-MDR activity.

Though most studies of verapamil use a racemic mixture of the drug, only the S-enantiomer selectively binds to calcium channels [55], whereas the S- and R-enantiomers of verapamil are equally active chemosensitizers [56,57]. Similarly, stereoisomers of many other calcium channel blockers differed markedly in their calcium channel blocking activity but were equally effective as MDR chemosensitizers [58]. In particular, the (−) isomer of niguldipine displayed a 45-fold lower affinity for calcium channel binding sites than its (+) isomer, but retained similar anti-MDR activity. Therefore, the use of less cardiotoxic enantiomers of verapamil and its analogs may provide a means for reaching clinically effective anti-MDR levels in patients. Already this strategy has been incorporated into ongoing clinical trials [59].

Calmodulin antagonists

The second class of MDR chemosensitizers to be identified includes drugs previously known for their ability to inhibit calmodulin-mediated processes and is represented by the phenothiazine calmodulin antagonist, trifluoperazine [45,46,60–62]. The examination of a series of phenothiazine derivatives and related drugs for potentiation of doxorubicin activity in MDR human breast cancer cells led to the identification of the thioxanthene class of calmodulin antagonist chemosensitizers, which possess significantly greater activity than phenothiazines against MDR [62] (Figure 1–3). The thioxanthenes exist as stereoisomers, and the *trans*-isomer of each in a series of 16 thioxanthenes showed greater activity than the *cis*-isomer for reversing MDR [37]. The lead compound, *trans*-flupenthixol, reversed MDR in a number of human and murine MDR cell lines, and in sensitive cells transfected with the *mdr*1 gene increased doxorubicin accumulation to a greater extent than either its stereoisomer *cis*-flupenthixol or verapamil (see Figure 1–3), and inhibited photoactive azidopine binding to P-gp [37].

The clinical pharmacology and toxicology of *trans*-flupenthixol suggests it may be uniquely suited for in vivo use. Clinical trials of the antipsychotic effects of thioxanthenes in humans showed the *cis*-flupenthixol was more effective and toxic than *trans*-flupenthixol [63]. This observation is explained by biochemical and crystallographic evidence that *cis*-flupenthixol is a potent antagonist of dopamine

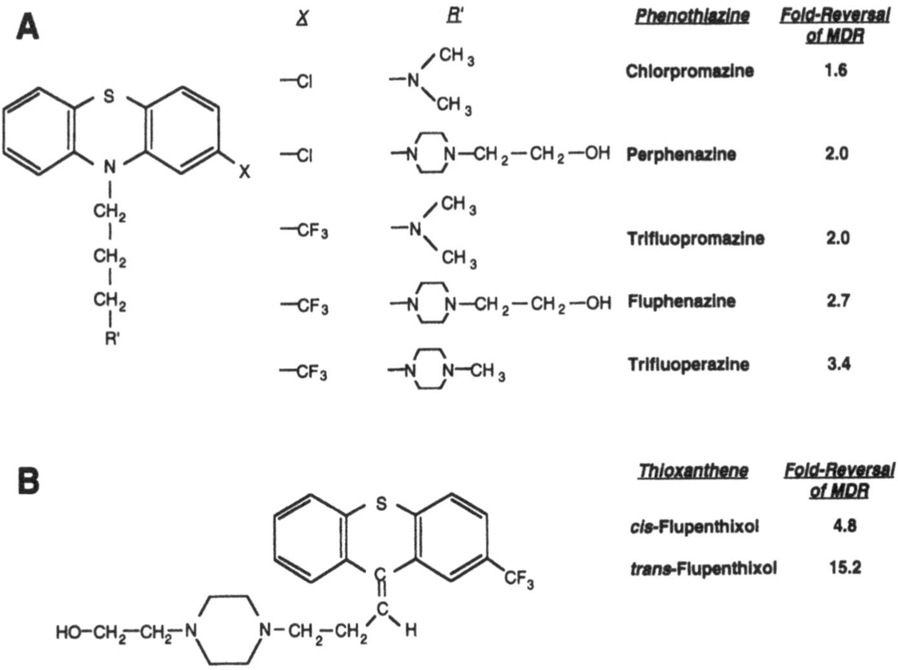

A

	X	R'	Phenothiazine	Fold-Reversal of MDR
	—Cl	—N(CH$_3$)(CH$_3$)	Chlorpromazine	1.6
	—Cl	—N⏜N—CH$_2$—CH$_2$—OH	Perphenazine	2.0
	—CF$_3$	—N(CH$_3$)(CH$_3$)	Trifluopromazine	2.0
	—CF$_3$	—N⏜N—CH$_2$—CH$_2$—OH	Fluphenazine	2.7
	—CF$_3$	—N⏜N—CH$_3$	Trifluoperazine	3.4

B

	Thioxanthene	Fold-Reversal of MDR
	cis-Flupenthixol	4.8
	trans-Flupenthixol	15.2

HO—CH$_2$—CH$_2$—N⏜N—CH$_2$—CH$_2$—C—H

Figure 1–3. Structures and anti-MDR activity of calmodulin antagonists with chemosensitizing activity. The fold-reversal of MDR was determined by measuring the relative ability of similar concentrations (3–5 μM) of phenothiazines (A) or thioxanthenes (B) to sensitize MCF-7/DOX human MDR breast cancer cells to doxorubicin. (Data from Ford et al. (1989), with permission [Reference 62].)

receptors [64,65], whereas *trans*-flupenthixol has virtually no activity as a dopamine antagonist, resulting in its apparent lack of extrapyramidal side effects [66].

Cyclosporines

Several immunosuppressive drugs, peptides with distinctly different pharmacologic and structural properties than other known chemosensitizing agents, have been found to possess unique and potent activities for modulating MDR. Cyclosporin A (CsA), a hydrophobic cyclic peptide of 11 amino acids that is widely used in human organ transplantation, was found to reverse resistance in MDR but not sensitive cells [67,68], although cytotoxic drug potentiation by CsA has been noted in certain sensitive cell lines [69–72]. Cyclosporin A also was found to affect MDR at concentrations lower than those necessary for most previously identified chemosensitizers (0.5–3 μM) [73].

The chemosensitizing effect of CsA on MDR appears complex. Cyclosporin A is accumulated less in P-gp–expressing cells [74] and is transported in a saturable manner across the apical surface of proximal tubule cell epithelium expressing a *mdr*1 cDNA [75]. Detailed kinetic analyses of the effect of CsA on drug accumulation and resistance in MDR Chinese hamster cells revealed CsA enhanced vincristine toxicity and accumulation in both sensitive and vincristine-resistant MDR cells, but by a 10-fold greater degree in the MDR cells [42]. Furthermore, CsA was a potent, competitive inhibitor of vincristine uptake by MDR cell membranes. Taken together, these results suggest the CsA may serve as a P-gp substrate and antagonize MDR, at least in part through competitive inhibition of P-gp–mediated outward transport of cytotoxic drugs, but also implies that CsA modulates cytotoxicity by other mechanisms. Thus, CsA appears to possess complex pharmacologic properties for modulating drug sensitivity, in accord with its known activity as an inhibitor of many important cellular enzymes.

There has been great interest in exploring the anti-MDR activity of other, less immunosuppressive or nephrotoxic cyclosporine analogs. Indeed, initial studies of several non-immunosuppressive analogs demonstrated modulation of MDR [67,68,71]. Numerous non-immunosuppressive cyclosporine analogs have now been studied for anti-MDR activity, and the cyclosporin D analog, PSC 833, was found to be 10-fold more potent than CsA, effective at a dose of 0.1 µM [76]. One micromole of PSC 833 has been shown to cause nearly complete reversion of drug resistance to taxol in rodent cells and was 30-fold more potent than verapamil [77]. A second non-immunosuppressive hydrophobic peptide being studied is SDZ 280–446, which appears similarly potent to PSC 833 for antagonism of MDR [78].

In summary, the cyclosporines sensitize MDR cells to a variety of chemotherapeutic drugs, either through a direct effect on P-gp, through alternative mechanisms of potentiation of chemotherapeutic drug toxicity, or a combination of these. This leads to the important possibility that CsA, in combination with other more P-gp–specific chemosensitizing agents, may act synergistically to antagonize MDR. The newly developed non-immunosuppressive cyclosporine analogs, particularly PSC 833, appear to be excellent candidates for the clinical reversal of drug resistance, due to their increased potency and specificity for P-gp–mediated MDR.

Steroids and hormonal analogs

The expression of high levels of P-gp in human adrenal cortex and placenta [79] suggests a possible role for the pump in physiologic transport of steroid hormones. In fact, cortisol and aldosterone are substrates for P-gp transport, though progesterone is not [10]. However, progesterone inhibits cytotoxic drug transport and binding to membranes from MDR cells and functions as a potent chemosensitizer [10,80–82]. These data suggest that the ability of a compound to act as a chemosensitizer and to inhibit transport of other drugs by P-gp is not necessarily related to its own ability to function as a substrate.

An orally active congener of progesterone, megesterol acetate (Megace), functioned as a chemosensitizer in human MDR cells and increased vincristine accumulation with two- to threefold greater potency than progesterone [83]. Paradoxically, Megace increased the binding of a photoactive calcium channel blocker to P-gp by up to twofold, while inhibiting labeled *Vinca* alkaloid binding to P-gp by 50%. These results strongly suggest that separate drug binding sites exist on P-gp for certain chemosensitizing compounds and drug substrates. Megace may be a poten-

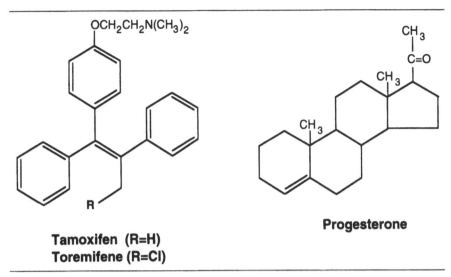

Figure 1–4. Structures of steroids and hormonal analogs with chemosensitizing activity.

tially useful clinical chemosensitizer, since high oral doses producing plasma levels of up to $2\,\mu M$ have been safely administered in trials of its anticachexia properties [84].

Synthetic steroid analogs have demonstrated particular promise for clinical use (Figure 1–4). Tamoxifen and the related antiestrogen toremifene are active chemosensitizers in a number of human P-gp–expressing MDR cell lines, independent of their effect on estrogen receptors [85–89]. For example, isobologram analyses demonstrate that tamoxifen synergistically potentiates vinblastine cytotoxicity and cellular accumulation in MDR human breast cancer cells [90]. Tamoxifen appears to act as a chemosensitizer by directly interacting with P-gp, as it has been shown to bind in a specific, saturable, and inhibitable manner to P-gp–enriched plasma membranes, and a photoactivatable analog irreversibly labels P-gp [91]. Like progesterone, however, transport of tamoxifen by P-gp was not detected.

The clinical pharmacology of antiestrogens makes them attractive for clinical use as chemosensitizers. Because of their relative lack of side effects, high serum concentrations have been achieved [87,92]. The major metabolite of toremifene, desmethyl-toremifene, possesses significant chemosensitizing activity itself. Thus, the in vitro and clinical pharmacokinetics of these antiestrogens suggest they may be well tolerated, effective chemosensitizers for use in combination with other chemotherapeutic agents in clinical drug resistance.

Dipyridamole

The antithrombotic drug dipyridamole has been shown to be a unique biochemical modulator of a variety of cytotoxic drugs of both MDR and non-MDR classes (Figure 1–5). Dipyridamole is a potent inhibitor of the salvage pathway for repletion of cellular nucleotide pools by nucleoside transport across cell membranes, and thus

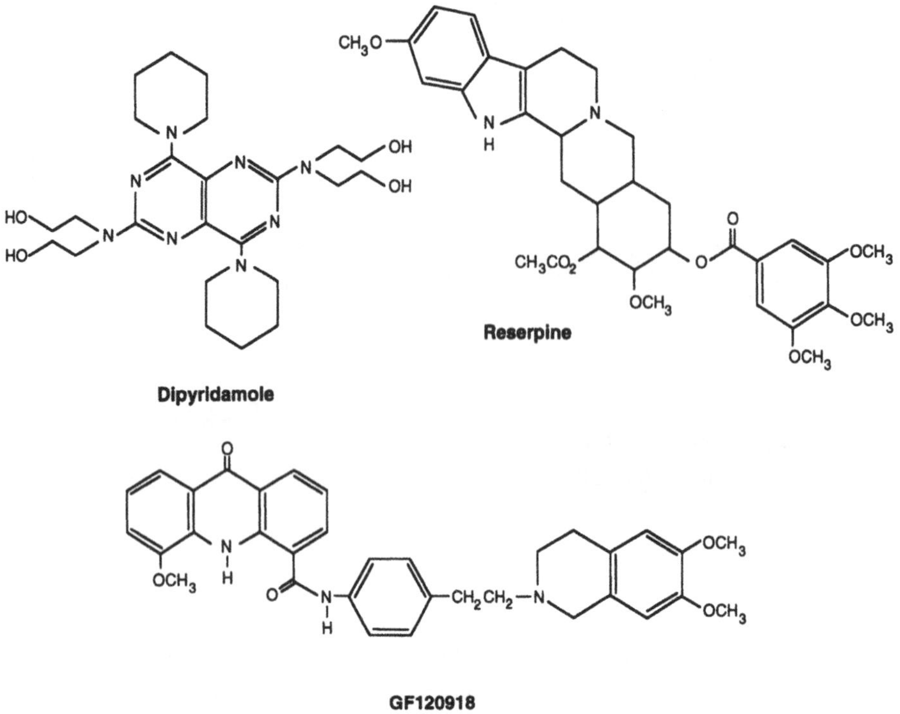

Figure 1–5. Structures of other compounds with chemosensitizing activity.

potentiates the activity of antimetabolites such as methotrexate [93] and 5-fluorouracil [94]. Dipyridamole also appears to modulate the cytotoxicity of cisplatin in various cell lines, although the mechanism remains obscure [95]. Recently, dipyridamole has been found to enhance the effects of several MDR-related drugs against both sensitive and resistant cell lines, potentially through multiple mechanisms, including inhibition of P-gp function. For example, nontoxic concentrations of dipyridamole interacted in a synergistic manner with VP-16, doxorubicin, and vinblastine in drug-resistant and -sensitive human ovarian carcinoma cells [96,97].

Recently, Cheng and coworkers described an analog of dipyridamole, BIBW 22, which displays markedly increased potency for the reversal of MDR and inhibition of nucleoside transport [98]. BIBW 22 was 10-fold more potent than dipyridamole in reversing vinblastine resistance in human MDR cells and completely inhibited photoactive azidopine binding to P-gp at concentrations of 1 μM. Furthermore, BIBW 22 was a 7-fold more potent inhibitor of nucleoside transport than dipyridamole, and resulted in a 20-fold enhancement of 5-fluorouracil cytotoxicity at 1 μM concentrations. Thus, this compound may have unique clinical properties as a "bifunctional modulator" in trials of combination chemotherapy employing both antimetabolites and *Vinca* alkaloids (reviewed in detail in Chapter VIII-16).

Miscellaneous compounds

The search for agents to circumvent MDR has led to the identification of numerous compounds not belonging to the previously discussed classes of chemosensitizers and not otherwise pharmacologically related (see Figure 1–5). Most of these compounds are lipophilic in nature and share a broad structural similarity that includes a heterocyclic ring nucleus separated at a distance from a cationic, amino group. This diverse group of chemosensitizing agents includes: antiarrythmics, such as amiodarone [99] and quinidine [100]; the quinoline amines, such as chloroquine [101]; the antimalarial, quinacrine [101]; the indole alkaloids, reserpine and yohimbine [102,103]; and the nonsedating antihistamine, terfenadine (Seldane®) [104]. Most have been reported to partially overcome resistance to cytotoxic drugs, and to increase drug accumulation and retention in various MDR cell lines.

Several newly identified calsses of chemosensitizers are of particular interest. The acridone carboxamide derivative, GF120918, possesses remarkable potency for reversing MDR, with concentrations as low as $0.02\mu M$ displaying similar in vitro activity as $5\mu M$ verapamil [105]. The triazinoaminopiperadine derivative, S 9788, has displayed potent in vitro activity [50,106], and increased intracellular daunorubicin accumulation in P-gp–positive clinical samples from patients with hematological malignancies more effectively than verapamil or CsA, as assessed by flow cytometry [107].

A novel class of compounds active against MDR has been identified by screening natural products extracted from strains of cyanobacteria (blue-green algae). Two such compounds, tolytoxin and cryptophycin, displayed significant cytotoxicity alone to both sensitive and MDR cells [108,109]. They did not effect vinblastine accumulation and were poor substrates for P-gp, and their activity for modulating *Vinca* alkaloid cytotoxicity appeared to be through microfilament depolymerization, and thus to be independent of P-gp. However, another cyanobacterial isolate, termed tolyporphin, functioned as a potent chemosensitizer [110]. This agent sensitized MDR cells to daunomycin, vinblastine, VP-16, and taxol at doses of $0.1\mu M$ and inhibited labeled vinblastine and azidopine binding to P-gp.

Structure–activity relationships among chemosensitizers

Although the broad specificity of P-gp for substrates and inhibitors has enabled the successful identification of many agents with chemosensitizing activity through screening efforts, rational drug development may uncover more potent and effective agents. Unfortunately, the lack of detailed crystallographic structural information of membrane-bound P-gp, or even detailed knowledge of the important protein binding sites of inhibitors, impedes a purely molecular approach to drug design for this target. Therefore, structure-based studies have been aimed at model chemosensitizer *pharmacophores* for P-gp inhibition. Most data suggest that while different chemosensitizers produce a wide variety of cellular effects and have multiple cellular targets, they share a common target site for reversal of MDR. Thus, these compounds must share certain structural features important for their chemosensitizing activity. It may be possible to define structural features that enhance the interaction of chemosensitizers with these target(s) by studying the anti-MDR activity of drugs within a single pharmacological class.

For example, critical structure–activity relationships were identified for a series of phenothiazines with individual molecular alterations for their ability to sensitize a human MDR breast cancer cell line to doxorubicin and included a hydrophobic tricyclic ring, a positively charged tertiary amine, and incorporation of the amino moiety into a cyclic structure [62] (see Figure 1–3). The structural principles derived from this study allowed the identification of the thioxanthenes, a structurally similar class of chemosensitizers that differ from the phenothiazines only by a carbon substitution for the nitrogen in the tricyclic ring, and by an exocyclic double bond to the side chain, creating stereoisomers for each thioxanthene analog. Similar to the phenothiazines, thioxanthenes with halogenated tricyclic rings and piperazinyl amino side groups were particularly effective chemosensitizers [37], and the *trans*-isomer of each thioxanthene pair was a more effective chemosensitizer than the *cis*-isomer. Ramu and Ramu subsequently studied a total of 543 phenothiazines and structurally related compounds, and came to similar conclusions regarding the structural features important for activity [111,112]. Pearce and colleagues found similar features for chemosensitizing compounds of different chemical classes, such as indole alkaloids [101].

A computer-aided approach to identifying structural features important for antagonism of MDR utilized chemical and pharmacologic information from 137 various compounds with documented chemosensitizing activity [113]. The computer program identified several *biophores*, which contributed to activity, and *biophobes*, which lessened activity. In fact, four novel compounds were designed and synthesized based on these predictions, and two were found to possess anti-MDR activity, demonstrating the validity of this approach.

Thus, systematic analyses of the structure–activity relationships of chemosensitizers such as the phenothiazines and thioxanthenes have defined particular structural features and spatial relationships important for anti-MDR activity. These imply a P-gp binding site with more stringent structural requirements for effective antagonism or partial agonist activity than previously imagined and should help to more precisely define this protein domain. Based on our data with MDR and the structural requirements found important for the binding of phenothiazines to calmodulin [114], we have proposed a model incorporating the importance of hydrophobicity and molecular structure for the interaction of phenothiazines or thioxanthenes with P-gp [115]. In this schema, the P-gp drug binding site is contained within a transmembrane α-helical segment containing a hydrophobic region separated by one-half turn of the helix from a hydrophilic region [116]. The hydrophobic pocket is produced by two aromatic phenylalanines residues, which are separated by two or three amino acids, and are oriented by the α-helix in such a way as to form a charge transfer complex with the aromatic, tricyclic groups in the phenothiazines or thioxanthenes. In fact, such phenylalanine repeat motifs exist in several transmembrane regions of human and murine P-gp [22,23], which are known to be labeled by azidopine [117].

NEW APPROACHES FOR MODULATION OF MULTIDRUG RESISTANCE

Although the most promising chemosensitizers to emerge from in vitro studies have not yet been adequately tested in clinical trials, alternative approaches to the reversal of MDR are also of interest. The increased understanding of the molecular biology of MDR has revealed alternative ways in which to affect P-gp function through novel pharmacologic, immunologic, and molecular means.

Combination chemosensitizers

The major limiting factor for achieving what are thought to be adequate human serum concentrations of chemosensitizers to reverse MDR are their intrinsic side effects. Therefore, a similar strategy to that originally proposed for combination chemotherapy may prove effective for the pharmacologic use of chemosensitizers; that is, by combining several chemosensitizing agents with nonoverlapping toxicities to achieve an overall anti-MDR effect greater than that possible with individual agents at higher doses. Studies of the pharmacologic affects of chemosensitizers have revealed that two agents, when used in combination, often result in additive [1], and occasionally supra-additive [118,119] activity for sensitizing MDR cells to cytotoxic drugs. Although determining the precise effects of combination chemosensitizers together with chemotherapeutic drugs on clinical pharmacokinetic parameters will prove challenging, the ability of this strategy to influence endpoints such as tumor growth and survival are awaited with great interest.

Modulating the post-translational modification of P-glycoprotein

By understanding the factors that regulate the function of P-gp, it should be possible to identify additional ways to modify its actions. Post-translational modification of P-gp through phosphorylation has been appreciated for many years, and a functional role has been suggested [120–126]. Exposure of cells to substrates for P-gp, including chemotherapeutic drugs and chemosensitizers, produces phosphorylation of the molecule above the basal levels [122,127], suggesting that means to interfere with this reaction could sensitize cells to chemotherapy.

P-gp can be phosphorylated by a variety of serine/threonine kinases and contains serine residues that resemble the consensus phosphorylation sites of protein kinase C (PKC), cAMP-dependent protein kinase, and calmodulin-dependent protein kinase II [125,126,128,129]. It has recently been shown that the major phosphorylation site on the murine *mdr*1b gene product was serine 669 when phosphorylated by PKC and serine 681 when phosphorylated by protein kinase A [130]. Similarly, the major phosphorylation site on human P-gp was a serine located within the linker region of the molecule [131]. Whether PKC or other kinases are the physiologic mediators of phosphorylation in human cancers remains unknown.

Protein kinase C has been shown to phosphorylate P-gp in cell membranes [132] and in immunoprecipitates [133,134], and is translocated to cell membranes in response to phorbol 12-myristate 13-acetate (PMA) in a manner temporally consistent with changes in drug accumulation [135]. PKC forms a stable complex with P-gp in intact cells as measured by co-immunoprecipitation with antibodies against both PKC and P-gp [134]. Treatment of sensitive cells with activators of PKC, such as phorbol esters, decreased the accumulation of chemotherapeutic drugs [136,137] and mimicked the MDR phenotype [123,137]. Treatment of MDR cells with PKC activators further increased drug resistance [122,123].

Just as activators of PKC seemed to augment the MDR phenotype, inhibitors of PKC appear to diminish it [138,139]. In fact, many of the commonly used chemosensitizers, including phenothiazines, thioxanthenes, tamoxifen, and CsA, are inhibitors, albeit weak ones, of the enzyme [37,44,140–143]. However, most studies of PKC inhibitors are complicated by the fact that many of these drugs interact directly with P-gp as well [37,143–145]. Using concentrations of staurosporine (300 nM) well below those required to inhibit azidopine binding to P-gp, Aftab et al. found that the phosphorylation of P-gp was increased and that the accumulation of vinblastine was decreased in MCF-7 MDR cells [134].

Evidence from our studies and others suggests that PKC may be a physiologic regulator of P-gp–mediated drug transport. In addition, the activity of this enzyme would be upregulated in MDR cell lines selected for resistance by chronic exposure to chemotherapeutic drugs if the drugs were inhibitors of the enzyme [146]. In fact, *Vinca* alkaloids and anthracyclines inhibited the activity of PKC purified from MDR cells [146], and PKC activity is increased in a variety of MDR cells compared with that of parental lines [123,145,147–149]. Furthermore, phosphorylation of P-gp is associated with marked changes in drug transport kinetics [43].

PKC exists as a family of at least eight isozymes that are differentially expressed in tissues [150], suggesting the selective alteration of PKC activity in tumor MDR cells may be possible. The isozymes are divided into two subfamilies: α, β (I/II), and γ, which depend on calcium for activity [151,152], and δ, ε, ζ, and η/Λ [153,154], which do not. The expression of individual isozymes in MDR cell lines has been recently investigated. PKC γ is upregulated in human HL-60 MDR cells [147], while PKC α and β are overexpressed in murine P388 MDR cells [155]. Recently, Blobe et al. [156] examined PKC in MCF-7 MDR cells and found a 10-fold increase in enzymic activity due to a selective increase in the expression of PKC α. To determine whether overexpression of a single PKC isoenzyme could affect the MDR phenotype, Glazer and colleagues cotransfected MCF-7 cells with cDNAs for MDR1 and PKC α, and found overexpression of this isozyme increased both drug resistance and phosphorylation of P-gp [157]. Therefore, phosphorylation of P-gp may be a fundamental control point for the activity of the transporter. Drugs that inhibit the activity of this enzyme may sensitize cells to chemotherapy and act synergistically with modulators that displace drugs from P-gp.

Despite the intense interest in PKC in MDR, surprisingly little is known about the role of phospholipase C (PLC), an enzyme that is critical to the activity of this kinase in drug resistance. PLCs are a family of enzymes that, among other functions, catalyze the conversion of PtdIns(4,5)P_2 to Ins(1,4,5)P_3 and 1,2 sn-diacylglycerol. These two second messengers mediate the release of intracellular calcium and the activation of PKC, respectively [150]. There is reason to believe that the activation of PLC in MDR cells may be responsible for the cascade of events leading to the activation of PKC and phosphorylation of P-gp. For example, phosphoinositide turnover is increased in MDR cells [158], and growth factor receptors known to be linked to PLC are overexpressed in MDR lines of epithelial origin [159]. In fact, doxorubicin has been shown to increase phosphoinositide turnover and to increase the membrane concentration of diacylglycerol [160], and we found this to be associated with phosphorylation of P-gp [Yang, Chin, and Hait, unpublished].

Phosphorylation of P-gp by PKC may be a response to a variety of cellular stress mechanisms. Heat shock, a cellular stress mechanism that actives PLC [161], increased the phosphorylation of P-gp in MCF-7 MDR cells to a degree similar to that seen when PKC was directly activated by phorbol esters [162]. In fact, the PKC inhibitor, staurosporine, blocked the phosphorylation of P-gp induced by heat shock. These experiments provide evidence that the phosphorylation of P-gp can be regulated by cellular stress responses that activate PLC.

Since stimulation of phosphorylation of P-gp increased its function, then inhibition of dephosphorylation of P-gp may have similar effects. Therefore, we have studied the effects of phosphatase inhibitors on the phosphorylation and function of P-gp and have found that okadaic acid resulted in an up to 300% increase in phosphorylation of P-gp, associated with a rapid decrease in drug accumulation [Aftab, unpublished]. Relatively little is known about the enzyme(s) responsible for the dephosphorylation of P-gp, though protein phosphatase 1 and 2a are implicated from our okadaic acid results. The potential role of phosphatase 2b (calcineurin), a calcium/calmodulin-dependent enzyme that is known to form a triplex with cyclosporin and cyclophilin and may also play a role in the pharmacological actions of cyclosporin A.

Based on the work discussed earlier, we have developed a model for the regulation of P-gp by phosphorylation (Figure 1–6). Upon exposure of MDR cells to chemotherapeutic drugs, the phosphorylation of P-gp and its transport functions are increased. Through the activation of PLC, the generation of diacylglycerol leads to the translocation of PKC to its target, P-gp, in the cell membrane. We now have evidence that P-gp forms a complex with PKC, since both proteins are seen in co-immunoprecipitation experiments [134]. The phosphorylation of P-gp activates drug efflux, diminishes cellular stress, and returns the activity of PLC to the basal state. Following the metabolism of diacylglycerol, PKC relocates to the cytosol, thereby decreasing the rate of phosphorylation of P-gp. The dephosphorylation of P-gp by protein phosphatase(s) returns the transporter to its basal state.

Monoclonal antibodies against P-glycoprotein

Monoclonal antibodies recognizing P-gp have been explored as potential inhibitors of P-gp that may lack the side effects associated with pharmacologic agents. For example, both of the monoclonal antibodies MRK-16 and UIC2, which recognize distinct external epitopes on human P-gp, increase the intracellular accumulation and cytotoxicity of various chemotherapeutic drugs in MDR cells [163,164]. In addition, MRK-16 alone induced regression of tumors [165] and enhanced the in

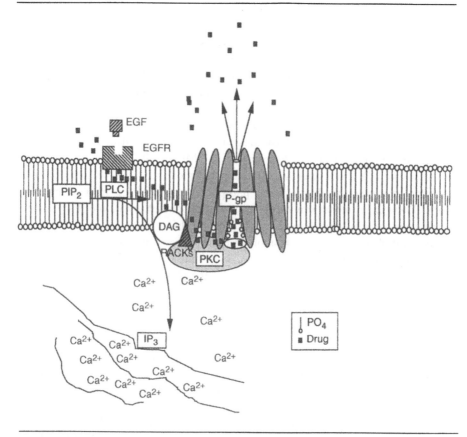

Figure 1–6. A role for phospholipase C in MDR. In this model, the activation of phospholipase C (PLC) by cellular stress, such as exposure to chemotherapeutic drugs or to certain growth factors, such as the epidermal growth factor (EGF), catalyzes the breakdown of phosphatidyl inositols (PIP2) to diacylglycerol (DAG) and Ins(1,4,5)P_3. The increased membrane DAG leads to the translocation of protein kinase C (PKC) to the plasma membrane, where it binds to the receptor for activated C kinase (RACKs) and phosphorylates P-gp. The production of Ins(1,4,5)P_3 causes the release of intracellular calcium. The phosphorylation of P-gp activates drug efflux, diminishes cellular stress, and returns the activity of PLC to the basal state. Following the metabolism of diacylglycerol, PKC relocates to the cytosol. Finally, the dephosphorylation of P-gp by protein phosphatases returns the transporter to its basal level of activity.

vivo activity of vincristine [166] in MDR xenografts in nude mice. Another provocative approach is the combination of the MRK-16 monoclonal antibody together with pharmacologic chemosensitizers, which has shown synergy with CsA but not verapamil [167]. Further investigation revealed that MRK-16 also caused an increased intracellular accumulation of CsA, but not verapamil, perhaps explaining this result.

Modification of monoclonal antibodies against P-gp have been made to enhance their antitumor activity. For example, MRK-16 antibodies coupled to *Pseudomonas* exotoxin exhibit increased activity for killing P-gp–expressing bone marrow cells in transgenic mice compared with the native monoclonal antibody alone [168]. Others have fused an anti–P-gp monoclonal antibody to doxorubicin-containing liposomes and have found an enhanced cytotoxic effect against P-gp–expressing cells compared with doxorubicin alone or liposomal doxorubicin without antibodies [169].

Thus, P-gp may serve as a target for potential immunologic therapies. The therapeutic use of antibodies in humans remains challenging. However, this approach to the treatment of MDR tumors may play a role alone or in combination with drug therapies.

Regulation of MDR1 gene expression

Studies of *mdr*1 promoter sequences provide insight into the mechanism of the regulation of *mdr*1 gene expression in normal tissue and tumor cells [170,171], and the presence of putative *cis*- and *trans*-activating transcriptional regulatory mechanisms suggests that modulation of P-gp expression may be possible at the genetic level. Numerous agents have been identified that increase the expression of the *mdr*1 gene, such as certain chemotherapeutic drugs [172], carcinogens [173], the differentiating agent sodium butyrate [174,175], ionizing radiation [176], progesterone [177], and oncogenes and tumor suppressor genes [178]. Therefore, agents may be identified that either block the induction of *mdr*1 gene expression or inhibit its promoter activity and downregulate P-gp expression. In fact, the cAMP analog, 8-Cl-cAMP, appears to possess this latter ability [179]. Preliminary results using a *mdr*1-CAT reporter construct also showed that 8-Cl-cAMP inhibits *mdr*1 promoter activity and downregulates P-gp expression [179]. The ability of this agent to specifically enhance cytotoxic drug activity or to alter drug accumulation in P-gp–expressing MDR cells has not been reported.

Phospholipase C may also contribute to the regulation of transcription of the *MDR*1 gene. For example, phorbol esters and diacylglycerol increased *MDR*1 gene expression in normal human peripheral blood lymphocytes, potentially by the activation of an AP-1 consensus sequence in the promoter region of the *MDR*1 gene [180]. In addition, potent activators of PLC, such as heat shock, arsenite, and cadmium, regulate *MDR*1 gene expression in a human kidney cell line [181]. These results raise the possibility that *MDR*1 expression might be induced by a variety of agents producing cellular stress, and that this stress response is mediated through PLC. Activators of PKC, such as phorbol esters, regulate the transcription of many genes, including c-*fos* and c-*jun*, which encode for proteins containing leucine zipper regions that form a heterodimeric transcription factor, AP-1. However, the mechanism underlying these observations remains unclear since the genomic sequences in the human *MDR*1 promoter are of limited homology with known AP-1 sites.

Ribozymes

An alternative strategy to disrupt the expression of P-gp and to potentially modulate MDR is through the molecular targeting of *MDR*1 mRNA using catalytic RNA endonucleases or ribozymes [182]. Several groups have now designed hammerhead ribozymes containing short sequences of *MDR1* mRNA that target GUC sequences near important P-gp functional domains [183–185]. In one study, such ribozymes site-specifically cleaved *MDR1* mRNA at sites near those coding for the P-gp codon 185 drug binding site. When cloned into a mammalian expression vector and introduced into a MDR tumor cell line, this ribozyme reduced the 700-fold vincristine resistance by 30-fold, concomitant with the decreased expression of *MDR1* mRNA and P-gp [183,186]. Other investigators have reported similar results using this strategy [184,185], which appears more efficient than previously attempted antisense RNA approaches. As with all gene therapy strategies, vector targeting and tissue-specific expression must be addressed to allow this technology to become clinically effective.

CLINICAL STUDIES OF MULTIDRUG RESISTANCE

The extensive experimental analysis of the function of P-gp in vitro has allowed for the investigation of its physiological role in humans and its potential relevance as a mechanism of drug resistance in human tumors. Strategies to reverse clinical MDR using P-gp chemosensitizers have also been translated into the clinic. The following section discusses the clinical relevance of P-gp and reviews clinical trials designed to reverse its function (also see [7,8]).

Expression of P-glycoprotein in normal human tissues

The expression and distribution of P-gp in normal human tissues suggests a variety of possible physiologic functions for this protein. For example, high levels of P-gp are found in the adrenal cortex, the proximal tubules of kidney, the apical biliary surface of hepatocytes, and epithelial cells of colon and jejunum [187–190]. The polarized expression of P-gp on the luminal surface of these tissues suggests either a physiologic role in secreting substances from these tissues, such as bilirubin [191] or steroid hormones [10], or a protective role by excluding potentially toxic xenobiotics or mutagenic chemicals [192]. P-glycoprotein is also expressed by endothelial cells of human capillary blood vessels at the blood–brain barrier and blood–testis barrier [193,194], suggesting that P-gp may serve to exclude various toxic compounds from the central nervous system and other pharmacologic sanctuaries.

Certain subsets of hematopoietic and lymphoid cells also express P-gp, including progenitor stem cells in the bone marrow [195], CD8+ T-suppressor cells, and CD56+ natural killer cells in peripheral blood lymphocytes [196,197]. The potential role for P-gp in the physiology of hematopoietic cells, possibly through secretion or presentation of specific peptide signals, remains obscure. However, the implication of this finding is profound with regard to the potential cytotoxic effect on stem cells and resultant myelosuppression in clinical trials of chemosensitizers in combination with cytotoxic drugs.

The recent generation of transgenic "knock-out" mice with homozygous disruptions of *mdr* genes provides additional information regarding the physiologic role of P-gp. Two genes homologous to human *MDR1* exist in mice, *mdr*1a and *mdr*1b, both of which exhibit drug transport capabilities. Mice lacking the *mdr*1a gene were hypersensitive to the effects of a neurotoxin and displayed significantly increased tissue concentrations of vinblastine following drug treatment in brain, muscle, and small intestine [198]. The phenotype of *mdr*1b-deficient mice has not yet been reported. Generation of mice with both *mdr*1a and *mdr*1b disruptions will provide the most relevant model for complete inhibition of human P-gp function. Similar experiments with mice lacking the *mdr*2 gene (homologous to human *MDR3*, which does not confer MDR) demonstrate that its protein product is essential for the secretion of phospholipids into bile [199]. Taken together, these data suggest that P-gp plays a critical role in a number of normal physiologic functions in human tissues, many of which may be related to secretion and/or protection of tissues from various naturally occurring toxins or commonly encountered xenobiotics.

Expression of P-glycoprotein in human tumors

Detection of *MDR1* expression in clinical tumor samples has been extensively studied to determine its potential role as a predictor of drug responsiveness. A clear relationship between the development of clinical drug resistance to MDR-related drugs and increased expression of *MDR1* mRNA or P-gp would argue favorably for the use of chemosensitizers in treating such patients. However, most studies to date have not been able to separate the role of increased P-gp expression as a poor prognostic factor, in general, from that of a specific determinate for chemoresistance to particular drugs.

In general, those cancers derived from tissues that normally express P-gp also constitutively express high levels of *MDR1*, such as colorectal cancers, renal cell carcinomas, hepatomas, and adrenocortical carcinomas [200–202]. In contrast, there are several tumor types that do not express *MDR1* in most cases, but often exhibit elevated P-gp levels following treatment with chemotherapeutic drugs, such as leukemias, lymphomas, breast cancers, and ovarian carcinomas [201,203,204]. Expression of P-gp in acute myeloid leukemias, in particular, appears to correlate with poor therapeutic outcome [205–207]. The potential clinical significance of *MDR1* tumor expression has been best documented in the studies of Chan et al., demonstrating a strong association between P-gp expression and both lack of chemotherapeutic response and poor survival in childhood soft-tissue sarcomas and neuroblastomas [208,209].

Recently, studies have begun to probe the role of P-gp in acquired drug resistance by measuring levels at diagnosis and at relapse after treatment with MDR-related drugs. For instance, in multiple myeloma, which initially responds to chemotherapy with vinblastine, doxorubicin, and dexamethasone in 70% of patients but nearly always relapses, quantitative immunohistochemical staining for P-gp in individual cells has shown that the myeloma cells of most patients express P-gp after relapse [210,211] and that the percentage of cells expressing P-gp in treated patients is significantly greater than in untreated patients [212,213].

Whether P-gp plays a functional role in the failure of initial chemotherapy in intrinsically resistant tumors or in the development of acquired resistance is not known. It is important to note that renal cell, adrenal, and colon carcinoma are also clinically resistant to drugs that are not known to be affected by P-gp, such as alkylating agents, antimetabolites, and bleomycin, and redundant or overlapping mechanisms of drug resistance in addition to P-gp–mediated MDR are likely to be present. Though P-gp is often increased in acquired drug resistance, many of these patients are also resistant to non-MDR classes of drugs. This suggests several possibilities: (1) that *MDR*1 overexpression reflects a general response of cells to toxic stress, (2) that P-gp is one of many cellular defense mechanisms produced by exposure to toxins, or (3) that P-gp expression is a specific response to chemotherapy and its antagonism could produce sensitivity to natural product chemotherapeutics.

At this time one can conclude that for certain tumors increased P-gp appears to be a marker for the existence of multiple mechanisms of drug resistance. To prove an association between intrinsic or acquired drug resistance and P-gp expression, careful analyses of the possible correlations between tumor P-gp levels and treatment responses to specific drugs must be performed, and prospective sampling of pre-treatment and post-treatment P-gp levels from individual patients must be determined. Finally, controlled trials designed to detect increased clinical response of tumors with intrinsic or acquired resistance to chemotherapeutic regimens containing inhibitors of P-gp function will be critical to understanding the therapeutic importance of clinical MDR.

Effects of chemosensitizers in human trials

The presence of detectable P-gp in many clinically drug-resistant tumors suggests that the addition of a chemosensitizer at appropriate doses may sensitize human tumors to chemotherapy regimens employing MDR-related drugs. Since P-gp is also expressed in many normal tissues, careful analysis of the toxicities encountered by combining P-gp inhibitors with cytotoxic drugs will be required to determine if a therapeutic advantage is achievable. A number of phase I and phase II trials of various chemosensitizers have now been reported [214].

Early attempts to combine verapamil with single-agent chemotherapy were hindered by cardiovascular toxities encountered at levels of verapamil nearing the effective anti-MDR range (3–6 µM) [48,215]. The use of verapamil with combination chemotherapy for lymphoma and myeloma has also been reported. In this trial, eight patients with multiple myeloma and non-Hodgkin's lymphoma, all refractory to standard treatment with 4 days of infusional vincristine and doxorubicin, and oral dexamethasone, were studied for tumor expression of P-gp and for response to treatment with the identical regimen plus verapamil [216]. Tumor cells from 6 out of 8 patients were shown to express P-gp by immunoperoxidase staining of bone marrow biopsies or node biopsies. Continuous infusion verapamil resulted in transient, objective remissions in 3 of 6 P-gp–positive patients. The two P-gp negative patients did not respond, nor did 3 of 6 P-gp–positive patients. Reversible cardiotoxicity was observed, but no increase in myelosuppression was noted with the addition of verapamil. A recent update of this study included 22 myeloma patients treated with this same regimen and showed 4 responses within a subset of 10 patients who had myeloma cells that expressed P-gp, whereas no responses were seen in 5 P-gp–negative patients [217].

These phase I/II trials suggest that clinical modulation by verapamil of an anthracycline/*Vinca* alkaloid–based chemotherapeutic regimen in tumors known to express P-gp may be possible. However, the toxic effects of verapamil at relevant anti-MDR concentrations have led to the clinical testing of other, potentially less toxic chemosensitizers.

The antiestrogens, tamoxifen and toremifene, have potential for clinical use in modulating MDR due to the expectation of minimal side effects at relevant doses [1]. A phase I study of high-dose tamoxifen (40–260 mg/m^2 twice a day for 12 days) combined with continuous infusion vinblastine in 53 patients resulted in serum tamoxifen concentrations of 6 μM without toxicity for most patients [218]. Reversible, dose-limiting toxicities were neurologic and occurred mostly at high dose levels.

Many current studies of clinical MDR modulation have employed CsA and its non-immunosuppressive analog, PSC 833, and several have now been published [214]. The Stanford trial of CsA plus VP-16 demonstrated that serum CsA levels of 2–4 μM could be achieved with acceptable toxicities, which included nausea, vomiting, myelosuppression, and reversible hyperbilirubinemia [219]. Pharmocokinetic studies demonstrated a marked increase of the area under the curve for VP-16 at target levels of CsA as a result of a decrease in both renal and nonrenal clearance mechanisms [220], and similar effects of CsA on the pharmacokinetics of doxorubicin [221], daunorubicin [222], and taxol [214] have been observed.

The CsA analogue PSC 833 has received considerable interest as a potential clinical modulator of MDR due to its nonimmunosuppresive and non-nephrotoxic profile, and 5- to 10-fold greater potency than CsA for reversing MDR in vitro. Preliminary results using PSC 833 in combination with VP-16 [223] and with taxol [224] have been reported. Serum concentrations greater than 1 μM have been achieved with an oral formulation of PSC 833, and the dose-limiting toxicity was neurologic, predominantly reversible cerebellar ataxia. Similar to CsA, marked pharmacokinetic effects of PSC 833 on chemotherapeutic drugs were observed, requiring approximately twofold reduction in VP-16 and taxol administered doses when combined with the chemosensitizer due to increased myelosuppression. Several apparent responses to either combination were observed in patients with cancers previously clinically resistant to VP-16 and taxol, respectively.

A single, randomized, placebo-controlled phase III study of clinical MDR modulation has been completed [225]. In this study, 223 women with metastatic breast cancer were randomized to receive epirubicin alone or epirubicin with quinidine. The median quinidine serum levels achieved was 5.5 μM, a chemosensitizer concentration less than that required to reverse P-gp–mediated MDR in vitro [1]. No significant differences were seen in the overall response rate or toxicity in the two treatment arms. There were also no detectable differences in the pharmacokinetics of epirubicin when administered with or without the chemosensitizer. Expression of MDR1 was not assessed. Therefore, it is difficult to draw strong conclusions from this study, which points out the complexities in carrying out large-scale, phase III trials to test this approach.

Other chemosensitizers that have been used in clinical trials to attempt to modulate MDR include trifluoperazine [226], quinine [227], progesterone [228], and the calcium channel blockers nifedipine [229] and bepridil [230]. Few conclusions can be drawn from these and other published phase I and II trials regarding the potential efficacy of chemosensitizers for reversing clinical drug resistance mediated by P-gp. Few of the studies thoroughly sampled tumors for the presence of increased P-gp expression, and even fewer prospectively selected patients proven to be MDR1 positive before entry into trials. Often, the concentration of chemosensitizer achieved in the serum without incurring significant toxicity was lower than that required for maximum activity in vitro. Although the serum concentration may not accurately reflect the concentration of these lipophilic drugs at their target sites, this will remain a question until more accurate assesments of in vivo chemomodulation are available. Finally, whether tumor P-gp can be selectively inhibited without unexceptable toxicities to normal tissue and whether effective inhibition of P-gp in vivo will result in improvements in clinical outcome remain important and unanswered questions.

The selection of appropriate tumors for studying MDR and its clinical modulation in future trials will be critical to testing the potential relevance of MDR. Criteria include selecting tumors that (1) consistently overexpresses P-gp but do not harbor multiple other mechanisms of resistance, (2) are either intrinsically resistant to drugs included in the MDR phenotype or acquire resistance to such drugs after initial treatment response, (3) are accessible for sequential biopsies, (4) result in reasonable life expectancy despite relatively early relapse, and (5) occur with relative frequency. As more specific and potent chemosensitizers with less clinical toxicity and side effects enter early clinical trials, it will be critical to carefully plan and coordinate prospective therapeutic trials and diagnostic procedures by measuring MDR markers at enrollment and relapse, achieving adequate serum chemosensitizer levels, and analyzing both tumor and plasma chemosensitizer and cytotoxic drug pharmacokinetics.

MDR1 and human gene therapy

Several strategies have been suggested for the use of the MDR1 gene in clinical trials of human gene therapy. For example, introduction and expression of MDR1 to confer drug resistance to progenitor stem cells from bone marrow of patients undergoing autologous stem-cell transplantation might allow for more intensive use of MDR chemotherapeutic drugs in patients with cancer while limiting the degree of myelosuppression. Alternatively, vectors may be constructed containing MDR1 in addition to another, nonselectable gene whose product would be beneficial, allowing for the in vivo selection of genetically modified cells containing this vector by treatment with an MDR drug. Initial attempts at such strategies have successfully demonstrated high-level and long-term expression of functional P-gp in transduced bone marrow stem cells engrafted into mice, and the level of drug resistance was substantially enriched following treatment with taxol [231–233]. Similar studies transducing CD34+ early human precursor cells with a replication-incompetent retrovirus carrying an MDR1 cDNA resulted in cells overexpressing P-gp and resistant to taxol when grown in cell culture [234]. Clinical trials reinfusing such genetically modified human stem cells into patients with advanced solid tumors following a marrow-ablative preparative chemotherapy regimen are currently underway, with the goal of delivering multiple cycles of dose-escalated MDR drugs (such as taxol) following re-engraftment [235,236]. Such studies will determine if genetic modification with MDR1 can protect a graft from chemotherapy-induced myelotoxicity and whether in vivo selection of the modified cells will increase their proportion and level of resistance.

SUMMARY

The study of the cellular, biochemical, and molecular biology and pharmacology of MDR has provided one of the most active and exciting areas within cancer research and one that holds great promise for translation into clinical benefit. While convincing evidence for the functional role of P-gp in mediating clinical drug resistance in humans remains elusive, studies of the clinical expression of P-gp and trials of chemosensitizers with cancer chemotherapy suggest "resistance modification" strategies may be effective in some tumors with intrinsic or acquired drug resistance. However, even if P-gp–associated MDR proves to be a relevant and reversible cause of clinical drug resistance, numerous problems remain to be solved before effective clinical chemosensitization may be achieved. Such factors as absorption, distribution, and metabolism; the effect of chemosensitizers on chemotherapeutic drug clearance; toxicity to normal tissues expressing P-gp; and the most efficacious modulator regimens all remain to be defined in vivo. Clearly, the identification of more specific, potent, and less clinically toxic chemosensitizers for clinical use remains critical to the possible success of this approach. Nonetheless, the finding that a number of pharmacological agents can antagonize a well-characterized form of experimental drug resistance provides promise for potential clinical applications. Further study of chemosensitizers in humans and the rational design of novel chemosensitizers with improved activity should define the importance of MDR in clinically resistant cancer.

REFERENCES

1. Ford JM, Hait WN (1990) Pharmacology of drugs that alter multidrug resistance in cancer. Pharmacol Rev 42:156–199.
2. Biedler JL, Richm H (1970) Cellular resistance to actinomycin D in Chinese hamster cells in vitro: Cross-resistance, radioautographic and cytogenetic studies. Cancer Res 30:1174–1184.
3. Dano K (1973) Active outward transport of daunomycin in resistant Ehrlich ascites tumour cells. Biochim Biophys Acta 323:466–483.

4. Pastan I, Gottesman MM (1987) Multiple-drug resistance in human cancer. N Engl J Med 316:1388–1393.
5. Moscow JA, Cowan KH (1988) Multidrug Resistance. J Natl Cancer Inst 80:14–20.
6. Ford JM, Hait WN (1993) Pharmacologic circumvention of multidrug resistance. Cytotechnology 12:171–212.
7. Clynes M (ed.) (1993) Multiple Drug Resistance in Cancer: Cellular, Molecular and Clinical Approaches. Dordrecht: Kluwer Academic Press, 396 pp.
8. Fisher GA, Sikic BI (eds.) (1995) Drug resistance in clinical oncology and hematology. In Hematology/Oncology Clinics of North America, Vol. 9, Philadelphia: WB Saunders, 511 pp.
9. Yeh GC, Lopaczynska J, Poore CM, Phang JM (1992) A new functional role for P-glycoprotein: Efflux pump for benzo(a)pyrene in human breast cancer MCF-7 cells. Cancer Res 52:6692–6695.
10. Ueda K, Okamura N, Hirai M, Tanigawara Y, Saeki T, Kioka N, Komano T, Hori R (1992) Human P-glycoprotein transports cortisol, aldosterone, and dexamethasone, but not progesterone. J Biol Chem 267:24248–24252.
11. Juliano RL, Ling V (1976) A surface glycoprotein modulating drug permeability in Chinese hamster ovary cell mutants. Biochim. Biophys. Acta 455:152–162.
12. Skovsgaard T (1978) Mechanisms of resistance to daunorubicin in Ehrlich ascites tumour cells. Cancer Res 38:1785–1791.
13. Kartner N, Riordan JR, Ling V (1983) Cell surface P-glycoprotein is associated with multidrug resistance in mammalian cell lines. Science 221:1285–1288.
14. Gerlach JH, Kartner N, Bell DR, Ling V (1986) Multidrug resistance. Cancer Surv 5:25–46.
15. Gros P, Neriah BY, Croop JM, Housman DE (1986) Isolation and expression of a complementary DNA that confers multidrug resistance. Nature 323:728–731.
16. Ueda K, Cardarelli C, Gottesman MM, Pastan I (1987) Expression of a full-length cDNA for the human mdr1 gene confers resistance to colchicine, doxorubicin, and vinblastine. Proc Natl Acad Sci USA 84:3004–3008.
17. Hammond JR, Johnstone RM, Gros P (1989) Enhanced efflux of [³H]vinblastine from Chinese hamster ovary cells transfected with a full-length complementary DNA clone for the mdr1 gene. Cancer Res 49:3867–3871.
18. Bibi E, Gros P, Kaback HR (1993) Functional expression of mouse mdr1 in Escherichia coli. Proc Natl Acad Sci USA 90:9209–9213.
19. Ruetz S, Raymond M, Gros P (1993) Functional expression of p-glycoprotein encoded by the mouse mdr3 gene in yeast cells. Proc Natl Acad Sci USA 90:11588–11592.
20. Raymond M, Ruetz S, Thomas DY, Gros P (1994) Functional expression of P-glycoprotein in Saccharomyces cerevisiae confers cellular resistance to tahe immunosuppressive and antifungal agent FK520. Mol Cell Biol 14:277–286.
21. Ruetz S, Gros P (1994) Functional expression of P-glycoproteins in secretory vesicles. J Biol Chem 269:12277–12284.
22. Gros P, Croop J, Housman D (1986) Mammalian multidrug resistance gene: Complete cDNA sequence indicates strong homology to bacterial transport proteins. Cell 47:371–380.
23. Chen CJ, Chin E, Ueda K, Clark CP, Pastan I, Gottesman MM, Roninson IB (1986) Internal duplication and homology with bacterial transport proteins in the mdr1 (P-glycoprotein) gene from multidrug resistant human cells. Cell 47:381–389.
24. Gros P, Shustik C (1991) Multidrug resistance: A novel class of membrane-associated transport proteins is identified. Cancer Invest 9:563–569.
25. Sharom FJ, Yu X, Doige CA (1993) Functional reconstitution of drug transport and ATPase activity in proteoliposomes containing partially purified P-glycoprotein. J Biol Chem 268:24197–24202.
26. Shapiro AB, Ling V (1994) ATPase activity of purified and reconstituted P-glycoprotein from Chinese hamster ovary cells. J Biol Chem 269:3745–3754.
27. Cornwell MM, Pastan I, Gottesman MM (1987) Certain calcium channel blockers bind specifically to multidrug resistant human KB carcinoma membrane vesicles and inhibit drug binding to P-glycoprotein. J Biol Chem 262:2166–2170.
28. Loo TW, Clarke DM (1994) Functional consequences of glycine mutations in the predicted cytoplasmic loops of P-glycoprotein. J Biol Chem 269:7243–7248.
29. Loo TW, Clarke DM (1994) Functional consequences of phenylalanine mutations in the predicted transmembrane domains of P-glycoprotein. J Biol Chem 268:19965–19972.
30. Morris DI, Greenberger LM, Bruggemann EP, Cardarelli C, Gottesman MM, Pastan I, Seamon KB

(1994) Localization of the forskolin labeling sites to both halves of P-glycoprotein: Similarity of the sites labeled by forskolin and prazosin. Mol Pharmocol 46:329–337.

31. Tsuruo T, Iida H, Tsukagoshi S, Sakurai Y (1981) Overcoming of vincristine resistance in P388 leukemia in vivo and in vitro through enhanced cytotoxicity of vincristine and vinblastine by verapamil. Cancer Res 41:1967–1972.

32. Naito M, Tsuruo T (1989) Competitive inhibition by verapamil of ATP-dependent high affinity vincristine binding to the plasma membrane of multidrug-resistant K562 cells without calcium ion involvement. Cancer Res 49:1452–1455.

33. Safa AR, Glover CJ, Sewell JL, Meyers MB, Biedler JL, Felsted RL (1987) Identification of the multidrug resistance-related membrane glycoprotein as an acceptor for calcium channel blockers. J Biol Chem 262:7884–7888.

34. Safa AR (1988) Photoaffinity labeling of the multidrug-resistance-related P-glycoprotein with photoactive analogs of verapamil. Proc Natl Acad Sci USA 85:7187–7191.

35. Safa AR (1988) Inhibition of azidopine binding to the multidrug resistance related gp 150–180 (P-glycoprotein) by modulators of multidrug resistance. Proc Am Assoc Cancer Res 29:1160.

36. Yang CH, Mellado W, Horwitz SB (1988) Azidopine photoaffinity labeling of multidrug resistance-associated glycoproteins. Biochem Pharmacol 37:1417–1421.

37. Ford JM, Bruggeman E, Pastan I, Gottesman MM, Hait WN (1990) Cellular and biochemical characterization of thioxanthenes for reversal of multidrug resistance in human and murine cell lines. Cancer Res 50:1748–1756.

38. Kajiji S, Dreslin JA, Grizzuti K, Gros P (1994) Structurally distinct MDR modulators show specific patterns of reversal against P-glycoproteins bearing unique mutations at serine[939/941]. Biochemistry 33:5041–5048.

39. Cardarelli CO, Aksentijevich I, Pastan I, Gottesman MM (1995) Differential effects of P-glycoprotein inhibitors on NIH3T3 cells transfected with wild-type (G185) or mutant (V185) multidrug transporters. Cancer Res 55:1086–1091.

40. Bruggemann EP, Currier SJ, Gottesman MM, Pastan I (1992) Characterization of the azidopine and vinblastine binding site of P-glycoprotein. J Biol Chem 267:21020–21026.

41. Yusa K, Tsuruo T (1989) Reversal mechanism of multidrug resistance by verapamil: Direct binding of verapamil to P-glycoprotein on specific sites and transport of verapamil outward across the plasma membrane of K562/ADM cells. Cancer Res 49:5002–5006.

42. Tamai I, Safa A (1991) Azidopine noncompetitively interacts with vinblastine and cyclosporin A binding to P-glycoprotein in multidrug resistant cells. J Biol Chem 266:16796–16800.

43. Aftab DT, Yang JM, Hait WN (1994) Functional role of phosphorylation of the multidrug transporter (P-glycoprotein) by protein kinase C in multidrug resistant MCF-7 cells. Oncol Res 6:59–70.

44. Aftab DT, Ballas LM, Loomis CR, Hait WN (1991) Structure-activity relationships of phenothiazines and related drugs for inhibition of protein kinase C. Mol Pharmacol 40:798–805.

45. Tsuruo T, Iida H, Tsukagoshi S, Sakurai Y (1982) Increased accumulation of vincristine and Adriamycin in drug-resistant P388 tumor cells following incubation with calcium antagonists and calmodulin inhibitors. Cancer Res 42:4730–4733.

46. Tsuruo T, Iida H, Tsukagoshi S, Sakurai Y (1983) Potentiation of vincristine and Adriamycin in human hematopoietic tumor cell lines by calcium antagonists and calmodulin inhibitors. Cancer Res 43:2267–2272.

47. Akiyama S, Cornwell MM, Kuwano M, Pastan I, Gottesman MM (1988) Most drugs that reverse multidrug resistance inhibit photoaffinity labeling of P-glycoprotein by a vinblastine analog. Mol Pharmacol 33:144–147.

48. Ozols RF, Cunnion RE, Klecker RW, Hamilton TC, Ostchega Y, Parrillo JE, Young RC (1987) Verapamil and Adriamycin in the treatment of drug-resistant ovarian cancer patients. J Clin Oncol 5:641–647.

49. Kessel D, Wilberding C (1985) Promotion of daunorubicin uptake and toxicity by the calcium antagonist tiapamil and its analogs. Cancer Treat Rep 69:673–676.

50. Plumb JA, Wishart GC, Setanoians A, Morrison JG, Hamilton T, Bicknell SR, Kaye SB (1994) Identification of a multidrug resistance modulator with clinical potential by analysis of synergistic activity in vitro, toxicity in vivo and growth delay in a solid human tumor xenograft. Biochem Pharmacol 47:257–266.

51. Tsuruo T, Iida H, Nojiri M, Tsukagoshi S, Sakurai Y (1983) Circumvention of vincristine and Adriamycin resistance in vitro and in vivo by calcium influx blockers. Cancer Res 43:2905–2910.

52. Ramu A, Spanier R, Rahamimoff H, Fuks Z (1984) Restoration of doxorubicin responsiveness in doxorubicin-resistant P388 murine leukaemia cells. Br J Cancer 50:501–507.
53. Tsuruo T, Kawabata H, Nagumo N, Iida H, Kitatani Y, Tsukagoshi S, Sakurai Y (1985) Potentiation of antitumor agents by calcium channel blockers with special reference to cross-resistance patterns. Cancer Chemother. Pharmacol 15:16–19.
54. Niwa K, Yamada K, Furukawa T, Shudo N, Seto K, Matsumoto T, Takao S, Akiyama S, Shimazu H (1992) Effect of a dihydropyridine analogue, 2-[benzyl(phenyl)amino]ethyl-1,4-dihydro-2,6-dimethyl-5-(5,5-dimethyl-2-oxo-1,3,2-dioxaphosphorinan-2-yl)-1-(2-morpholino-ethyl)-4-(3-nitrophenyl)-3-pyridinecarboxylate on reversing in vivo resistance of tumor cells to adriamycin. Cancer Res 52:3655–3660.
55. Weir MR, Peppler R, Gomolka D, Handwerger BS (1992) Evidence that the antiproliferative effect of verapamil on afferent and efferent immune responses is independent of calcium channel inhibition. Transplantation 54:681–685.
56. Gruber A, Peterson C, Reizenstein P (1988) D-verapamil and L-verapamil are equally effective in increasing vincristine accumulation in leukemic cells in vitro. Int J Cancer 41:224–226.
57. Plumb JA, Milroy R, Kaye SB (1990) The activity of verapamil as a resistance modifier in vitro in drug resistant human tumor cell lines is not stereospecific. Biochem Pharmacol 39:787–792.
58. Hollt V, Kouba M, Dietel M, Vogt G (1992) Stereoisomers of calcium antagonists which differ markedly in their potencies as calcium blockers are equally effective in modulating drug transport by P-glycoprotein. Biochem Pharmacol 43:2601–2608.
59. Wilson WH, Bates S, Kang YK, Fojo A, Bryant G, Wittes R, Stevenson MA, Steinberg S, Chabner BA (1993) Reversal of multidrug resistance with R-verapamil and analysis of mdr-1 expression in patients with lymphoma refractory to EPOCH chemotherapy. Proc Am Assoc Cancer Res 34:1266.
60. Ganapathi R, Grabowski D, Rouse W, Riegler F (1984) Differential effect of the calmodulin inhibitor trifluoperazine on cellular accumulation, retention, and cytotoxicity of anthracyclines in doxorubicin (Adriamycin)-resistant P388 mouse leukemia cells. Cancer Res 44:5056–5061.
61. Ganapathi R, Grabowski D, Schmidt H (1986) Factors governing the modulation of vinca-alkaloid resistance in doxorubicin-resistant cells by the calmodulin inhibitor trifluoperazine. Biochem Pharmacol 35:673–678.
62. Ford JM, Prozialeck WC, Hait WN (1989) Structural features determining activity of phenothiazines and related drugs for inhibition of cell growth and reversal of multidrug resistance. Mol Pharmacol 35:105–115.
63. Johnstone EC, Crow TJ, Frith CD, Carney MWD, Price JS (1978) Mechanism of the antipsychotic effect in the treatment of acute schizophrenia. Lancet 1:848–851.
64. Post ML, Kennard U, Horn AS (1975) Stereoselective blockade of the dopamine receptor and the X-ray structures of alpha and beta-flupenthixol. Nature 256:342–343.
65. Huff RM, Molinoff B (1984) Assay of dopamine receptors with [α-3H] flupenthixol. J Pharmacol Exp Ther 232:57–61.
66. Nielsen IM, Pedersen V, Nymark M, Franch KF, Boeck V, Fjalland B, Christensen AV (1973) Comparative pharmacology of flupenthixol and some reference neuroleptics. Acta Pharmacol Toxicol (Copenh) 33:353–362.
67. Twentyman PR, Fox NE, White DJG (1987) Cyclosporin A and its analogues as modifiers of Adriamycin and vincristine resistance in a multi-drug resistant human lung cancer cell line. Br J Cancer 56:55–57.
68. Hait WN, Stein JM, Koletsky AJ, Harding MW, Handschumacher RE (1989) Activity of cyclosporin A and a non-immunosuppressive cyclosporin on multidrug resistant leukemic cell lines. Cancer Commun 1:35–43.
69. Slater LM, Sweet P, Stupecky M, Wetzel MW, Gupta S (1986) Cyclosporin A corrects daunorubicin resistance in Ehrlich ascites carcinoma. Br J Cancer 54:235–238.
70. Osieka R, Seeber S, Pannenbacker R, Soll D, Glatte P, Schmidt CG (1986) Enhancement of etoposide-induced cytotoxicity by cyclosporin A. Cancer Chemother Pharmacol 18:198–202.
71. Chambers SK, Hait WN, Kacinski BM, Keyes SR, Handschumacher RE (1989) Enhancement of anthracycline growth inhibition in parent and multidrug-resistant Chinese hamster ovary cells by cyclosporin A and its analogues. Cancer Res 49:6275–6279.
72. Gaveriaux C, Boesch D, Boilsterli JJ, Bollinger P, Eberle MK, Hiestand P, Payne T, Traber R, Wenger R, Loor F (1989) Overcoming multidrug resistance in Chinese hamster ovary cells in vitro by cyclosporin A (Sandimmune) and non-immunosuppressive derivatives. Br J Cancer 60:867–871.

73. Silbermann MH, Boersma AWM, Janssen ALW, Scheper RJ, Herweijer H, Nooter K (1989) Effects of cyclosporin A and verapamil on the intracellular daunorubicin accumulation in Chinese hamster ovary cells with increasing levels of drug-resistance. Int J Cancer 44:722–726.
74. Goldberg H, Ling V, Wong PY, Skorecki K (1988) Reduced cyclosporin accumulation in multidrug-resistant cells. Biochem Biophys Res Commun 152:552–558.
75. Saeki T, Ueda K, Tanigawara Y, Hori R, Komano T (1993) Human P-glycoprotein transports cyclosporin A and FK506. J Biol Chem 268:6077–6080.
76. Boesch D, Muller K, Pourtier-Manzanedo A, Loor F (1991) Restoration of daunomycin retention in multidrug-resistant P388 cells by submicromolar concentrations of SDZ PSC 833, a nonimmunosuppressive cyclosporin derivative. Exp Cell Res 196:26–32.
77. Jachez B, Nordmann R, Loor F (1993) Restoration of taxol sensitivity of multidrug-resistant cells by the cyclosporine SDZ PSC 833 and the cyclopeptolide SDZ 280–446. J Natl Cancer Inst 85:478–483.
78. Loor F, Boesch D, Gaveriaux C, Jachez B, Dourtier-Manzanedo A, Emmer G (1992) SDZ 280–446, a novel semisynthetic cyclopeptide: In vitro and in vivo circumvention of P-glycoprotein mediated tumor cell multidrug resistance. Br J Cancer 65:11–18.
79. Arceci RJ, Croop JM, Horwitz SB, Housman D (1988) The gene encoding multidrug resistance is induced and expressed at high levels during pregnancy in the secretory epithelium of the uterus. Proc Natl Acad Sci USA 85:4350–4354.
80. Yang C-PH, DePinho SH, Greenberger LM, Arceci RJ, Horwitz SB (1989) Progesterone interacts with P-glycoprotein in multidrug-resistant cells and in the endometrium of gravid uterus. J Biol Chem 264:782–788.
81. Yang CPH, Cohen D, Greenberger LM, Hsu SH, Horwitz SB (1990) Differential transport properties of two mdr gene products are distinguished by progesterone. J Biol Chem 265:10282–10288.
82. Naito M, Yusa K, Tsurou T (1989) Steroid hormones inhibit binding of *Vinca* alkaloid to multidrug resistance related P-glycoprotein. Biochem Biophys Res Commun 158:1066–1071.
83. Fleming GF, Amato JM, Agresti M, Safa AR (1992) Megestrol acetate reverses multidrug resistance and interacts with P-glycoprotein. Cancer Chemother Pharmacol 29:445–449.
84. Aisner J, Tchekmedyian NS, Tait N, Parnes H, Novak M (1988) Studies of high-dose megestrol acetate: Potential applications in cachexia. Semin Oncol 15S:68–75.
85. Ramu A, Glaubiger D, Fuks Z (1984) Reversal of acquired resistance to doxorubicin in P388 murine leukemia cells by tamoxifen and other triparanol analogues. Cancer Res 44:4392–4395.
86. Foster BJ, Grotzinger KR, McKoy WM, Rubinstein LV, Hamilton TC (1988) Modulation of induced resistance to Adriamycin in two human breast cancer cell lines with tamoxifen or perhexiline maleate. Cancer Chemother Pharmacol 22:147–152.
87. DeGregorio MW, Ford JM, Benz CC, Wiebe VJ (1989) Toremifene: Pharmacologic and pharmacokinetic basis of reversing multidrug resistance. J Clin Oncol 7:1359–1364.
88. Chatterjee M, Harris A (1990) Enhancement of adriamycin cytotoxicity in a multidrug resistant Chinese hamster ovary (CHO) subline, CHO-Adr', by toremifene and its modulation by alpha 1 acid glycoprotein. Eur J Cancer 26:432–436.
89. Kirk J, Houlbrook S, Stuart NSA, Stratford IJ, Harris AL, Carmichael J (1993) Differential modulation of doxorubicin toxicity to multidrug and intrinsically drug resistant cell lines by antioestrogens and their major metabolites. Br J Cancer 67:1189–1195.
90. Leonessa F, Jacobson M, Boyle B, Lippman J, McGarvey M, Clarke R (1994) Effect of tamoxifen on the multidrug-resistant phenotype in human breast cancer cells: Isobologram, drug accumulation, and M_r 170,000 glycoprotein binding studies. Cancer Res 54:441–447.
91. Callaghan R, Higgins CF (1995) Interaction of tamoxifen with the multidrug resistance P-glycoprotein. Br J Cancer 71:294–299.
92. Jordan VC, Bain RR, Brown RR, Gosden B, Santos MA (1983) Determination and pharmacology of a new hydroxylated metabolite of tamoxifen observed in patient sera during therapy for advanced breast cancer. Cancer Res 43:1446–1450.
93. Nelson JA, Drake S (1984) Potentiation of methotrexate toxicity by dipyridamole. Cancer Res 44:2493–2496.
94. Grem JL, Fischer PH (1985) Augmentation of 5-flourouracil cytotoxicity in human colon cancer cells by dipyridamole. Cancer Res 45:2967–2972.
95. Jekunen A, Vick J, Sanga R, Chan TCK, Howell SB (1992) Synergism between dipyridamole and cisplatin in human ovarian carcinoma cells in vitro. Cancer Res 52:3566–3571.

96. Howell SB, Hom D, Sanga R, Vick JS, Abramson IS (1989) Comparison of the synergistic potentiation of etoposide, doxorubicin and vinblastine cytotoxicity by dipyridamole. Cancer Res 49:3178–3183.
97. Howell SB, Hom DK, Sanga R, Vick JS, Chan TCK (1989) Dipyridamole enhancement of etoposide sensitivity. Cancer Res 49:4147–4153.
98. Chen HX, Bamberger U, Heckel A, Guo X, Cheng YC (1993) BIBW 22, a dipyridamole analogue, acts as a bifunctional modulator on tumor cells by influencing both P-glycoprotein and nucleoside transport. Cancer Res 53:1974–1977.
99. Chauffert B, Martin M, Hammann A, Michel MF, Martin F (1986) Amiodarone-induced enhancement of doxorubicin and 4′-deoxydoxorubicin cytotoxicity to rat colon cancer cells in vitro and in vivo. Cancer Res 46:825–830.
100. Tsuruo T, Iida H, Kitatani Y, Yokota K, Tsukagoshi S, Yakurai Y (1984) Effects of quinidine and related compounds on cytotoxicity and cellular accumulation of vincristine and Adriamycin in drug-resistant tumor cells. Cancer Res 44:4303–4307.
101. Zamora JM, Pearce HL, Beck WT (1988) Physical-chemical properties shared by compounds that modulate multidrug resistance in human leukemic cells. Mol Pharmacol 33:454–462.
102. Beck WT, Cirtain MC, Glover CJ, Felsted RL, Safa AR (1988) Effects of indole alkaloids on multidrug resistance and labeling of P-glycoprotein by a photoaffinity analog of vinblastine. Biochem Biophys Res Comm 153:959–966.
103. Pearce HL, Safa AR, Bach NJ, Winter MA, Cirtain MC, Beck WT (1989) Essential features of the P-glycoprotein pharmacophore as defined by a series of reserpine analogs that modulate multidrug resistance. Proc Natl Acad Sci USA 86:5128–5132.
104. Hait WN, Gesmonde JF, Murren JR, Yang JM, Chen HX, Reiss M (1993) Terfenadine (Seldane): A new drug for restoring sensitivity to multidrug resistant cancer cells. Biochem Pharmacol 45:401–406.
105. Hyafil F, Vergely C, Du Vignaud P, Grand-Perret T (1993) In vitro and in vivo reversal of multidrug resistance by GF120918, an acridonecarboxamide derivative. Cancer Res 53:4595–4602.
106. Pierre A, Dunn TA, Kraus-Berthier L, Leonce S, Saint-Dizier D, Regnier G, Dhainaut A, Berlion M, Bizzari JP, Atassi G (1992) In vitro and in vivo circumvention of multidrug resistance by Servier 9788, a novel triazinoaminopiperidine derivative. Invest New Drugs 10:137–148.
107. Merlin JL, Guerci A, Marchal S, Missoum N, Ramacci C, Humbert JC, Tsuruo T, Guerci O (1994) Comparaitive evaluation of S9788, verapamil, and cyclosporine A in K562 human leukemia cell lines and in P-glycoprotein-expressing samples from patients with hematologic malignancies. blood 84:262–269.
108. Smith CD, Carmeli S, Moore RE, Patterson GML (1993) Scytophycins, novel microfilament-depolymerizing agents which circumvent P-glycoprotein-mediated multidrug resistance. Cancer Res 53:1343–1347.
109. Smith CD, Zhang X, Mooberry SL, Patterson GML, Moore RE (1994) Cryptophycin: A new antimicrotubule agent active against drug-resistant cells. Cancer Res 54:3779–3784.
110. Smith CD, Prinsep MR, Caplan FR, Moore RE, Patterson GM (1994) Reversal of multiple drug resistance by tolyporphin, a novel cyanobacterial natural product. Oncol Res 6:211–218.
111. Ramu A., Ramu N (1992) Reversal of multidrug resistance by phenothiazines and structurally related compounds. Cancer Chemother Pharmacol 30:165–173.
112. Ramu A, Ramu N (1994) Reversal of multidrug resistance by bis(phenylalkyl) amines and structurally related compounds. Cancer Chemother Pharmacol 34:423–430.
113. Klopman G, Srivastava S, Kolossvary I, Epand RF, Ahmed N, Epand RM (1992) Structure-activity study and design of multidrug-resistant reversal compounds by a computer automated structure evaluation methodology. Cancer Res 52:4121–4129.
114. Prozialeck WC, Weiss B (1982) Inhibition of calmodulin by phenothiazines and related drugs: Structure-activity relationships. J Pharmacol Exp Ther 222:509–516.
115. Hait WN, Aftab DT (1992) Rational design and pre-clinical pharmacology of drugs for reversing multidrug resistance. Biochem Pharmacol 43:103–107.
116. Reid RE (1983) Drug interactions with calmodulin: The binding site. J Theor Biol 105:63–76.
117. Bruggemann EP, Germann UA, Gottesman MM, Pastan I (1989) Two different regions of phosphoglycoprotein are photoaffinity-labeled by azidopine. J Biol Chem 264:15483–15488.
118. Hu XF, Martin TJ, Bell DR, Luise M, Zalcberg JR (1990) Combined use of cyclosporin A and verapamil in modulating multidrug resistance in human leukemia cell lines. Cancer Res 50:2953–2957.

119. Osann K, Sweet P, Slater LM (1992) Synergistic interaction of cyclosporin A and verapamil on vincristine and daunorubicin resistance in multidrug-resistant human leukemia cells in vitro. Cancer Chemother Pharmacol 30:152–154.
120. Carlsen SA, Till JE, Ling V (1977) Modulation of drug permeability in Chinese hamster ovary cells—possible role for phosphorylation of surface glycoproteins. Biochim Biophys Acta 467:238–250.
121. Center MS (1983) Evidence that Adriamycin resistance in Chinese hamster lung cells is regulated by phosphorylation of a plasma membrane glycoprotein. Biochem Biophys Res Commun 115:159–166.
122. Hamada H, Hagiwara K-I, Nakajima T, Tsuruo T (1987) Phosphorylation of the M_r 170,000 to 180,000 glycoprotein specific to multidrug-resistant tumor cells: Effects of verapamil, trifluoperazine, and phorbol esters. Cancer Res 47:2860–2865.
123. Fine RL, Patel JA, Chabner BA (1988) Phorbol esters induce multidrug resistance in human breast cancer cells. Proc Natl Acad Sci USA 85:582–586.
124. Ma L, Marquardt D, Takemoto L, Center MS (1991) Analysis of P-glycoprotein phosphorylation in HL-60 cells isolated for resistance to vincristine. J Biol Chem 266:5593–5599.
125. Meyers MB (1989) Protein phosphorylation in multidrug resistant Chinese hamster cells. Cancer Commun 1:233–241.
126. Mellado W, Horwitz SB (1987) Phosphorylation of the multidrug resistance associated glycoprotein. Biochemistry 26:6900–6904.
127. Center MC (1985) Mechanisms regulating cell resistance to Adriamycin—evidence that drug accumulation in resistant cells is modulated by phosphorylation of a plasma membrane glycoprotein. Biochem Pharmacol 34:1471–1476.
128. Kemp BE, Pearson RB (1990) Protein kinase recognition sequence motifs. Trends Biochem Sci 15:342–346.
129. Kennelly PJ, Krebs EG (1991) Consensus sequences as substrate specificity determinants for protein kinases and protein phosphatases. J Biol Chem 266:15555–15558.
130. Orr GA, Han EK, Browne PC, Nieves E, O'Connor BM, Yang CP, Horwitz SB (1993) Identification of the major phosphorylation domain of murine mdr1b P-glycoprotein: Analysis of the protein kinase A and protein kinase C phosphorylation sites. J Biol Chem 268:25054–25062.
131. Chambers TC, Pohl J, Raynor RL, Kuo JF (1993) Identification of specific sites in human P-glycoprotein phophoyrlated by protein kinase C. J Biol Chem 268:4592–4595.
132. Chambers TC, McAvoy EM, Jacobs JW, Eilon G (1990) Protein kinase C phosphorylates P-glycoprotein in multidrug resistant human KB carcinoma cells. J Biol Chem 265:7679–7686.
133. Aftab DT, Hait WN (1992) Effects of phorbol 12-myristate 13-acetate on drug accumulation and P-glycoprotein phosphorylation in sensitive and multidrug resistant MCF-7 cells. Proc Am Assoc Cancer Res 33:2821.
134. Yang JM, Chin KY, Hait WN (1996) Interaction of P-glycoprotein with protein kinase C in human multidrug resistant carcinoma cells. Cancer Res (in press).
135. Chambers TC, Chalikonda I, Eilon G (1990) Correlation of protein kinase C translocation, P-glycoprotein phosphorylation and reduced drug accumulation in multidrug resistant human KB cells. Biochem Biophys Res Commun 169:253–259.
136. Ido M, Asao T, Sakurai M, Inagaki M, Saito M, Hidaka H (1986) An inhibitor of protein kinase C, 1-(5-isoquinolinylsulfonyl)-2-methylpiperazine (H-7) inhibits TPA-induced reduction of vincristine uptake from P388 murine leukemic cells. Leuk Res 10:1063–1069.
137. Ferguson PF, Cheng Y (1987) Transient protection of cultured human cells against antitumor agents by 12-O-tetradecanoylphorbol-13-acetate. Cancer Res 47:433–441.
138. Dong Z, Ward NE, Fan D, Gupta KP, O'Brian CA (1991) In vitro model for intrinsic drug resitance: Effects of protein kinase C activators on the chemosensitivity of cultured human colon cancer cells. Mol Pharmacol 39:563–569.
139. O'Brian CA, Fan C, Ward NE, Dong Z, Iwamoto L, Gupta KP, Earnest LE, Fidler IJ (1991) Transient enhancement of multidrug resistance by the bile acid deoxycholate in murine fibrosarcoma cells in vitro. Biochem Pharmacol 41:797–806.
140. Mori T, Takai Y, Minakuchi R, Yu B, Nishizuka Y (1980) Inhibitory action of chlorpromazine, dibucaine, and other phospholipid-interacting drugs on calcium-activated, phospholipid-dependent protein kinase. J Biol Chem 255:8378–8380.
141. Schatzman RC, Wise BC, Kuo JF (1981) Phospholipid-sensitive calcium-dependent protein kinase: Inhibition by anti-psychotic drugs. Biochem Biophys Res Commun 98:669–676.

142. O'Brian CA, Liskamp RM, Solomon DH, Weinstein IB (1985) Inhibition of protein kinase C by tamoxifen. Cancer Res 45:2462–2465.
143. Walker RJ, Lazzaro VA, Duggin GG, Horvath JS, Tiller DJ (1989) Cyclosporin A inhibits protein kinase C activity: A contributing mechanism in the development of nephrotoxicity? Biochem Biophys Res Commun 160:409–415.
144. Foxwell BMJ, Mackie A, Ling V, Ryffel B (1989) Identification of the multidrug resistance-related P-glycoprotein as a cyclosporin binding protein. Mol Pharmacol 36:543–546.
145. Posada JA, McKeegan EM, Worthington KF, Morin MJ, Jaken S, Tritton TR (1989) Human multidrug resistant KB cells overexpress protein kinase C: Involvement in drug resistance. Cancer Commun 1:285–292.
146. Palayoor ST, Stein JM, Hait WN (1987) Inhibition of protein kinase C by antineoplastic agents: Implications for drug resistance. Biochem Biophys Res Commun 148:718–725.
147. Aquino A, Hartman KD, Knode MC, Grant S, Huang K-P, Niu C-H, Glazer RI (1988) Role of protein kinase C in phosphorylation of vinculin in Adriamycin-resistant HL-60 leukemia cells. Cancer Res 48:3324–3329.
148. O'Brian CA, Fan D, Ward NE, Seid C, Fidler IJ (1989) Level of protein kinase C activity correlates directly with resistance to Adriamycin in murine fibrosarcoma cells. FEBS Lett 246:78–82.
149. Anderson L, Cummings J, Bradshaw T, Smyth JF (1991) The role of protein kinase C and the phosphatidylinositol cycle in multidrug resistance in human ovarian cancer cells. Biochem Pharmacol 42:1427–1432.
150. Nishizuka Y (1988) The molecular heterogeneity of protein kinase C and its implications for cellular regulation. Nature 334:661–665.
151. Ono Y, Fujii T, Ogita K, Kikkawa U, Igarashi K, Nishizuka Y (1988) The stucture, expression, and properties of additional members of the protein kinase C family. J Biol Chem 263:6927–6932.
152. Ono Y, Fujii T, Ogita K, Kikkawa U, Igarashi K, Nishizuka Y (1989) Protein kinase C ζ subspecies from rat brain: Its structure, expression and properties. Proc Natl Acad Sci 86:3099–3103.
153. Osada S, Mizuno K, Saido TC, Akita Y, Suzuki K, Kuroki T, Ohno S (1990) A phorbol ester receptor/protein kinase, PKCη, a new member of the protein kinase C family predominantly expressed in lung and skin. J Biol Chem 265:22434–22440.
154. Bacher N, Zisman Y, Berent E, Livneh E (1991) Isolation and characterization of PKC-Λ, a new member of the protein kinase C-related gene family specifically expressed in lung, skin, and heart. Mol Cell Biol 11:126–133.
155. Gollapudi S, Patel K, Jain V, Gupta S (1992) Protein kinase C isoforms in multidrug resistant P388/ADR cells: A possible role in daunorubicin transport. Cancer Lett 62:69–75.
156. Blobe GC, Sachs CW, Khan WA, Fabbro K, Stabel S, Wetsel W, Obeid LM, Fine RL, Hannun YA (1993) Selective regulation of expression of protein kinase C isoenzymes in multidrug-resistant MCF-7 cells: Functional significance of enhanced expression of PKC α. J Biol Chem 268:658–664.
157. Yu G, Ahmad S, Aquino A, Fairchild CR, Trepel JB, Ohno S, Suzuki K, Tsuruo T, Cowan KH, Glazer RI (1991) Transfection with protein kinase C α confers increased multidrug resistance to MCF-7 cells expressing P-glycoprotein. Cancer Commun 3:181–189.
158. Tritton TR (1991) Cell surface actions of adriamycin. Pharmacol Ther 49:293–309.
159. Meyers MB, Merluzzi VJ, Spengler BA, Biedler JL (1986) Epidermal growth factor receptor is increased in multidrug-resistant Chinese hamster and mouse tumor cells. Proc Natl Acad Sci USA 83:5521–5525.
160. Posada J, Vichi P, Tritton TR (1989) Protein kinase C in Adriamycin action and resistance in mouse sarcoma 180 cells. Cancer Res 49:6634–6639.
161. Calderwood SK, Stevenson MA (1993) Inducers of the heat shock response stimulate phospholipase C and phospholipase A2 activity in mammalian cells. J Cell Physiol 155:248–256.
162. Yang JM, Chin KY, Hait WN (1995) Involvement of Phospholipase C in heat-shock induced phosphorylation of P-glycoprotein in multidrug resistant human breast cancer cells. Biochem Biophys Res Commun 210:21–30.
163. Hamada H, Tsuruo T (1986) Functional role for the 170- to 180-kDa glycoprotein specific to drug-resistant tumor cells as revealed by monoclonal antibodies. Proc Natl Acad Sci USA 83:7785–7789.
164. Mechetner EB, Roninson IB (1992) Efficient inhibition of P-glycoprotein-mediated multidrug resistance with a monoclonal antibody. Proc Natl Acad Sci USA 89:5824–5828.
165. Tsuruo T, Hamada H, Sata S, Heike Y (1987) Inhibition of multidrug-resistant human tumor growth in athymic mice by anti-P-glycoprotein monoclonal antibodies. Jpn J Cancer Res 80:627–631.

166. Pearson JW, Fogler WE, Volker K, Usui N, Goldenberg SK, Gruys E, Riggs CW, Domschlies D, Wiltrout RH, Tsuruo T, Pastan I, Gottesman MM, Longo DL (1991) Reversal of drug resistance in a human colon cancer xenograft expressing MDR1 complementary DNA by in vivo administration of MRK-16 monoclonal antibody. J Natl Cancer Inst 83:1386–1391.

167. Naito M, Tsuge H, Kuroko C, Koyama T, Tomida A, Tatsuta T, Heike Y, Tsuruo T (1993) Enhancement of cellular accumulation of cyclosporine by anti-P-glycoprotein monoclonal antibody MRK-16 and synergistic modulation of multidrug resistance. J Natl Cancer Inst 85:311–316.

168. Mickisch GH, Pai LH, Gottesman MM, Pastan I (1992) Monoclonal antibody MRK16 reverses the multidrug resistance of multidrug-resistant transgenic mice. Cancer Res 52:4427–4432.

169. Ahmad I, Allen TM (1992) Antibody-mediated specific binding and cytotoxicity of liposome-entrapped doxorubicin to lung cancer cells in vitro. Cancer Res 52:4817–4820.

170. Goldsmith ME, Madden MJ, Morrow CS, Cowan KH (1993) A Y-box consensus sequence is required for basal expression of the human multidrug resistance (mdr1) gene. J Biol Chem 268:5856–5860.

171. Madden MJ, Morrow CS, Nakagawa M, Goldsmith ME, Fairchild CR, Cowan KH (1993) Identification of 5′ and 3′ sequences involved in the regulation of transcription of the human mdr1 gene in vivo. J Biol Chem 268:8290–8297.

172. Chaudhary PM, Roninson IB (1993) Induction of multidrug resistance in human cells by transient exposure to different chemotherapeutic drugs. J Natl Cancer Inst 85:632–639.

173. Burt RK, Thorgeirsson SS (1988) Coinduction of MDR-1 multidrug resistance and cytochrome P-450 genes in rat liver by xenobiotics. J Natl Cancer Inst 80:1383–1386.

174. Mickley LA, Bates SE, Richert ND, Currier S, Tanaka S, Foss F, Rosen N, Fojo AT (1989) Modulation of the expression of a multidrug resistance gene by differentiating agents. J Biol Chem 264:18031–18040.

175. Morrow CS, Nakagawa M, Goldsmith ME, Madden MJ, Cowan KH (1994) Reversible transcriptional activation of mdr1 by sodium butyrate treatment of human colon cancer cells. J Biol Chem 269:10739–10746.

176. Hill BT, Deuchars K, Hosking LK, Ling V, Whelan KDH (1990) Overexpression of P-glycoprotein in mammalian tumor cell lines after fractionated X-irradiation in vitro. J Natl Cancer Inst 82:607–612.

177. Piekarz RL, Cohen D, Horwitz SB (1993) Progesterone regulates the murine multidrug resistance mdr1b gene. J Biol Chem 268:7613–7616.

178. Chin KV, Pastan I, Gottesman MM (1993) Function and regulation of the human multidrug resistance gene. Adv Cancer Res 60:157–180.

179. Budillon A, Kelly K, Cowan K, Cho-Chung YS (1993) 8-Cl-cAMP, a site-selective cAMP analog as a novel agent that inhibits the promoter activity of multidrug-resistance gene. Proc Am Assoc Cancer Res 34:1940.

180. Chaudhary PM, Roninson IB (1992) Activation of MDR-1 (P-glycoprotein) gene expression in human cells by protein kinase C agonists. Oncol Res 4:281–290.

181. Chin KV, Tanaka S, Darlington G, Pastan I, Gottesman MM (1990) Heat shock and arsenite increase expression of the multidrug resistance (MDR1) gene in human renal carcinoma cells. J Biol Chem 265:221–226.

182. Cech TR (1988) Ribozymes and their medical implications. JAMA 260:3030–3034.

183. Kobayashi H, Dorai T, Holland JF, Ohnuma T (1994) Reversal of drug sensitivity in multidrug-resistant tumor cells by an MDR1 (PGY1) ribozyme. Cancer Res 54:1271–1275.

184. Scanlon KJ, Ishida H, Kashani-Sabet M (1994) Ribozyme-mediated reversal of the multidrug-resistant phenotype. Proc Natl Acad Sci USA 91:11123–11127.

185. Kiehntopf M, Brach MA, Licht T, Petschauer S, Karawajew L, Kirshning C, Herrmann F (1994) Ribozyme-mediated cleavage of the MDR1 transcript restores chemosensitivity in previously resistant cancer cells. EMBO J 13:4645–4652.

186. Kobayashi H, Dorai T, Holland JF, Ohnuma T (1993) Cleavage of human MDR1 mRNA by a hammerhead ribozyme. FEBS Lett 319:71–74.

187. Sugawara I, Kataoka I, Morishita Y, Hamada H, Tsuruo T, Itoyama S, Mori S (1988) Tissue distribution of P-glycoprotein encoded by a multidrug-resistant gene as revealed by a monoclonal antibody, MRK 16. Cancer Res 48:1926–1929.

188. Sugawara I, Nakahama M, Hamada H, Tsuruo T, Mori S (1988) Apparent stronger expression in the human adrenal cortex than in the human adrenal medulla of Mr 170,000–180,000 P-glycoprotein. Cancer Res 48:4611–4614.

189. Thiebaut F, Tsuruo T, Hamada H, Gottesman MM, Pastan I, Willingham, MD (1987) Cellular

localization of the multidrug-resistance gene product P-glycoprotein in normal human tissues. Proc Natl Acad Sci USA 84:7735–7738.

190. Lieberman DM, Reithmeier RAF, Ling V, Charuk JHM, Goldberg H, Skorecki KL (1989) Identification of P-glycoprotein in renal brush border membranes. Biochem Biophys Res Commun 162:244–252.

191. Gosland MP, Vore M, Goodin S, Tsuboi C (1993) Estradiol-17β-(β-D-glucuronide): A cholestatic organic anion and substrate for the multidrug resistance transporter. Proc Am Assoc Cancer Res 34:1842.

192. Ferguson LR, Baguley BC (1993) Multidrug resistance and mutagenesis. Mutat Res 285:79–90.

193. Cordon-Cardo C, O'Brien JP, Casals D, Rittman-Grauer L, Biedler JL, Melamed MR, Bertino JR (1989) Multidrug-resistance gene (P-glycoprotein) is expressed by endothelial cells at blood-brain barrier sites. Proc Natl Acad Sci USA 86:695–698.

194. Thiebaut F, Tsuruo T, Hamada H, Gottesman MM, Pastan I, Willingham MC (1989) Immuno-histochemical localization in normal tissues of different epitopes in the multidrug transport protein P170: Evidence for localization in brain capillaries and crossreactivity of one antibody with a muscle protein. J Histochem Cytochem 37:159–164.

195. Chaudhary PM, Roninson IB (1991) Expression and activity of P-glycoprotein, a multidrug efflux pump, in human hematopoietic stem cells. Cell 66:85–94.

196. Chaudhary PM, Mechetner EB, Roninson IB (1992) Expression and activity of the multidrug resistance P-glycoprotein in human peripheral blood lymphocytes. Blood 80:2735–2739.

197. Klimecki WT, Futscher BW, Grogan TM, Dalton WS (1994) P-glycoprotein expression and function in circulating blood cells from normal volunteers. Blood 83:2451–2458.

198. Schinkel AH, Smit JJM, van Tellingen O, Beijnen JH, Wagenaar E, van Deemter L, Mol CAAM, van der Valk MA, Robanus-Maandag EC, te Riele HPJ, Berns AJM, Borst P (1994) Disruption of the mouse mdr1a P-glycoprotein gene leads to a deficiency in the blood-brain barier and to increased sensitivity to drugs. Cell 77:491–502.

199. Smit JJM, Schinkel AH, Elferink RPJO, Groen AK, Wagenaar E, van Deemter L, Mol CAAM, Ottenhoff R, van der Lugt NMT, van Roon MA, van der Valk MA, Offerhaus GJA, Berns AJM, Borst P (1993) Homozygous disruption of the murine mdr2 P-glycoprotein gene leads to a complete absence of phospholipid from bile and to liver disease. Cell 75:451–462.

200. Fojo AT, Ueda K, Slamon DJ, Poplack DG, Gottesman MM, Pastan I (1987) Expression of a multidrug-resistance gene in human tumors and tissues. Proc Natl Acad Sci USA 84:265–269.

201. Goldstein LJ, Galski H, Fojo A, Willingham M, Lai S-L, Gazdar A, Pirker R, Green A, Crist W, Brodeur GM, Lieber M, Cossman J, Gottesman MM, Pastan I (1989) Expression of a multidrug resistance gene in human cancers. J Natl Cancer Inst 81:116–124.

202. Nooter K, Herwijer H (1991) Multidrug resistance (MDR) in human cancers. Br J Cancer 63:663–669.

203. Holzmayer TA, Hilsenbeck S, Von Hoff DD, Roninson IB (1992) Clinical correlates of MDR1 (P-glycoprotein) gene expression in ovarian and small-cell lung carcinomas. J Natl Cancer Inst 84:1486–1491.

204. Marie JP (1995) P-glycoprotein in adult hematologic malignancies. Hematol Oncol Clin North Am 9:239–249.

205. Pirker R, Wallner J, Geissler K, Linkesh W, Haas OA, Bettelheim P, Hopfner M, Scherrer R (1991) MDR1 gene expression and treatment outcome in acute myeloid leukemia. J Natl Cancer Inst 83:708–712.

206. Marie JP, Zittoun R, Sikic BI (1991) Multidrug resistance (mdr1) gene expression on adult acute leukemias: Correlations with treatment outcome and in vitro drug sensitivity. Blood 78:586–592.

207. Campos L, Guyout D, Archimbaud E, Calmard-Oriol P, Tsuruo T, Troncy J, Treille D, Fiere D (1992) Clinical significance of multidrug resistance P-glycoprotein expression on acute nonlymphoblastic leukemia cells at diagnosis. Blood 79:473–476.

208. Chan HSL, Haddad B, Thorner PS, DeBoer G, Lin YP, Oncrusek N, Yeger H, Ling V (1991) P-glycoprotein expression as a predictor of the outcome of therapy for neuroblastoma. N Engl J Med 325:1608–1614.

209. Chan HSL, Thorner PS, Haddad G, Ling V (1990) Immunohistochemical detection of P-glycoprotein: Prognostic correlation in soft tissue sarcoma of childhood. J Clin Oncol 8:689–704.

210. Dalton WS, Grogan TM, Rybski JA, Scheper RJ, Richter W, Kailey J, Broxterman HJ, Pinedo HM, Salmon SE (1989) Immunohistochemical detection and quantitation of P-glycoprotein in multiple drug-resistant human myeloma cells: Association with level of drug resistance and drug accumulation. Blood 73:747–752.

211. Salmon SE, Grogan TM, Miller T, Scheper R, Dalton WS (1989) Prediction of doxorubicin resistance in vitro in myeloma, lymphoma, and breast cancer by P-glycoprotein staining. J Natl Cancer Inst 81:696–701.
212. Epstein J, Barlogie B (1989) Tumor resistance to chemotherapy associated with expression of the multidrug resistance phenotype. Cancer Bull 41:41–44.
213. Epstein J, Xiao H, Oba BK (1989) P-glycoprotein expression in plasma-cell myeloma is associated with resistance to VAD. Blood 74:913–917.
214. Fisher GA, Sikic BI (1995) Clinical studies with modulators of multidrug resistance. Hematol Oncol Clin North Am 9:363–382.
215. Benson AB, Trump DL, Koeller JM, Egorin MI, Olman EA, Wittes RS, Davis TE, Tormey DC (1985) Phase I study of vinblastine and verapamil given by concurrent iv infusion. Cancer Treat Rep 69:795–799.
216. Dalton WS, Grogan TM, Meltzer PS, Scheper RJ, Durie BGM, Taylor CW, Miller TP, Salmon SE (1989) Drug-resistance in multiple myeloma and non-Hodgkin's lymphoma: Detection of P-glycoprotein and potential circumvention by addition of verapamil to chemotherapy. J Clin Oncol 7:415–424.
217. Salmon SE, Dalton WS, Grogan TM, Plezia P, Lehnert M, Roe DJ, Miller TP (1991) Multidrug-resistant myeloma: Laboratory and clinical effects of verapamil as a chemosensitizer. Blood 78:44–50.
218. Trump DL, Smith DC, Ellis PG, Rogers MP, Schold SC, Winer EP, Panella TJ, Jordan VC, Fine RL (1992) High-dose oral tamoxifen, a potential multidrug-resistance-reversal agent: Phase I trial in combination with vinblastine. J Natl Cancer Inst 84:1811–1816.
219. Yahanda AM, Adler KM, Fisher GM, Brophy NA, Halsy J, Hardy RI, Gosland MP, Lum BL, Sikic BI (1992) Phase I trial of etoposide with cyclosporine as a modulator of multidrug resistance. J Clin Oncol 10:1624–1634.
220. Lum BL, Kaubisch S, Yahanda AM, Adler KM, Jew L, Ehsan MN, Brophy NA, Halsey J, Gosland MP, Sikic BI (1992) Alteration of etoposide pharmacokinetics and pharmacodynamics by cyclosporine in a phase I trial to modulate multidrug resistance. J Clin Oncol 10:1635–1642.
221. Bartlett NL, Lum BL, Fisher GA, Brophy NA, Ehsan MN, Halsey J, Sikic BI (1994) Phase I trial of doxorubicin with cyclosporine as a modulator of multidrug resistance. J Clin Oncol 12:835–842.
222. List AF, Spier CS, Greer J, Wolff S, Hutter J, Dorr R, Salmon S, Futscher B, Baier M, Dalton W (1993) Phase I/II trial of cyclosporine as a chemotherapy-resistance modifier in acute leukemia. J Clin Oncol 11:1652–1660.
223. Hausdorff J, Fisher GA, Halsey J, Collins HL, Lum BL, Brophy NA, Duran GE, Nix D, Pearce T, Sikic BI (1995) A phase I trial of etoposide with the oral cyclosporin SDZ PSC 833, a modulator of multidrug resistance (MDR). Proc Am Soc Clin Oncol 14:181.
224. Collins HL, Fisher GA, Hausdorff J, Lum BL, Pearce T, Halsey J, Sikic BI (1995) Phase I trial of paclitaxel in combination with SDZ PSC 833, a multidrug resistance modulator. Proc Am Soc Clin Oncol 14:181.
225. Wishart GC, Bisset D, Paul J, Jodrell D, Harnett A, Habeshaw T, Kerr DJ, Macham MA, Soukop M, Leonard RCF, Knepil J, Kaye SB (1994) Quinidine as a resistance modulator of epirubicin in advanced breast cancer: Mature results of a placebo-controlled randomized trial. J Clin Oncol 12:1771–1777.
226. Miller RL, Bukowski RM, Budd GT, Purvis J, Weick JK, Shepard K, Midha KK, Ganapathi R (1988) Clinical modulation of doxorubicin resistance by the calmodulin-inhibitor, trifluoperazine: A phase I/II trial. J Clin Oncol 6:880–888.
227. Solary E, Caillot D, Chauffert B, Casanovas RO, Dumas M, Maynadie M, Guy H (1992) Feasability of using quinine, a potential multidrug resistance-reversing agent, in combination with mitoxantrone and cytarabine for the treatment of acute leukemias J Clin Oncol 10:1730–1736.
228. Christen RD, McClay EF, Plaxe SC, Yen SSC, Kim S, Kirmani S, Wilgus LL, Heath DD, Shalinsky DR, Freddo JL, Braly PS, O'Quigley J, Howell SB (1993) Phase I/pharmacokinetic study of high-dose progesterone and doxorubicin. J Clin Oncol 11:2417–2426.
229. Philip PA, Joel S, Monkman SC, Dolega-Ossowski E, Tonkin K, Carmichael J, Idle IR, Harris AL (1992) A phase I study on the reversal of multidrug resistance (MDR) in vivo: Nifedipine plus etoposide. Br J Cancer 65:267–270.
230. Linn SC, van Kalken CK, an Tellingen O, van der Valk P, van Groeningen CJ, Kuiper CM, Pinedo HM, Giaccone G (1994) Clinical and pharmacologic study of multidrug resistance reversal with vinblastine and bepridil. J Clin Oncol 12:812–819.
231. Podda S, Ward M, Himelstein A, Richardson C, de la Flor-Weiss E, Smith L, Gottesman M,

Pastan I, Bank A (1992) Transfer and expression of the human multiple drug resistance gene into live mice. Proc Natl Acad Sci USA 89:9676–9680.

232. Sorrentino BP, Brandt SJ, Bodine D, Gottesman M, Pastan I, Cline A, Nienhuis AW (1992) Selection of drug-resistant bone marrow cells in vivo after retroviral transfer of human *MDR*1. Science 257:99–103.

233. Hanania E, Deisseroth A (1994) Serial transplantation shows that early hematopoietic precursor cells are transduced by MDR-1 retroviral vector in a mouse gene therapy model. Cancer Gene Ther 1:21–25.

234. Hanania EG, Fu S, Zu Z, Hegewisch-Becker S, Korbling M, Hester I, Durett A, Andreeff M, Mechetner E, Roninson IB, Giles RE, Berenson R, Heimfeld S, Deisseroth AB (1995) Chemotherapy resistance to taxol in clonogenic progenitor cells following transduction of CD34 selected marrow and peripheral blood cells with a retrovirus that contains the MDR-1 chemotherapy resistance gene. Gene Ther 2:285–294.

235. O'Shaughnessy JA, Cowan KH, Nienhuis AW, McDonogh KT, Sorrentino BP, Dunbar CE, Chiang Y, Wilson W, Goldspiel B, Kohler D (1994) Retroviral mediated transfer of the human multidrug resistance gene (MDR-1) into hematopoietic stem cells during autologous transplantation after intensive chemotherapy for metastatic breast cancer. Hum Gene Ther 5:891–911.

236. Deisseroth AB, Kavanagh J, Champlin R (1994) Use of safety-modified retroviruses to introduce chemotherapy resistance sequences into normal hematopoietic cells for chemoprotection during therapy of ovarian cancer: A pilot trial. Hum Gene Ther 5:1507–1522.

2. MULTIDRUG RESISTANCE ASSOCIATED WITH OVEREXPRESSION OF MRP

SUSAN P.C. COLE, Ph.D. AND ROGER G. DEELEY, Ph.D.

Drug resistance occurs with all classes of chemotherapeutic agents and is a major cause of treatment failure in many human malignancies. In some types of tumors, such as non–small cell lung carcinomas, this resistance is inherent, while in others (e.g., acute myelogenous leukemia) it is acquired during treatment. The problem of drug resistance has been studied in the laboratory primarily by using drug-selected, cultured tumor cell lines as model systems. These cell lines are typically derived by exposure of cells to a single chemotherapeutic agent. When the selecting drug is a natural product, the resistant cells frequently acquire simultaneous crossresistance to structurally unrelated compounds that exert their cytotoxicity through a number of different subcellular targets. Such cells are commonly referred to as displaying a *multidrug resistance phenotype*. The spectrum of drugs encompassed by this experimental phenotype are almost always natural products and their semisynthetic derivatives, and they include agents such as VP-16 (etoposide), doxorubicin, mitoxantrone, and vincristine. Since many of these drugs are therapeutically very useful, elucidation of the mechanisms responsible for causing resistance to these agents is of considerable interest and potential clinical importance.

In experimental systems, multidrug resistance is now known to be conferred by two proteins, the 170 kDa P-glycoprotein (encoded by the *MDR*1 gene) [1,2] and the 190 kDa multidrug resistance protein, MRP (encoded by the *MRP* gene) [3–6]. Although both of these proteins belong to the ATP-binding cassette (ABC) superfamily of transport proteins, they share less than 15% amino acid identity. At present, they are the only known human members of the ABC superfamily that can confer resistance to anticancer drugs.

P-glycoprotein was first described nearly 20 years ago [7], and since then it has been the focus of much basic and clinical research. Despite these investigative efforts, however, there remains some uncertainty regarding the mechanism(s) by which P-glycoprotein mediates drug resistance and how its broad substrate specificity is achieved. Furthermore, its normal cellular function and its clinical relevance are still not completely understood. MRP was first identified in 1992 [3], and thus it is not surprising that far less is known about MRP than P-glycoprotein. Nevertheless, with the knowledge gained in the past few years, it has become clear that these two drug resistance proteins differ significantly in their structure, physiological function(s), and possibly their mode of action. The mammalian P-glycoproteins and their cognate genes have been reviewed extensively by others [8–19]. The major focus of this chapter is the multidrug resistance associated with overexpression of MRP; P-glycoprotein–mediated multidrug resistance will only be referred to in a comparative context.

ISOLATION OF MRP AND ASSOCIATION WITH
NON–P-GLYCOPROTEIN–MEDIATED MULTIDRUG RESISTANCE

It has long been established that P-glycoprotein is frequently overexpressed in multidrug-resistant cell lines and in some human tumors. However, studies of clinical samples made it clear some time ago that not all multidrug resistance is associated with P-glycoprotein [20,21], suggesting that additional resistance mechanisms must exist. Experimental evidence of other causes of multidrug resistance was first provided by reports of cell lines that displayed multidrug resistance but did not overexpress P-glycoprotein [22–30]. One of the most extensively characterized non–P-glycoprotein multidrug resistant cell lines is H69AR, a small cell lung cancer cell line originally described in 1987. This cell line was derived by repeated in vitro exposure of its parental H69 cell line to doxorubicin [22,31,32]. As has been shown for many other non–P-glycoprotein cell lines, reduced levels of the drug target topoisomerase II α and β [33,34], and alterations in levels of enzymes associated with glutathione-mediated drug detoxification [35] were found in H69AR cells, but none of these changes could completely account for the resistance phenotype observed. Evidence of additional changes in gene expression acquired during the development of drug resistance was obtained by differential hybridization of an H69AR cDNA library. These experiments identified clones derived from a novel 6.5 kb mRNA that was highly overexpressed in H69AR cells but not in drug-sensitive parental H69 or revertant H69PR cells [3]. Sequencing of these cloned cDNAs demonstrated that the mRNA encoded a 1531 amino acid protein, which was named *multidrug resistance protein* (MRP). The deduced amino acid sequence and domain organization of MRP indicated that, like P-glycoprotein, it belonged to the superfamily of ABC transporter proteins [3,4].

The overexpression of MRP in H69AR cells was associated with amplification of its cognate gene. This raised the possibility that the MRP gene itself did not confer multidrug resistance but was simply coamplified with the gene that did [3]. However, this possibility was eliminated when a MRP expression vector was transfected into HeLa cells, and resistance to multiple chemotherapeutic agents was observed along with elevated levels of a 190 kDa *N*-glycosylated protein that reacted with MRP-specific antisera [5,36]. These studies firmly established that MRP overexpression was sufficient to cause multidrug resistance, and these findings were subsequently confirmed in other laboratories [37,38]. The MRP cDNA transfection studies also suggested that a previously unidentified 190 kDa protein overexpressed in several other non–P-glycoprotein multidrug resistant cell lines was almost certain to be MRP [39,40]. Since the original characterization of MRP mRNA in H69AR cells, elevated levels of its expression or the 190 kDa protein it encodes have been found in many "non–P-glycoprotein" drug-selected multidrug resistant cell lines (Table 2–1). These cell lines have been derived not only from lung carcinoma cell lines [41–44], but also leukemia [6,45,46], breast [47,48], bladder [49], prostate [50], and cervical [3,51,52] carcinoma cell lines, and a fibrosarcoma cell line [53]. Many of these cell lines overexpressing MRP have been selected in doxorubicin (or similar anthracycline), but several human cell lines selected in VP-16, as well as a murine erythroleukemia cell line selected in vincristine, also express elevated levels of MRP [43,47,52,54]. Thus MRP may be overexpressed in cell lines from a variety of tumor types that have been selected with drugs from several chemical classes (Table 2–1). There have also been reports of substantial levels of MRP mRNA in nonselected cell lines derived from gliomas, neuroblastomas, non–small cell lung carcinomas, and thyroid carcinomas [3,55–58] (Table 2–2). Because these tumor

Table 2–1. MRP expression in drug-selected tumor cell lines from various tissues

Tumor type	Name	Selecting drug	Reference
Human			
Small cell lung	H69AR	Doxorubicin	Cole et al., 1992 [3]
	GLC₄/ADR	Doxorubicin	Zaman et al., 1993 [41]
	H69/VP	VP-16	Brock et al., 1995 [43]
	POGB/DX	Doxorubicin	Binaschi et al., 1995 [44]
Non–small cell lung	MOR/R	Doxorubicin	Barrand et al., 1994 [42]
	CORL23/R		
Cervical	HeLa/J2	Doxorubicin	Cole et al., 1992 [3]
	KB/C-A	Doxorubicin[a]	Sumizawa et al., 1994 [51]
	KB/7d	VP-16	Gaj et al., 1995 [52]
Fibrosarcoma	HT1080/DR4	Doxorubicin	Slovak et al., 1993 [53]
Leukemia	HL60/ADR	Doxorubicin	Krishnamachary and Center, 1993 [6]
	U-937/A	Doxorubicin	Slapak et al., 1994 [45]
	CEM/E	Epirubicin	Davey et al., 1995 [46]
Breast	MCF7/VP	VP-16	Schneider et al., 1994 [47]
	MCF7/GLᴿ	Geldanamycin	Benchekroun et al., 1994 [48]
Bladder	T24/ADM	Doxorubicin	Hasegawa et al., 1995 [49]
	KK47/ADM	Doxorubicin	
Prostate	P/VP20	VP-16	Tasaki et al., 1995 [50]
Mouse			
Erythroleukemia	PC-V	Vincristine	Slapak et al., 1994 [54]

[a] With cepharanthine and mezerein.

Table 2–2. Expression of MRP in nonselected human tumor cell lines

Tumor type	Reference
Non–small cell lung	Cole et al., 1992 [3]
Neuroblastoma	Bordow et al., 1994 [56]
Thyroid	Sugawara et al., 1994 [57]
Glioma	Abe et al., 1994 [55]

types are generally considered to be poorly responsive to chemotherapy from the outset, these findings suggest a role for MRP in intrinsic drug resistance. What determines whether cells will acquire resistance through overexpression of P-glycoprotein (*MDR*1) or MRP is not yet known, but it is apparent that overexpression of P-glycoprotein and MRP are not mutually exclusive. Co-overexpression of MRP and *MDR*1 has been demonstrated in a number of cell lines [43,45,49]. Furthermore, in several series of cell lines displaying increasing levels of resistance, overexpression of MRP preceded the elevation of P-glycoprotein. This observation has led to the suggestion that MRP expression may be more relevant to the levels of resistance observed clinically than is P-glycoprotein, at least in some tumor types [43,45,49].

MRP IS AN ATP-BINDING *N*-GLYCOSYLATED INTEGRAL MEMBRANE PHOSPHOPROTEIN

There is considerable structural diversity among the proteins belonging to the ABC superfamily, but they all contain at least one hydrophobic multispanning transmembrane region and a cytoplasmic nucleotide binding domain (NBD) that preferentially binds ATP [59]. More than 50 eukaryotic and prokaryotic ABC proteins have been described, and they are all involved in the transport of molecules or ions across cellular membranes [59,60]. There is broad variation in the chemical nature of the substrates for the ABC proteins, and in mammalian cells alone they range from simple ions, such as chloride, transported by the cystic fibrosis transmembrane conductance regulator (CFTR) [61,62], to relatively complex peptides conveyed by transporters involved in antigen processing (TAP1/TAP2) [63–65], to xenobiotics transported by P-glycoprotein. Human MRP appears to be in a different branch of the superfamily from P-glycoproteins [3]. The two protein share less than 15% amino acid sequence identity, and much of this similarity is attributable to their NBDs, which are generally conserved in members of the ABC superfamily.

Computer-assisted hydropathy and consensus motif analyses suggest that MRP has a secondary structure quite distinct from the proposed secondary structures of P-glycoprotein and several other eukaryotic ABC proteins (i.e., a tandemly duplicated molecule with six transmembrane segments and a NBD in each half [59]). The original topological model proposed for MRP was predicted to contain eight transmembrane segments in the NH_2-proximal half of the molecule and only four in the COOH-proximal half, and both halves of MRP were *N*-glycosylated (Figure

A. "8 + 4" model

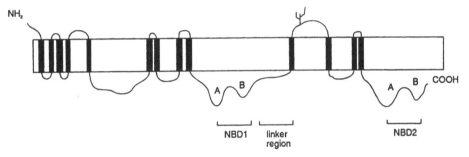

B. "9 + 4" model

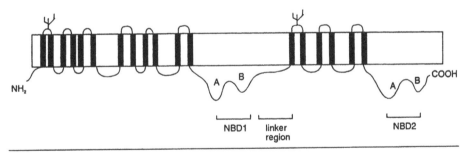

C. "11-12 + 6" model

Figure 2–1. Predicted secondary structures of human MRP. This 190kDa N-glycosylated integral membrane phophoprotein of 1,531 amino acids is encoded by the *MRP* gene located on chromosome 16. MRP has a domain organization common to many ATP-binding cassette transporter proteins, including P-glycoprotein, in that each half of the molecule contains a hydrophobic membrane spanning domain followed by a hydrophilic nucleotide binding domain (NBD). The two halves of the molecule are joined by a "linker" region and, in contrast to P-glycoprotein, are not symmetrically duplicated. Potential N-glycosylation sites predicted to be on the noncytoplasmic side of a membrane are indicated. Several possible topological models of MRP suggested by various hydropathy analyses are shown. The first model proposed (A) indicates that the transmembrane segments of MRP could be in an "8 + 4" configuration [3]. A second model (B) was developed using methods that rely on comparison with model proteins [67]. However, it has been experimentally demonstrated that both halves of the MRP molecule are N-glycosylated [Hipfner et al., unpublished results], suggesting this configuration is incorrect. The most recent analyses predict a structure as shown in (C), which is based on a sequence comparison of human and murine MRP and other members of a subfamily of ABC proteins [68].

2–1A) [3,66]. A second model was developed based on methods that rely on comparison with model proteins [67]. This analysis suggests a "9 + 4" configuration for MRP (Figure 2–1B) and predicts that only the COOH-proximal half of the protein is N-glycosylated. Finally, a third model has been suggested in which MRP is postulated to contain 11–12 transmembrane segments in the NH₂-proximal half and 6 transmembrane segments in the COOH-proximal half (Figure 2–1C) and, like the first model, both halves are predicted to be N-glycosylated [68]. This latter model is based on comparative analyses of the deduced amino acid sequences of human and murine MRP, and other recently identified proteins that appear to belong to an MRP "branch" of the superfamily tree (see later) [68]. Elucidation of the correct topology of MRP in vivo (and there may be more than one) will require further analyses and experimental studies, similar to those carried out with respect to P-glycoprotein [69–75]. At the present time, however, it is clear that MRP and P-glycoprotein are structurally very different molecules, despite the fact that they are both ABC proteins that confer multidrug resistance in mammalian cells.

MRP shares significantly greater sequence identity with members of a branch of the ABC superfamily, which, in addition to MRP, currently includes CFTR (19% amino acid identity), which mediates chloride conductance [61]; *ltpgpA* (32% amino acid identity), a leishmania gene that confers resistance to heavy metal oxyanions [76,77]; *YCF1* (43% amino acid identity), a yeast gene that mediates cadmium resistance [78]; and the rat β cell sulfonylurea receptor (SUR) gene (29% amino acid identity), which is postulated to play a role in insulin release [79]. One intriguing structural characteristic conserved in MRP and several other members of this branch of the superfamily resides within their NH₂-proximal nucleotide binding domains, NBD1 [3,78]. A NBD is comprised of two highly conserved elements, referred to as the *Walker A and B motifs* [80]. In the NBD1 of MRP, CFTR, *YCF1*, and *ltpgpA* (but not SUR), 11 amino acids present in the P-glycoproteins are absent from the comparable location in these proteins, which significantly shortens the distance between the Walker A and B motifs. The precise conservation of this structural feature in proteins spanning such an evolutionary distance suggests some as yet unidentified functional importance. Intriguingly, SUR has an extra 25 amino acids (rather than 11) at this location. Another distinguishing feature of MRP, *YCF1*, *ltpgpA*, CFTR, and SUR is that there is considerably less similarity between the first and second NBDs of these five proteins than there is between the two NBDs of the P-glycoproteins. Perhaps the most striking difference between most members of the MRP cluster and the P-glycoproteins and CFTR is the presence of an extremely hydrophobic NH₂-terminal extension of approximately 230 amino acids that may contain as many as six transmembrane segments (see Figure 2–1C) [68]. The functional significance of the various structural characteristics shared by MRP, *YCF1*, CFTR, SUR, and *ltpgpA* relative to other ABC proteins (including the P-glycoproteins) is currently under investigation.

On the basis of its deduced amino acid sequence, MRP was predicted to be an ATP-binding, integral membrane N-glycosylated phosphoprotein with a calculated polypeptide molecular weight of 171 kDa. Experimental evidence supporting many of these structural predictions has been obtained [6,66,81]. Thus a 190 kDa N-glycosylated phosphoprotein present in H69AR cells and MRP-transfected HeLa cells, and that reacts with MRP-specific antibodies, can be labelled with a photoaffinity analog of ATP. However, the protein has not yet been formally demonstrated to exhibit ATPase activity.

The primary amino acid sequence of human MRP contains 14 consensus sequences (Asn-X-Thr/Ser) for N-linked glycosylation, but the number of sites exposed to the lumen of the endoplasmic reticulum, and thus accessible for glycosylation, varies according to the secondary structure of the molecule (see Figure 2–1). In both drug-selected MRP overexpressing cells and in MRP-transfected cells, human MRP has been shown to be N-glycosylated on both halves of the molecule with complex oligosaccharides [Hipfner et al., unpublished observations], indicating that it has been processed through the Golgi apparatus. Furthermore, when deglycosylated, the electrophoretic mobility of the 190 kDa MRP is reduced to 170 kDa, in good agreement with the molecular mass predicted from its cDNA sequence [6,66]. Studies using inhibitors of glycosylation such as tunicamycin indicate that the reduced drug accumulation observed in intact MRP-transfected cells is unaffected by N-glycosylation [66]. However, whether or not N-glycosylation affects the routing or sorting efficiency of MRP and thus affects its subcellular compartmentalization remains to be determined. N-glycosylation may also help or stabilize correct folding of MRP or protect it from proteolytic degradation en route to the plasma membrane [82]. These aspects of MRP N-glycosylation await a thorough investigation.

Regulation via phosphorylation and dephosphorylation has been demonstrated to be essential for the function of some ABC proteins, such as CFTR, and may also be important in the function of P-glycoprotein [61,83–88]. The primary amino acid sequence of human MRP contains multiple phosphorylation consensus sequences, but which of these, if any, are functionally significant is currently unknown. We and others have shown that MRP is phosphorylated in vivo, primarily on serine residues [66,81] [Almquist et al., unpublished], but the specific amino acids in MRP that are phosphorylated and the kinases responsible have not yet been identified. The murine and human MRP sequences do not share conserved protein kinase C phosphorylation consensus sites in the region that connects the two halves of the molecule [68]. This is in contrast to the murine and human CFTR and P-glycoprotein sequences, and raises the possibility that, unlike CFTR and P-glycoprotein, phosphorylation of this region of MRP by protein kinase C may not be functionally significant.

Treatment of P-glycoprotein–overexpressing cells with protein kinase C inhibitors (e.g., staurosporine, H-7, calphostin C) has been reported to decrease drug resistance, to enhance drug accumulation, and to reduce P-glycoprotein phosphorylation [89–92]. These data have been interpreted as evidence for the existence of an interaction between protein kinase C and the drug efflux activity of P-glycoprotein. However, the results of these studies need to be viewed with some caution because the majority of chemicals that stimulate or inhibit protein kinase C and other protein kinases are not highly specific [93] and are known to have effects on other biomolecules. In addition, some are actually transported by P-glycoprotein. Similarly, the apparent effects on MRP-associated drug accumulation and efflux detected after treatment of drug-selected HL60/Adr cells with inhibitors of protein kinase C may also be indirect [81]. More extensive studies are required to establish whether or not phosphorylation plays a role in regulating MRP activity and drug resistance.

MPR GENE STRUCTURE AND REGULATION

The human *MRP* gene has been mapped to chromosome 16 at band p13.13-13.12, but the structure and organization of the gene has only been partially elucidated [3,53,94,95]. Elevated protein levels resulting from increased gene expression may be achieved by gene amplification or transcriptional activation, or by post-transcriptional events such as stabilization of mRNA and increased translational efficiency. Amplification of the *MRP* gene appears to occur relatively often in multidrug resistant cell lines, but the cytogenetic manifestations associated with this amplification vary among different cell lines [3,41,42,53,95–97]. Fluorescence in situ hybridization studies of H69AR cells have shown that multiple copies of the *MRP* gene are localized both to homogeneously staining regions on chromosomes other than 16 and to multiple double-minute chromosomes [53]. In contrast, the *MRP* gene in another multidrug resistant cell line, HT1080/DR4, has been amplified at its native location [53]. These findings differ from resistance associated with overexpression of human P-glycoprotein, in which amplification of the human *MDR1* gene occurs relatively infrequently [98,99]. It has been suggested that the presence of chromosome-specific repetitive sequences in the vicinity of the *MRP* gene might contribute to the apparently greater ease with which this gene is amplified [94,95]. It is of interest to note, in this regard, that the *MRP* gene maps very close to the short-arm breakpoint of the pericentric inversion of chromosome 16 associated with the M4Eo subclass of acute myelogenous leukemia [94]. In a proportion of leukemias with this inversion, part of the *MRP* gene is actually deleted (see later).

In addition to gene amplification, there is evidence that MRP expression may be upregulated by other mechanisms in certain cells. For example, in H69AR cells the level of *MRP* amplification is less than the level of overexpression of MRP mRNA. Moreover, MRP mRNA in low-level resistant "revertant" H69PR cells is severalfold more abundant than in sensitive parental cells, despite retention of only a single MRP allele in the revertant cells [3,53]. To determine whether transcriptional activation is involved with increased expression of *MRP* in H69PR cells, knowledge of the structure of the promoter region of *MRP* gene and the factors that interact with this region is necessary. A 2.2 kb genomic DNA fragment encompassing the 5' end of the human MRP gene from the HL60/Adr leukemia cell line has been isolated, sequenced, and partially characterized [100]. A similar region has been cloned from the parental H69, resistant H69AR, and revertant H69PR cells, as well as DNA from normal lymphocytes [101].

Sequence analyses of the MRP promoter from these different sources of DNA show that, like the promoter of the human *MDR1* gene [102], it contains no TATA element and appears to have multiple transcriptional start sites. It has also been determined that the core promoter region resides in an extremely GC-rich segment of about 200 bp located approximately 100–300 nucleotides upstream of the ATG translational start codon [100,101]. The one major difference between the sequences of the different MRP promoters occurs in the 5' untranslated region of MRP mRNA, which in HL60/ADR cells contains a triplet repeat of seven GCCs [100], while in the small cell lung cancer cell lines and in normal DNA, the promoter contains a repeat of 13–14 GCCs [101]. It is unclear whether variation in this region is of functional significance as it is in other genes with similar triplet repeats. The MRP promoter also contains consensus recognition sequences for the ubiquitous *trans*-acting factor, Sp1 [103], as well as Ap-1 and many other known *trans*-activating factors. However, which of these potential regulatory elements are functionally important remains to be established.

The *MDR1* promoter has been shown to be responsive to a variety of stimuli, including cytotoxic drugs [104–107] and environmental stresses, such as heat shock [108], serum deprivation [109], and ultravioltet irradiation [106]. More recently, *MDR1* expression has also been reported to be influenced by factors involved in the regulation of cell proliferation, such as c-Ha-*ras*, p53, and c-*raf* [110–112]. Whether or not the *MRP* promoter is similarly responsive is not yet known. Finally, there is evidence that *MDR* gene expression may be activated and regulated in a species and cell-specific fashion, and this is also likely to be the case with *MRP* [113–116].

MECHANISM OF MRP-MEDIATED MULTIDRUG RESISTANCE

Precisely how MRP confers multidrug resistance is not known. P-glycoprotein is believed to mediate multidrug resistance by binding cytotoxic drugs and exporting them to the outside of the cell. ATP hydrolysis by P-glycoprotein is presumed to provide the energy for this process. Some biochemical evidence in support of such a transport mechanism includes the demonstration that P-glycoprotein can be labeled with photoactive analogues of cytotoxic drugs [117–120]. ATP-dependent binding and transport of drugs at relevant concentrations have not yet been demonstrated in membrane vesicles from cells that overexpress MRP [121]. Moreover, in contrast to cell lines that overexpress P-glycoprotein, membrane proteins of a doxorubicin-selected leukemia cell line, which is now known to overexpress MRP, could not be labeled with photoaffinity analogs of vinblastine [6,39]. Similarly, MRP in H69AR cells could not be labeled with a photoaffinity analog of doxorubicin [66]. Thus, there is at present no direct evidence that MRP acts in a manner analogous to P-glycoprotein. To establish unequivocally whether or not MRP functions directly as a drug efflux pump, purification and reconstitution studies similar to those carried out with P-glycoprotein are required [122,123].

Reduced drug accumulation and enhanced drug efflux are usually observed in drug-selected cells that overexpress MRP, as it is with cells overexpressing P-glycoprotein. However, there is some variation in the pharmacokinetic profiles of different drug-selected MRP cell lines, the basis of which is presently not understood [33,44,47,124–127]. In cells transfected with MRP cDNA expression vectors,

ATP-dependent reduced drug accumulation and enhanced drug efflux are observed, although the degree to which accumulation is reduced is less than the degree of resistance [36,38]. Alterations in intracellular distribution of fluorescent anthracyclines have been detected in a number of drug-selected MRP-overexpressing cell lines, and in some cases have been shown to be energy dependent [40,44,45,127–132]. This has led to the suggestion that MRP may participate, either directly or indirectly, in sequestering drugs away from their cellular target [3]. Differences in the subcellular distribution of MRP have also been detected. In some cell lines, MRP has been reported to be predominantly in the endoplasmic reticulum [133], while in others, including MRP-transfected HeLa cells, the protein was found predominantly on the plasma membrane [66,134]. What governs these apparent differences in subcellular localization is unknown, but they may reflect cell type specific variations in trafficking of membrane proteins such as MRP. Although there is as yet no evidence that MRP is directly involved in the vesicular sequestration of drugs, the possibility remains that this might contribute to the variation in transport phenomena observed in different MRP-overexpressing cell lines.

The recent demonstration that MRP can transport the glutathione conjugate leukotriene C_4 (see later) has led to the speculation that while MRP does not appear to transport unmodified drugs directly, it may instead transport drug conjugates. However, there is little evidence that conjugations to glutathione or other endogenous small molecules are important pathways for phase II biotransformation of chemotherapeutic agents to which MRP confers resistance, particularly the anthracycline antibiotics [135] (see Chapter ••). Moreover, there are little data indicating that these processes occur to any significant extent in extrahepatic tissues or cells. Clearly much work remains to be done to understand precisely how MRP confers resistance.

PHYSIOLOGICAL FUNCTION OF MRP

Initial reports have indicated that MRP mRNA is expressed at low levels in many tissues, including hematopoietic cells. At present, it appears that the highest levels of expression are in lung, testes, and muscle [3,41,68,136]. Studies of MRP expression in normal tissues are still preliminary, and in many cases the type and location of the cells expressing the protein are not known. Consequently, studies that include the immunohistochemical detection of the protein are clearly needed. Of relevance to the possible physiological role(s) of MRP is the demonstration that it can function as an ATP-dependent transporter of leukotriene C_4 (LTC_4) in membrane vesicles [121,137,138] (Figure 2–2). LTC_4 is a potent arachidonic acid derivative involved in a number of receptor-mediated signal transduction pathways controlling vascular permeability and smooth muscle contraction [138]. It is synthesized from the precursor LTA_4 by conjugation with glutathione, a reaction catalyzed by the microsomal enzyme LTC_4 synthase [EC 2.5.1.37] [139,140]. After synthesis, it is exported from the cell in an ATP-dependent manner and converted extracellularly by peptidases to the cysteinyl leukotrienes, LTD_4 and LTE_4. Together, LTC_4, LTD_4, and LTE_4 make up the slow-reacting substance of anaphylaxis and play an important

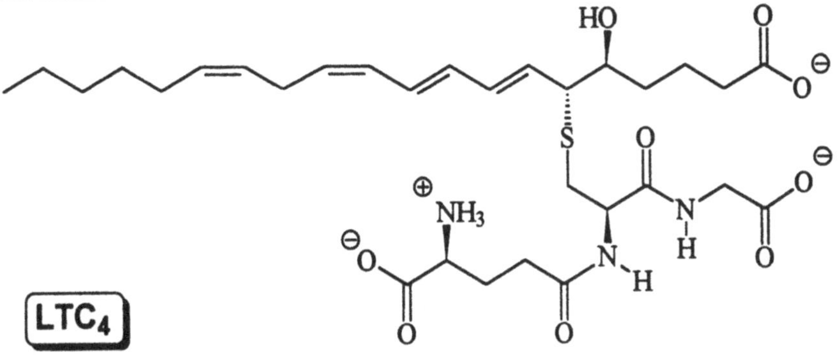

Figure 2–2. Structure of leukotriene C$_4$. Leukotriene C$_4$ (LTC$_4$) is a potent glutathione-conjugated arachidonic acid derivative involved in a number of receptor-mediated signal transduction pathways controlling vascular permeability and smooth muscle contraction. LTC$_4$ is transported from cells in which it is synthesized in an ATP-dependent manner. Membrane vesicles containing MRP transport LTC$_4$ and some other glutathione conjugates with high affinity, and specific photoaffinity labeling of MRP with LTC$_4$ has been demonstrated [137]. These data suggest a possible physiological role for MRP as an ATP-dependent transporter of LTC$_4$ and other cysteinyl leukotrienes.

role in the pathogenesis of human bronchial asthma.

The demonstration of ATP-dependent transport of LTC$_4$ in membrane vesicles prepared from MRP-transfected cells, and the ability of an inhibitor of leukotriene C$_4$ transport to suppress the photoaffinity binding of LTC$_4$ to MRP, have provided the strongest evidence for the involvement of MRP in cysteinyl leukotriene transport [137]. MRP can also transport some other glutathione conjugates, which has prompted the speculation that MRP may be the glutathione conjugate export carrier or so-called GS-X pump [141,142], or some other type of organic anion transporter [36,143]. Evidence for these roles of MRP is still circumstantial, but it is of interest to note that MRP confers resistance to heavy metal oxyanions in addition to chemotherapeutic drugs [36]. Investigation of the specificity of MRP for other endogenous substrates, together with identification of the individual cell types that express this protein, should provide important information regarding the physiological function(s) of MRP. A complementary approach will be to generate mice in which the MRP gene has been "knocked-out." Such mice will provide in vivo models for elucidating the physiological function of this protein, a strategy that has been very informative with respect to understanding the normal function(s) of the P-glycoprotein [144–146]. Our recent cloning of the murine MRP mRNA represents the first step in these important experiments [68].

REVERSAL OF MRP-ASSOCIATED DRUG RESISTANCE

It was first demonstrated in 1981 that resistance associated with overexpression of P-glycoprotein could be reversed by verapamil [147]. Since then a large number of structurally diverse chemicals have been reported to "chemosensitize" drug resistant cells in vitro [148,149]. These observations have resulted in considerable clinical interest in using these so-called reversing agents as adjuncts to conventional chemo-therapy [150–152]. In some instances, chemicals that reverse resistance have been shown to bind to P-glycoprotein, leading to the suggestion that they interact directly with the protein and interfere with its function [153–155]. Unfortunately, most of these agents have been found to be considerably less effective at reversing resistance in non–P-glycoprotein multidrug resistant cell lines now known to overexpress MRP [40,156].

Attempts to reverse MRP-associated resistance have yielded somewhat variable results, overall assessment of which is complicated by differences in methodologies as well as the choice of chemotherapeutic agent(s) and "chemosensitizer" in the individual studies. In some cases, reversal has been measured as the ability of the agent to increase cellular drug accumulation, while in others the ability to enhance chemosensitivity has been measured directly. Compounds reported to increase drug accumulation, to alter drug distribution, and/or to modulate resistance in MRP-overexpressing cells (at least to some degree) include the phenylalkylamine calcium channel blocker verapamil [24,44,46,156], the dihydropyridines nicardipine [156] and NIK250 [50,58], the tiapamil analog DMDP [27], the bisindolylmaleimide protein kinase C inhibitor GF109203X [157], the anionic quinolone LTD_4 receptor antagonist MK571 [158], the cyclosporin analog PSC 833 [159], the isoflavanoid tyrosine kinase inhibitor genistein [160], the quinolone difloxacin [161], and the diiodinated benzofuran amiodarone [159]. Some of these compounds restore accumulation only at concentrations that are by themselves highly toxic, which will presumably preclude their use in vivo.

In addition, most of these agents are unable to completely restore drug accumulation or drug sensitivity to levels comparable with sensitive cells. Moreover, the extent to which resistance to different drugs is reversed can vary significantly, even within the same cell lines. This variability is not entirely surprising, given that most studies to date have been carried out using drug-selected cell lines. Although known to overexpress MRP, there is also evidence for the presence of additional mecha-nisms of resistance in many of these cell lines, such as co-overexpression of P-glycoprotein or alterations in topoisomerase II [25,29,33,34,47,162,163]. Con-sequently, it is not possible to attribute the effects of potential reversing agents exclusively to their action on MRP. Only a few studies have been carried out on MRP-transfected cells, and these suggest that agents such as verapamil and cyclosporin A do not specifically inhibit the action of MRP [36,38]. Consistent with this conclusion is the finding that it has not been possible to label MRP with a photoaffinity analog of verapamil [39], suggesting that, in contrast to P-glycoprotein, the effect of verapamil on MRP-mediated resistance does not involve direct interac-tion with the protein.

The recent demonstration that membrane vesicles containing MRP can transport the cysteinyl leukotrienes (as described earlier) has led to the suggestion that compounds that alter cellular glutathione levels (and thus alter ability to form glutathione conjugates) may have the potential to modulate MRP-mediated resis-tance. The most common agent used experimentally to deplete glutathione in cultured cells is buthionine sulfoximine (BSO), an irreversible inhibitor of γ-glutamylcysteine synthetase that is the rate-limiting enzyme of the glutathione biosynthetic pathway [164]. In resistant H69AR cells, glutathione levels were found to be six-fold lower than in parental cells, and the resistant cells displayed a collateral sensitivity to BSO [35]. Further depletion of glutathione by BSO, however, did not alter doxorubicin resistance in H69AR cells [35]. On the other hand, BSO has been reported to enhance anthracycline and/or vincristine sensitivity in other MRP-overexpressing cell lines [46,158,165–167]. Thus, as with the more conventional chemosensitizing agents described earlier, there is considerable variability in the effects of BSO in different model systems, again probably due to the confounding effects caused by the presence of multiple resistance mechanisms in drug-selected cell lines. The effects of BSO on resistance to chemotherapeutic agents in MRP-transfected cells are under investigation, and these studies should help to clarify the extent to which this interferes with the ability of MRP to confer resistance to particular classes of drugs.

DETECTION OF MRP AND CLINICAL RELEVANCE

The evaluation of MRP as a prognostic indicator and as a therapeutic target for chemosensitizing agents has only just begun. However, the increasing availability of biological reagents for detection of MRP mRNA and protein should facilitate rapid progress in this area. Validation of methods for detecting expression of this gene and its encoded protein in clinical samples is still in progress. The detection of P-glycoprotein in human tissues should serve as a paradigm for these studies. However, it should be noted that a consensus regarding the most useful, relevant, and standardized method of P-glycoprotein measurement has still not been established [168]. In most studies to date, tissue levels of MRP mRNA have been measured by various methods, including northern blot analyses [3], RT-PCR [169,170], and RNAse protection assays [41,171]. Such methods of bulk analysis provide no indication of the heterogeneity of MRP expression within a tissue or clinical sample, and precise quantitation of mRNA levels can be difficult. A further concern is the possibility that there may not always be a good correlation between levels of MRP mRNA and protein [5,36]. For these reasons, there is considerable need to establish reliable methods for detection of the 190kDa protein product of the *MRP* gene [172]. Both polyclonal antisera raised against MRP-derived synthetic peptides and more recently derived MRP-specific monoclonal antibodies (MAbs) have been used to detect MRP protein in drug-selected and transfected multidrug resistant cell lines. They have also provided the means to examine MRP structure, biosynthesis, and subcellular distribution [5,6,36,42,66,134,173,174]. These immunoreagents are essential tools for ongoing and future investigations of the clinical relevance of MRP.

Detection of MRP mRNA or even MRP itself is not necessarily indicative of the levels of functional protein. For this reason, there is considerable interest in developing methods for the specific detection of MRP activity. P-glycoprotein has been shown to be capable of extruding a number of commonly used lipophilic fluorescent dyes [175,176]. The fluorescent properties of some of these chemicals permits the use of flow cytometry or fluorescence microscopy with live cells to measure their cellular accumulation, distribution, and efflux, thus providing information about functional levels of P-glycoprotein. Although convenient for examining P-glycoprotein function, there is some evidence that such assays may not be suitable for measuring MRP function. For example, accumulation of rhodamine 123 (the dye most often used in studies of P-glycoprotein) is reportedly not reduced in some MRP-overexpressing cell lines [177–179] and so may not be an appropriate substrate. Other dyes, such as calcein acetoxymethyl ester, look more promising [178; Lautier et al., unpublished results]. To provide an indication of the extent to which active transport contributes to the rate of dye efflux, these assays are frequently carried out in the presence and absence of agents such as verapamil or cyclosporin A (which are effective reversers of P-glycoprotein–mediated resistance); the difference between the two measurements is then attributed to the presence of a functional transport protein [180,181]. However, as discussed earlier, verapamil and cyclosporin A are generally poor reversers of MRP-associated resistance and truly specific inhibitors of MRP function have not been identified as yet. Consequently, MRP may be underestimated or escape detection in such assays. Finally, measurement of total cellular drug accumulation or efflux does not provide any indication of differences in intracellular drug distribution that may contribute to resistance, which could be particularly important in the case of cells overexpressing MRP [131,182–184]. As has been the case for P-glycoprotein, it is unlikely that evaluation of the clinical significance of MRP will be conclusive until reliable, specific, and standardized assays to detect the presence and activity of MRP are established.

Although methods for analyzing MRP levels and activity are still being developed, a number of studies of its expression in malignant cells from patients with various tumor types have been reported (Table 2–3). Several early clinical studies indicate that MRP is frequently expressed in some forms of leukemia and may play a role in resistance (see Table 2–3 and references therein). In contrast, in one study decreased MRP expression was associated with increased chemosensitivity. Samples from 13 patients with the M4Eo subclass of acute myeloid leukemia associated with an inversion on chromosome 16 [inv(16)(p13q22)] were examined for the presence of the MRP gene by in situ hybridization and by gene dosage analysis [94]. The MRP allele on chromosome (inv)16 was deleted in leukemic samples from five of the patients, and the deletions were associated with a significantly longer time from diagnosis until death or relapse from complete remission. These data, while very preliminary, suggest the possibility that loss of an MRP allele may serve to increase sensitivity to daunorubicin, the anthracycline most commonly used in the treatment of this form of leukemia. There are fewer reports of MRP expression in solid tumors, but the most intriguing to date is the neuroblastoma study by Haber and coworkers [56]. At present, amplification of the N-myc oncogene is the strongest negative prognostic indicator of both response to chemotherapy and outcome in neuroblastoma patients. When expression of MRP was examined in 25 primary tumors, a highly significant correlation was found with expression of the N-myc gene. These observations suggest a potential link between the molecular mechanisms

Table 2–3. MRP expression in human tumors

Tumor type	MRP expression	Test	Reference
Anaplastic thyroid (11)	+	mRNA	Sugawara et al., 1994 [57]
Neuroblastoma (25)	+	mRNA	Bordow et al., 1994 [56]
Leukemias			
Acute myelocytic	+	mRNA	Burger et al., 1994 [171]
Chronic lymphocytic	+		
B-chronic lymphocytic (32)	+	mRNA	Burger et al., 1994 [185]
B-prolymphocytic (10)	+		
Hairy cell (7)	−		
Non–Hodgkin's (13)	−		
Myeloma (18)	−		
Acute myelocytic (12)	−	mRNA	Abbaszadegan et al., 1994 [136]
Myeloma (12)	−		
B-chronic lymphocytic (11)	+	mRNA	Beck et al., 1994 [186]
Acute lymphoblastic	+	mRNA	Hart et al., 1994 [187]
Acute myeloid	−		
Acute myeloid	+	mRNA	Schuurhuis et al., 1995 [188]
Acute lymphoblastic (60)	+	mRNA	Beck et al., 1995 [189]
Acute myeloid		DNA[a]	Kuss et al., 1994 [94]

[a] In this study clinical samples were tested for the presence of the *MRP* gene. See text for more details.

mediating tumor progression and chemoresistance in neuroblastoma. Further studies comparing levels of *MRP* expression in neuroblastoma tumors before and after treatment with cytotoxic drugs, as well as determination of the independent correlation of *MRP* expression with clinical outcome, are unquestionably warranted. These studies should clarify the role of MRP in this highly chemoresistant pediatric malignancy.

CONCLUSIONS

In the past two decades, multidrug resistance has been a major focus of basic and clinical oncological research, initially prompted largely by the discovery and characterization of P-glycoprotein. The recent identification of MRP as a second integral membrane protein that can confer resistance to multiple chemotherapeutic agents provides molecular evidence that this phenotype is complex and will continue to present a therapeutic challenge. While the properties of MRP and P-glycoprotein are similar in many respects, they clearly differ in others, most notably in their structure, physiological function, and possibly their modes of action. Although much has been learned about MRP in the past 3 years, the significance of this novel drug resistance protein in malignant disease and its role in normal cellular function remain to be established.

ACKNOWLEDGMENTS

The authors are indebted to the members of their research laboratories for their past and ongoing contributions to the studies described. We also wish to thank Dr. J.H.

Gerlach for sequence analyses and insightful discussions. We are grateful to the many individuals who made available to us information on MRP prior to publication. S.P.C. Cole is a Career Scientist of the Ontario Cancer Foundation, and R.G. Deeley is the Stauffer Research Professor of Queen's University. Research in the authors' laboratories has been supported by grants from the Medical Research Council of Canada, the National Cancer Institute of Canada with funds from the Canadian Cancer Society, the Ontario Cancer Foundation, the Cancer Research Society, and the Clare Nelson Bequest of Kingston General Hospital.

REFERENCES

1. Ueda K, Cardarelli C, Gottesman MM, Pastan I (1987) Expression of a full-length cDNA for the human "*MDR1*" gene confers resistance to colchicine, doxorubicin, and vinblastine. Proc Natl Acad Sci USA 84:3004–3008.
2. Gros P, Neriah YB, Croop JM, Housman DE (1986) Isolation and expression of a complementary DNA that confers multidrug resistance. Nature 323:728–731.
3. Cole SPC, Bhardwaj G, Gerlach JH, Mackie JE, Grant CE, Almquist KC, Stewart AJ, Kurz EU, Duncan AMV, Deeley RG (1992) Overexpression of a transporter gene in a multidrug-resistant human lung cancer cell line. Science 258:1650–1654.
4. Cole SPC, Deeley RG (1993) Multidrug resistance-associated protein: Sequence correction. Science 260:879.
5. Grant CE, Valdimarsson G, Hipfner DR, Almquist KC, Cole SPC, Deeley RG (1994) Overexpression of multidrug resistance-associated protein (MRP) increases resistance to natural product drugs. Cancer Res 54:357–361.
6. Krishnamachary N, Center MS (1993) The MRP gene associated with a non-P-glycoprotein multidrug resistance encodes a 190-kDa membrane bound glycoprotein. Cancer Res 53:3658–3661.
7. Juliano RL, Ling V (1976) A surface glycoprotein modulating drug permeability in Chinese hamster ovary cell mutants. Biochim Biophys Acta 455:152–162.
8. Bradley G, Juranka PF, Ling V (1988) Mechanism of multidrug resistance. Biochim Biophys Acta 948:87–128.
9. Gerlach JH, Kartner N, Bell DR, Ling V (1986) Multidrug resistance. Cancer Surv 5:25–46.
10. Gottesman MM, Pastan I (1988) The multidrug transporter, a double-edged sword. J Biol Chem 263:12163–12166.
11. Juranka PF, Zastawny RL, Ling V (1989) P-glycoprotein: Multidrug-resistance and a superfamily of membrane-associated transport proteins. FASEB J 3:2583–2592.
12. Georges E, Sharom FJ, Ling V (1990) Multidrug resistance and chemosensitization: Therapeutic implications for cancer chemotherapy. Adv Pharmacol 21:185–220.
13. Roninson IB (1992) From amplification to function: The case of the MDR1 gene. Muta Res 276:151–161.
14. Tsuruo T (1988) Mechanisms of multidrug resistance and implications for therapy. Jpn J Cancer Res 79:285–296.
15. Endicott JA, Ling V (1989) The biochemistry of P-glycoprotein–mediated multidrug resistance. Annu Rev Biochem 58:137–171.
16. Gerlach JH (1989) Structure and function of P-glycoprotein. In RF Ozols, ed. Drug Resistance in Cancer Therapy. Boston: Kluwer Academic, pp 37–53.
17. Gottesman MM, Pastan I (1993) Biochemistry of multidrug resistance mediated by the multidrug transporter. Annu Rev Biochem 62:385–427.
18. Chin K-V, Pastan I, Gottesman MM (1993) Function and regulation of the human multidrug resistance gene. Adv Cancer Res 60:157–180.
19. Leveill-Webster CR, Arias IM (1995) The biology of the P-glycoproteins. J Membr Biol 143:89–102.
20. Goldstein LJ, Galski H, Fojo A, Willingham M, Lai S-L, Gazdar A, Pirker R, Green A, Crist W, Brodeur GM, Lieber M, Cossman J, Gottesman MM, Pastan I (1989) Experession of a multidrug resistance gene in human cancers. J Natl Cancer Inst 81:116–124.

21. Lai S-L, Goldstein LJ, Gottesman MM, Pastan I, Tsai C-M, Johnson BE, Mulshine JL, Ihde DC, Kayser K, Gazdar AF (1989) MDR1 gene expression in lung cancer. J Natl Cancer Inst 81:1144–1150.
22. Mirski SEL, Gerlach JH, Cole SPC (1987) Multidrug resistance in a human small cell lung cancer cell line selected in adriamycin. Cancer Res 47:2594–2598.
23. McGrath T, Center MS (1987) Adriamycin resistance in HL60 cells in the absence of detectable P-glycoprotein. Biochem Biophys Res Commun 145:1171–1176.
24. Slovak ML, Hoeltge GA, Dalton WS, Trent JM (1988) Pharmacological and biological evidence for differing mechanisms of doxorubicin resistance in two human tumor cell lines. Cancer Res 48:2793–2797.
25. de Jong S, Zijlstra JG, de Vries EGE, Mulder NH (1990) Reduced DNA topoisomerase II activity and drug-induced DNA cleavage activity in an Adriamycin-resistant human small cell lung carcinoma cell line. Cancer Res 50:304–309.
26. Reeve JG, Rabbitts PH, Twentyman PR (1990) Non-P-glycoprotein-mediated multidrug resistance with reduced EGF receptor expression in a human large cell lung cancer cell line. Br J Cancer 61:851–855.
27. Cole SPC (1992) The 1991 Merck Frosst Award. Multidrug resistance in small cell lung cancer. Can J Physiol Pharmacol 70:313–329.
28. Hill BT (1993) Differing patterns of cross-resistance resulting from exposures to specific antitumour drugs or to radiation in vitro. Cytotechnology 12:265–288.
29. Ferguson PJ, Fisher MH, Stephenson J, Li D-H, Zhou B-S, Cheng Y-C (1988) Combined modalities of resistance in etoposide-resistant human KB cell lines. Cancer Res 48:5956–5964.
30. Eijdems EWH, Borst P, Jongsma APM, de Jong S, de Vries EGE, van Groenigen M, Versantvoort CHM, Nieuwint AWM, Baas F (1992) Genetic transfer of non-P-glycoprotein-mediated multidrug resistance (MDR) in somatic cell fusion: Dissection of a compound MDR phenotype. Proc Natl Acad Sci USA 89:3498–3502.
31. Cole SPC (1986) Rapid chemosensitivity testing of human lung tumor cells using the MTT assay. Cancer Chemother Pharmacol 17:259–263.
32. Gazdar AF, Carney DN, Russell EK, Sims HL, Baylin SB, Bunn PA, Guccion JG, Minna JD (1980) Establishment of continuous, clonable cultures of small-cell carcinoma of the lung which have amine precursor uptake and decarboxylation cell properties. Cancer Res 40:3502–3507.
33. Cole SPC, Chanda ER, Dicke FP, Gerlach JH, Mirski SEL (1991) Non-P-glycoprotein-mediated multidrug resistance in a small cell lung cancer cell line: Evidence for decreased susceptibility to drug-induced DNA damage and reduced levels of topoisomerase II. Cancer Res 51:3345–3352.
34. Evans CD, Mirski SEL, Danks MK, Cole SPC (1994) Reduced levels of topoisomerase II α and β in a multidrug resistant small cell lung cancer cell line. Cancer Chemother Pharmacol 34:242–248.
35. Cole SPC, Downes HF, Mirski SEL, Clements DJ (1990) Alterations in glutathione and glutathione-related enzymes in a multidrug resistant small cell lung cancer cell line. Mol Pharmacol 37:192–197.
36. Cole SPC, Sparks KE, Fraser K, Loe DW, Grant CE, Wilson GM, Deeley RG (1994) Pharmacological characterization of multidrug resistant MRP-transfected human tumor cells. Cancer Res 54:5902–5910.
37. Kruh GD, Chan A, Myers K, Gaughan K, Miki T, Aaronson SA (1994) Expression complementary DNA library transfer establishes *mrp* as a multidrug resistance gene. Cancer Res 54:1649–1652.
38. Zaman GJR, Flens MJ, Van Leusden MR, de Haas M, Mulder HS, Lankelma J, Pinedo HM, Scheper RJ, Baas F, Broxterman HJ, Borst P (1994) The human multidrug resistance-associated protein MRP is a plasma membrane drug-efflux pump. Proc Natl Acad Sci USA 91:8822–8826.
39. McGrath T, Latoud C, Arnold ST, Safa AR, Felsted RL, Canter MS (1989) Mechanisms of multidrug resistance in HL60 cells: Analysis of resistance associated membrane proteins and levels of *mdr* gene expression. Biochem Pharmacol 38:3611–3619.
40. Barrand MA, Rhodes T, Center MS, Twentyman PR (1993) Chemosensitisation and drug accumulation effects of cyclosporin A, PSC-833 and verapamil in human MDR large cell lung cancer cells expressing a 190k membrane protein distinct from P-glycoprotein. Eur J Cancer 29:408–415.
41. Zaman GJR, Versantvoort CHM, Smit JJM, Eijdems EWHM, de Haas M, Smith AJ, Broxterman HJ, Mulder NH, de Vries EGE, Baas F, Borst P (1993) Analysis of the expression of *MRP*, the gene for a new putative transmembrane drug transporter, in human multidrug resistant lung cancer cell lines. Cancer Res 53:1747–1750.

42. Barrand MA, Heppell-Parton AC, Wright KA, Rabbitts PH, Twentyman PR (1994) A 190-kilodalton protein overexpressed in non-P-glycoprotein-containing multidrug-resistant cells and its relationship to the MRP gene. J Natl Cancer Inst 86:110–117.

43. Brock I, Hipfner DR, Nielsen BE, Jensen PB, Deeley RG, Cole SPC, Sehested M (1995) Sequential co-expression of the multidrug resistance genes, MRP and mdr1 and their products in VP-16 (etoposide) selected H69 small cell lung cancer cells. Cancer Res 55:459–462.

44. Binaschi M, Supino R, Gambetta RA, Giaccone G, Prosperi E, Capranico G, Cataldo I, Zunino F (1995) MRP gene overexpression is a human doxorubicin-resistant SCLC cell line: Alterations in cellular pharmacokinetics and in pattern of cross-resistance. Int J Cancer 61:1, 84–89.

45. Slapak CA, Mizunuma N, Kufe DW (1994) Expression of the multidrug resistance associated protein and P-glycoprotein in doxorubicin-selected human myeloid leukemia cells. Blood 84:3113–3121.

46. Davey RA, Longhurst TJ, Davey MW, Belov L, Harvie RM, Hancox D, Wheeler H (1995) Drug resistance mechanisms and MRP expression in response to epirubicin treatment in a human leukaemia cell line. Leuk Res 17:1–8.

47. Schneider E, Horton JK, Yang C-H, Nakagawa M, Cowan KH (1994) Multidrug resistance-associated protein gene overexpression and reduced drug sensitivity of topoisomerase II in a human breast carcinoma MCF7 cell line selected for etoposide resistance. Cancer Res 54:152–158.

48. Benchekroun MN, Schneider E, Safa AR, Townsend AJ, Sinha BK (1994) Mechanisms of resistance to ansamycin antibiotics in human breast cancer cell lines. Mol Pharmacol 46:677–684.

49. Hasegawa S, Abe T, Naito S, Kotoh S, Kumazawa J, Hipfner DR, Deeley RG, Cole SPC, Kuwano M (1995) Expression of multidrug resistance-associated protein (MRP), MDR1 and DNA topoisomerase II in human multidrug-resistant bladder cancer cell lines. Br J Cancer 71:907–913.

50. Tasaki Y, Nakagawa M, Ogata J, Kiue A, Tanimura H, Kuwano M, Nomura Y (1995) Reversal by a dihydropyridine derivative of non-P-glycoprotein-mediated multidrug resistance in etoposide-resistant human prostatic cancer cell lines. J Urol, 154:1210–1216.

51. Sumizawa T, Chuman Y, Sakamoto H, Iemura K, Almquist KC, Deeley RG, Cole SPC, Akiyama S-i (1994) Non-P-glycoprotein-mediated multidrug resistant human KB cells selected in medium containing Adriamycin, cepharanthine and mezerein. Soma Cell Mol Genet 20:423–435.

52. Gaj CL, Anyanwutaku IO, Cole SC, Chang Y, Cheng YC (1995) Reversal of multidrug resistance associated protein mediated multidrug resistance in a human carcinoma cell line by the l/-enantiomer of verapamil (abstr). Proc Am Assoc Cancer Res 36:346.

53. Slovak ML, Ho JP, Bhardwaj G, Kurz EU, Deeley RG, Cole SPC (1993) Localization of a novel multidrug resistance-associated gene in the HT1080/DR4 and H69AR human tumor cell lines. Cancer Res 53:3221–3225.

54. Slapak CA, Fracasso PM, Martell RL, Toppmeyer DL, Lecerf J-M, Levy SB (1994) Overexpression of the multidrug resistance-associated protein (MRP) gene in vincristine but not doxorubicin-selected multidrug resistant murine erythroleukemia cells. Cancer Res 54:5607–5613.

55. Abe T, Hasegawa S, Taniguchi K, Yokomizo A, Kuwano T, Ono M, Mori T, Hori S, Kohno K, Kuwano M (1994) Possible involvement of multidrug-resistance-associated protein (MRP) gene expression in spontaneous drug resistance to vincristine, etoposide and adriamycin in human glioma cells. Int J Cancer 58:860–864.

56. Bordow SB, Haber M, Madafiglio J, Cheung B, Marshall GM, Norris MD (1994) Expression of the multidrug resistance-associated protein (MRP) gene correlates with amplification and overexpression of the N-myc oncogene in childhood neuroblastoma. Cancer Res 54:5036–5040.

57. Sugawara I, Arai T, Yamashita T, Yoshida A, Masunaga S, Itoyama S (1994) Expression of multidrug resistance-associated protein (MRP) in anaplastic carcinoma of the thyroid. Cancer Lett 82:185–188.

58. Abe T, Koike K, Ohga T, Kubo T, Wada M, Kohno K, Mori T, Hidaka K, Kuwano M (1995) Chemosensitization of spontaneous multidrug resistance by a 1,4-dihydropyridine analog and verapamil in human glioma cell lines overexpressing MRP or MDR1. Br J Cancer 72:418–423.

59. Higgins CF (1992) ABC transporters: From microorganisms to man. Ann Rev Cell Biol 8:67–113.

60. Fath MJ, Kolter R (1993) ABC transporters: Bacterial exporters. Microbiol Rev 57:995–1017.

61. Riordan JR, Rommens JM, Kerem B-S, Alon N, Rozmahel R, Grzelczak Z, Zielenski J, Lok S, Plasvsic N, Chou J-L, Drumm ML, Iannuzzi MC, Collins FS, Tsui L-C (1989) Identification of the cystic fibrosis gene: Cloning and characterization of complementary DNA. Science 245:1066–1073.

62. Welsh MJ, Smith AE (1993) Molecular mechanisms of CFTR chloride channel dysfunction in cystic fibrosis. Cell 73:1251–1254.

63. Kelly A, Powis SH, Kerr L-A, Mockridge I, Elliott T, Bastin J, Uchanska-Ziegler B, Ziegler A, Trowsdale J, Townsend A (1992) Assembly and function of the two ABC transporter proteins

encoded in the human major histocompatibility complex. Nature 355:641–644.

64. Neefjes JJ, Momburg F, Hammerling GJ (1993) Selective and ATP-dependent translocation of peptides by the MHC-encoded transporter. Science 261:769–771.

65. Heemels M-T, Schumacher TNM, Wonigeit K, Ploegh HL (1993) Peptide translocation by variants of the transporter associated with antigen processing. Science 262:2059–2063.

66. Almquist KC, Loe DW, Hipfner DR, Mackie JE, Cole SPC, Deeley RG (1995) Characterization of the 190 kDa multidrug resistance protein (MRP) in drug-selected and transfected human tumor cells. Cancer Res 55:102–110.

67. Jones DT, Taylor WR, Thornton JM (1994) A model recognition approach to the prediction of all-helical membrane protein structure and topology. Biochemistry 33:3038–3049.

68. Stride BD, Valdimarsson G, Gerlach JH, Wilson G, Cole SPC, Deeley RG (1996) Structure and expression of the mRNA encoding the murine multidrug resistance protein (MRP), an ATP-binding cassette transporter. Mol Pharmacol, in press.

69. Yoshimura A, Kuwazuru Y, Sumizawa T, Ichikawa M, Ikeda S-I, Uda T, Akiyama S-I (1989) Cytoplasmic orientation and two-domain structure of the multidrug transporter, P-glycoprotein, demonstrated with sequence-specific antibodies. J Biol Chem 264:16282–16291.

70. Georges E, Tsuruo T, Ling V (1993) Topology of P-glycoprotein as determined by epitope mapping of MRK-16 monoclonal antibody. J Biol Chem 268:1792–1798.

71. Georges E, Bradley G, Gariepy J, Ling V (1990) Detection of P-glycoprotein isoforms by gene-specific monoclonal antibodies. Proc Natl Acad Sci USA 87:152–156.

72. Skach WR, Lingappa VR (1994) Transmembrane orientation and topogenesis of the third and fourth membrane-spanning regions of human P-glycoprotein (MDR1). Cancer Res 54:3202–3209.

73. Skach WR, Calayag MC, Lingappa VR (1993) Evidence for an alternate model of human P-glycoprotein structure and biogenesis. J Biol Chem 268:6903–6908.

74. Zhang J-T, Ling V (1991) Study of membrane orientation and glycosylated extracellular loops of mouse P-glycoprotein by in vitro translation. J Biol Chem 266:18224–18232.

75. Zhang J-T, Lee CH, Duthie M, Ling V (1995) Topological determinants of internal transmembrane segments in P-glycoprotein sequences. J Biol Chem 270:1742–1746.

76. Callahan HL, Beverley SM (1991) Heavy metal resistance: A new role for P-glycoproteins in *Leishmania*. J Biol Chem 266:18427–18430.

77. Papadopoulou B, Roy G, Dey S, Rosen BP, Ouellette M (1994) Contribution of the *Leishmania* P-glycoprotein-related gene *ltpgpA* to oxyanion resistance. J Biol Chem 269:11980–11986.

78. Szczypka MS, Wemmie JA, Moye-Rowley WS, Thiele DJ (1994) A yeast metal resistance protein similar to human cystic fibrosis transmembrane conductance regulator (CFTR) and multidrug resistance-associated protein. J Biol Chem 269:22853–22857.

79. Aguilar-Bryan L, Nichols CG, Wechsler SW, Clement JP, Boyd AE, Gonzalez G, Herrera-Sosa H, Nguy K, Bryan J, Nelson DA (1995) Cloning of the β cell high-affinity sulfonylurea receptor: A regulator of insulin secretion. Science 268:423–426.

80. Walker JE, Saraste M, Runswick MJ, Gay NJ (1982) Distantly related sequences in the α- and β-subunits of ATP synthase, myosin, kinases and other ATP-requiring enzymes and a common nucleotide binding fold. EMBO J 1:945–951.

81. Ma L, Krishnamachary N, Center MS (1995) Phosphorylation of the multidrug resistance associated protein gene encoded protein P190. Biochemistry 34:3338–3343.

82. Lis H, Sharon N (1993) Protein glycosylation. Structural and functional aspects. Eur J Biochem 218:1–27.

83. Becq F, Jensen TJ, Chang X-B, Savoia A, Rommens JM, Tsui L-C, Buchwald M, Riordan JR, Hanrahan JW (1994) Phosphatase inhibitors activate normal and defective CFTR chloride channels. Proc Natl Acad Sci USA 91:9160–9164.

84. Chambers TC, Pohl J, Ryanor RL, Kuo JF (1993) Identification of specific sites in human P-glycoprotein phosphorylated by protein kinase C. J Biol Chem 268:4592–4595.

85. Orr GA, Han EK-H, Browne PC, Nieves E, O'Connor BM, Yang C-PH, Horwitz SB (1993) Identification of the major phosphorylation domain of murine *mdr*1b P-glycoprotein. Analysis of the protein kinase A and protein kinase C phosphorylation sites. J Biol Chem 268:5054–25062.

86. Picciotto MR, Cohn JA, Bertuzzi G, Greengard P, Nairn AC (1992) Phosphorylation of the cystic fibrosis transmembrane conductance regulator. J Biol Chem 267:12742–12752.

87. Chang X-B, Tabcharani JA, Hou Y-X, Jensen TJ, Kartner N, Alon N, Hanrahan JW, Riordan JR (1993) Protein kinase A (PKA) still activates CFTR chloride channel after mutagenesis of all 10 PKA consensus phosphorylation sites. J Biol Chem 268:11304–11311.

88. Cheng SH, Rich DP, Marshall J, Gregory RJ, Welsh MJ, Smith AE (1991) Phosphorylation of the R domain by cAMP-dependent protein kinase regulates the CFTR chloride channel. Cell

66:1027–1036.

89. Chambers TC, Zheng B, Kuo JF (1992) Regulation of phorbol ester and protein kinase C inhibitors, and by a protein phosphatase inhibitor (okadaic acid), of P-glycoprotein phosphorylation and relationship to drug accumulation in multidrug-resistant human KB cells. Mol Pharmacol 41:1008–1015.

90. Bates SE, Lee JS, Dickstein B, Spolyar M, Fojo AT (1993) Differential modulation of P-glycoprotein transport by protein kinase inhibition. Biochemistry 32:9156–9164.

91. Sato W, Yusa K, Naito M, Tsuruo T (1990) Staurosporine, a potent inhibitor of C-kinase, enhances drug accumulation in multidrug-resistant cells. Biochem Biophys Res Commun 173:1252–1257.

92. Sampson KE, Wolf CL, Abraham I (1993) Staurosporine reduces P-glycoprotein expression and modulates resistance. Cancer Lett 68:7–14.

93. Epand RM, Stafford AR (1993) Protein kinases and multidrug resistance. Cancer J 6:154–158.

94. Kuss BJ, Deeley RG, Cole SPC, Willman CL, Kopecky KJ, Wolman SR, Eyre HJ, Lane SA, Nancarrow JK, Whitmore SA, Callen DF (1994) Deletion of gene for multidrug resistance in acute myeloid leukaemia with inversion in chromosome 16: Prognostic implications. Lancet 343:1531–1534.

95. Eijems EWHM, de Haas M, Coco-Martin JM, Ottenheim CPE, Zaman GJR, Dauwerse GH, Breuning MH, Twentyman PR, Borst P, Baas F (1995) Mechanisms of MRP over-expression in four human lung-cancer cell lines and analysis of the MRP amplicon. Int J Cancer 60:676–684.

96. Ray ME, Guan X-Y, Slovak ML, Trent JM, Meltzer PS (1994) Rapid detection, cloning and molecular cytogenetic characterisation of sequences from an MRP-encoding amplicon by chromosome microdissection. Br J Cancer 70:85–90.

97. Slovak ML, Ho J, Deeley RG, Cole SPC, de Vries EGE, Broxterman H, Scheffer GL, Scheper RJ (1995) The drug resistance related protein LRP maps proximal to MRP on the short arm of chromosome 16 (abstr). Proc Am Assoc Cancer Res 36:114.

98. Shen D-W, Fojo A, Chin JE, Roninson IB, Richert N, Pastan I, Gottesman MM (1986) Human multidrug-resistant cell lines: Increased mdr1 expression can precede gene amplification. Science 232:643–645.

99. Baas F, Jongsma APM, Broxterman HJ, Arceci RJ, Housman D, Scheffer GL, Riethorst A, van Groenigen M, Nieuwint AWM, Joenje H (1990) Non-P-glycoprotein mediated mechanism for multidrug resistance precedes P-glycoprotein expression during in vitro selection for doxorubicin resistance in a human lung cancer cell line. Cancer Res 50:5392–5398.

100. Zhu Q, Center MS (1994) Cloning and sequence analysis of the promoter region of the MRP gene of HL60 cells isolated for resistance to Adriamycin. Cancer Res 54:4488–4492.

101. Kurz EU, Grant CE, Vasa MZ, Burtch-Wright RA, Cole SPC, Deeley RG (1995) Analysis of the proximal promoter region of the multidrug resistance protein (MRP) gene in three small cell lung cancer cell lines (abstr). Proc Am Assoc Cancer Res 36:1917.

102. Ueda K, Pastan I, Gottesman MM (1987) Isolation and sequence of the promoter region of the human multidrug-resistance (P-glycoprotein) gene. J Biol Chem 262:17432–17436.

103. Dynan WS, Tjian R (1985) Control of eukaryotic messenger RNA synthesis by sequence-specific DNA-binding proteins. Nature 316:774–778.

104. Kohno K, Sato S-i, Uchiumi T, Takano H, Tanimura H, Miyazaki M, Matsuo K-i, Hidaka K, Kuwano M (1992) Activation of the human multidrug resistance 1 (MDR1) gene promoter in response to inhibitors of DNA topoisomerases. Int J Oncol 1:73–77.

105. Chaudhary PM, Roninson IB (1993) Induction of multidrug resistance in human cells by transient exposure to different chemotherapeutic drugs. J Natl Cancer Inst 85:632–639.

106. Uchiumi T, Kohno K, Tanimura H, Hidaka K, Asakuno K, Abe H, Uchida Y, Kuwano M (1993) Involvement of protein kinase in environmental stress-induced activation of human multidrug resistance 1 (MDR1) gene promoter. FEBS Lett 326:11–16.

107. Kohno K, Sato S-i, Takano H, Matsuo K-i, Kuwano M (1989) The direct activation of human multidrug resistance gene (MDR1) by anticancer agents. Biochem Biophys Res Commun 165:1415–1421.

108. Miyazaki M, Kohno K, Uchiumi T, Tanimura H, Matsuo K-i, Nasu M, Kuwano M (1992) Activation of human multidrug resistance-1 gene promoter in response to heat shock stress. Biochem Biophys Res Commun 187:677–684.

109. Tanimura H, Kohno K, Sato S-i, Uchiumi T, Miyazaki M, Kobayashi M, Kuwano M (1992) The human multidrug resistance 1 promoter has an element that responds to serum starvation. Biochem Biophys Res Commun 183:917–924.

110. Zastawny RL, Salvino R, Chen J, Benchimol S, Ling V (1993) The core promoter region of the P-glycoprotein gene is sufficient to confer differential responsiveness to wild-type and mutant p53. Oncogene 8:1529–1535.

111. Chin K-V, Ueda K, Pastan I, Gottesman MM (1992) Modulation of activity of the promoter of the human *MDR*1 gene by ras and p53. Science 255:459–462.

112. Cornwell MM, Smith DE (1993) A signal transduction pathway for activation of the *mdr*1 promoter involves the proto-oncogene c-*raf* kinase. J Biol Chem 268:15347–15350.

113. Cohen D, Piekarz RL, Hsu SI-H, DePinho RA, Carrasco N, Horwitz SB (1991) Structural and functional analysis of the mouse *mdr*1b gene promoter. J Biol Chem 266:2239–2244.

114. Brown PC, Thorgeirsson SS, Silverman JA (1993) Cloning and regulation of the rat *mdr*2 gene. Nucleic Acids Res 21:3885–3891.

115. Hsu SI-H, Cohen D, Kirschner LS, Lothstein L, Hartstein M, Horwitz SB (1990) Structural analysis of the mouse *mdr*1a (P-glycoprotein) promoter reveals the basis for differential transcript heterogeneity in multidrug-resistant J774.2 cells. Mol Cell Biol 10:3596–3606.

116. Raymond M, Gros P (1990) Cell-specific activity of cis-acting regulatory elements in the promoter of the mouse multidrug resistance gene *mdr*1. Mol Cell Biol 10:6036–6040.

117. Safa AR, Glover CJ, Meyers MB, Biedler JL, Felsted RL (1986) Vinblastine photoaffinity labeling of a high molecular weight surface membrane glycoprotein specific for multidrug-resistant cells. J Biol Chem 261:6137–6140.

118. Safa AR, Mehta ND, Agresti M (1989) Photoaffinity labeling of P-glycoprotein in multidrug resistant cells with photoactive analogs of colchicine. Biochem Biophys Res Commun 162:1402–1408.

119. Beck WT, Cirtain MC, Glover CJ, Felsted RL, Safa AR (1988) Effects of indole alkaloids on multidrug resistance and labeling of P-glycoprotein by a photoaffinity analog of vinblastine. Biochem Biophys Res Commun 153:959–966.

120. Busche R, Tummler B, Riordan JR, Cano-Gauci DF (1989) Preparation and utility of a radioiodinated analogue of daunomycin in the study of multidrug resistance. Mol Pharmacol 35:414–421.

121. Muller M, Meijer C, Zaman GJR, Borst P, Scheper RJ, Mulder NH, de Vries EGE, Jansen PLM (1994) Overexpression of the gene encoding the multidrug resistance-associated protein results in increased ATP-dependent glutathione S-conjugate transport. Proc Natl Acad Sci USA 91:13033–13037.

122. Shapiro AB, Ling V (1995) Using purified P-glycoprotein to understand multidrug resistance. J Bioenerg Biomenbr 27:7–13.

123. Sharom FJ (1995) Characterization and functional reconstitution of the multidrug transporter. J Bioenerg Biomembr 27:15–22.

124. Coley HM, Workman P, Twentyman PR (1991) Retention of activity by selected anthracyclines in a multidrug resistant human large cell lung carcinoma line without P-glycoprotein hyperexpression. Br J Cancer 63:351–357.

125. McGrath T, Center MS (1988) Mechanisms of multidrug resistance in HL60 cells: Evidence that a surface membrane protein distinct from P-glycoprotein contributes to reduced cellular accumulation of drug. Cancer Res 48:3959–3963.

126. Marsh W, Sicheri D, Center MS (1986) Isolation and characterization of adriamycin-resistant HL-60 cells which are not defective in the initial intracellular accumulation of drug. Cancer Res 46:4053–4057.

127. Marquardt D, Center MS (1992) Drug transport mechanisms in HL60 cells isolated for resistance to adriamycin: Evidence for nuclear drug accumulation and redistribution in resistant cells. Cancer Res 52:3157–3163.

128. Cole SPC (1992) Drug resistance and lung cancer. In J Wood, ed. Cancer: Concept to Clinic. Fairlawn, NJ: Medical Publishing Enterprises, pp 15–21.

129. Cole SPC, Bhardwaj G, Gerlach JH, Almquist KC, Deeley RG (1993) A novel ATP-binding cassette transporter gene overexpressed in multidrug-resistant human lung tumour cells (abstr). Proc Am Assoc Cancer Res 34:579.

130. Coley HM, Amos WB, Twentyman PR, Workman P (1993) Examination by laser scanning confocal fluorescence imaging microscopy of the subcellular localisation of anthracyclines in parent and multidrug resistant cell lines. Br J Cancer 67:1316–1323.

131. Gervasoni JE Jr, Fields SZ, Krishna S, Baker MA, Rosado M Thuraisamy K, Hindenburg AA, Taub RN (1991) Subcellular distribution of daunorubicin in P-glycoprotein-positive and -negative drug-resistant cell lines using laser-assisted confocal microscopy. Cancer Res 51:4955–4963.

132. Hindenburg AA, Gervasoni JE Jr, Krishna S, Stewart VJ, Rosado M, Lutzky J, Bhalla K, Baker MA, Taub RN (1989) Intracellular distribution and pharmacokinetics of daunorubicin in anthracycline-sensitive and -resistant HL-60 cells. Cancer Res 49:4607–4614.

133. Marquardt D, McCrone S, Center MS (1990) Mechanisms of multidrug resistance in HL60 cells: Detection of resistance-associated proteins with antibodies against synthetic peptides that correspond to the deduced squence of P-glycoprotein. Cancer Res 50:1426–1430.

134. Flens MJ, Izquierdo MA, Scheffer GL, Fritz JM, Meijer CJLM, Scheper RJ, Zaman GJR (1994) Immunochemical detection of the multidrug resistance-associated protein MRP in human multidrug-resistant tumor cells by monoclonal antibodies. Cancer Res 54:4557–4563.

135. Tew KD (1994) Glutathione-associated enzymes in anticancer drug resistance. Cancer Res 54:4313–4320.

136. Abbaszadegan MR, Futscher BW, Klimecki WT, List A, Dalton WS (1994) Analysis of multidrug resistance-associated protein (MRP) messenger RNA in normal and malignant hematopoietic cells. Cancer Res 54:4676–4679.

137. Leier I, Jedlitschky G, Buchholz U, Cole SPC, Deeley RG, Keppler D (1994) The MRP gene encodes an ATP-dependent export pump for leukotriene C_4 and structurally related conjugates. J Biol Chem 269:27807–27810.

138. Keppler D (1992) Leukotrienes: Biosynthesis, transport, inactivation and analysis. Rev Physiol Biochem Pharmacol 121:2–30.

139. Nicholson DW, Ali A, Vaillancourt JP, Calaycay JR, Mumford RA, Zamboni RJ, Ford-Hutchinson AW (1993) Purification to homogeneity and the N-terminal sequence of human leukotriene C_4 synthase: A homodimeric glutathione S-transferase composed of 18-kDa subunits. Proc Natl Acad Sci USA 90:2015–2019.

140. Combates NJ, Rzepka RW, Chen Y-NP, Cohen D (1994) NF-IL6, a member of the C/EBP family of transcription factors, binds and trans-activates the human MDR1 gene promoter. J Biol Chem 269:29715–29719.

141. Ishikawa T (1992) The ATP-dependent glutathione S-conjugate export pump. Trends Biochem Sci 17:463–468.

142. Ishikawa T, Wright CD, Ishizuka H (1994) GS-X pump is functionally overexpressed in cis-diamminedichloroplatinum (II)-resistant human leukemia HL-60 cells and down-regulated by cell differentiation. J Biol Chem 269:29085–29093.

143. Oude Elferink RPJ, Jansen PLM (1994) The role of the canalicular multispecific organic anion transporter in the disposal of endo- and xenobiotics. Pharmacol Ther 64:77–97.

144. Smit JJM, Schinkel AH, Oude Elferink RPJ, Groen AK, Wagenaar E, van Deemter L, Mol CAAM, Ottenhoff R, van der Lugt NMT, van Roon MA, van der Valk MA, Offerhaus GJA, Berns AJM, Borst P (1993) Homozygous disruption of the murine mdr2 P-glycoprotein gene leads to a complete absence of phospholipid from bile and to liver disease. Cell 75:451–462.

145. Schinkel AH, Smit JJM, van Tellingen O, Beijnen JH, Wagenaar E, van Deemter L, Mol CAAM, van der Valk MA, Robanus-Maandag EC, te Riele HPJ, Berns AJM, Borst P (1994) Disruption of the mouse mdr1a P-glycoprotein gene leads to a deficiency in the blood-brain barrier and to increased sensitivity to drugs. Cell 77:491–502.

146. Reutz S, Gros P (1994) Phosphatidylcholine translocase: A physiological role for the mdr2 gene. Cell 77:1071–1081.

147. Tsuruo T, Iida H, Tsukagoshi S, Sakurai Y (1981) Overcoming of vincristine resistance in P388 leukemia in vivo and in vitro through enhanced cytotoxicity of vincristine and vinblastine by verapamil. Cancer Res 41:1967–1972.

148. Ford JM, Hait WN (1991) Pharmacology of drugs that alter multidrug resistance in cancer. Pharmacol Rev 42:155–199.

149. Ford JM, Hait WN (1993) Pharmacologic circumvention of multidrug resistance. Cytotechnology 12:171–212.

150. Raderer M, Scheithauer W (1993) Clinical trials of agents that reverse multidrug resistance. A literature review. Cancer 72:3553–3563.

151. Gottesman MM, Pastan I (1989) Clinical trials of agents that reverse multidrug-resistance. J Clin Oncol 7:409–411.

152. Sikic BI (1993) Modulation of multidrug resistance: At the threshold. J Clin Oncol 11:1629–1635.

153. Foxwell BMJ, Mackie A, Ling V, Ryffel B (1989) Identification of the multidrug resistance-related P-glycoprotein as a cyclosporine binding protein. Mol Pharmacol 36:543–546.

154. Safa AR (1988) Photoaffinity labeling of the moltidrug-resistance-related P-glycoprotein with photoactive analogs of verapamil. Proc Natl Acad Sci USA 85:7187–7191.

155. Rao US, Scarborough GA (1994) Direct demonstration of high affinity interactions of immunosuppressant drugs with the drug binding site of the human P-glycoprotein. Mol Pharmacol 45:773–776.

156. Cole SPC, Downes HF, Slovak ML (1989) Effect of calcium antagonists on the chemosensitivity of two multidrug resistant human tumour cell lines which do not overexpress P-glycoprotein. Br J Cancer 59:42–46.

157. Gekeler V, Boer R, Ise W, Sanders KH, Schachtele C, Beck J (1995) The specific bisindolylmaleimide PKC-inhibitor GF 109203X efficiently modulates MRP-associated multiple drug resistance. Biochem Biophys Res Commun 206:119–126.

158. Gekeler V, Ise W, Sanders KH, Ulrich W-R, Beck J (1995) The leukotriene LTD$_4$ receptor antagonist MK571 specifically modulates MRP associated multidrug resistance. Biochem Biophys Res Commun 208:345–352.

159. van der Graaf WTA, de Vries EGE, Timmer-Bosscha H, Meersma GJ, Mesander G, Vellenga E, Mulder NH (1994) Effects of amiodarone, cyclosporin A, and PSC 833 on the cytotoxicity of mitroxantrone, doxorubicin, and vincristine in non-P-glycoprotein human small cell lung cancer cell lines. Cancer Res 54:5368–5373.

160. Versantvoort CHM, Schuurhuis GJ, Pinedo HM, Eekman CA, Kuiper CM, Lankelma J, Broxterman H (1993) Genistein modulates the decreased drug accumulation in non-P-glycoprotein mediated multidrug resistant tumour cells. Br J Cancer 68:939–946.

161. Gollapudi S, Thadepalli F, Kim CH, Gupta S (1995) Difloxacin reverses multidrug resistance in HL-60/AR cells that overexpress the multidrug resistance-related protein (MRP) gene. Oncol Res 7:73–85.

162. Zwelling LA, Slovak ML, Hinds M, Chan D, Parker E, Mayes J, Sie KL, Meltzer PS, Trent JM (1990) HT1080/DR4: A P-glycoprotein-negative human fibrosarcoma cell line exhibiting resistance to topoisomerase II-reactive drugs despite the presence of a drug-sensitive topoisomerase II. J Natl Cancer Inst 82:1553–1561.

163. de Jong S, Zijlstra JG, Mulder NH, de Vries EGE (1991) Lack of cross-resistance to fostriecin in a human small-cell lung carcinoma cell line showing topoisomerase II-related drug resistance. Cancer Chemother Pharmacol 28:461–464.

164. Griffith OW, Meister A (1979) Potent and specific inhibition of glutathione synthesis by buthionine sulfoximine (S-n-butyl homocysteine sulfoximine). J Biol Chem 254:7558–7560.

165. Versantvoort CHM, Broxterman HJ, Bagrij T, Scheper RJ, Twentyman PR (1995) Regulation by glutathione of drug transport in multidrug-resistant human lung tumour cell lines overexpressing multidrug resistance-associated protein. Br J Cancer 72:82–89.

166. Meijer C, Mulder NH, Timmer-Bosscha H, Peters WHM, de Vries EGE (1991) Combined in vitro modulation of adriamycin resistance. Int J Cancer 49:582–586.

167. Lutzky J, Astor MB, Taub RN, Baker MA, Bhalla K, Gervasoni JE Jr, Rosado M, Stewart V, Krishna S, Hindenburg AA (1989) Role of glutathione and dependent enzymes in anthracycline-resistant HL60/AR cells. Cancer Res 49:4120–4125.

168. Brophy NA, Marie JP, Rojas VA, Warnke RA, McFall PJ, Smith SD, Sikic BI (1994) *Mdr*1 gene expression in childhood acute lymphoblastic leukemias and lymphomas: A critical evaluation by four techniques. Leukemia 8:327–335.

169. Futscher BW, Abbaszadegan MR, Domann F, Dalton WS (1994) Analysis of *MRP* mRNA in mitoxantrone-selected, multidrug-resistant human tumor cells. Biochem Pharmacol 47:1601–1606.

170. Lazaruk LC, Campling BG, Baer KA, Lam Y-M, Cole SPC, Deeley RG, Gerlach JH (1995) Drug resistance and expression of MRP and MDR1 in small cell lung cancer cell lines (abstr). Proc Am Assoc Cancer Res 36:1953.

171. Burger H, Nooter K, Zaman GJR, Sonneveld P, van Wingerden KE, Oostrum RG, Stoter G (1994) Expression of the multidrug resistance-associated protein (*MRP*) in acute and chronic leukemias. Leukemia 8:990–997.

172. Chan HSL, Haddad G, Hipfner DR, Deeley RG, Cole SPC (1995) Sensitive detection of the multidrug resistance protein (MRP) in malignant cells (abstr). Proc Am Assoc Cancer Res 36:1941.

173. Krishnamachary N, Ma L, Zheng L, Safa AR, Center MS (1994) Analysis of MRP gene expression and function in HL60 cells isolated for resistance to adriamycin. Oncol Res 6:119–127.

174. Hipfner DR, Gauldie SD, Deeley RG, Cole SPC (1994) Detection of the M_r 190,000 multidrug resistance protein, MRP, with monoclonal antibodies. Cancer Res 54:5788–5792.

175. Lalande ME, Ling V, Miller RG (1981) Hoechst 33342 dye uptake as a probe of membrane permeability changes in mammalian cells. Proc Natl Acad Sci USA 78:363–367.

176. Neyfakh AA (1988) Use of fluorescent dyes as molecular probes for the study of multidrug

resistance. Exp Cell Res 174:168–176.
177. de Jong S, Holtrop M, de Vries H, de Vries EGE, Mulder NH (1992) Increased sensitivity of an adriamycin-resistant human small cell lung carcinoma cell line to mitochondrial inhibitors. Biochem Biophys Res Commun 182:877–885.
178. Feller N, Kuiper CM, Lankelma J, Ruhdal JK, Scheper RJ, Pinedo HM, Broxterman HJ (1995) Functional detection of *MDR*1/P170 and *MRP*/P190 mediated multidrug resistance in tumor cells by flow cytometry. Br J Cancer 72:543–549.
179. Twentyman PR, Rhodes T, Rayner S (1994) A comparison of rhodamine 123 accumulation and efflux in cells with P-glycoprotein-mediated and MRP-associated multidrug resistance phenotypes. Eur J Cancer 30A:1360–1369.
180. Nooter K, Sonneveld P, Oostrum R, Herweijer H, Hagenbeek T, Valerio D (1990) Overexpression of the *mdr*1 gene in blast cells from patients with acute myelocytic leukemia is associated with decreased anthracycline accumulation that can be restored by cyclosporin-A. Int J Cancer 45:263–268.
181. Ross DD, Wooten PJ, Tong Y, Cornblatt B, Levy C, Sridhara R, Lee EJ, Schiffer CA (1994) Synergistic reversal of multidrug-resistance phenotype in acute myeloid leukemia cells by cyclosporin A and cremophor EL. Blood 83:1337–1347.
182. Schuurhuis GJ, Broxterman HJ, Cervantes A, van Heijningen THM, de Lange JHM, Baak JPA, Pinedo HM, Lankelma J (1989) Quantitative determination of factors contributing to doxorubicin resistance in multidrug-resistant cells. J Natl Cancer Inst 81:1887–1892.
183. Rutherford AV, Willingham MC (1993) Ultrastructural localization of daunomycin in multidrug-resistant cultured cells with modulation of the multidrug transporter. J Histochem Cytochem 41:1573–1577.
184. Hindenburg AA, Baker MA, Gleyzer E, Stewart VJ, Case N, Taub RN (1987) Effect of verapamil and other agents on the distribution of anthracyclines and on reversal of drug resistance. Cancer Res 47:1421–1425.
185. Burger H, Nooter K, Sonneveld P, van Wingerden KE, Zaman GJR, Stoter G (1994) High expression of the multidrug resistance-associated protein (MRP) in chronic and prolymphocytic leukaemia. Br J Haematol 88:348–356.
186. Beck J, Niethammer D, Gekeler V (1994) High mdr1 and mrp-, but low topoisomerase IIα-gene expression in B-cell chronic lymphoycytic leukaemias. Cancer Lett 86:135–142.
187. Hart SM, Ganeshaguru K, Hoffbrand AV, Prentice HG, Mehta AB (1994) Expression of the multidrug resistance-associated protein (MRP) in acute leukemia. Leukemia 8:2163–2168.
188. Schuurhuis GJ, Broxterman HJ, Ossenkoppele GJ, Baak JPA, Eekman CA, Kuiper CM, Feller N, van Heijningen THM, Klumper E, Pieters R, Lankelma J, Pinedo HM (1995) Functional multidrug resistance phenotype associated with combined overexpression of Pgp/*MDR1* and *MRP* together with 1-β-D-arabinofuranosylcytosine sensitivity may predict clinical response in acute myeloid leukemia. Clin Cancer Res 1:81–93.
189. Beck J, Handgretinger R, Dopfer R, Klingebiel T, Niethammer D, Gekeler V (1995) Expression of mdr1, mrp, topoisomerase IIα/β, and cyclin A in primary or relapsed states of acute lymphoblastic leukaemias. Br J Haematol 89:356–363.

II. RESISTANCE TO ALKYLATING AGENTS

3. MECHANISMS OF RESISTANCE TO ALKYLATING AGENTS

PHILIP G. PENKETH, KRISHNAMURTHY SHYAM, AND ALAN C. SARTORELLI

A major problem in cancer chemotherapy is the frequently encountered rapid loss in responsiveness to therapeutic agents [1]. Drug resistance can be the result of the induction of a variety of protective mechanisms or the result of the selection of resistant clones. In some cases, neoplastic cells may also have a high intrinsic level of resistance [2]. Alkylating agents, particularly agents that alkylate preferentially at the O^6 position of guanine, are highly mutagenic [3], and this greatly increases the genetic variability of the neoplasm and provides a heterogeneous population from which resistant mutants can be selected, in a manner akin to the in vitro treatment of cells with N-methyl-N'-nitro-N-nitrosoguanidine (MNNG) to produce experimentally useful mutations. Moreover, since the therapeutic indices of most alkylating agents are low, sublethal drug exposure is frequently encountered, and this produces an ideal selection environment.

The cumulative host toxicity of many agents may result in the host becoming less able to tolerate the agent, while the neoplasm becomes more tolerant. Both of these effects can contribute to the narrowing of an already low therapeutic index. Since alkylating agents act on many sites and lack a specific target, multiple mechanisms of resistance may be involved. It is therefore possible, in view of the low therapeutic index of alkylating agents, that a number of subtle changes within a cell can increase resistance to these agents sufficiently to negate any beneficial value. There are many well-documented mechanisms of acquired drug resistance, and some of the major mechanisms include: (a) changes in drug transport; (b) modified metabolism, such as elevated levels of detoxification enzymes, reduced levels of drug-activating enzymes,

65

or changes in the kinetic parameters of drug metabolism or related pathways so as to minimize deleterious events; (c) increased or decreased levels of primary or secondary targets (depending upon whether the interaction of the drug with the target creates a toxic event directly or an inactivation of the target); (d) enhanced levels of repair enzymes; and (e) decreased activation of cell suicide pathways (apoptosis) [4–7].

Most current chemotherapeutic regimens involve the use of multiple agents. One of the major rationales behind such treatments is to use drugs with nonoverlapping dose-limiting toxicities so as to spread the overall toxicity over several normal tissues while maximizing the toxicity directed against the tumor. An advantage of this type of treatment is that it is unlikely that a single change is capable of conferring resistance to all of the agents involved, although some changes can give rise to resistance to multiple agents or structurally diverse agents with similar electrophilicity. A large number of studies have been carried out to study the cellular changes involved in the acquisition of resistance to many anticancer drugs. The ultimate goal of such studies is to achieve the reversal of resistance through interference with the protective mechanism involved, resulting in increased toxicity to the tumor without an equivalent change in host toxicity. Several successful modulatory therapies have arisen from such studies [8,9]. In this chapter we discuss the mechanisms involved in the resistance of neoplastic cells to alkylating agents and describe how some of these changes may be circumvented or exploited.

MODIFICATION OF TRANSPORT MECHANISMS

Role of the MDR phenotype

The multidrug resistance (MDR) phenotype has been intensively studied since the early 1970s [6,10]. The MDR phenotype is characterized by a pleiotropic cross-resistance after selection by a single agent [6]. There may be multiple mechanisms that are capable of conferring cross-resistance to multiple agents. However, the term *MDR* has become synonymous with the overexpression of a 170 kDa protein, known as the P-glycoprotein, encoded by the *mdr*1 gene. This transmembrane protein mediates an energy-dependent drug efflux mechanism [6]. The P-glycoprotein pump appears to be most active against natural product anticancer drugs, presumably because this efflux system favors weakly basic hydrophobic molecules with molecular weights greater than 600 Da [6]. As a consequence, the P-glycoprotein has little relevance in mediating resistance to most alkylating agents, with mitomycin C being a notable exception [11]. Typically, alkylating agents have relatively low molecular weights, are at least moderately hydrophilic, and are frequently nonbasic. The role of MDR in the resistance of malignant cells to anticancer drugs has been extensively reviewed recently [12].

Role of amino acid and other transporters

A modified amino acid carrier has been linked to increased resistance to melphalan [13]. In the resistant cell line, both a lower velocity of drug uptake and a lower intracellular accumulation of drug at equilibrium occurred than in the sensitive parental cell line, while drug efflux remained unchanged. The uptake of melphalan was susceptible to inhibition by amino acids such as L-leucine and DL-β-2-aminobicyclo[2,2,1]heptane-2-carboxylic acid, a specific inhibitor of the low-affinity L-system. The melphalan-resistant cell line, which had been maintained in continuous passage in mice treated with melphalan for 1 year, was extremely resistant to melphalan. Therefore, it is likely that the reduced intracellular steady-state levels of melphalan (70% of the sensitive cell line) were only partially responsible for the observed resistance, and a multitude of changes probably contribute to the overall resistance of these cells to the alkylating agent.

In nitrogen mustard (mechlorethamine) resistant L5178Y lymphoblasts, changes in the choline transporter have been linked to the resistant phenotype [14]. Resistance to cis-diamminedichloroplatinum (II) (cDDP) in L1210 cells has similarly been associated with changes in transport via an amino acid carrier [15]. The low molecular weight and moderate hydrophilicity of many alkylating agents would, however, suggest that transport mechanisms do not play a major role in the mechanisms of resistance to agents of this kind.

ROLE OF THIOLS AND ASSOCIATED ENZYMES IN RESISTANCE TO ALKYLATING AGENTS

Chemistry of alkylation

Alkylating agents replace hydrogen atoms of a molecule by an alkyl group. The mechanism usually involves the reaction of an electrophilic species (i.e., the alkylating agent) with a nucleophilic site on the target molecule (e.g., DNA). The preference of electrophiles for various nucleophiles depends on several factors [16]. The concept of hard and soft electrophiles and nucleophiles is a useful qualitative method for predicting the reactivity of various structurally diverse electrophiles and nucleophiles toward each other. Electrophiles and nucleophiles are classified as hard or soft depending upon the distribution of the electronic charge. Hard electrophiles and nucleophiles are charged, or are at least highly polarized, having high local positive or negative charge densities, respectively. Soft electrophiles and nucleophiles, on the other hand, have weakly polarized or easily polarizable groups with low positive and negative charge densities, respectively. The activation energy for the reaction of electrophiles with nucleophiles is the lowest when they react with molecules of similar hardness/softness [16].

A common misconception is that as electrophiles become more reactive (harder), their reactions with nucleophiles increase in range. This is because they are now able to react with harder nucleophiles (more weakly nucleophilic sites), with which soft electrophiles would not readily react. It is, however, only a shift in range and not an extension of range that is being observed [16]. Of the many biological nucleophilic sites available, the softest are the thiols, followed by nitrogen-based sites such as amino groups, which, in turn, are softer than oxygen-based centers, such as hydroxyl groups, which are relatively hard in nature. The major nucleophilic sites in DNA in the order of increasing hardness are N^7 of guanine $<$ other amino functionalities of purine/pyrimidine bases $<$ oxygen functionalities of purine/pyrimidine bases (O^6 of guanine being one of the hardest) $<$ O^- of the phosphate groups in the sugar phosphate backbone. From a purely chemical point of view, thiols would be expected to protect the N^7 group of guanine from alkylation by relatively soft electrophiles, which prefer to alkylate thiols and the N^7 of guanine, by acting as competing nucleophiles but offer little protection to the O^6 group of guanine (or phosphate) against alkylation by relatively hard alkylating agents, which would prefer alkylation at this site.

Importance of GSH and GSTs in resistance mechanisms

Early studies have indicated that several alkylating agents react preferentially with tissue sulfhydryl groups [17] and that changes in the thiol status of cells can be an important factor in the resistance/cross-resistance to alkylating agents [18]. Since virtually all cells (prokaryote and eukaryote) contain glutathione (GSH) [19], or in some cases an alternative low molecular weight thiol [20], GSH probably represents an early evolutionary development that protects cells from electrophilic assault. However, GSH is restricted by its chemistry to offer effective protection only against relatively soft alkylating agents unless present at extremely high concentrations. Glutathione S-transferases (GSTs) probably represent a later evolutionary development that serves to extend the range of protection afforded by GSH. GSTs are a supergene family of dimeric enzymes with a dimeric molecular weight of 48–52 kDa that function as homodimers or heterodimers [21]. Microsomal GSTs, being functional trimers with trimeric molecular weights of 51 kDa, differ significantly from this pattern and may be a product of convergent functional evolution. They are subject to 10- to 15-fold activation upon the covalent modification of an enzymatic thiol by an electrophilic xenobiotic [22]. The GSTs catalyze the reaction of GSH with a wide range of electrophiles, ranging from soft to very hard species.

GSTs have been purified from a large number of species, ranging from *E. coli* to humans [21]. Different GSTs favor reaction with different classes of electrophiles. Most of the GST isoenzymes have relatively low substrate affinities and overlapping broad substrate specificities, which afford protection against a variety of electrophiles [21]. However, some GSTs may have evolved to have more specific functions, such as the inactivation of specific insecticides in organisms facing a frequent onslaught by the same or similar toxins [23]. Some of the protective action attributed to elevated levels of GSH may be mediated in part by GSTs; therefore, in some tissues not all GSTs may be fully saturated by normal levels of GSH. Furthermore, some GSH conjugates of anticancer drugs are competitive inhibitors of GST [24]. Thus, elevation of GSH levels would counter this product inhibition, since elevation of intracellular levels of GSH will accelerate the conjugation of reactive electrophiles by both nonenzymatic and enzymatic mechanisms.

Over the years, several different nomenclature schemes have been used to describe GSTs, and this subject has been extensively reviewed [21]. In mammals, four major cytosolic classes of GSTs exist that all contain a short sequence of homology, suggesting evolution from a common primordial gene [25]. Within each class, regions of high sequence identity are shared. In humans, these classes have been named α, μ, π, and θ [25]. Only one GST π class enzyme appears to be expressed in humans and rats, but multiple α and μ classes are known with characteristic patterns of tissue distribution. In the rat, Ya and Yc correspond to the human α class; Yb1, Yb2, and Yb3 correspond to μ class enzymes; and Yp and Yrs correspond to π and θ class enzymes, respectively. It is believed that the primordial protein was θ-like in structure [26].

Enzymes in the α class have isoelectric points in the 7.5–9.0 range and are described as basic, the μ class of enzymes have isoelectric points around 6.6 and are described as neutral, while the π class of catalysts have isoelectric points close to 4.8 and are acidic. The basic α class human GSTs have high peroxidase activity with organic peroxides and high isomerase activity with Δ^5-androstene-3,17 dione, but are not as active against 1-chloro-2,4-dinitrobenzene (CDNB) as the μ and π classes, although they still have high activity with this electrophilic substrate. The near neutral μ class has the highest activity with CDNB and high activity with styrene-7,8-oxide. The μ class enzyme appears to be absent in 40% of individuals, and this deficiency is associated with increased lung cancer rates in smokers [27]. The π class enzyme shows high activity against ethacrynic acid and 1,2-epoxy-5-(p-nitrophenoxy)propane and is frequently expressed at high levels in neoplastic tissues [21,28].

In view of the properties of GSH/GSTs and their inducibility by xenobiotics via AP-1–like regulatory elements [29], it is not surprising that they play a role not only in the metabolism of electrophilic carcinogens but also in the inactivation of alkylating agents [28]. Thus, there is a vast body of literature attributing resistance to various antineoplastic agents to the overexpression of GSTs, particularly GST π. However, since numerous changes are probably involved in the acquisition of drug resistance and GST π is both inducible and frequently overexpressed in neoplastic tissues [28,29], great care must be taken when ascribing differences in sensitivity or increases in resistance to differences or changes in the expression of GST.

Relatively few studies have been sufficiently well controlled to make this point unambiguously. A series of experiments carried out in the laboratory of W. Fahl conclusively show that increases in the expression of GST following transfection of various GST cDNAs does impart some resistance to many alkylating agents [30,31]. In these studies, mouse C3H/10T1/2 fibroblasts stably transfected with GST π, Ya, or Yb, and monkey COS cells transfected with the same GST genes, were compared with equivalent cells transfected with vector alone with respect to their resistance to the cytotoxic actions of a number of alkylating agents. GST Ya produced the greatest degree of resistance to the nitrogen mustards, with up to a 2.9-fold increase in the observed LD_{90} for chlorambucil; Yb1 conferred the greatest degree of resistance to cisplatin (1.5-fold), and π gave the highest level of resistance against doxorubicin (1.3-fold). Statistically significant increases in the LD_{90} values were also reported for a number of other agents, including melphalan and benzo(a)pyrene ($\pm$)-anti-diol epoxide [30,31]. The degree of drug resistance appeared to be proportional to the level of expression of GST, and reversion of the transiently expressing cells resulted in a complete loss of enhanced drug resistance [31]. The relatively modest increases in drug resistance observed in GST transfected cell lines are similar to those observed in the clinic and represent significant changes with respect to attainment of successful therapy. It should be noted that the parental cell line contained significant GST activity, and only a relatively modest fold change in the level of resistance of GST transfected lines would therefore be anticipated as a consequence.

A large body of additional literature exists showing strong associations between elevated GST activity and resistance to a number of other clinically used alkylating agents. In the case of 1,3-bis(2-chloroethyl)-1-nitrosourea (BCNU), direct biochemical evidence exists for drug denitrosation catalyzed by GST μ [32]. This action would preclude the generation of any alkylating species by the known routes of activation. GST can also offer protection from chloroethylnitrosoureas by a second detoxification mechanism that involves dechlorination as a result of the attack of the sulfur at the chloro-bearing carbon atom and the formation of a drug-GSH conjugate [33]. Typically, crosslinking nitrosoureas are approximately 50- to 100-fold more potent than their monofunctional counterparts, so loss of bifunctionality represents a significant reduction in cytotoxicity [34]. Furthermore, the nitroso group may then leave, resulting in a total loss of alkylating activity [33]. Rodent liver GST preparations have been proposed to catalyze the detoxification of BCNU via this route [33]. Direct biochemical evidence also exists for the inactivation of nitrogen mustard drugs by α class GSTs [35].

GSH itself can offer significant protection to cells and organisms from alkylating agents, and this action should not be overlooked in view of the fact that many resistant cells also show elevated thiol levels [18]. Such elevated levels are due to increased expression of γ-glutamylcysteine synthetase (γ-GCS), the rate-limiting enzyme in GSH synthesis, which together with γ-glutamyltranspeptidase (γ-GT) supplies cysteine for γ-GCS [36,37].

Protection by protein thiols and metallothioneins

Any abundant thiol species within cells can act as a soft electrophilic sink and spare DNA and crucial proteins from alkylation. If the thiol species is relatively dispensable or alkylation of the thiol group does not greatly impair its function, elevation of this species can primarily serve a protective function. GSTs may also offer some protection via this mechanism since these enzymes contain cysteine residues [26], the alkylation of which in the case of microsomal GSTs greatly increases their enzymatic activity [22] and in some cells constitute up to 10% of the cytosolic protein [38].

Metallothioneins are small 6–7 kDa cysteine-rich proteins that appear to protect cells from the toxicity of heavy metals such as copper, zinc, mercury, and cadmium [39]. Seven heavy metal atoms can be bound to each metallothionein molecule via thiolate bonds [39]. In humans, five isoforms are known. The functional significance of metallothioneins may extend beyond their ability to protect cells by binding electrophilic heavy metal ions, since they can also be induced by factors other than heavy metals. Metallothionein synthesis can be induced by steroids and other hormones, stress, x-rays, high O_2 tension, and alkylating agents. Thus, met-allothioneins may play a role in oxygen radical scavenging and protection from other electrophilic species, as well as their proposed function in Zn^{2+} and Cu^{2+} homeostasis. The protective role of metallothioneins against heavy metal toxicity promoted the study of these proteins in the resistance of cells to cDDP [40]. It was found that Cd^{2+}-resistant cells, which expressed high levels of metallothionein, were cross-resistant to cDDP. Changes in the uptake of cDDP were not involved in the acquisition of resistance in these cells, since the resistant cell line accumulated more drug than the sensitive wild-type parental cell line. In the cDDP-resistant subline, a greater proportion of the platinum was associated with metallothionein [40].

High levels of metallothionein are also associated with resistance to other alkylat-ing agents, with both monofunctionality and bifunctionality [41]. Much of this activity is probably a consequence of the high abundance and high thiol content of metallothionein. Calculations for horse kidney, a particularly rich source of metallothionein, based upon the assumption that 100% of the cadmium in the kidney cortex is bound to metallothionein, making it approximately 1–2% of the kidney cortex dry weight [42]; that the kidney cortex dry weight is approximately 25% of its wet weight; and that 20 of the 61–62 amino acids of metallothionein are cysteines [39], puts the net molarity of the thiol groups from metallothionein at 5–10 mM, which is comparable to the contribution of GSH to the total thiol pool. Owing to the different local environments of the cysteines in this protein, the nucleophilicities of these residues are likely to vary and, therefore, may offer a broader degree of protection than GSH alone. In support of these concepts, a human squamous cell carcinoma that is stably resistant to cDDP was found to be cross-resistant to a number of alkylating agents and to Cd^{2+}, and to have normal nonprotein sulfhydryl levels but elevated metallothionein, which resulted in an approximate doubling of the protein sulfhydryl level [43]. This cell line contained an elevated level of GST, which also may have contributed to the resistance of this squamous cell carcinoma to some chemotherapeutic agents [43].

Resistant cell lines with both elevated nonprotein sulfhydryl and protein sulfhy-dryl groups have also been isolated [44]. Not all findings, however, fit the concept that metallothionein can protect cells from alkylating agent toxicity. Thus, pretreat-ment of CHO cells with 0.1 M Zn^{2+} for several hours before exposure to melphalan resulted in the induction of considerable resistance to melphalan; however, Cd^{2+}-resistant mutants of the same cell line that had a 40-fold increased capacity to induce metallothionein in response to Zn^{2+} did not show any enhanced resistance to melphalan [45]. Moreover, the only cell line tested that did not show a protective effect induced by pretreatment with Zn^{2+} was a cell line that readily expressed elevated metallothionein levels in response to heavy metals. Clearly, factors other than the induction of metallothionein are involved in the effects produced by Zn^{2+}. It is also surprising that elevated levels of metallothionein did not afford protection in these cell lines. One possible explanation for this phenomenon is that when the thiol groups of metallothionein are saturated with Zn^{2+}, they are not readily available to act as competing nucleophiles, thereby negating the protective role of the metallothionein in these instances. Such a possibility could also explain the protective action of Zn^{2+}, since imidazole-like nitrogen atoms are excellent ligands for zinc and could likewise be protected from alkylation if they are involved in the coordination of Zn^{2+}. Therefore, it is possible that Zn^{2+} could directly protect sites such as the N^7 of guanine from alkylation by coordination of this site.

MODIFICATIONS OF DRUG METABOLISM

Advantages and disadvantages of prodrugs

Changes in drug metabolism may be important factors in the resistance of cells to alkylating agents [5]. Many alkylating agents are administered as prodrugs that require activation by cellular enzymes to generate the ultimate alkylating species. Drugs in this category include mitomycin C, cyclophosphamide, 5-(3,3-dimethyl-1-triazenyl)-1H-imidazole-4-carboxamide (DTIC), and procarbazine. While alternative metabolic pathways may circumvent the generation of the alkylating species or inactivate the generated electrophile, biologically activated prodrugs can have several potential advantages over the direct administration of the ultimate alkylating species. The administration of a prodrug may allow the successful distribution of the drug to the target site of an otherwise very short-lived agent and also prevent or minimize local toxicity. It is also possible to design prodrugs that are activated to a greater degree within tumor cells than in host cells, thereby producing some degree of preferential targeting, and as a consequence an increase in the therapeutic index. Potential disadvantages of using biologically activated prodrugs include: (a) the extended half-life of the drug allows more time for metabolism by alternative inactivating pathways, and (b) resistance can be readily attained by a decrease in the levels of activating enzymes or increases in the levels of enzymes that metabolize the prodrug to inactive products. Many examples of these phenomena are documented in the literature [5], and GST- and metallothionein-mediated inactivation mechanisms have been discussed.

Resistance to cyclophosphamide

Cytochrome P-450–mediated mixed function oxidoreductases play a significant role in the activation of several anticancer drugs [46]. Cyclophosphamide is a P-450 mixed function oxidoreductase activated prodrug of phosphoramide mustard; thus, cyclophosphamide itself has no alkylating activity. The enzymatic hydroxylation of this prodrug results in the formation of 4-hydroxycyclophosphamide, which can spontaneously decompose to generate acrolein and the active alkylating species, phosphoramide mustard. The parent compound can be inactivated by N-dechloroethylation, and the 4-hydroxy metabolite may be inactivated by oxidation via aldehyde dehydrogenase [47].

Both of the above mechanisms can potentially result in the attainment of resistance by neoplastic cells. Increased resistance to cyclophosphamide has also been reported to occur in cells as a result of decreased levels of P-450 mixed function oxidoreductase activity, which led to a decrease in the formation of phosphoramide mustard [48,49]. Increased resistance to cyclophosphamide has been reported in L1210/CPA cells, which express a 200-fold increase in aldehyde dehydrogenase activity and, thereby, convert 4-hydroxycyclophosphamide to the inactive 4-ketocyclophosphamide metabolite [47]. These cells specifically express resistance to cyclophosphamide and oxazaphosphorine analogs, but not to other alkylating agents. Thus, when exposed to cyclophosphamide, L1210/CPA cells accumulate carboxyphosphamide and are restored to parental sensitivity by inhibitors of aldehyde dehydrogenase.

Resistance to chloroethylnitrosoureas

The 2-chloroethylnitrosoureas may also be inactivated by a P-450–mediated pathway, as well as a GST-mediated route [32,50], and significant metabolic inactivation of these agents can occur [51]. 1-(2-Chloroethyl)-3-cyclohexyl-1-nitrosourea (CCNU), BCNU, and possibly other related drugs can be metabolized by liver microsomal enzymes in an NADPH-dependent reaction to yield the corresponding urea, which is devoid of alkylating activity [50]. The reductive denitrosation reaction is carried out by components of the cytochrome P-450 system. CCNU may also be hydroxylated on the cyclohexane ring by the P-450–mediated pathway; such a change does not negate the alkylating activity of this molecule and may mediate much of the antitumor activity of CCNU. This modification may also result in a compound with an extended biological half-life, since the product is more resistant to denitrosation [52].

ENHANCED DNA REPAIR

Several nitrosoureas have been evaluated clinically and have been shown to possess significant antineoplastic activity against brain tumors, colon cancer, and lymphomas [53,54]. Characterization of the decomposition products of the nitrosoureas employed clinically has resulted in the identification of several reactive products, including alkylating [55,56] and carbamoylating [55–57] species. The two major classes of nitrosoureas used clinically, that is, the chloroethylnitrosoureas or CNUs (e.g., BCNU and CCNU) and the methylnitrosoureas (e.g., streptozotocin), are activated by similar decomposition mechanisms. However, while the methylnitrosoureas generate methyldiazohydroxide, a monofunctional alkylating agent, as the electrophilic species, the CNUs generate the bifunctional alkylating species, the 2-chloroethyldiazohydroxide [55].

The key site of DNA alkylation for the nitrosoureas appears to be the O^6 position of guanine [58,59]. In the case of the CNUs, alkylation of the O^6 position of guanine is followed by an intramolecular nucleophilic substitution reaction, resulting in the formation of 1,O^6-ethanoguanine. The latter compound reacts with the N^3 position of a cytosine residue on an opposite strand of DNA to form a 1-(N3-deoxycytidinyl)-2-(N1-deoxyguanosinyl)ethane DNA crosslink [60,61]. In general,

DNA repair becomes considerably more difficult once crosslinks are formed. This may explain the increased cytotoxicity of the CNUs compared with the methylnitrosoureas. However, there is a considerable time lag (e.g., 6–12 hours) between monoadduct formation, that is, the generation of O^6-chloroethylguanine or $1,O^6$-ethanoguanine, and the appearance of crosslinks [58]. Any cellular mechanism that effectively interferes with the formation of DNA crosslinks should confer resistance to the CNUs.

Regeneration of guanine from O^6-chloroethylguanine by the repair enzyme, O^6-alkylguanine-DNA alkyltransferase (AGT), is one such mechanism. AGT was originally found to cause demethylation of O^6-methylguanine in DNA [62]. Subsequently, this enzyme was found to be capable of removing a variety of alkyl groups from the O^6-position of guanine [63]. The presence of high levels of this enzyme in human tumors compared with their murine counterparts appears to explain, at least in part, the therapeutic efficacy of the nitrosoureas in the treatment of murine tumors and their comparative lack of success in the clinic [9].

O^6-Alkylation of guanine residues in DNA is repaired by AGT, which acts by, transferring the offending alkyl group to a cysteine residue in the active site of the enzyme [62,64–67]. The mechanism of action is thought to be an S_N^2 reaction in which the active site cysteine, perhaps as its thiolate, attacks the α-carbon of the O^6-alkyl group [68]. The cysteine is part of a highly conserved polypeptide sequence, Pro-Cys-His-Arg-Val/Ileu, present in all AGT proteins [69]. The histidine residue may facilitate the reaction by deprotonating the thiol group of cysteine to generate the highly nucleophilic thiolate group [69,70]. The proline may serve to bend the protein chain in such a way as to correctly position the cysteine moiety [69,70]. The end result of the reaction of AGT is the restoration of a normal guanine residue at the site of the modified base. Gonzaga et al. [71] have provided convincing evidence that $1,O^6$-ethanoguanine is also a substrate for AGT. In an in vitro study, these authors showed that reaction of AGT with $1,O^6$-ethanoguanine resulted in the protein becoming covalently bound to DNA via the 1-position of guanine, thereby preventing the production of an N^1-guanine, N^3-cytosine DNA crosslink. The significance of this reaction in vivo is unknown.

The O^6-dealkylation reaction is both irreversible and stoichiometric, with one damaged base being repaired by one protein molecule. The cysteine acceptor site in the enzyme is not regenerated, and the alkyl group remains covalently bound to the protein. Since no regeneration of the acceptor site occurs, the number of O^6-alkylguanine adducts that can be repaired is limited to the number of available molecules of AGT protein. Furthermore, there is a significant time lag between enzyme inhibition and enzyme resynthesis, which a number of laboratories have sought to exploit [72].

Mammalian cell lines can be classified according to their capacity to repair O^6-alkylguanine in DNA [73]. Cells that express AGT, and therefore have the capacity to repair this lesion are termed Mer⁺. For practical purposes, cells with fewer than 200 molecules of AGT are designated as Mer⁻ [73]. In general, Mer⁻ cells are particularly sensitive to the cytotoxic effects of chloroethylating agents (e.g., BCNU,

CCNU, and clomesone) and methylating agents that target the O^6 position of guanine (e.g., dacarbazine, streptozotocin, and temozolomide). The ability of CNUs to produce DNA crosslinks varies widely in cell lines. In general, there appears to be a good correlation between the number of DNA crosslinks and the cytotoxicity produced by the CNUs.

Erickson et al. [58] have measured the DNA interstrand crosslinks produced by 1-(2-chloroethyl)-1-nitrosourea in 13 human cell lines characterized as having the Mer$^+$ or the Mer$^-$ phenotype. Six strains deficient in the capacity to repair the O^6-alkylation of guanine in DNA, that is, the Mer$^-$ phenotype, produced consistently higher levels of interstrand crosslinks than 5 of 7 Mer$^+$ strains examined. Furthermore, when DNA of CNU-resistant Mer$^+$ cells was transfected into CNU-sensitive Mer$^-$ cells, a clone with greater AGT activity and increased resistance to the nitrosoureas was obtained [74]. A correlation between the content of AGT and the sensitivity of cells to CNUs was also obtained in six human rhabdomyosarcoma lines transplanted in nude mice [75]. The cytotoxicity of methylating agents such as 5-(3-methyl-1-triazenyl)-1H-imidazole-4-carboxamide (MTIC), the active metabolite of DTIC, and temozolomide also correlates well with the level of AGT in cells, with Mer$^-$ cells once again being more sensitive than Mer$^+$ cells [76–78]. The above findings suggest that the level of AGT in neoplastic cells can be a significant determinant in the efficacy of cancer chemotherapeutic agents that function through alkylation, such as the CNUs and the methyltriazenes that are used clinically.

APOPTOSIS

Other mechanisms that are not directly related to drug transport, drug metabolism, or the repair of drug-induced damage may be involved in resistance to cytodestructive agents. One such mechanism is impaired apoptosis [79]. In multicellular organisms a balance normally exists between cellular proliferation, differentiation, and death. Cell death is frequently genetically programmed and involves the production of proteins required for death and the optimum destruction of dead cells. This programmed cell death is called *apoptosis*. During this process cells shrink, hydrolyze their genome into oligonucleosome-sized fragments, and finally lose membrane integrity. The resultant fragments are readily taken up by surrounding cells [80]. Apoptosis plays a role in normal development, where the elimination of certain cell populations may be required [81]. Apoptosis can be triggered by many mechanisms; of particular relevance to cancer chemotherapy is the triggering of apoptosis by DNA damage [82]. This may represent a cell suicide phenomenon that protects multicellular organisms from aberrant cells generated by insufficient genetic damage to directly cause their destruction but sufficiently damaged such that repair would result in the production of cells that could compromise the organism as a whole. Many alkylating agents may exert their effects by inducing apoptosis rather than due to direct lethal damage to DNA [83]. The very frequent occurrence of tumors in mice lacking the p53 gene suggests that apoptosis plays an important role in the self-destruction of DNA-damaged cells that would otherwise lead to the development of tumors [84]. In view of these findings, cells that have an impaired ability to undergo apoptosis or are incapable of undergoing apoptosis would be expected to be relatively resistant to both chemotherapeutic agents and x-irradiation. The overexpression of the *bcl*-2 oncogene has been shown to inhibit apoptosis in several cell types, and also to produce cells that are less sensitive to alkylating and other cytotoxic agents [82]. Therefore, overexpression of *bcl*-2 or other mechanisms by which apoptosis may be suppressed can represent important mechanisms by which resistance to alkylating agents can be expressed.

CONCLUSIONS

Studies on mechanisms of resistance to alkylating agents have been quite fruitful, defining specific properties that lead to tumor insensitivity, thereby providing a number of targets for therapeutic circumvention. These findings have led to the preclinical and clinical evaluation of a number of agents with the potential to circumvent the resistant phenotype. The MDR phenotype appears to be of relatively little importance in conferring resistance to alkylating agents, with the notable exception of mitomycin C. The protection of cells via elevated cellular levels of thiols and/or GSTs also lends itself to exploitation. Thus, buthionine sulfoximine (BSO), an irreversible inhibitor of γ-GCS, which produces marked reductions in cellular concentrations of GSH [85], is in clinical trial [9]. BSO has been shown to reverse acquired resistance to alkylating agents that occurs as a consequence of elevations in GSH in a moderately selective manner [86]. The greater reliance on GSH as a protectant in resistant tumor cells results in a greater sensitization of these cells than of host cells. Conversely, the use of thiols such as S-2-(3-aminopropylamino)ethylphosphorothioic acid (WR-2721) or the glutathione prodrug, glutathione monoethyl ester, to supplement the endogenous thiol levels of the host so as to offer additional protection of the host against electrophilic agents is being studied [87]. These agents are taken up at differential rates by different tissues and do not seem to protect tumor tissue to the same extent that they spare critical normal tissues [87]. Inhibitors of GST are also being studied for their capacity to reverse drug resistance caused by elevated GST activity. In this regard, ethacrynic acid has been found to sensitize drug-resistant tumor cells to chlorambucil at low nontoxic concentrations [88]. This inhibitor has now progressed into phase I clinical trial [89]. More specific inhibitors of GST are currently under development [90].

An additional approach to the exploitation of elevated levels of GSH and/or GST is to develop prodrugs of hard alkylating agents that are activated by thiolysis, preferably catalyzed specifically by GST. MNNG is a thiol-activated alkylating agent that has been successfully used to select for cells with a reduced content of GSH, as a consequence of being selectively toxic to cells with a relatively high content of thiols [91]. However, this agent is not suitable for use as a chemotherapeutic agent due to its high carcinogenicity and mutagenicity [65]. Attempts are now underway to synthesize thiol/GSH- and GST-activated agents more suitable for clinical use [92,93].

Attempts have also been made to increase the clinical effectiveness of current agents against cells rich in AGTs. Since a high level of AGT activity protects against the cytotoxic effects of CNUs and methyltriazenes, approaches that reduce the activity of AGT in neoplastic cells prior to exposure to CNUs have been tested. Several approaches have been tried, including pretreatment with (a) methylating agents such as DTIC and streptozotocin [94], (b) O^6-methylguanine [95], and (c) O^6-benzylguanine and its derivatives [96,97]. Of these, the most promising results have been obtained with O^6-benzylguanine and analogs thereof. It is to be expected that continued studies on the mechanisms of drug resistance to alkylating agents will lead to further improvement in therapeutic regimens that employ these reactive agents for the treatment of neoplastic diseases.

REFERENCES

1. Woolley PV, Tew KD (1988) Mechanisms of Drug Resistance in Neoplastic Cells. San Diego, CA: Academic Press, pp 1–390.
2. Waxman DJ (1990) Glutathione S-transferases: Role in alkylating agent resistance and possible target for modulation chemotherapy—a review. Cancer Res 50:6449–6454.
3. Loveless A (1969) Possible relevance of O-6 alkylation of deoxyguanosine to the mutagenicity and carcinogenicity of nitrosamines and nitrosamides. Nature 223:206–207.
4. Arrick BA, Nathan CF (1984) Glutathione metabolism as a determinant of therapeutic efficacy: A review. Cancer Res 44:4224–4232.
5. LeBlanc GA, Waxman DJ (1989) Interaction of anticancer drugs with hepatic monooxygenase enzymes. Drug Metab Rev 20:395–439.
6. Ford JM, Hait WN (1990) Pharmacology of drugs that alter multidrug resistance in cancer. Pharm Rev 42:155–199.
7. Collins MKL, Lopez-Rivas A (1993) The control of apoptosis in mammaliam cells. Trends Biol Sci 18:307–309.
8. Miller RL, Bukowski RM, Budd GT, et al. (1988) Clinical modulation of doxorubicin resistance by calmodulin-inhibitor trifluoperazine: A phase I/II trial. J Clin Oncol 6:880–888.
9. Tew KD, Houghton JA, Houghton PJ (1993) Preclinical and Clinical Modulation of Anticancer Drugs. Boca Raton, FL: CRC Press.
10. Bielder JL, Riehm H (1970) Cellular resistance to actinomycin D in cross resistance, radioautographic, and cytogenic studies. Cancer Res 30:1174–1184.
11. Giavazzi R, Kartner N, Hart IR (1984) Expression of cell surface P-glycoprotein by an Adriamycin-resistant murine fibrosarcoma. Cancer Chemother Pharmacol 13:145–147.
12. Bates SE, Zhan Z, Dickstein B, et al. (1994) Reversal of multidrug resistance. J Hematother 3:219–223.
13. Redwood WR, Colvin M (1980) Transport of melphalan by sensitive and resistant L1210 cells. Cancer Res 40:1144–1149.
14. Goldenberg GJ, Vanstone CL, Israels LG, Ilse D, Bihler I (1970) Evidence for a transport carrier of nitrogen mustard in nitrogen mustard-sensitive and -resistant L5178Y lymphoblasts. Cancer Res 30:2285–2291.
15. Gross RB, Waxman S, Scanlon KJ (1986) Amino acid membrane transport properties of L1210 cells resistant to cisplatinum. Chemotherapia 5:37–43.
16. Coles B (1984–1985) Effects of modifying structure on electrophilic reactions with biological nucleophiles. Drug Metab Rev 15:1307–1334.
17. Roberts JJ, Warwick GP (1957) Mode of action of alkylating agents: Formation of S-ethylcysteine from ethyl methanesulphonate in vivo. Nature 179:1181–1182.
18. Hirono I (1960) Non-protein sulfhydryl group in the original strain and sub-line of the ascites tumour resistant to alkylating reagents. Nature 186:1059–1060.
19. Meister A (1988) On the discovery of glutathione. Trends Biol Sci 13:185–188.
20. Penketh PG, Kennedy WPK, Patton CL, Sartorelli AC (1987) Trypanosomatid hydrogen peroxide metabolism. FEBS Lett 221:427–431.
21. Mannervik B (1985) The isoenzymes of glutathione transferase. Adv Enzymol Relat Areas Mol Biol 57:357–417.

22. Morgenstern R, Depierre JW (1988) Membrane-bound glutathione transferase. In H Sies, B Ketterer, eds. Glutathione Conjugation. New York: Academic Press, pp 157–174.
23. Fournier D, Bride JM, Poirie M, Berge J-B, Plapp FW (1992) Insect glutathione S-transferase. Biochemical characteristics of the major forms from houseflies susceptible and resistant to insecticides. J Biol Chem 267:1840–1845.
24. Clark AG, Debnam P (1988) Inhibition of glutathione S-transferase from rat liver by S-nitroso-L-glutathione. Biochem Pharmacol 37:3199–3207.
25. Pickett CD, Lu AYH (1989) Glutathione S-transferases: Gene structure, regulation, and biological function. Annu Rev Biochem 58:743–764.
26. Taylor J, Pemble S, Harris J, Meyer D, Spencer S, Xia C-L, Ketterer B (1993) Evolution of GST genes. In KD Tew, CB Pickett, TJ Mantle, B Mannervik, JD Hayes, eds. Structure and Function of Glutathione Transferases. Boca Raton, FL: CRC Press, pp 163–173.
27. Zhong S, Hayes JD, Spurr NK, Wolf CR (1993) Molecular genetics of the human Mu class GST multigene family. In KD Tew, CB Pickett, TJ Mantle, B Mannervik, JD Hayes, eds. Structure and Function of Glutathione Transferases. Boca Raton, FL: CRC Press, pp 147–159.
28. Tew KD (1994) Glutathione-associated enzymes in anticancer drug resistance. Cancer Res 54:4313–4320.
29. Rushmore TH, Nguyen T, Pickett CB (1993) ARE and XRE mediated induction of the glutathione S-transferase Ya subunit gene: Induction by planar aromatic compounds and phenolic antioxidants. In KD Tew, CB Pickett, TJ Mantle, B Mannervik, JD Hayes, eds. Structure and Function of Glutathione Transferases. Boca Raton, FL: CRC Press, pp 119–128.
30. Manoharan TH, Puchalski RB, Burgess JA, Pickett CB, Fahl WE (1987) Promoter-glutathione S-transferase Ya cDNA hybrid genes. J Biol Chem 262:3739–3745.
31. Puchalski RB, Fahl WE (1990) Expression of recombinant glutathione S-transferase π, Ya, or Yb₁ confers resistance to alkylating agents. Proc Natl Acad Sci USA 87:2443–2447.
32. Berhane K, Hao X-Y, Egyházi S, Hansson J, Ringborg U, Mannervik B (1993) Contribution of glutathione transferase M3-3 to 1,3-bis(2-chloroethyl)-1-nitrosourea resistance in a human non-small cell lung cancer cell line. Cancer Res 53:4257–4261.
33. Smith MT, Evans CG, Doane-Setzer P, Castro VM, Tahir MK, Mannerik B (1989) Denitrosation of 1,3-bis(2-chloroethyl)-1-nitrosourea by mu glutathione transferases and its role in cellular resistance in rat brain tumor cells. Cancer Res 53:4257–4261.
34. Kohn KW, Ewig RAG, Erickson LC, Zwelling LA (1981) Measurement of strand breaks and cross-links by alkaline elution. In EC Friedberg, PC Hanawalt, eds. DNA Repair: A Laboratory Manual of Research Procedures. New York: Marcel Dekker, pp 379–401.
35. Hall AG, Matheson E, Hickson ID, Foster SA, Hogarth L (1994) Purification of an α class glutathione S-transferase from melphalan-resistant Chinese hamster ovary cells and demonstration of its ability to catalyze melphalan-glutathione adduct formation. Cancer Res:54:3369–3372.
36. Godwin AK, Meister A, O'Dwyer PJ, Huang CS, Hamilton TC, Anderson ME (1992) High resistance to cisplatin in human ovarian cancer cell lines is associated with marked increase of glutathione synthesis. Proc Natl Acad Sci USA 89:3070–3074.
37. Mulcahy RT, Bailey HH, Gipp JJ (1994) Up-regulation of γ-glutamylcysteine synthetase activity in melphalan-resistant human multiple myeloma cells expressing increased glutathione levels. Cancer Chemother Pharmacol 34:67–71.
38. Habig WH, Jakoby WB (1981) Glutathione S-transferases (rat and human). Methods Enzymol 77:218–231.
39. Hamer DH (1986) Metallothionein. Annu Rev Biochem 55:913–951.
40. Bakka A, Endresen L, Johnsen ABS, Edminson PD, Rugstand HE (1981) Resistance against cis-dichlorodiammineplatinum in cultured cells with a high content of metallothionein. Toxicol Appl Pharmacol 61:215–226.
41. Kelley SL, Basu A, Teicher BA, Hacker MP, Hamer DH, Lazo JS (1988) Over-expression of metallothionein confers resistance to anticancer drugs. Science 241:1813–1815.
42. Kägi JH, Vallee BL (1960) Metallothionein: A cadmium- and zinc-containing protein from equine renal cortex. J Biol Chem 235:3460–3465.
43. Teicher BA, Holden SA, Kelly MJ, Shea TC, Cucchi CA, Rosowsky A, Henner WD, Frei E III (1987) Characterization of a human squamous carcinoma cell line resistant to cis-diamminedichloroplatinum (II). Cancer Res 47:388–393.
44. Andrews PA, Murphy MP, Howell SB (1987) Metallothionein mediated cisplatin resistance in human ovarian carcinoma cells. Cancer Chemother Pharmacol 19:149–154.

45. Tobey RA, Enger MD, Griffith JK, Hildebrand CE (1982) Zinc-induced resistance to alkylating agent toxicity. Cancer Res 42:2980–2984.
46. Cox PJ, Phillip BJ, Thomas P (1975) The enzymatic basis of the selective action of cyclophosphamide. Cancer Res 35:3755–3761.
47. Sladek NE (1987) Oxazaphosphorines. In G Powis, RA Prough, eds. Metabolism and Action of Anticancer Drugs. London: Taylor and Francis, pp 48–90.
48. Sladek NE, Landkamer GL (1985) Restoration of sensitivity to oxazaphosphorines by inhibitors of aldehyde dehydrogenase activity in cultured oxazaphosphorine-resistant L1210 and crosslinking agent-resistant P388 cell lines. Cancer Res 45:1549–1555.
49. Hilton J (1984) Role of aldehyde dehydrogenase in cyclophosphamide-resistant L1210 leukemia. Cancer Res 44:5156–5160.
50. Weber GF, Waxman DJ (1993) Denitrosation of the anticancer drug 1,3-bis(2-chloroethyl)-1-nitrosourea catalyzed by microsomal glutathione S-transferase and cytochrome P450 monooxygenases. Arch Biochem Biophys 307:369–378.
51. Lemoine A, Lucas C, Ings RMJ (1991) Metabolism of the chloroethylnitrosoureas. Xenobiotica 21:775–791.
52. Potter DW, Levin W, Ryan DE, Thomas PE, Reed DJ (1984) Stereoselective monooxygenation of carcinostatic 1-(2-chloroethyl)-3-(cyclohexyl)-1-nitrosourea and 1-(2-chloroethyl)-3-(trans-4-methylcyclohexyl)-1-nitrosourea by purified cytochrome P-450 isozymes. Biochem Pharmacol 33:609–613.
53. DeVita VT, Carbone PP, Owens AH Jr, Gold GL, Krant MJ, Edmonson J (1965) Clinical trials with 1,3-bis(2-chloroethyl)-1-nitrosourea, NSC-409962. Cancer Res 25:1876–1881.
54. Nissen NI, Pajak TF, Glidewell O, et al. (1979) Comparative study of a BCNU containing 4-drug program versus MOPP versus 3-drug combinations in advanced Hodgkin's disease. Cancer 43:31–40.
55. Montgomery JA, James R, McCaleb GS, Johnston TP (1967) The modes of decomposition of 1,3-bis(2-chloroethyl)-1-nitrosourea and related compounds. J Med Chem 10:668–674.
56. Montgomery JA, James R, McCaleb GS, Kirk MC, Johnston TP (1975) Decomposition of N-(2-chloroethyl)-N-nitrosoureas in aqueous media. J Med Chem 18:568–571.
57. Weinkam RJ, Lin H-S (1979) Reactions of 1,3-bis(2-chloroethyl)-1-nitrosourea and 1-(2-chloroethyl)-3-cyclohexyl-1-nitrosourea in aqueous solution. J Med Chem 22:1193–1198.
58. Erickson LC, Laurent G, Sharkey NA, Kohn KW (1980) DNA cross-linking and monoadduct repair in nitrosourea-treated human tumor cells. Nature 288:727–729.
59. Lown JW, McLaughlin LW, Chang YM (1978) Mechanism of action of 2-haloethylnitrosoureas on DNA and its relation to their antileukemic properties. Bioorg Chem 7:97–110.
60. Tong WP, Kirk MC, Ludlum DB (1982) Formation of the crosslink 1-[N^3-deoxycytidyl],2-[N^1-deoxyguanosinyl]ethane in DNA treated with N,N'-bis(2-chloroethyl)-N-nitrosourea. Cancer Res 42:3102-3105.
61. Tong WP, Kirk MC, Ludlum DB (1983) Mechanism of action of the nitrosoureas. V. Formation of O^6-(2-fluoroethyl)guanine and its probable role in the crosslinking of deoxyribonucleic acid. Biochem Pharmacol 32:2011-2015.
62. Pegg AE (1983) Alkylation and subsequent repair of DNA after exposure to dimethylnitrosamine and related carcinogens. Rev Biochem Toxicol 5:83–133.
63. Pegg AE, Scicchitano D, Dolan ME (1984) Comparison of the rates of repair of O^6-alkylguanines in DNA by rat liver and bacterial O^6-alkylguanine-DNA alkyltransferase. Cancer Res 44:3806–3811.
64. Demple B, Karran P (1983) Death of an enzyme: Suicide repair of DNA. Trends Biol Sci 8:137–139.
65. Yarosh DB (1985) The role of O^6-methylguanine-DNA methyltransferase in cell survival, mutagenesis and carcinogenesis. Mutat Res 145:1–16.
66. Lindhal T, Sedgwick B, Sekiguchi M, Nakabeppu Y (1988) Regulation and expression of the adaptive response to alkylating agents. Annu Rev Biochem 57:133–157.
67. Demple B (1990) Self-methylation by suicide DNA repair enzymes. In WM Paik, S Kim, eds. Protein Methylation. Boca Raton, FL: CRC Press, pp 285–304.
68. Pegg AE, Boosalis M, Samson L, Moschel RC, Byers T, Swenn K, Dolan ME (1993) Mechanism of inactivation of human O^6-alkylguanine-DNA alkyltransferase by O^6-benzylguanine. Biochemistry 32:11998–12006.
69. Pegg AE, Byers TL (1992) Repair of DNA containing O^6-alkylguanine. FASEB J 6:2302-2310.
70. Arris CE, Bleasdale C, Calvert AH, et al. (1994) Probing the active site and mechanism of action of

O^6-methylguanine-DNA methyltransferase and substrate analogues (O^6-substituted guanines). Anticancer Drug Des 9:401–408.

71. Gonzaga PE, Harris L, Margison GP, Brent TP (1990) Evidence that covalent complex formation between BCNU-treated oligonucleotides and *E. coli* alkyltransferases requires the O^6-alkylguanine function. Nucleic Acids Res 18:3961–3966.

72. Pegg AE (1990) Mammalian O^6-alkylguanine-DNA alkyltransferase: Regulation and importance in response to alkylating carcinogenic and therapeutic agents. Cancer Res 50:6119–6129.

73. Day RS III, Ziolkowski CHJ, Scudiero DA, Meyer SA, Lubiniecki AS, Girardi AJ, Galloway SM, Bynum GD (1980) Defective repair of alkylated DNA by human tumor and SV-40-transformed human cell strains. Nature 288:724–727.

74. Yarosh DB, Foote RS, Mitra S, Day RS III (1983) Repair of O^6-methylguanine in DNA by demethylation is lacking in Mer− human tumor strains. Carcinogenesis 4:199–205.

75. Brent TP, Houghton PJ, Houghton JA (1985) O^6-Alkylguanine-DNA alkyltransferase activity correlates with the therapeutic response to human rhabdomyosarcoma xenografts to 1-(2-chloroethyl)-3-(trans-4-methylcyclohexyl)-1-nitrosourea. Proc Natl Acad Sci USA 82:2985–2989.

76. Gibson NW, Hartley J, La France RJ, Vaughan K (1986) Differential cytotoxicity and DNA-damaging effects produced in human cells of the Mer+ and Mer− phenotypes by a series of alkyltriazenylimidazoles. Carcinogenesis 7:259–265.

77. Catapano CV, Broggini M, Erba E, Ponti M, Mariani L, Citti L, D'Incalci M (1987) In vitro and in vivo methazolastone-induced DNA damage and repair in L-1210 leukemia sensitive and resistant to chloroethylnitrosoureas. Cancer Res 47:4884–4889.

78. Lunn JM, Harris AL (1988) Cytotoxicity of 5-(3-methyl-1-triazeno)imidazole-4-carboxamide (MTIC) on Mer+, Mer+Rem− and Mer− cell lines: Differential potentiation by 3-acetamidobenzamide. Br J Cancer 57:54–58.

79. Wyllie AH (1980) Glucocorticoid induced thymocyte apoptosis is associated with endogenous endonuclease activation. Nature 284:555–556.

80. Savill J, Dransfield I, Hogg N, Haslett C (1990) Vitronectin receptor-mediated phagocytosis of cells undergoing apoptosis. Nature 343:170–173.

81. Raff MC (1993) Social controls on cell survival and cell death. Nature 356:397–400.

82. Collins MKL, Marvel J, Malde P, Lopez-Rivas A (1992) Interleukin 3 protects murine bone marrow cells from apoptosis induced by DNA damaging agents. J Exp Med 176:1043–1051.

83. Vaux DL, Aguila HL, Weissman IL (1992) Bcl-2 prevents death of factor-deprived cells but fails to prevent apoptosis in targets of cell mediated killing. Int Immunol 4:821–824.

84. Lane DP (1993) A death in the life of p53. Nature 362:786–787.

85. Griffith OW, Meister A (1979) Potent and specific inhibition of glutathione synthesis by buthionine sulfoximine (S-n-butyl homocysteine sulfoximine). J Biol Chem 254:7558–7560.

86. Russo A, DeGraff W, Friedman N, Mitchell JB (1986) Selective modulation of glutathione levels in human normal versus tumor cells and subsequent differential response to chemotherapy drugs. Cancer Res 46:2845–2848.

87. Teicher BA, Crawford JM, Holden SA, Lin Y, Cathcart KNS, Luchette CA, Flatow J (1988) Glutathione monoethyl ester can selectively protect liver from high dose BCNU or cyclophosphamide. Cancer 62:1275–1281.

88. Tew KD, Bomber AM, Hoffman SJ (1988) Ethacrynic acid and piriprost as enhancers of cytotoxicity in drug resistant and sensitive cell lines. Cancer Res 48:3622–3625.

89. Lacreta FP, Brennan JM, Nash SL, Comis RL, Tew KD, O'Dwyer PJ (1994) Pharmacokinetics and bioavailability study of ethacrynic acid as a modulator of drug resistance in patients with cancer. J Pharmacol Exp Ther 270:1186–1191.

90. Lyttle MH, Hocker MD, Hui HC, Caldwell CG, Aaron DT, Ergqvist-Goldstein A, Flatgaard JE, Bauer K (1994) Isozyme-specific glutathione S-transferase inhibitors: Design and synthesis. J Med Chem 37:189–194.

91. Lawley P, Thatcher CJ (1970) Methylation of deoxyribonucleic acid in cultured mammalian cells by N-methyl-N'-nitro-N-nitrosoguanidine. Biochem J 116:693–707.

92. Shyam K, Penketh PG, Divo AA, Loomis RH, Rose WC, Sartorelli AC (1993) Synthesis and evaluation of 1-acyl-1,2-bis(methylsulfonyl)-2-(2-chloroethyl)hydrazines as antineoplastic agents. J Med Chem 36:3496–3502.

93. Lyttle MH, Satyam A, Hocker MD, Bauer KE, Caldwell CG, Hui HC, Morgan AS, Mergia A, Kauvar LM (1984) Glutathione S-transferase activates novel alkylating agents. J Med Chem 37:1501–1507.

94. Zlotogorski WJ, Erickson LC (1984) Pretreatment of human colon tumor cells with DNA methylating agents inhibits their ability to repair chloroethyl monoadducts. Carcinogenesis 5:83–87.
95. Gerson SL, Trey JE (1988) Modulation of nitrosourea resistance in myeloid leukemias. Blood 71:1487–1494.
96. Dolan ME, Moschel RC, Pegg AE (1990) Depletion of mammalian O^6-alkylguanine-DNA alkyltransferase activity by O^6-benzylguanine provides a means to evaluate the role of this protein in protection against carcinogenic and therapeutic alkylating agents. Proc Natl Acad Sci USA 87:5368–5372.
97. Chae M, Swenn K, Kanugula S, Dolan ME, Pegg AE, Moschel RC (1995) 8-Substituted O^6-benzylguanine, substituted 6(4)-(benzyloxy)pyrimidine, and related derivatives as inactivators of human O^6-alkylguanine-DNA alkyltransferase. J Med Chem 38:359–365.

4. GLUTATHIONE S-TRANSFERASES

ABHIJIT RAHA AND KENNETH D. TEW

Glutathione (GSH), the most ubiquitous and abundant nonprotein thiol, is essential in numerous detoxification reactions and is therefore considered a chemoprotectant. In the human, levels of GSH range from $30\,\mu M$ in plasma to $3\,mM$ in kidney proximal tubules; tumors of various organs can contain up to $10\,mM$ GSH [1]. GSH is synthesized via the γ-glutamyl cycle (Figure 4–1). The rate-limiting step is catalyzed by γ-glutamylcysteine synthetase (γ-GCS) to form γ-glutamylcysteine. The following step is catalyzed by glutathione synthetase, which forms GSH. The glyoxalase system, which consists of glyoxalase I and II, converts methylglyoxal to D-lactate and replenishes GSH. Glutathione that is oxidized by oxidants (GSSG), such as hydrogen peroxide, and in response to oxidant stress is converted back to the reduced form of glutathione (GSH) by glutathione reductase. Glutathione is broken down into cysteinyl glycine by γ-glutamyltranspeptidase; GSH, as a nucleophile, is utilized as a cofactor in a variety of detoxification reactions. Among the enzymes that employ GSH in this manner are the glutathione S-transferases.

The glutathione S-transferases (GSTs; EC 2.5.1.18) comprise a family of multi-functional isoenzymes with broad substrate specificities that catalyze the phase II nucleophilic addition of the sulfur atom of reduced glutathione to electrophilic centers of a variety of compounds to render them more water soluble and less toxic, and to enhance their elimination [2–7]. In this manner, GSTs protect cellular macromolecules against attack by reactive electrophiles, which are mutagens, carcinogens, and other toxic compounds. The GSH-dependent, selenium-independent peroxidase activity of GSTs protects tissues against damage caused by endogenous

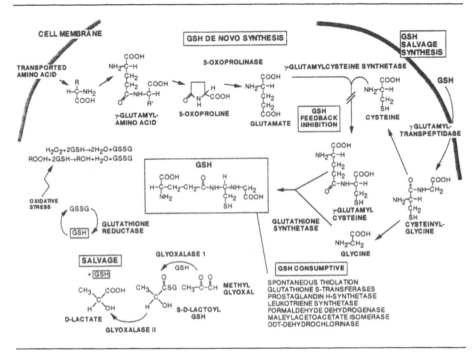

Figure 4-1. Summary schema of interrelated GSH-producing and utilizing pathways. GSSG = oxidized glutathione; DDT = 1,1,1-trichloro-2,2-bis(P-chlorophenyl)-ethane. (From Tew [320], with permission.)

organic hydroperoxides that are formed during oxidative stress [8–12]. These enzymes also bind a variety of hydrophobic compounds, such as bilirubin, heme, and hormones, which indicate that they can act as intracellular transport proteins or carriers [13]. Because GSTs can bind to a variety of ligands, they were also called *ligandins*. In certain invertebrates, the GSTs function as crystalline lens proteins [14]. These enzymes coexist with glutathione in a variety of aerobic organisms, such as fish [15], plants [16], insects [17,18], parasites, yeast [19], fungi [20,21], and bacteria [22–25].

On the basis of evolutionary considerations, substrate and inhibitor specificities, antibody crossreactivities, and primary structures, the mammalian GSTs are a multigene family and can be grouped into five classes, designated alpha, mu, pi, theta, and microsomal [5,26–29]. Recently, leukotriene C_4 synthase, which is involved in the synthesis of leukotrienes, has been identified as a new class of GST [30].

The cytosolic GSTs are fairly abundant and are differentially distributed in human, rat, and mouse tissue. The initial characterization and those most thoroughly studied have been the GSTs in rat liver [4]. In human liver, they comprise up to 5% of total cytosolic protein. Expression of the various isozymes is highly tissue specific. Among the GST isozymes, the pi form is the most widely distributed and usually the most abundant [31]; this isozyme is prevalent in blood cells and other tissues, including erythrocytes, lung, breast, placenta, and prostate [32]. The alpha class enzymes are primarily localized in liver and kidney [4,32]. The cytosolic GSTs are ubiquitous among aerobic organisms.

PHYSICOCHEMICAL PROPERTIES OF GST ISOENZYMES

In terms of physicochemical structure, cytosolic GSTs are heterogenous and are each approximately 50 kDa homodimers or heterodimers, which consist of 24–28 kDa monomeric subunits. Heterodimers have yet to be identified between isoenzymes of different classes. However, monomeric subunits of a specific class of GST share a 60–80% amino acid sequence identity, yet exhibit distinct substrate specificity. Allelic variants have also been identified among each class of GSTs [33]. The heterogeneity of GSTs may be complicated by the existence of covalent post-translational modifications, such as glycosylation [34]. The cytosolic GSTs represent multigene products. For example, the human alpha-, mu-, and pi-class GSTs are products of at least six gene loci, which include the A1 and A2 (alpha), M1–M5 (mu), and P1 (pi) [28,35,36]. From an evolutionary standpoint, the cytosolic GSTs may have evolved from a common ancestral gene; the membrane-bound or microsomal GST shows no apparent sequence relationship to any of the cytosolic enzymes [37]. It has been suggested that the alpha, mu, and pi enzymes originated from a theta gene duplication and that the class mu diverged before the alpha and pi divergence [38]. Because the exon–intron boundaries appear to be similar in the alpha, mu, and pi classes of GSTs, the diversification of GSTs is thought to be due in part to exon shuffling [7].

The GSTs range from 210 to 300 amino acids in length. In all known amino acid sequences of the GSTs, six residues are conserved: Tyr-7, Pro-53, Asp-57, Ile-68, Gly-145, and Asp-152. X-ray crystallography studies have clearly established a role for the former two amino acids; they make up part of the GSH binding site. The other conserved residues may be important in protein folding. All GSTs contain the motif Ser/Thr-Arg/Asn-Ala-Ileu-Leu centered about residue 67. However, this motif is not exclusive to GSTs. When amino acid sequences are compared for homologies (Figure 4–2) [7], several conclusions about GST classification can be drawn. Chicken GST sequences can be classified as alpha and mu. Liver fluke GSTs can be classified as mu. Certain bacteria, fish, and insect GSTs can be classified as theta. Squid lens proteins, which have been identified as GSTs [14,42], are placed in the sigma class by one group of investigators [41]. When comparing GST amino acid sequences, there are sequence homologies to other proteins that have been noted. These include some dehalogenases [43–45], a stringent starvation protein [46] in certain species of bacteria, and an ethylene-responsive flower senescence–related protein [47]. The significances of these matches are as yet unclear [7]. After taking into consideration conservative amino acid substitutions, a comparison of sequence homologies between various species and classes of GSTs is presented in Table 4–1 [7].

On the basis of the primary amino acid sequences, hydropathy plots of the cytosolic GSTs predicted secondary structures for the GST chains in alternating α-

Figure of multiple sequence alignment of GST amino acid sequences with rows labeled: pi, mu, alpha, theta, octopus, insect, plant, fluke, bacteria, and G/H site annotations. Secondary structure elements (β1, α1, β2, α2, β3, β4, α3, α4, α5, α6, α7, α8) are indicated across residue positions 1 through 209+.

Figure 4–2. Alignment of consensus GST amino acid sequences. The alignments of intraclass sequences were performed using the PILEUP program in the GCG package (gap weight = 3.0, gap length weight = 0.10) [39]. Consensus sequences were calculated with PRETTY from the GCG package [39]. Sequences were extracted from the SWISSPROT database [40]. Invariant residues are shown boxed. The locations of alpha-helices (denoted α) and beta-strands (denoted β) are indicated. Residues located in the GSH and substrate binding sites are marked by the letters G and H, respectively. (From Wilce et al. [7], with permission.).

Table 4–1. Comparison of sequence homologies

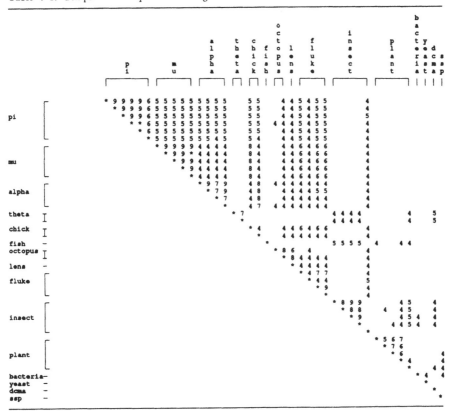

Sequences were extracted from the SWISSPROT database [40] and initially aligned using the PILEUP program of the GCG package [39]. The alignment was subsequently optimized with LINEUP [39]. Sequence homology was calculated using DISTANCES (match threshold 0.6) [39]. The homology values take into account conservative substitutions and thus are more sensitive indicators of structural relatedness. Each number in the table refers to the pairwise percentage sequence homology, divided by 10 and rounded to the nearest integer.

*Sequence identities between 95% and 100%. Only values above 35% are shown.

pi = pi-class GSTs from human, bovine, pig, mouse, rat and nematode; mu = mu-class GSTs from human, mouse, hamster, guinea pig, and rat; alpha = human, rabbit, rat, and mouse; theta = theta-class GSTs from rat; fish = plaice GST; lens = GST from octopus lens; fluke = fluke GSTs from *Fasciola* and *Schistosoma*; insect = *Drosophila*, house fly, blowfly, mosquito; plant = maize, tobacco, silene, wheat, carnation; bacteria = *Proteus mirabilis*; dcma = dichloromethane dehalogenase; ssp = starvation stringent protein.

From Wilce et al. [7], with permission.

helices and β-sheets [48,49], similar to the TIM barrel-fold character determined for triosephosphate isomerase [50] and 15 other enzymes [51]. However, these secondary structure predictions were proven false once the first GST's three-dimensional crystal structure was analyzed [52], reflecting the danger of interpreting secondary structures on the basis of algorithms alone.

The first GST for which a three-dimensional structure was described was a pi enzyme from porcine lung [52] complexed with the inhibitors glutathione sulfonate and S-hexyl GSH [52,53]. This pi homodimer was a globular protein with unit cell dimensions of 45 × 55 × 60 Å. Each subunit of the homodimer existed as a polypeptide fold composed of two domains. The first (N-terminal) domain (amino acids 1–76) consists of four strands of a mixed β-sheet (β1–β4) flanked and packed on one side by two α-helices (α1, α3), and the other side by another helix (α2), which faces the solvent. The second (C-terminal) domain (amino acids 81–209) is made up of five α-helices (α4–α8). The α4 and α5 helices are greater than 40 Å long, pack in an antiparallel fashion, and are crescent shaped. The bent appearance of the α5 helix is due to the presence of Pro-123 and Pro-128 in the helix. The two domains are linked by a short peptide (amino acids 77–82). The interface between these two domains is roughly V-shaped and represents a surface area of 1,500 Å², which is buried between the monomeric subunits. This GST is only active as a homodimer; monomers by themselves were discovered to have no activity [54,55].

The GSH binding site (G-site) is fairly conserved in all forms of GSTs. The G-site of the pi homodimer was identified because it was crystallized with the competitive inhibitor, glutathione sulfonate. In each GST monomer of the homodimer, the G-site was localized between the two domains in a 15 Å V-shaped cleft, with the N-terminal domain comprising most of the site. The distance between the G-sites of each monomer in the homodimer is at least 14 Å. The competitive inhibitor, glutathione sulfonate, and reduced glutathione [56] bind to the G-site of the GSTs and some other GSH binding enzymes [57,58] in an extended conformation, with the γ-glutamyl portion pointing toward the dimer interface and the glycine pointing toward the N-terminal domain. When GSH binds to the G-site, its sulfur atom interacts with Tyr-7, which is conserved in all GSTs and plays some role in the catalytic mechanism. This G-site is lined with the side chains of Tyr-7, Gly-12, Arg-13, Trp-38, Lys-42, Gln-49, Pro-51, Gln-62, Ser-63, and Glu-95. The consensus motif Ser/Thr-Arg/Asn-Ala-Ileu-Leu centered about residue 67 in α-helix 3 contributes to the G-site and the domain interface. Once GSH is bound to its site, there are at least 21 potential hydrogen bonding interactions with the GSH, which may explain the stereospecificity of GSTs for GSH.

The site to which electrophilic substrates (H-site) bind in the pi-class GST was determined only when this GST enzyme from human placenta was complexed with the competitive inhibitor, S-hexyl GSH, and was isolated and characterized [53]. This H-site was shown to be within a hydrophobic cleft on top of the loop connecting β1 to α-helix 1 adjacent to the G-site for GSH. This cleft is lined by the side chains contributed by Tyr-7, Phe-8, Pro-9, Val-10, Val-35, and Tyr-106. Besides the G-site and this one H-site, the possibility that additional H-sites may exist cannot be completely ruled out [7].

Currently, one of the mu class GSTs from rat liver (rat GST 3-3) is the only one to have been crystallized in the presence of glutathione [59–61]. Although there is only a 31% sequence identity when the mu and pi class GSTs are compared, the folding topology of these two classes of GSTs is similar overall [61]. The class mu GSTs are globular, with unit cell dimensions of 53 × 62 × 56 Å. The N-terminal domain spans residues 1–82, containing four β-strands and three α-helices arranged in a βαβαββα motif; the C-terminal domain spans residues 90–217, which are arranged in five α-helices. Only the mu class GSTs contain a long loop between β-strand 2 and α-helix 2 (mu loop), which results in a deeper active site cleft, that is not present in the pi-GSTs. However, as is the case in the pi-class GSTs, the GSH also binds to the mu enzyme in an extended manner, and hydrogen bonding interaction is observed between the sulfur atom in GSH and the hydroxyl group in the Tyr-7 residue. Seven amino acid residues that contact GSH in the pi enzymes also play the same role in the mu GSTs.

The electrophilic substrate binding site has not been identified in the mu-class GSTs by x-ray crystallography, but some progress has been made using nuclear magnetic resonance (NMR) spectroscopy. The H-site of a human muscle GST has been localized in the C-terminal domain using a spin-labelled probe conjugated to GSH, and this site is comprised of, or close to, Met-35, Ala-38, Met-105, Met-109, Ala-112, Tyr-116, Met-212, and Ala-213 [62].

Crystals for the human α-GSTs have been isolated in association with methylmercuric chloride [60] and S-(2-iodobenzyl) glutathione [63]. The structure for the human α-GST (A1-1) [64] reveals that it consists of a polypeptide fold similar to the pi-class enzymes. The α-GSTs do not contain the mu loop. However, the major difference in the α-GST exists due to the additional amino acid residues at the C-terminus, which fold into an additional alpha helix (α9) that partially blocks the substrate binding site from the solvent. There is approximately 20% and 32% amino acid sequence identity between the α-GSTs and μ- and π-GSTs, respectively [64]. In the α-GSTs, the G-site also lies in domain I and the hydroxyl group of the conserved tyrosine (Tyr-9) interacts with the sulfur atom of glutathione. In addition, Arg-15 interacts with the GSH sulfur atom. The same interactions exist for GSH within the elements of the G-site. GSTs from nonmammalian species have been recently characterized. X-ray crystallographic studies of GSTs from *Schistosoma mansoni* [65] and the Australian sheep blowfly [7] suggest that these GSTs belong to the pi [66,67] and theta class, respectively.

The location of the non–substrate binding site that is involved in binding heme, bilirubin, and bile acids has not been ascertained for any of the GSTs. The first studies suggested that a single GST dimer possesses a single non–substrate binding site [68], which consists of regions of low and high binding affinity [69]. When the C-terminal region of GSTs was truncated, the resulting mutants could bind bromosulfophthalein equally as well as regular GSTs, whereas the ability of ligands to bind the substrate binding site was drastically curtailed, indicating that the non–substrate binding site was closer to the N-terminal region of GSTs [70]. Photoaffinity labeling studies suggest that a tryptophan-containing peptide in the N-terminal region is involved in this binding site [71]. Electron paramagnetic resonance (EPR) studies that titrated a nitroxide-labeled human placental enzyme with hemin suggest that this non–substrate binding site is approximately 10 Å away from Cys-47, which is 10.7 Å away from the sulfur atom of GSH [72]. With the use of fluorescence labeling techniques, a binding site, which accomodates C-12 to C-18 fatty acids [73] and bilirubin [74] in a rat pi-GST enzyme, has been traced to a region between residues 141 and 188. Therefore, large, fairly hydrophobic ligands may bind in this site, which is a V-shaped cleft at the subunit interface.

Because most ligands that bind the active site are fairly hydrophobic in nature, in the absence of ligand this site is shielded from solvent. A number of studies have suggested that the active site is shielded by a lid and this lid opens in response to ligand binding [75–78]. The flexibility of the substrate binding site in terms of its ability to accomodate substrates is due to the existence of flexible regions within the site. These include regions around α-helix 2, which partially lines the G-site, the mu-loop, and the part of the C-terminus that buries itself into the substrate binding site. There is evidence showing that in the absence of ligand, the substrate binding site is shielded from the solvent and the C-terminus is involved. In the pi-GSTs, it has been estimated on the basis of thermodynamic considerations that there would be a lowering of the free energy for protein folding when the active site is buried in the absence of ligand because apolar side chains would be less exposed to the water solvent; exposure of these side chains to solvent increases the free energy for protein folding by decreasing the entropy of water [79,80]. There are approximately seven hydrophobic residues from the C-terminus that line and bury the substrate binding site in the pi-class GSTs. This is also the case in the alpha GSTs. In the mu class GSTs, without ligand binding a portion of the C-terminus has been demonstrated to fold over and bury the substrate binding site [7].

Chemical modification studies were conducted before the x-ray crystallographic studies but proved to be misleading. The catalytic activity of the pi-class GST was thought to be due to cysteine residues residing in the active site because thiol-reactive agents caused enzyme inhibition [66,81–84]. Chemical modifying agents, such as N-ethylmaleimide, used with various cysteine mutants of these GSTs traced the enzymatic inhibition to Cys-47. However, there were no cysteine residues detected in the glutathione or substrate binding site in any class of GST using site-directed mutagenesis studies [85–91] or x-ray crystallography [52,53]. Chemical modification studies have also implicated histidine, tryptophan, arginine, and aspartic residues in the catalytic mechanism of the GSTs [92–96], but site-directed mutagenesis studies have ruled out the possibility that histidine [85–88,97–100], tryptophan [91,101], arginine [101], or aspartic acid residues [101] are involved in the catalytic mechanism of the GST enzymes. Other residues implicated in the catalytic mechanism, but then later excluded from playing a role, include His-15 for the mu-class GSTs [100] and Lys-127 for the pi-class GSTs [102].

CATALYTIC MECHANISM OF THE GSTS

Several mechanisms of catalysis for the various classes of GSTs have been proposed, including random, sequential, and ping-pong mechanisms [103–105]. A number of kinetic studies suggest that the S-conjugation reaction between glutathione and hydrophobic electrophiles occurs in a sequential manner [5,27,106,107]. Under physiological conditions, because intracellular concentrations of reduced glutathione are between 1 and 10 mM and this range of concentrations is about three orders of magnitude higher than the K_d of GSH for GSTs (K_d = 10–200 μM), GSH would bind to the G-site of the GSTs first. Early studies have demonstrated the specificity of the G-site for GSH. Through a series of binding studies with synthetic GSH analogues [108–110], the orientations of both the γ-glutamyl and thiol groups of GSH at the G-site were shown to be critical for substrate recognition. The γ-glutamyl group, in particular, interacts at a number of contact points at the G-site. Because cysteine and histidine residues are lacking at the active site of GSTs, as demonstrated by site-directed mutagenesis studies [62,85–87,91,97,98,111], acid-base catalysis by these amino acids has been excluded. Rather, once GSH is bound to the G-site, the thiol group of GSH has been demonstrated to be ionized to form the thiolate anion [107] with the aid of a conserved tyrosine residue [Tyr-7 (pi); Tyr-6 (mu); Tyr-8 (alpha)] residing within the G-site.

As demonstrated by kinetic, spectroscopic, and x-ray crystallography studies [52,53,61,62,64,91,112–119], this conserved tyrosine residue is directly involved in the catalytic activation of GSH by favoring the formation and stabilization of the thiolate anion by donating a hydrogen bond to the sulfur of GSH. Site-directed mutagenesis studies [62,91,99,115–118,120] have investigated the role of this conserved tyrosine residue and have also confirmed that it is directly involved in the catalytic activation of GSH. When GSH is bound to a GST's G-site, there is a lowering of the pK_a from 9 in aqueous solution down to between 5.7 and 7.0 [91,113,114,117,118,121]. More recent studies [122–124] have shown that the hydroxyl groups of the conserved tyrosine residues have unusually lowered pK_a values that are approximately two units lower than normal (pKa–Tyr OH = 2.2); this is attributed to the electrostatic environment at the active site. This conserved tyrosine residue may also be responsible for the proper orientation of GSH at the G-site, such that the thiol proton may easily migrate out of this site [118]. An on-face hydrogen bond between the side chain hydroxyl group of threonine-13 and the conserved tyrosine has also been demonstrated to be an additional factor that stabilizes the thiolate anion [125]. Other residues implicated in the stabilization of the thiolate anion include Arg-15 and Asp-98 in the alpha GSTs [116,117] and Tyr-115 in the mu GSTs [126]. However, Tyr-106 of the pi enzymes and Val-110 of the alpha enzymes has been implicated in participating catalytically in nucleophilic substitution reactions with 1-chloro-2, 4-dinitrobenzene [62,126].

SUBSTRATE BINDING SITE—BASIS FOR SUBSTRATE SELECTIVITY

The GSTs are capable of binding a wide variety of substrates. This is partly because there are multiple isoenzymes within each class of GSTs. The shape and size of the substrate binding site between each class can vary considerably, and these factors can determine specificity. Studies conducted with various GSTs for their substrate specificities with regard to 4-hydroxyalkenals showed that the substrate binding site can occupy compounds with a specified carbon side chain length and hydrophobicity, thus reflecting the steric constraints at these sites [127–129]. Differences in substrate specificities of the various classes of GSTs have been partly attributed to interclass differences in the structures of the C-terminal residues. Studies using photoaffinity labeling techniques [130] and those involving deletion mutants [70] suggest that the C-terminal portion of the GSTs is involved in their substrate selectivity. Differences in the composition of the residues that make up the substrate binding site and the flexibility of the C-terminal tail that projects into this site also contribute to the broad substrate specificity [64].

GST GENE STRUCTURE

A number of laboratories [131–137] have studied the rat cDNA clones for the Y_a (GST 1-1) and Y_c (GST 2-2) [5] subunits of the alpha-GSTs. When Y_a and Y_c mRNA sequences were compared, the protein coding regions were 75% identical [137]. The resultant protein from the rat Y_a cDNA yielded a 222 amino acid protein. When the mouse Y_a subunit, which yielded a 223 amino acid protein, was compared with that of a rat Y_a cDNA, there was a 94% homology between the two proteins [138]. The mouse Y_a gene has been localized to chromosome 9 [139–141]. Comparison of the human Ha subunit and the rat Y_a and Y_c subunits revealed a close relationship in the amino acid sequence and a >80% identity in cDNA sequences [142,143]. Using a Y_a cDNA probe, Southern blot hybridization studies indicated that the mouse and rat subunits are encoded by a multigene family [139], and that multiple Y_a and Y_c genes exist [144]. The nucleotide sequences of three human alpha GST genes have been reported [139,142,143,145–151] and have been localized to chromosome 6 [145].

Structural aspects of the Y_a gene have been elucidated for the mouse [138,152], rat [153], and human [148]. The mouse and rat Y_a gene is 11 kb long and consists of seven exons and six introns. Comparison of these genes showed that there is up to an 80% sequence identity with respect to their introns at exon–intron junctions and in the regions beyond the polyadenylation site [138]. The human gene spans 12 kb, but also consists of seven exons [148]. However, only the regulatory elements of the 5′-flanking regions of the mouse [154,155] and rat [156] Y_a genes have been localized and well characterized. On the basis of sequence analysis and functional assays, there was no evidence for the existence of xenobiotic- or antioxidant-response elements in the 5′-flanking region of the human GSTA1 gene between −1,300 and +500 bp from the transcription start site [150]. However, there was a negative regulatory element between −694 and −336 bp in this gene, which may play a significant role in the developmental and tissue-specific expression of the alpha GSTs in humans. There was a 95% nucleotide sequence identity between the GST A1 and GST A2 genes within the −1,300 and +500 bp region of the genes. It is most likely that regulatory elements do exist beyond −1,300 bp in the distal 5′-flanking region of these alpha GST genes, which can explain their differences in expression [150].

Several of the mu GST genes have been isolated and characterized [157–160]; the earliest work involved the isolation and characterization of the Y_b cDNA clones in the rat [157,161–164]. Sequence comparisons of cDNA clones for the subunit Y_{b1}, Y_{b2}, and Y_{b3} indicate an 80% identity of the protein-coding regions and the greatest divergence at the 3'-untranslated mRNA regions [164], but little sequence homology between Y_b cDNA and the Y_a and Y_c nucleotide sequences [133,136,163]. Southern blot hybridization studies with Y_b cDNA probes conducted with rat genomic DNA indicate that the rat Y_b family is multigenic [157,159]. The isolation and characterization of the Y_{b1}, Y_{b2}, and Y_{b4} genes have been described [157,159]. The Y_{b3} gene has not been isolated, but studies conducted with its cDNA indicate that it is only highly expressed in brain tissue [165]. The rat Y_b gene is 5 kb in length and contains eight exons and seven introns. When comparing the nucleotide sequence, three of the seven introns share a >88% identity [157,159]. Reports of homologous regions in the introns of human GST genes have also been described [160]. Because sequence identity in introns exists across species, this is considered evidence of gene conversion, which is thought to have played a role in the evolution of the GST Y_b genes, and it may be due to the presence of regulatory elements within these regions [166].

In the human, there are currently five mu isoenzymes (GSTM1-1 through GSTM5-5) that have been identified [151]. Of the six GST loci (GST 1 through GST 6) that have been studied, only GST 1, GST 4, and GST 5 encode mu class enzymes [31,167–169]. GST 1 is a polymorphic locus that consists of three alleles, a null allele, GST 1-1, and GST 1-2. Individuals homozygous for the null allele lack mu GST activity, as characterized by assays conducted with *trans*-stilbene oxide [170]. Approximately 50% of the human population is homozygous for the null allele, and this has been correlated with an increase in susceptibility to lung cancer [170–172]. GST 1-1 and GST 1-2 mRNAs and cDNAs have been isolated and characterized [158,173]. The resulting proteins differ only at residue 172 in that GST 1-1 encodes an asparagine resulting in GST ψ [174] and GST 1-2 encodes a lysine resulting in GST μ [168], respectively. Genomic DNA hybridization studies conducted with mouse–human somatic cell hybrids have localized the mu GST genes in humans to chromosomes 1, 6, and 13. The gene localized to chromosome 13, the GST ψ gene, the expression of which is polymorphic in the human population, is thought to have been created by a recombination event; a lack of this event plus a gene deletion may have resulted in the null phenotype [175]. GSTM1-1 (two alleles) is expressed primarily in the liver and peripheral blood [168]. Other class μ GST genes have been isolated and characterized [159,160], but most of the μ GST genes' regulatory 5'-flanking regions have not been characterized, so little information is available about regulation of gene expression. These GST isoenzymes are expressed in other tissues. GSTM2-2 is expressed in muscle [176]. GSTM3-3 and GSTM4-4 are both expressed primarily in the testes [177,178]. GSTM5-5 is expressed in the brain [179].

cDNA clones and the structural genes, that encode the rat [180–182] and human [183–185] pi GST enzymes have been isolated and characterized. The genes expressing GST-P in the rat and GST π in the human span 3 kb and consist of seven exons and six introns. The resulting protein in both species is approximately 210 amino acids long, and each protein is only encoded by a single gene [182,184]. Genomic organization of these genes in both species is similar [184,186,187]. In a recent study, three human GST π gene variants were isolated from λgt 11 libraries of human malignant glioma cells [Ali-Osman, personal communication]. These variants were demonstrated to be the result of A→G and C→T transitions at +313 and +341; this was the first conclusive evidence for polymorphism of the human GST π gene locus.

cDNA clones, which encode both rat and human microsomal GST enzymes, have been isolated and characterized [188]. Both clones encode a 154 amino acid protein and share a 95% amino acid sequence identity to each other. However, they share little sequence identity to cytosolic GSTs, with the exception of amino acids 57–63 [37,188]. Southern blot hybridization studies conducted with mouse–human somatic cell hybrids demonstrated that the microsomal GST gene is a low copy number gene in both the rat and human, and has been localized to chromosome 12 in the human [189].

GST GENE REGULATION

The GST pi gene's 5'-flanking regulatory region has been well characterized. Transfection studies of the rat gene [190] utilizing CAT constructs of this region detected two elements, which are similar to the antioxidant response element, GPE-I and GPE-II, approximately 2.5 and 2.0 kb upstream, respectively, from the transcription start site. GPE-I contains an AP-1 motif, which is also a TPA-responsive region. Further point mutation studies localized two TPA-response elements (TRE) toward the 3'-end. Each of these TREs had no effect, but together they acted cooperatively to form a strong enhancer element [191,192]. Several transcription factors, including the fos/jun heterodimeric protein complex, were demonstrated to bind to the GPE-I element [193,194] and to mediate transcription. GPE-II consists of two SV-40 enhancer-like elements and one polyoma-like element. A silencer element, which is responsible for the negative regulation of this gene, has been localized 400 bp upstream from the transcription start site that binds at least three *trans*-acting factors. One of these proteins, silencer factor B, was later identified as the IL-6–inducible LAP–IL-6–DBP [195]. Around the proximal promoter region is an AP-1 binding site at −61 bp and a GC box at −40 bp, which together regulate basal expression of the rat GST pi gene [190,191,196]. The human GST pi gene consists of four regulatory motifs, a TATA box (29 base pairs upstream from the transcription start site), two SP-1 recognition sequences (at −46 to −41 bp and −56 to −51 bp), and an AP-1 recognition sequence at −69 to −63 bp [184,185]. However, unlike the rat gene, there is no GPE-I enhancer element [186,187]. The human GST pi gene contains an additional *cis*-acting element between +8 and +72 bp, which is essential for maximal basal activity of the promoter; within this region is an additional AP-1 binding site between +35 and +41 bp [197].

Analysis of the 5'-flanking regulatory region of a hamster GST mu gene by deletion analysis detected two glucocorticoid-inducible regions [198,199]. Neither contained classical glucocorticoid response elements, but four potential helix-loop-helix domains were identified within this region. Transcriptional activation of the hamster GST mu gene by glucocorticoids was demonstrated to be dependent upon protein synthesis and, therefore, an induction event by glucocorticoids.

At least 2 kb of the 11 kb rat GST Y_a subunit gene constitutes the 5'-flanking region. Using deletion constructs made of this region that were transfected into HepG2 cells and CAT assays conducted in the absence and presence of various inducers, at least five distinct regulatory subunits have been identified to date [153,156,200–202]. The first cis-acting element spans −860 to −850 bp and has been demonstrated to be essential for maximal basal level expression; it consists of a recognition motif for the liver-specific transcription factor, HNF-1 (hepatocyte nuclear factor 1) [200,201]. An HNF-4 recognition motif was localized between −775 to −755 bp [200]. Using computer-aided sequence examination, a xenobiotic response element (XRE) core sequence was identified upstream from the HNF-1 binding site between −908 and −899 bp [200,201], and a glucocorticoid response element (GRE) was localized between −1,609 and −1,595 bp [201].

The XRE of the GST Y_a gene has been shown to be responsible for the regulation of basal and inducible expression. As in the case of the cytochrome P-4501A1 gene [203–206], the XRE of the GST Y_a gene has been shown to be recognized by the ligand-bound Ah receptor [207]. This receptor complex binds planar aromatic compounds with high affinity, translocates into the nucleus, and activates transcription of the genes containing the XRE motif, including the GST Y_a gene [207]. In addition, the C/EBP liver-specific transcription factor and like factors have also been demonstrated to interact with the GST Y_a gene XRE [200,207–209]. The fifth cis-acting element of the rat GST Y_a gene is localized between −722 and −682 bp, and does not resemble the XRE motif. It also plays a role in regulating basal and inducible expression, and mediates the induction by Ah receptor ligands, such as 3-methylcholanthrene (3-MC) and β-naphthoflavone, and phenolic antioxidants, such as tert-butylhydroquinone. Talalay and his coworkers suggest that the latter group of compounds induce phase II drug-metabolizing enzymes, such as the GST Y_a isoenzyme, by an Ah receptor-independent mechanism [210–213]. Because antioxidants can transactivate the GST Y_a gene via this cis-acting element, it is termed the antioxidant response element (ARE) or electrophile responsive element (EpRE).

Employing deletion studies of this region, the specific core sequence within the ARE shown to be required for inducible activity is 5'-GTGACAAAGC-3' [214]. More specifically, point mutation studies have shown that the TGAC tetramer is absolutely critical for regulating basal and inducible expression of the GST Y_a gene. Methylation interference and protection assays have shown that there is an interaction of trans-acting factors with the ARE [200,201,215]. With regard to the identity of these proteins, gel mobility shift assays conducted with in-vitro translated c-fos and c-jun proteins have shown that they interact specifically with the ARE sequence of the mouse GST Y_a gene [216,217], but this has not been demonstrated to be the case for the ARE of the rat GST Y_a gene [218].

The AP-1 complex of proteins as well as a 160 kDa protein have been demonstrated to bind to the human ARE within the 5'-flanking region of the NAD(P)H:

quinone oxidoreductase gene [219]. Nuclear extracts derived from HeLa cells have shown that a 160 kDa protein is unrelated to the AP-1 complex because binding of this protein was not affected by anti-fos or anti-jun antibodies in gel mobility shift assays.

There is a growing body of evidence implicating genes with AREs, including the GST Y_a gene, as part of the defense system against oxidative stress. When cells either deficient in the Ah receptor or cytochrome P-4501A1 are exposed to phenolic antioxidants, CAT constructs made solely of the ARE can be activated [202]. Hydrogen peroxide and superoxide anion have been implicated as byproducts of phenolic antioxidants; hydrogen peroxide has been shown to directly activate the transcription of the GST Y_a gene through the ARE [214]. NAD(P)H-quinone reductase has been shown to protect cells against reactive oxidants generated by redox cycling of endogenous and exogenous quinones [220]; the rat [221] and human [222,223] NAD(P)H-quinone reductase genes have been demonstrated to have functional AREs in their 5'-flanking regulatory regions. Antioxidant response elements (AREs) within the GST Y_a and NAD(P)H:quinone oxidoreductase (NQO_1) genes consist of TRE (perfect AP-1) and TRE-like (imperfect AP-1) elements, which mediate basal and inducible expression of these genes in response to xenobiotics and antioxidants [218,222,223]. Mutations in the 3'-TRE of the human NQO_1 gene hARE eliminated binding of nuclear proteins to this element and resulted in a loss of basal and inducible expression; mutations in the 5'-TRE of this gene's hARE decreased inducible expression mediated by xenobiotics [224].

ROLE OF INDUCTION IN CHEMOPROTECTION

Induction of the phase II drug-metabolizing enzymes, including glutathione S-transferases, glucuronosyl transferases, and NAD(P)H:quinone oxidoreductase, by multiple structurally diverse compounds is considered one major chemoprotective mechanism against chemical or oxidative stress and carcinogenesis [225–227]. The induction of GSTs has been correlated directly with the extent of the increase in mRNA levels and enhanced enzymatic synthesis and activities [228]; the induction of the phase II drug-metabolizing enzymes has provided a basis for screening naturally occurring and synthetic compounds [229–232]. Compounds that induce both phase I and phase II metabolizing enzymes include the planar aromatic compounds, such as polycyclic aromatic hydrocarbons, dioxins, flavonoids, and azo dyes. Compounds that solely induce phase II enzymes include the phenolic antioxidants, coumarins, isothiocyanates [233], thiocarbamates, and 1,2-dithiol-3-thiones [234], such as Oltipraz.

Talalay and his coworkers consider the former compounds as bifunctional inducers and the latter compounds as monofunctional inducers [226]. On the bases of multiple pieces of evidence derived from their studies on NAD(P)H:quinone reductase in the Hepa 1c1c7 mouse hepatoma cell line and its Ah receptor-defective variants [210–212], they proposed a model to explain the mechanisms of induction of phase I and phase II drug-metabolizing enzymes. NAD(P)H:quinone oxidoreductase was chosen for study because it is well expressed in a number of hepatoma cell lines and also coordinately regulated with the GST isoenzymes. Only the induction of NAD(P)H:quinone oxidoreductase caused by many planar aromatic hydrocarbons required a functional Ah receptor. Induction of this enzyme caused by the phenolic antioxidants and other monofunctional inducers occurred through an Ah receptor-independent mechanism. Talalay and his coworkers also showed that there is a one-to-one correspondence in the levels of NADPH:quinone oxidoreductase, cytochrome P_1-450, and GSTs in AHH-responsive and AHH-nonresponsive mice strains. In C57BL/6J (AHH-responsive) mice, which contain high-affinity Ah receptors, all three enzymes exist at high levels; in DBA/2J (AHH-nonresponsive) mice, which contain low-affinity Ah receptors, these enzymes exist at much lower levels. On the basis of these findings, they concluded that these enzymes are all coordinately regulated [226]. Because of the coordinate regulation of the phase I and phase II drug-metabolizing enzymes, planar aromatic hydrocarbons have been proposed to induce the phase II enzymes by binding to the Ah receptor and inducing cytochrome P_1-450. Their redox labile metabolites, the diphenols, aminophenols, and quinones, induce phase II drug-metabolizing enzymes [226]. An alternate model proposes that these compounds bind the Ah receptor, the receptor-ligand complex translocates, and it binds to XREs localized within the 5'-regulatory flanking region of various phase II enzymes' genes to upregulate their transcription [212].

Although there is great structural diversity among inducers of phase II enzymes, one common structural feature most of them share is some α,β–unsaturated system adjacent to an electron-withdrawing group and, therefore, act as electrophilic Michael acceptors in classical Michael reactions [213]. The better a compound is as a Michael acceptor, the more potent it is as an inducer of phase II enzymes. The electron-withdrawing groups in these Michael acceptors render their unsaturated systems electrophilic. GST substrates can be considered Michael acceptors, and the glutathione conjugation reaction catalyzed by the GSTs could be considered a nucleophilic thiol addition to an electrophilic β-carbon on α,β–unsaturated compounds [5]. GST substrates, such as α,β–unsaturated aldehydes, esters, ketones, lactones, nitroalkenes, quinones, sulfones, ethacrynic acid, and other compounds, also induce phase II enzymes, exemplified by NAD(P)H:quinone oxidoreductase. For a series of compounds, there is a strong positive correlation between the potencies of inducers of quinone reductase and their efficacies as substrates for GST isoenzymes [235]. Among other classes of compounds that participate in phase II enzyme induction, the diphenols and phenylenediamines with amino or hydroxyl group substituents in the ortho- and para-positions are the greatest inducers; meta-substituted compounds are not inducers. These observations are explained because 1,2- and 1,4-diphenols can be oxidized to quinones; 1,3-diphenols cannot be oxidized to quinones.

Another structural feature that many phase II enzyme inducers share in common is that these xenobiotics have quinoid structures, which are metabolized to active oxygen species and are known to activate GST and NAD(P)H:quinone oxidoreductase genes. These xenobiotics include the phenolic antioxidants, such as the diphenol compounds, and the planar aromatic hydrocarbons, such as 3-methyl-cholanthrene, benzo[a]pyrene, β-naphthoflavone, and the azo dyes [212]. Many of these compounds are bioactivated by the cytochrome P-450s and are metabolized to quinoid structures.

ROLE OF THE AP-1 COMPLEX IN THE REGULATION OF GST EXPRESSION

The fos and jun proteins, which comprise the AP-1 protein complex, have been demonstrated to act as heterodimers and to activate the transcription of the mouse GST Y_a gene through adjacent AP-1 binding sites in the promoter region between −714 to −754 bp [236–240]. Two of the AP-1 binding sites combined make up the electrophile response element (EpRE). The jun homodimers [241] and fos-jun heterodimers have both been demonstrated to activate transcription. The fos-jun heterodimers undergo enhanced AP-1 binding and cooperative transcriptional activation of genes containing EpREs [236,242–247]. The expression of fos and jun is induced by a wide spectrum of biological, physical, and chemical mediators, such as serum [248], growth factors [249], neurotransmitters [250,251], calcium and potassium channel activators and membrane depolarization [252–255], neoplastic transformation [256,257], transforming oncogenes [258,259], and agents that cause oxidative and chemical stress. Many members of this latter group, which include phenobarbital [260], 2,3,7,8-tetrachlorodibenzo-p-dioxin (TCDD) [261], phorbol esters, polycyclic aromatic hydrocarbons, tert-butylhydroquinone, and hydrogen peroxide [262], act as mediators of GST Y_a gene transcription and are Michael acceptors. De novo synthesis of the AP-1 complex has been shown to be required for GST Y_a gene transactivation through the AP-1 binding site [257,258]. The protein synthesis inhibitor, cycloheximide, also could inhibit enhanced GST Y_a gene expression by tert-butylhydroquinone in H4II hepatoma cells [262], indicating that de novo protein synthesis of the fos and jun proteins was required for the induction process.

After the binding of trans-acting factors to AP-1 motifs occurs, the mechanisms by which genes containing the AP-1 motifs are activated by a wide spectrum of environmental signals is unclear. One possibility is that there is a transduction signal in common with these various stimuli. Currently, the best candidates to play such a role are reactive oxygen species, such as superoxide anion, hydrogen peroxide, hydroxyl radicals, organic peroxides, and radicals produced as a result of metabolic reactions, including those involving many inducers of GSTs and NAD(P)H: quinone oxidoreductase. These enzymes are affected by quinones, which are the reactive intermediates that form as a result of the metabolism of phenolic antioxidants [214,226], and polycyclic aromatic hydrocarbons [212]. Among the phenolic antioxidants, only the ortho- and para-diphenols were demonstrated to be inducers of the GST Y_a gene through the ARE because these compounds are solely oxidized to quinones [226]. Planar aromatic hydrocarbons, such as 3-methyl-cholanthrene and benzo(a)pyrene, have been shown to form quinones by the action of cytochrome P450 enzymes and dihydrodiol dehydrogenase [212,263,264].

TCDD has been shown to inhibit mitochondrial respiration by binding to cytochrome b and partial uncoupling of oxidative phosphorylation, thereby causing the formation of the oxidants hydrogen peroxide and superoxide anion [262]. Therefore, these findings may explain why TCDD, although not metabolized by the cytochrome P450 enzymes [265], can still induce the expression of fos and jun proteins, increase AP-1 activity, and activate the GST Y_a gene via the EpRE [216,261]. Heat shock, arsenite, and arsenate have also been demonstrated to disrupt mitochondrial oxidative phosphorylation and to cause increased formation of active oxygen species [266–268]. Inhibition of antioxidant enzymes, such as superoxide dismutase, by diethyldithiocarbamate also causes oxidative stress and has been shown to potentiate the effects of ozone and paraquat [269]. The tumor promoter phorbol-12-myristate-13-acetate (PMA), which induces GST Y_a gene expression through the EpRE [217], has been shown to decrease the levels of superoxide dismutase (SOD) and catalase [270] and to cause alterations in membrane conformation, thereby forming reactive oxygen species via the activation of the arachidonic acid cascade [271,272].

CLINICAL SIGNIFICANCE, ROLE IN DRUG RESISTANCE, AND THERAPEUTIC IMPLICATIONS OF GSTS

The peptidoleukotriene LTD_4 has been implicated as a causative agent in human bronchial asthma. The leukotrienes are metabolic products derived from arachidonic acid, which is released from membranes by the action of phospholipase A_2 [273,274]. As a result and via the action of 5′-lipooxygenase, LTA_4, an unstable epoxide intermediate, forms. LTA_4 is then converted to LTC_4, a sulfidopeptide, by the action of leukotriene C_4 synthase, which has been demonstrated to be a glutathione S-transferase [275,276]. Recently, photoaffinity labeling experiments conducted with radioiodinated LTC_4 in protein fractions that have been purified up to 10^4-fold suggest that LTC_4 synthase is an 18 kDa membrane protein [277,278]. LTD_4 and LTE_4 are synthesized during the next two steps by γ-glutamyl transpeptidase and cysteinylglycine dipeptidase, respectively. Collectively, LTC_4, LTD_4, and LTE_4 comprise the slow-reacting substance of anaphylaxis (SRS-A). These metabolic intermediates bind to the high-affinity LTD_4 receptor sites and produce effects characteristic of the leukotrienes in the lungs, such as pulmonary smooth muscle contraction, vasoconstriction, changes in vascular permeability, and mucous hypersecretion [279]. Therefore, development of antagonists of LTC_4 synthesis and those against the high-affinity LTD_4 receptor would prove clinically useful. As a matter of fact, such drugs have already been developed, are currently in clinical trial, and have proven to be efficacious against human bronchial asthma [280,281]. A future direction for research in this area includes development of new drugs or suicide substrates that are targeted against LTC_4 synthase as a means for treating human bronchial asthma.

Role of GSTs in cancer and anticancer drug resistance

There are several lines of evidence implicating GSTs in intrinsic and acquired drug resistance. These include the following: (1) overexpression of GSTs in cancers; (2)

acquired resistance of cell lines caused by selection with specific chemotherapeutic agents that overexpress GST isoenzymes; (3) transfection of specific GST cDNAs into cells conferring drug resistance; (4) anticancer drugs being demonstrated to be substrates for GST isoenzymes; and (5) inhibition of GST isoenzymes proving to be efficacious in combating drug resistance.

Overexpression of GST isoenzymes in cancer

The GST isoenzymes are induced in preneoplastic foci and in tumors isolated from organisms exposed to carcinogens or alkylating agents, and this induction occurs even after a single in vivo exposure to carcinogen [282–287]. The pi isoenzyme is primarily expressed in these preneoplastic foci as well as in tumors [288–292]. Although the overexpression of the GST pi isoenzyme in a variety of preneoplastic foci and tumors suggests that this isozyme may be directly involved in chemotherapeutic drug resistance, there is evidence suggesting that the overexpression of these isoenzymes may be due to a pleiotropic response to chemical or oxidative stress in that cytotoxic agents have been shown to cause similar alterations in GSH-dependent enzymes in both normal and drug-resistant cells [293,294].

A recent study, however, has reported that the π-class GST isoenzymes are not expressed in most human prostate cancers; this was accompanied by hypermethylation of cytidine nucleotides in GSTP1 regulatory sequences [295]. Immunohistochemical staining with anti-GSTP1 antibodies did not detect this isoenzyme in >90% of prostatic carcinomas. GSTP1 expression was only limited to human prostatic cell lines, normal tissues, or prostatic tissues exhibiting benign hyperplasia. In each case, GSTP1 expression was accompanied by hypomethylation of regulatory sequences in the π-class glutathione S-transferase GSTP1 promoter region.

Cell lines derived directly from various human tumors also overexpressed GST isoenzymes as well as other GSH-dependent enzymes [296], such as glutathione peroxidase, glutathione reductase, and glyoxalase I. In most cases, the pi GST isoenzyme was predominantly expressed with lower, but detectable, levels of the alpha and mu GST isoenzymes. However, in comparison with normal prostate or samples derived from benign prostatic hypertrophy, human prostatic carcinoma cell lines exhibited substantially less glutathione S-transferase activities, including that for the π-isoenzyme [297]. Cell lines derived from various human tumors included the $CaCO_2$ colon adenocarcinoma [298], small cell lung cancer cell lines [299], and others [296], with the exception of Raji cells derived from Burkitt's lymphoma. Time-dependent alterations in the GST isoenzyme profile were also reported for the $CaCO_2$ colon adenocarcinoma cells, indicating that cell culture conditions can influence the outcome of GST expression [298]. In this cell line, the pi and alpha GST isoenzymes were predominantly expressed in 4 and 20 days, respectively.

There are examples of positive or inverse clinical correlations between the expression of GST isoenzymes and the onset of chemotherapeutic drug resistance. Lymphocytes derived from CLL patients clinically refractory to nitrogen mustards showed a twofold increase in GST activity over those derived from untreated CLL patients, which was attributed primarily to the expression of the pi GST isoenzyme [300]. Before and after the onset of clinical resistance to chlorambucil, cisplatin, and 5-fluorouracil, ovarian adenocarcinoma cell lines derived from the same patients showed that, after the onset of drug resistance, there were 1.8-, 2.2-, 1.3-, and 4.1-fold elevations in GSH, GST, GSH peroxidase, and γ-glutamyltranspeptidase activities, respectively, over those cells taken from the same patients prior to chemotherapy [301]. There are epidemiological studies involving the use of *trans*-stilbene oxide as a substrate for the detection of GST mu isoenzyme activity that suggest that there is an inverse correlation between GST mu expression and lung cancer susceptibility [170,171].

DRUG-RESISTANT CELL LINE STUDIES

The first evidence to suggest that GSTs were directly involved in drug resistance came from reports of the overexpression of the pi and alpha GST isoenzymes in drug-resistant cell lines [302–313]. Overexpression of the GST alpha isoenzyme has been more strongly implicated in resistance against alkylating agents, more specifically, nitrogen mustards [301,302,305,314–316]. Overexpression of the GST mu isoenzymes has been implicated in resistance against another subset of the alkylating agents, the nitrosoureas. One study involving rat 9L gliosarcoma cells resistant to 1,3-bis(2-chloroethyl)-1-nitrosourea (BCNU) attributes this resistance to an overexpression of GST mu isoenzymes [306]. In a human non–small cell lung cancer cell line resistant to BCNU, overexpression of the GST mu isoenzyme 3-3 has been shown to be responsible for this resistance [317].

Overexpression of the pi GST has frequently been linked to the MDR phenotype. In MCF-7 human breast carcinoma cells, overexpression of this GST and the MDR protein [303,304] has also been directly associated with the coordinate expression of selenium-dependent glutathione peroxidase and superoxide dismutase [318]. In addition, the oncogenes v-H-*ras* and v-*raf* also confer resistance to cytotoxic agents, such as Adriamycin, by causing the overexpression of the MDR-1 gene product and GST pi [319]. However, it is unclear whether GST pi is directly responsible for much of the drug resistance since no drug has yet been clearly established as a substrate for this isoenzyme [320]. There is a growing body of evidence that an increase in GST pi in drug-resistant cells and tumors is more likely the result of a pleiotropic stress response and is not directly responsible for the production of the MDR phenotype. One study that is an exception involved an Adriamycin-resistant FLC cell line in which GST alpha was overexpressed and, unlike other MDR phenotypes, did not overexpress glutathione peroxidase [311].

There is a more direct link between overexpression of the alpha GST isoenzyme and the acquisition of the nitrogen mustard–resistant phenotypes. Human ovarian adenocarcinoma cells derived from patients resistant to chlorambucil primarily overexpressed the GST alpha isoenzyme [321]. The Walker-256 rat mammary carcinoma cells resistant to chlorambucil were also shown to be resistant to other nitrogen mustards [302,305]. Among the phenotypic differences noted in the Walker resistant cells relative to the wild-type cells, the 29.5 kD Y_c subunit of the GST alpha isoenzyme was detected [305,314,315]. The resistant cell line exhibited a 10- to 15-fold resistance against chlorambucil [305], and a 4-fold increase in activity using 1-chloro-2,4-dinitrobenzene as the substrate [314] over the wild-type Walker cell line. Chinese hamster ovary (CHO) cells made resistant to bifunctional nitrogen mustards were shown to express enhanced levels of Y_c GST, γ-glutamyltranspeptidase, and glutathione [301]. There was amplification of the Y_c gene and enhanced expression of the Y_c mRNA and protein. In another study, the same cell line, but resistant to chlorambucil, was also cross-resistant to melphalan [316]. These cells also overexpressed the GST alpha protein; gene amplification was also demonstrated. Although there was enhanced Y_c mRNA and protein expressed, amplification of the Y_c gene in the chlorambucil-resistant cells could not be demonstrated [315]. It was reasoned that chlorambucil resistance was unstable and reversible, and that these cells would periodically have to be placed under selection pressure by exposing them to chlorambucil in order to maintain this resistance.

TRANSFECTION STUDIES

Because the acquisition of drug-resistant phenotypes almost certainly involves multiple factors, including the overexpression of various GST isoenzymes, cDNAs encoding various GST isoenzymes have been transfected into mammalian and yeast cells in order to define the role of a specific GST isoenzyme in drug resistance [322–328]. In general, results of these studies indicate that GST isoenzymes can confer some drug resistance, particularly in relation to overexpression of the GST alpha isoenzymes and nitrogen mustard resistance.

The role of GST pi in conferring drug resistance appears to be minor. Transfection of human GST pi cDNA expression vectors into NIH3T3 [329] and MCF-7 [322] cells conferred only up to a fourfold level of resistance against ethacrynic acid and a low level of resistance against Adriamycin [329]. Chinese hamster ovary cells transfected with a GST pi expression vector conferred a two- to threefold level of resistance against cisplatin and carboplatin [325].

What weakens the link between the overexpression of pi GSTs and the acquisition of drug-resistance phenotypes are two observations. None of the above-mentioned studies have clearly demonstrated that the drugs studied are substrates for this isoenzyme. Secondly, although there is a suggested link between GST pi overexpression and the MDR phenotype, some studies have shown that GST pi plays a minor role in drug resistance [330]. In this study, transfection of the mdr-1 gene cDNA expression vector into MCF-7 cells was shown to cause up to 16-, 71-, and 24-fold resistance against Adriamycin, actinomycin D, and vinblastine, respectively. But transfection of these cells with a GST pi expression vector alone conferred low levels of resistance against these cytotoxic agents. Cotransfection of these two expression vectors did not enhance mdr-1–induced drug resistance caused by transfection of the mdr-1 gene cDNA expression vector alone. Cos cells also transfected with a GST pi expression vector showed only a 1.5-fold increase in resistance against Adriamycin over nontransfected cos cells [331].

The causal link between the overexpression of the GST alpha isoenzyme and nitrogen mustard resistance phenotypes is more convincing. Transfection of Mat B rat mammary carcinoma cells with GST Y_c cDNA expression vectors conferred up to a 30-, 16-, and 12-fold resistance to chlorambucil, mechlorethamine, and mephalan, respectively, over nontransfected cells [327]. The transfected cells showed up to a fourfold increase in GST activity and increased expression of the GST Y_c protein. Another study transfected a retroviral vector containing a Y_c cDNA in the reverse orientation into cells resistant to alkylating agents, and the Y_c antisense oligonucleotide was capable of reversing alkylating agent resistance [328]. An exception to this trend is one study in which CHO cells transfected with a GST alpha expression vector afforded protection against bleomycin [332].

It should be noted that because of the low level of GST expression and little conferred anticancer drug resistance after transfection of expression vectors into mammalian cells, there have been similar studies conducted in yeast cells [323] that have provided better evidence of the cause–effect relationship between overexpression of various GST isoenzymes and acquisition of drug-resistance phenotypes. Transfection of GST pi cDNA expression vectors into *Saccharomyces cerevisiae* cells conferred a 2- to 10-fold resistance to Adriamycin and a 2- to 5-fold resistance to chlorambucil. Cells transfected with a human GST alpha cDNA expression vector became resistant to chlorambucil (up to 8-fold) and Adriamycin (up to 16-fold), but not to BCNU.

ANTICANCER DRUGS ARE SUBSTRATES FOR GSTS

In the last several years, there has been direct evidence that specific GST isoenzymes can catalyze conjugation reactions with various anticancer drugs (Table 4-2). These GST-catalyzed conjugation reactions usually occur at rates and to such an extent that enough drug can be detoxified to protect cells against sublethal damage. In comparison with other GST isoenzymes, kinetic analysis has shown that the mu class GSTs are primarily responsible for catalyzing the denitrosation of BCNU [333] and nitrosoguanidinium compounds [334]. This has been further substantiated by detecting overexpression of the mu GST in BCNU-resistant 9L-rat gliosarcoma cells [306]. The GST mu isoenzyme 3-3 has been shown to catalyze the denitrosation of BCNU in BCNU-resistant human non–small cell lung cancer cell lines [317]. The specific mu GST isoenzymes involved in the denitrosation of nitrosoguanidinium compounds are the mouse, rat, and hamster 3–4 isoenzymes [334].

There have been reports suggesting that there is a direct association between increased GSH and GST pi isoenzyme levels and cisplatin resistance. Although no study has clearly shown that cisplatin is a GST pi substrate, there is evidence that GSH levels are inversely correlated with levels of cisplatin-induced cytotoxicity. Glutathione has been specifically shown to inhibit the interaction of cisplatin with DNA [335]. A more recent study using L-buthionine sulfoximine (BSO) to deplete ovarian adenocarcinoma cells of GSH showed that these cells were more susceptible to the action of cisplatin over those cells that were untreated by this inhibitor [336].

The best evidence to date that specific anticancer drugs serve as substrates for GSTs is for the alpha GST isoenzymes; the substrates are various alkylating agents.

Table 4–2. Anticancer drugs as substrates for glutathione S-transferases[a]

Convincing substrate/ kinetic data exist	No definitive proof of catalysis exists	Indirect evidence[b] exists
Chlorambucil[c]	Antimetabolites	Bleomycin
Melphalan[c]	Antimicrotubule drugs[d]	Hepsulfam
Nitrogen mustard[c]	Topoisomerase I and II inhibitors	Mitomycin C
Phosphoramide mustard[c,e]		Adriamycin
Acrolein[e]		Cisplatin
BCNU[f]		Carboplatin
Hydroxyalkenals[g]		
Ethacrynic acid		
Steroids[h]		

[a] The catalyzed reaction is assumed to involve conjugation with GSH through thioether bond formation.
[b] Indirect evidence can include low levels of resistance conveyed by transfection.
[c] The aziridinium intermediate of the nitrogen mustards is the main GST substrate.
[d] The antimicrotubule drug estramustine is an inhibitor of GST, but there is no direct evidence that it is a substrate.
[e] Metabolites of cyclophosphamide.
[f] GST catalyzes a denitrosation of BCNU.
[g] Most electrophilic anticancer drugs produce lipid peroxidation, degradation of which produces a variety of hydroxyalkenals.
[h] GST can act as transporter ligands for some steroids.
From Tew [320], with permission.

Table 4–3. Apparent kinetic constants for human and mouse GST-catalyzed formation of monochloromonoglutathionyl chlorambucil metabolite

Sample	Pool	pI	V_{max} (nmol/min/0.1 mg)	K_m (μM)	Efficiency (V_{max}/K_m)
Human liver GSTα	I	9.1	0.8	19	0.042
	II	8.8	1.9	150	0.013
	III	8.3, 7.9	3.4	220	0.016
Mouse liver GSTα	I	—	1.0	38	0.026
Human ovarian GSTπ	IV	4.6, 4.75, 4.81	1.6	830	0.002

Reaction mixtures consisted of 100 μg/ml purified GST, 1 mM GSH in 0.1 M potassium phosphate buffer, pH 6.5, and were permitted to run with varying concentrations of chlorambucil for 2.5 min. The determination of the monochloromonoglutathionyl chlorambucil adduct was performed by HPLC as described previously [337,338]. From Ciaccio et al. [338] and Ciaccio and Tew [363], with permission.

Both chlorambucil [337] and mephalan [316] have clearly been shown to be ligands for GST alpha isoenzymes. Mouse and human liver GST alpha and ovarian GST pi were demonstrated to conjugate glutathione to chlorambucil to form mono-chloromonoglutathionyl chlorambucil, but the alpha isoenzymes had at least a 22-fold greater affinity for chlorambucil (Table 4-3) [337,338]. Mouse liver GST alpha, rabbit, and human cytosolic and microsomal GST isoenzymes were demonstrated to conjugate melphalan [339,340]. When melphalan was incubated with glutathione and solubilized rabbit or human liver microsomal protein, the product mixtures contained monochloromonoglutathionyl melphalan and diglutathionyl melphalan [340]. The human glutathione S-transferase isoenzymes GST A1-1 (α)

and GST P1-1 (π) were demonstrated to conjugate thiotepa [tris(1-aziridinyl) phosphine sulfide], a trifunctional alkylating agent, and to form monoglutathionyl thiotepa. These isoenzymes also catalyzed the conversion of thiotepa to monoglutathionyl conjugates of TEPA [tris(1-aziridinyl) phosphine oxide] [341]. Purified cytosolic GSTs from CHO cells, which were made resistant to bifunctional nitrogen mustards, were shown to conjugate melphalan and to be of the alpha class [316]. The higher efficiencies of the GST alpha isoenzymes in performing these conjugation reactions with alkylating agents is consistent with the observation that GST alpha isoenzymes are overexpressed in cells expressing the alkylating agent phenotype. Some exceptions to this trend are that the 4-hydroxycyclophosphamide metabolite acrolein has been shown to be a good substrate for the pi, mu, and alpha GST isoenzymes [342] and cyclophosophamide has been shown to be metabolized by microsomal GSTs [343].

THERAPEUTIC STRATEGIES INVOLVING GST ISOENZYMES

Because of the evidence that GSTs are causally linked to drug resistance, therapeutic strategies involving the targeting of these isoenzymes that may reverse or attenuate drug-resistant phenotypes have been devised. However, at this time there have been a very limited number of these therapeutic strategies tried in the clinical setting.

Ethacrynic acid is an α,β–unsaturated plant phenolic acid, which conjugates glutathione via a Michael addition [344] and acts as a competitive and noncompetitive inhibitor of all three major classes of the GST isoenzymes [345,346]. At clinically achievable plasma concentrations, ethacrynic acid has been shown to inhibit the conjugation reaction between chlorambucil and glutathione mediated by alpha GST isoenzymes [337]. Ethacrynic acid, at nontoxic concentrations, has also been shown to increase the efficacy of chlorambucil in previously resistant cells derived from rats (Walker 256 mammary carcinoma) and humans (HT-29 colon carcinoma) [346]. Treatment with ethacrynic acid also increased the effects of melphalan in previously resistant RPN-1822 human melanoma cells [347] and the cytotoxic effects of BCNU in BCNU-resistant 9L gliosarcoma cells [306].

There have been clinical reports that indicate ethacrynic acid can increase the efficacy of alkylating agents. Clearance of thio-TEPA from patients was diminished in half when they were treated with a combination of thio-TEPA alone [349]. At the concentrations administered to patients, ethacrynic acid produced inhibition of the GST isoenzymes in peripheral lymphocytes and, yet, promoted manageable diuresis. Corroborating these findings was a report that ethacrynic acid altered the elimination kinetics of thio-TEPA in perfused rat livers [350]. A more recent clinical report cited that ethacrynic acid was able to reverse chlorambucil resistance in a chronic lymphocytic leukemia (CLL) patient [351].

However, ethacrynic acid should be administered in the clinical setting judiciously as there is in vitro evidence that prolonged exposure to this agent can lead to the development of ethacrynic acid–resistant phenotypes. One study has shown that chronic exposure of HT-29 colon carcinoma cells to ethacrynic acid leads to resistance to this drug, as was reflected by increased expression of glutathione [352] and the GST pi isoenzyme [352–355]. This enhanced expression was caused by both the enhanced rate of transcription [352] and the increased stabilization of the target GST isoenzyme mRNA and protein [352–354], but was readily reversed when the drug was withdrawn [354,355]. In these cells, resistance to ethacrynic acid was also associated with the overproduction of a 37.5 kDa enzyme [356], which was subsequently identified as dihydrodiol dehydrogenase [357].

There are a series of compounds, which are GSH analogues, that have been synthesized by Terrapin Technologies, Inc. that target specific human GST isoenzymes. These include the Ter-183, -199, -200, -206, and -317 GSH analogues [358–360]. Ter-286 appears to act like a prodrug as it is activated by a metabolic reaction catalyzed by GST isoenzymes [360]. The octyl GSH derivatives, Ter-143 [361] and Ter-183 [358], primarily inhibited the GST alpha isoenzyme A1-1. The compounds Ter-117 [361], Ter-135 [361], Ter-199 [358], Ter-286 [358], and Ter-317 [358] all primarily inhibited the GST pi isoenzyme P1-1. Ter-286 was demonstrated to be a substrate for this isoenzyme [360]. The β-alanine derivative, Ter-200 [358], and the naphthyl derivative, Ter-211 [361], were shown to be primarily inhibitors of the GST mu isoenzyme M1a1a. The compound Ter-199 could induce chloramphenicol acetyltransferase activity in Hepal cells that were stably transfected with NAD(P)H:quinone oxidoreductase NQO_1 hARE-tk-CAT chimeric gene constructs, suggesting a link between Ter-199 as a competive inhibitor of the pi isoenzyme and its ability to upregulate the γ-glutamylcysteine synthetase and DDH genes via the ARE [362]. Therefore, these compounds show promise as chemotherapeutic agents because GST isoenzymes are overexpressed in various tumors and drug-resistant cell lines relative to normal tissues and cells.

CONCLUDING REMARKS

The glutathione S-transferases (E.C.2.5.1.18) are a family of isoenzymes that catalyze the nucleophilic attack of the sulfur atom of glutathione upon the electrophilic center of a variety of compounds. Therefore, these enzymes participate in the thiol-mediated detoxification of anticancer drugs that produce toxic electrophilic intermediates. Because many of the GST isoenzymes are overexpressed in tumors and in drug-resistant cell types, the presence or absence of specific GST isoenzymes can be used as biomarkers to characterize certain disease states, such as lung cancer. Overexpression of these isoenzymes can also lead to rational approaches, which could enhance the therapeutic index by selective inhibition of various isoenzymes. Inhibitors of these various isoenzymes could be designed rationally upon better understanding of the GST protein structure, including the active site, and the catalytic mechanism of GST-mediated reactions. An enhanced comprehension of GST gene structure and regulation could be employed to design effective strategies with which to inhibit signaling pathways that lead to the overexpression of these isoenzymes. Understanding GST expression and polymorphisms within the human population could be a predictive tool in determining which individuals are susceptible to carcinogens and would benefit from specific drug regimens. However, caution should be maintained when attempting to determine cause–effect relationships between GST overexpression and drug resistance mechanisms, as these mechanisms can often involve multiple factors.

REFERENCES

1. Tew KD, Houghton JA, Houghton PJ (1993) Preclinical and Clinical Modulation of Anticancer Drugs. Boca Raton, FL: CRC Press.
2. Boyland E, Chasseaud LF (1969) The role of glutathione and glutathione S-transferases in mercapturic acid biosynthesis. Adv Enzymol Relat Areas Mol Biol 32:173–219.
3. Jakoby WB (1978) The glutathione S-transferases: A group of multifunctional detoxification proteins. Adv Enzymol Relat Areas Mol Biol 46:383–414.
4. Mannervik B (1985) The isoenzymes of glutathione transferase. Adv Enzymol Relat Areas Mol Biol 57:357–417.
5. Mannervik B, Danielson UH (1988) Glutathione S-transferases—structure and catalytic activity. CRC Crit Rev Biochem 23:283–337.
6. Daniel V (1993) Glutathione S-transferases: Gene structure and regulation of expression. CRC Crit Rev Biochem Mol Biol 28:173–207.
7. Wilce MCJ, Parker MW (1994) Structure and function of glutathione S-transferases. Biochim Biophys Acta 1205:1–18.
8. Mantle TJ, Pickett CB, Hayes JD (eds) (1987) Glutathione S-Transferases and Carcinogenesis. London: Taylor and Francis.
9. Sies H, Ketterer B (eds) (1988) Glutathione Conjugation: Mechanisms and Biological Significance. New York: Academic Press.
10. Hayes JD, Pickett CB, Mantle TJ (eds) (1990) Glutathione S-Transferases and Drug Resistance. London: Taylor and Francis.
11. Coles B, Ketterer B (1990) The role of glutathione and glutathione transferases in chemical carcinogenesis. CRC Crit Rev Biochem Mol Biol 25:47–70.
12. Jakoby WB, Ziegler DM (1990) The enzymes of detoxication. J Biol Chem 265:20715–20718.
13. Listowsky I (1993) Glutathione S-transferases: Intracellular binding, detoxification and adaptive responses. In N Tavoloni, PD Berk, eds. Hepatic and Bile Secretion Transport: Physiology and Pathophysiology. New York: Raven Press, p 397.
14. Tomarev SI, Zinovieva RD (1988) Squid major lens polypeptides are homologous to glutathione S-transferase subunits. Nature 336:86–88.
15. Ramage PI, Rae GH, Nimmo IA (1986) Purification and properties of the hepatic glutathione S-transferases of the Atlantic salmon (Salmo salar). Comp Biochem Physiol 83B:23–29.
16. Mozer TJ, Tiemeier DC, Jaworski EG (1983) Purification and characterization of corn glutathione S-transferase. Biochemistry 22:1068–1072.
17. Clark AG, Shamaan NA, Sinclair MD, Dauterman WC (1986) Insecticide metabolism by multiple glutathione S-transferases in two strains of the housefly, Musca domestica. Pestic Biochem Physiol 25:169–175.
18. Cochrane BJ, Morrisse JJ, LeBlanc GA (1987) The genetics of xenobiotic metabolism in Drosophila. 4. Purification and characterization of the major glutathione S-transferase. Insect Biochem 17:731–738.
19. Tamaki H, Kumagai H, Tochikura T (1989) Purification and properties of glutathione transferase from Issatchenkia orientalis. J Bacteriol 171:1173–1177.
20. Cohen E, Gamliel A, Katan J (1986) Glutathione and glutathione S-transferase in fungi—effect of pentachloronitrobenzene and 1-chloro-2,4-dinitrobenzene—purification and characterization of the transferase from Fusarium. Pestic Biochem Physiol 26:1–9.
21. Ando K, Honma M, Chiba S, Jahara S, Mizutani J (1988) Glutathione transferase from Mucor javanicus. Agric Biol Chem 52:135–139.
22. Di Ilio C, Aceto A, Piccolomini R, Allocati N, Faraone A, Cellini L, Ravagnan G, Federici G (1988) Purification and characterization of three forms of glutathione transferase from Proteus mirabilis. Biochem J 255:971–975.
23. Ilzuka M, Inoue Y, Murata K, Kimura A (1989) Purification and some properties of glutathione S-transferase from Escherichia coli B. J Bacteriol 171:6039–6042.
24. Piccolomini R, Di Ilio C, Aceto A, Allocati N, Faraone A, Cellini L, Ravagnan G, Federici G (1989) Glutathione transferase in bacteria: Subunit composition and antigenic characterization. J Gen Microbiol 135:3119–3125.

25. Arca P, Garcia P, Hardisson C, Suarez JE (1990) Purification and study of a bacterial glutathione S-transferase. FEBS Lett 263:77–79.
26. Mannervik B, Alin P, Guthenberg C, Jensson H, Tahir MK, Warholm M, Tornvall H (1985) Identification of three classes of cytosolic glutathione transferase common to several mammalian species: Correlation between structural data and enzymatic properties. Proc Natl Acad Sci USA 82:7202–7206.
27. Pickett CB, Lu AYH (1989) Glutathione S-transferases: Gene structure, regulation, and biological function. Ann Rev Biochem 58:743–764.
28. Board P, Coggan M, Johnston P, Ross V, Suzuki T, Webb G (1990) Genetic heterogeneity of the human glutathione S-transferases—a complex of gene families. Pharmacol Ther 48:357–369.
29. Meyer DJ, Coles B, Pemble SE, Gilmore KS, Fraser GM, Ketterer B (1991) Theta, a new class of glutathione transferases purified from rat and man. Biochem J 274:409–414.
30. Nicholson DW, Ali A, Vaillancourt JP, Calaycay JR, Mumford RA, Zamboni RJ, Ford-Hutchinson AW (1993) Purification to homogeneity and the N-terminal sequence of human leukotriene C₄ synthase: A homodimeric glutathione S-transferase composed of 18 kD subunits. Proc Natl Acad Sci USA 90:2015–2019.
31. Suzuki T, Coggan M, Shaw DC, Board PG (1987) Electrophoretic and immunological analysis of human glutathione S-transferase isozymes. Ann Hum Genet 51:95–106.
32. Di Ilio C, Aceto A, Bucciarelli T, Angelucci S, Felaco M, Grilli A, Federici G (1990) Glutathione transferase isoenzymes from human prostate. Biochem J 271:481–485.
33. Mannervik B, Awasthi YC, Board PG, Hayes JD, Di Ilio C, Ketterer B, Listowsky I, Morgenstern R, Muramatsu M, Pearson WR, Pickett CB, Sato K, Widersten M, Wolf CR (1992) Nomenclature for human glutathione transferases. Biochem J 282:305–308.
34. Kuzmich S, Vanderveer LA, Tew K (1991) Evidence for a glycoconjugate form of glutathione S-transferase pi. Int J Pept Protein Res 37:565–571.
35. Zhong S, Spurr NK, Hayes JD, Wolf CR (1993) Deduced amino acid sequence, gene structure, and chromosomal location of a novel human class mu glutathione S-transferase, GSTM4. Biochem J 291:41–50.
36. Takahashi Y, Campbell EA, Hirata Y, Takayama T, Listowsky I (1993) A basis for differentiating among the multiple human Mu-glutathione S-transferases and molecular cloning of brain GSTM5. J Biol Chem 268:8893–8898.
37. Morgenstern R, DePierre JW, Jornvall H (1985) Microsomal glutathione transferase: Primary structure. J Biol Chem 260:13976–13983.
38. Pemble SE, Taylor JB (1992) An evolutionary perspective on glutathione S-transferases inferred from class-theta glutathione transferase cDNA sequences. Biochem J 287:957–963.
39. Devereux J, Haeberli P, Smithies O (1984) A comprehensive set of sequence analysis programs for the VAX. Nucleic Acids Res 12:387–395.
40. Bairoch A, Boeckmann B (1991) The SWISS-PROT protein sequence data bank. Nucleic Acids Res 19:2247–2249.
41. Buetler TM, Eaton DL (1992) Glutathione S-transferases: Amino acid sequence comparison, classification, and phylogenetic relationship. Environ Carcinogen Ecotoxicol Rev C10:181–203.
42. Doolittle RF (1988) Lens proteins: More molecular opportunism. Nature 336:18.
43. Kohler-Staub D, Leisinger T (1985) Dichloromethane dehydrogenase of Hyphomicrobium sp. strain DM2. J Bacteriol 162:676–681.
44. Scholtz R, Wackett LP, Egli C, Cook AM, Leisinger T (1988) Dichloromethane dehalogenase with improved catalytic activity isolated from a fast-growing dichloromethane-utilizing bacterium. J Bacteriol 170:5698–5704.
45. LaRoche SD, Leisinger T (1990) Sequence analysis and expression of the bacterial dichloromethane dehalogenase structural gene, a member of the glutathione S-transferase supergene family. J Bacteriol 172:164–171.
46. Toung Y-PS, Tu C-PD (1992) Drosophila glutathione S-transferases have sequence homology to the stringent starvation protein of Escherichia coli. Biochem Biophys Res Commun 182:355–360.
47. Meyer RC, Goldsbrough PB, Woodson WR (1991) An ethylene-responsive flower senescence-related gene from carnation encodes a protein homologous to glutathione S-transferases. Plant Mol Biol 17:277–281.
48. Persson B, Jornvall H, Alin P, Mannervik B (1988) Structural classes of glutathione transferase: distinctions between isoenzymzes and enzymes. Protein Seq. Data Anal 1:183–186.

49. Ahmad H, Wilson DE, Fritz RR, Singh SV, Medh RD, Nagle GT, Awasthi YC, Kurosky A (1990) Primary and secondary structural analyses of glutathione S-transferase π form human placenta. Arch Biochem Biophys 278:398–408.
50. Banner DW, Bloomer AC, Petsko GA, Phillips DC, Pogson CI, Wilson IA, Corran PH, Furth AJ, Milman JD, Offord RE, Priddle JD, Waley SG (1975) Structure of chicken muscle triose phosphate isomerase determined crystallographically at 2.5 Å resolution using amino acid sequence data. Nature 255:609–614.
51. Branden C, Tooze T (1991) Introduction To Protein Structure. Chapter 4 Alpha-Beta Structures. New York: Garland, pp 43–48.
52. Reinemer P, Dirr HW, Ladenstein R, Schaffer J, Gallay O, Huber R (1991) The three-dimensional structure of class π glutathione S-transferase in complex with glutathione sulfonate at 2.3 Å resolution. EMBO J 10:1997–2005.
53. Reinemer P, Dirr HW, Ladenstein R, Huber R, LoBello M, Federici G, Parker MW (1992) Three-dimensional structure of class π glutathione S-transferase from human placenta in complex with S-hexylglutathione at 2.8 Å resolution. J Mol Biol 227:214–226.
54. Dirr HW, Reinemer P (1991) Equilibrium unfolding of class π glutathione S-transferase. Biochem Biophys Res Commun 180:294–300.
55. Aceto A, Caccuri M, Saccheta P, Bucciarelli T, Dragani B, Rosato N, Federici G, Di Ilio C (1992) Dissociation and unfolding of Pi-class glutathione transferase. Evidence for a monomeric inactive intermediate. Biochem J 285:241–245.
56. Wright WB (1958) The crystal structure of glutathione. Acta Crystallogr 11:632–663.
57. Rosevear PR, Sellin S, Mannervik B, Kuntz ID, Mildvan AS (1984) NMR and computer modeling studies of the conformations of glutathione derivatives at the active site of glyoxalase I. J Biol Chem 259:11436–11447.
58. Karplus PA, Pai EF, Schultz GE (1989) A crystallographic study of the glutathione binding site of glutathione reductase at 0.3 nm resolution. Eur J Biochem 178:693–703.
59. Sesay MA, Ammon HL, Armstrong RN (1987) Crystallization and a preliminary X-ray diffraction study of isoenzyme 3-3 of glutathione S-transferase from rat liver. J Mol Biol 197:377–378.
60. Fu J-H, Rose J, Chung Y-J, Tam MF, Wang B-C (1991) Crystals of isoenzyme 3-3 of rat liver glutathione S-transferase with and without inhibitor. Acta Crystallogr B47:813–814.
61. Ji X, Zhang P, Armstrong RN, Gilliland GL (1992) A three-dimensional structure of a glutathione S-transferase from the mu gene class. Structural analysis of the binary complex of isoenzyme 3-3 and glutathione at 2.2 Å resolution. Biochemistry 31:10169–10184.
62. Penington CJ, Rule GS (1992) Mapping the substrate-binding site of a human class mu glutathione transferase using nuclear magnetic resonance spectroscopy. Biochemistry 31:2912–2920.
63. Cowan SW, Bergfors T, Jones TA, Tibbelin G, Olin B, Board PG, Mannervik B (1989) Crystallization of GST 2, a human class alpha glutathione transferase. J Mol Biol 208:369–370.
64. Sinning I, Kleywegt GJ, Cowan SW, Reinemer P, Dirr HW, Huber R, Gilliland GL, Armstrong RN, Ji X, Board PG, Olin B, Mannervik B, Jones TA (1993) Structure determination and refinement of human class alpha glutathione S-transferase A1-1, and a comparison with the mu and pi class enzymes. J Mol Biol 232:192–212.
65. Trottein F, Vaney M-C, Bachet B, Pierce R-J, Colloc'h N, Lecocq J-P, Capron A, Mornon J-P (1992) Crystallization and preliminary X-ray diffraction studies of a protective cloned 28 kD glutathione S-transferase from Schistosoma mansoni. J Mol Biol 224:515–518.
66. Schaeffer T, Gallay O, Ladenstein R (1988) Glutathione transferase from bovine placenta. Preparation, biochemical characterization, crystallization, and preliminary crystallographic analysis of a neutral class pi enzyme. J Biol Chem 263:17405–17411.
67. Parker MW, LoBello M, Federici G (1990) Crystallization of glutathione S-transferase from human placenta. J Mol Biol 213:221–222.
68. Ketley JN, Habig WH, Jakoby WB (1975) Binding of nonsubstrate ligands to the glutathione S-transferases. J Biol Chem 250:8670–8673.
69. Caccuri AM, Aceto A, Piemonte F, Di Ilio C, Rosato N, Federici G (1990) Interaction of hemin with placental glutathione transferase. Eur J Biochem 189:493–497.
70. Board PG, Mannervik B (1991) The contribution of the C-terminal sequence to the catalytic activity of GST 2, a human alpha class glutathione transferase. Biochem J 275:171–174.
71. Bhargava MM, Dasgupta A (1988) Binding of sulfobromophthalein to rat and human ligandins: Characterization of a binding-site peptide. Biochim Biophys Acta 955:296–300.
72. Desideri A, Caccuri AM, Polizio F, Bastoni R, Federici G (1991) Electron paramagnetic resonance

identification of a highly reactive thiol group in the proximity of the catalytic site of human placenta glutathione S-transferase. J Biol Chem 266:2063–2066.

73. Nishihira J, Ishibashi T, Sakai M, Nishi S, Kondo H, Makita A (1992) Identification of the fatty acid binding site on glutathione S-transferase P. Biochem Biophys Res Commun 189:197–205.

74. Satoh K, Hatayama I, Tsuchida S, Sato K (1991) Biochemical characteristics of a preneoplastic marker enzyme glutathione S-transferase P-form (7-7). Arch Biochem Biophys 285:312–316.

75. Franken SM, Rozeboom HJ, Kalk KH, Dijkstra BW (1991) Crystal structure of haloalkane dehalogenase: An enzyme to detoxify halogenated alkanes. EMBO J 10:1297–1302.

76. Vrielink A, Lloyd LF, Blow DM (1991) Crystal structure of cholesterol oxidase from *Brevibacterium sterolicum* refined at 1.8 Å resolution. J Mol Biol 219:533–554.

77. Sharff AJ, Wilson DK, Chang Z, Quiocho FA (1992) Refined 2.5 Å structure of murine adenosine deaminase at pH 6.0. J Mol Biol 226:917–921.

78. Derewanda ZS, Sharp AM (1993) News from the interface: The molecular structures of triacylglyceride lipases. Trends Biochem Sci 18:20–25.

79. Derewanda U, Brzozowski AM, Lawson DM, Derewanda ZS (1992) Catalysis at the interface: The anatomy of a conformational change in a triglyceride lipase. Biochemistry 31:1532–1541.

80. Eisenberg D, McLachlan AD (1986) Solvation energy in protein folding and binding. Nature 319:199–203.

81. Ricci G, Del Boccio G, Pennelli A, Aceto A, Whitehead EP, Federici G (1989) Nonequivalence of the two subunits of horse erythrocyte glutathione transferase in their reaction with sulfhydryl reagents. J Biol Chem 264:5462–5467.

82. Van Ommen B, Ploemen JHTM, Ruven HJ, Vos RME, Bogaards JJP, Van Berkel WJH, Van Bladeren PJ (1989) Studies on the active site of rat glutathione transferase isoenzyme 4-4. Chemical modification by tetrachloro-1,4-benzoquinone and its glutathione conjugate. Eur J Biochem 181:423–429.

83. Lo Bello M, Petruzzelli R, De Stefano E, Tenedini C, Barra D, Federici G (1990) Identification of a highly, reactive sulphydryl group in human placental glutathione transferase by a site-directed fluorescent reagent. FEBS Lett 263:389–391.

84. Tamai K, Satoh K, Tsuchida S, Hatayama I, Maki T, Sato K (1990) Specific inactivation of glutathione S-transferases in class pi by SH-modifiers. Biochem Biophys Res Commun 167:331–338.

85. Kong K-H, Inoue H, Takahashi K (1991) Non-essentiality of cysteine and histidine residues for the activity of human class pi glutathione S-transferase. Biochem Biophys Res Commun 181:748–755.

86. Tamai K, Shen H, Tsuchida S, Hatayama I, Maki T, Sato K (1991) Role of cysteine residues in the activity of rat glutathione transferase P (7-7): Elucidation by oligonucleotide site-directed mutagenesis. Biochem Biophys Res Commun 179:790–797.

87. Widersten M, Holmstrom E, Mannervik B (1991) Cysteine residues are not essential for the catalytic activity of human class Mu glutathione transferase M1a-1a. FEBS Lett 293:156–159.

88. Hsieh J-C, Huang S-C, Chen W-L, Lai Y-C, Tam MF (1991) Cysteine-86 is not needed for the enzymic activity of glutathione S-transferase 3-3. Biochem J 278:293–297.

89. Chen W-L, Hsieh J-C, Hong J-L, Tsai S-P, Tam MF (1992) Site-directed mutagenesis and chemical modification of cysteine residues of rat glutathione S-transferase 3-3. Biochem J 286:205–210.

90. Nishihira J, Ishibashi T, Sakai M, Nishi S, Kumazaki T, Hatanaka Y, Tsuda S, Hikichi K (1992) Characterization of cysteine residues of glutathione S-transferase P: Evidence for steric hindrance of substrate binding by a bulky adduct to Cys-47. Biochem Biophys Res Commun 188:424–432.

91. Wang RW, Newton DJ, Pickett CB, Lu AY (1992) Site-directed mutagenesis of glutathione S-transferase Y_aY_a: Functional studies of histidine, cysteine, and tryptophan mutants. Arch Biochem Biophys 297:86–91.

92. Awasthi YC, Bhatnagar A, Singh SV (1987) Evidence for the involvement of histidine at the active site of glutathione S-transferase ψ from human liver. Biochem Biophys Res Commun 143:965–970.

93. Van Ommen B, den Besten C, Rutten ALM, Ploemen JHTM, Vos RME, Muller F, Van Bladeren PJ (1988) Active site-directed inhibition of glutathione S-transferases by the glutathione conjugate of tetrachloro-1,4-benzoquinone. J Biol Chem 263:12939–12942.

94. Van Ommen B, Ploemen JHTM, Bogaards JJP, Monks TJ, Gau SS, Van Bladeren PJ (1991) Irreversible inhibition of rat glutathione S-transferase 1-1 by quinones and their glutathione conjugates. Structure-activity relationship and mechanism. Biochem J 276:661–666.

95. Chang L-H, Wang L-Y, Tam MF (1991) The single cysteine residue on an alpha family chick liver

glutathione S-transferase CL 3-3 is not functionally important. Biochem Biophys Res Commun 180:323–328.

96. Ricci G, Del Boccio G, Pennelli A, Lo Bello M, Petruzzelli R, Caccuri AM, Barra D, Federici G (1991) Redox forms of human placenta glutathione transferase. J Biol Chem 266:21409–21415.

97. Wang RW, Newton DJ, Pickett CB, Lu AYH (1991) Site-directed mutagenesis of glutathione S-transferase Y_aY_a: Nonessential role of histidine in catalysis. Arch Biochem Biophys 286:574–578.

98. Zhang P, Graminski GF, Armstrong RN (1991) Are the histidine residues of glutathione S-transferase important in catalysis? An assessment by ^{13}C-NMR spectroscopy and site-specific mutagenesis. J Biol Chem 266:19475–19479.

99. Manoharan TH, Gulick AM, Puchalski RB, Servais AL, Fahl WE (1992) Structural studies on human glutathione S-transferase π. Substitution mutations to determine amino acids necessary for binding glutathione. J Biol Chem 267:18940–18945.

100. Widersten B, Mannervik B (1992) A structural role of histidine-15 in human glutathione transferase M1-1, an amino acid residue conserved in class Mu enzymes. Protein Eng 5:551–557.

101. Wang RW, Newton DJ, Huskey S-E, McKeever BM, Pickett CB, Lu AYH (1992) Site-directed mutagenesis of glutathione S-transferase Y_aY_a: Important roles of tyrosine 9 and aspartic acid 101 in catalysis. J Biol Chem 267:19866–19871.

102. Lo Bello M, Petruzzelli R, Reale L, Ricci G, Barra D, Federici G (1992) Chemical modification of human placental glutathione transferase by pyridoxal 5'-phosphate. Biochim Biophys Acta 1121:167–172.

103. Jakobson I, Askelof P, Warholm M, Mannervik B (1977) A steady-state kinetic random mechanism for glutathione S-transferase A from rat liver. A model involving kinetically significant enzyme-product complexes in the forward reaction. Eur J Biochem 77:253–262.

104. Schramm VL, McCluskey R, Emig FA, Litwack G (1984) Kinetic studies and active site-binding properties of glutathione S-transferase using spin-labeled glutathione, a product analogue. J Biol Chem 259:714–722.

105. Ivanetich KM, Goold RD (1989) A rapid equilibrium random sequential bi-bi mechanism for human placental glutathione S-transferase. Biochim Biophys Acta 998:7–13.

106. Armstrong RN (1987) Enzyme-catalyzed detoxication reactions: Mechanisms and stereochemistry. CRC Crit Rev Biochem Mol Biol 22:39–88.

107. Armstrong RN (1991) Glutathione S-transferases: Reaction mechanism, structure, and function. Chem Res Toxicol 4:131–140.

108. Adang AEP, Brussee J, Meyer DJ, Coles B, Ketterer B, Van Der Gen A, Mulder GJ (1988) Substrate specificity of rat liver glutathione S-transferase isoenzymes for a series of glutathione analogues, modified at the γ-glutamyl moiety. Biochem J 255:721–724.

109. Adang AEP, Brussee J, Van Der Gen A, Mulder GJ (1990) The glutathione binding site in glutathione S-transferases. Investigation of the cysteinyl, glycyl, and γ-glutamyl domains. Biochem J 269:47–54.

110. Chen W-J, Graminski GF, Armstrong RN (1988) Dissection of the catalytic mechanism of isoenzyme 4-4 of glutathione S-transferase with alternative substrates. Biochemistry 27:647–654.

111. Chang L-H, Tam MF (1993) Site-directed mutagenesis and chemical modification of histidine residues on an α-class chick liver glutathione S-transferase CL 3-3. Histidines are not needed for the activity of the enzyme and diethylpyrocarbonate modifies both histidine and lysine residues. Eur J Biochem 211:805–811.

112. Blundell TL, Johnson LN (1976) Protein Crystallography. New York: Academic Press.

113. Graminski GF, Zhang P, Sesay MA, Ammon HL, Armstrong RN (1989) Formation of the 1-(S-glutathionyl)-2,4,6-trinitrocyclohexadienate anion at the active site of glutathione S-transferase: Evidence for enzymatic stabilization of σ-complex intermediates in nucleophilic aromatic substitution reactions. Biochemistry 28:6252–6258.

114. Graminski GF, Kubo Y, Armstrong RN (1989) Spectroscopic and kinetic evidence for the thiolate anion of glutathione at the active site of glutathione S-transferase. Biochemistry 28:3562–3568.

115. Sternberg G, Board PG, Mannervik B (1991) Mutation of an evolutionary conserved tyrosine residue in the active site of a human class alpha glutathione transferase. FEBS Lett 293:153–155.

116. Kolm RH, Sroga GE, Mannervik B (1992) Participation of the phenolic hydroxyl group of Tyr-8 in the catalytic mechanism of human glutathione transferase P1-1. Biochem J 285:537–540.

117. Kong K-H, Nishida M, Inoue H, Takahashi K (1992) Tyrosine-7 is an essential residue for the catalytic activity of human class pi glutathione S-transferase: Chemical modification and site-directed mutagenesis studies. Biochem Biophys Res Commun 182:1122–1129.

118. Liu S, Zhang P, Ji X, Johnson WW, Gilliland GL, Armstrong RN (1992) Contribution of tyrosine

6 to the catalytic mechanism of isoenzyme 3-3 of glutathione S-transferase. J Biol Chem 267:4296–4299.

119. Manoharan TH, Gulick AM, Reinemer P, Dirr HW, Huber R, Fahl WE (1992) Mutational substitution of residues implicated by crystal structure in binding the substrate glutathione to human glutathione S-transferase π. J Mol Biol 226:319–322.

120. Kong K-H, Inoue H, Takahashi K (1992) Site-directed mutagenesis of amino acid residues involved in the glutathione binding of human glutathione S-transferase P1-1. Biochemistry (Tokyo) 112:725–728.

121. Huskey S-EW, Huskey WP, Lu AYH (1991) Contributions of thiolate desolvation to catalysis by glutathione S-transferase isoenzymes 1-1 and 2-2: Evidence from kinetic solvent isotope effects. J Am Chem Soc 113:2283–2290.

122. Atkins WM, Wang RW, Bird AW, Newton DJ, Lu AYH (1993) The catalytic mechanism of glutathione S-transferase (GST): Spectroscopic determination of the pKa of Tyr-9 in rat α1-1 GST. J Biol Chem 268:19188–19191.

123. Karshikoff A, Reinemer P, Huber R, Ladenstein R (1993) Electrostatic evidence for the activation of the glutathione thiol by Tyr-7 in π-class glutathione transferases. Eur J Biochem 215:663–670.

124. Meyer DJ, Xia C, Coles B, Chen H, Reinemer P, Huber R, Ketterer B (1993) Unusual reactivity of Tyr-7 of GSH transferase P1-1. Biochem J 293:351–356.

125. Liu S, Ji X, Gilliland GL, Stevens WJ, Armstrong RN (1993) Second-sphere electrostatic effects in the active site of glutathione S-transferase. Observation of an on-face hydrogen bond between the side chain of threonine-13 and the π-cloud of tyrosine 6 and its influence on catalysis. J Am Chem Soc 115:7910–7911.

126. Johnson WW, Liu S, Ji X, Gilliland GL, Armstrong RN (1993) Tyrosine-115 participates both in chemical and physical steps of the catalytic mechanism of a glutathione S-transferase. J Biol Chem 268:11508–11511.

127. Katusz RM, Colman RF (1991) S-(4-bromo-2,3-dioxobutyl) glutathione: A new affinity label for the 4-4 isoenzyme of rat liver glutathione S-transferase. Biochemistry 30:11230–11238.

128. Askelof P, Guthenberg C, Jakobson I, Mannervik B (1975) Purification and characterization of two glutathione S-aryltransferase activities from rat liver. Biochem J 147:513–522.

129. Danielson UH, Esterbauer H, Mannervik B (1987) Structure-activity relationships of 4-hydroxyalkenals in the conjugation catalysed by mammalian glutathione transferases. Biochem J 247:707–713.

130. Hoesch RM, Boyer TD (1989) Localization of a portion of the active site of two rat liver glutathione S-transferases using a photoaffinity label. J Biol Chem 264:17712–17717.

131. Kalinyak JE, Taylor JM (1982) Rat glutathione S-transferase. Cloning of double-stranded cDNA and induction of its mRNA. J Biol Chem 257:523–530.

132. Daniel V, Sarid S, Bar-Nun S, Litwack G (1983) Rat ligandin mRNA molecular cloning and sequencing. Arch Biochem Biophys 227:266–271.

133. Lai H-CJ, Li N-Q, Weiss MJ, Reddy CC, Tu C-PD (1984) The nucleotide sequence of a rat liver glutathione S-transferase subunit cDNA clone. J Biol Chem 259:5536–5542.

134. Pickett CB, Telakowski-Hopkins CA, Ding GJF, Aregenbright L, Lu AYH (1984) Rat liver glutathione S-transferases. Complete nucleotide sequence of a glutathione S-transferase mRNA and the regulation of the Y_a, Y_b and Y_c mRNAs by 3-methylcholanthrene and phenobarbital. J Biol Chem 259:5182–5188.

135. Taylor JB, Craig RK, Beale D, Ketterer B (1984) Construction and characterization of a plasmid containing complementary DNA to mRNA encoding the N-terminal amino acid sequence of the rat glutathione transferase Y_a subunit. Biochem J 219:223–231.

136. Tu CPD, Lai H-CJ, Li N-Q, Weiss MJ, Reddy CC (1984) The Y_c and Y_a subunits of rat liver glutathione S-transferases are the products of separate genes. J Biol Chem 259:9434–9439.

137. Telakowski-Hopkins CA, Rodkey JA, Bennett CD, Lu AYH, Pickett CB (1985) Rat liver glutathione S-transferases. Construction of a cDNA clone complementary to a Y_c mRNA and prediction of the complete amino acid sequence of a Y_c subunit. J Biol Chem 260:5820–5825.

138. Daniel V, Sharon R, Tichauer Y, Sarid S (1987) Mouse glutathione S-transferase Y_a subunit: gene structure and sequence. DNA 6:317–324.

139. Czonek H, Sarid S, Barker PE, Ruddle FH, Daniel V (1984) Glutathione S-transferase Ya subunit is coded by a multigene family located on a single mouse chromosome. Nucleic Acids Res 12:4825–4834.

140. Kingsley DM, Jenkins NA, Copeland NG (1989) A molecular genetic linkage map of mouse chromosome 9 with regional localizations for the Gsta, T3g, Ets-1, and Ldlr loci. Genetics 123:165–172.

141. Masanori K, Matsumura E, Webb G, Board PG, Figueroa F, Klein J (1990) Mapping of class alpha glutathione S-transferase 2 (Gst-2) genes to the vicinity of the d locus on mouse chromosome 9. Genomics 8:90–96.
142. Tu C-PD, Matsushima A, Li N-Q, Rhoads DM, Srikumar K, Reddy AP, Reddy CC (1986) Immunological and sequence interrelationships between multiple human liver and rat glutathione S-transferases. J Biol Chem 261:9540–9545.
143. Tu C-PD, Qian B (1986) Human liver glutathione S-transferases: Complete primary sequence of an H_a subunit cDNA. Biochem Biophys Res Commun 141:229–237.
144. Rothkopf GS, Telakowski-Hopkins CA, Stotish RL, Pickett CB (1986) Multiplicity of glutathione S-transferase genes in the rat and association with a type 2 Alu repetitive element. Biochemistry 25:993–1002.
145. Board PG, Webb GC (1987) Isolation of a cDNA clone and localization of human glutathione S-transferase 2 genes to chromosome band 6p12. Proc Natl Acad Sci USA 84:2377–2381.
146. Rhoads DM, Zarlengo RP, Tu C-PD (1987) The basic glutathione S-transferases from human livers are products of separate genes. Biochem Biophys Res Commun 145:474–481.
147. Hayes JD, Kerr LA, Cronshaw AD (1989) Evidence that glutathione S-transferases B1B1 and B2B2 are the products of separate genes and that their expression in human liver is subject to inter-individual variation. Molecular relationships between the B1 and B2 subunits and other alpha class glutathione S-transferases. Biochem J 264:437–445.
148. Rozen F, Nguyen T, Pickett CB (1992) Isolation and characterization of a human glutathione S-transferase Ha_1 subunit gene. Arch Biochem Biophys 292:589–593.
149. Suzuki T, Johnston PN, Board PG (1993) Structure and organization of the human alpha class glutathione S-transferase genes and related pseudogenes. Genomics 18:680–686.
150. Suzuki T, Smith S, Board PG (1994) Structure and function of the 5′-flanking sequences of the human alpha class glutathione S-transferase genes. Biochem. Biophys Res Commun 200:1665–1671.
151. Morel F, Schulz WA, Sies H (1994) Gene structure and regulation of expression of human glutathione S-transferases alpha. Biol Chem Hoppe Seyler 375:641–647.
152. Daniel V, Sharon R, Tichauer Y, Sarid S (1987) Mouse glutathione S-transferase Ya subunit: Gene structure and sequence. In G Fey, G Fuller, eds. In: Regulation of Liver Gene Expression Meeting. Cold Spring Harbor, NY: Cold Spring Harbor Laboratory Press, p 41.
153. Telakowski-Hopkins CA, Rothkopf GS, Pickett CB (1986) Structure analysis of a rat liver glutathione S-transferase Y_a gene. Proc Natl Acad Sci USA 83:9393–9397.
154. Daniel V, Tichauer Y, Sharon R (1988) 5′-flanking sequence of mouse glutathione S-transferase Y_a gene. Nucleic Acids Res 16:351.
155. Daniel V, Sharon R, Bensimon A (1989) Regulatory elements controlling the basal and drug-inducible expression of glutathione S-transferase Y_a subunit gene. DNA 8:399–408.
156. Telakowski-Hopkins CA, King RG, Pickett CB (1988) Glutathione S-transferase Y_a subunit gene: Identification of regulatory elements required for basal level and inducible expression. Proc Natl Acad Sci USA 85:1000–1004.
157. Lai HC-J, Qian B, Frove G, Tu C-PD (1988) Gene expression of rat glutathione S-transferases. Evidence for gene conversion in the evolution of the Y_b multigene family. J Biol Chem 263:11389–11395.
158. Seidegard J, Vorachek WR, Pero RW, Pearson WR (1988) Hereditary differences in the expression of the human glutathione transferase active on trans-stilbene oxide are due to a gene deletion. Proc Natl Acad Sci USA 85:7293–7297.
159. Morton MR, Bayney RM, Pickett CB (1990) Isolation and characterization of the rat glutathione S-transferase Y_{b1} subunit gene. Arch Biochem Biophys 277:56–60.
160. Taylor JB, Oliver J, Sherrington R, Pemble SE (1991) Structure of human glutathione S-transferase class Mu genes. Biochem J 274:587–593.
161. Ding GJ-F, Lu AYH, Pickett CB (1985) Rat liver glutathione S-transferases. Nucleotide sequence analysis of a Y_{b1} cDNA clone and prediction of the complete amino acid sequence of the Y_{b1} subunit. J Biol Chem 260:13268–13271.
162. Ding GJ-F, Ding VD-H, Rodkey JA, Bennett CD, Lu AYH, Pickett CB (1986) DNA sequence analysis of a Y_{b2} cDNA clone and regulation of the Y_{b1} and Y_{b2} mRNAs by phenobarbital. J Biol Chem 261:7952–7957.
163. Lai H-CJ, Grove G, Tu C-PD (1986) Cloning and sequence analysis of a cDNA for a rat liver glutathione S-transferase Y_b subunit. Nucleic Acids Res 14:6101–6114.
164. Lai H-CJ, Tu C-PD (1986) Rat glutathione S-transferases supergene family. Characterization of an anionic Y_b subunit cDNA clone. J Biol Chem 261:13793–13799.

165. Abramovitz M, Listowsky I (1987) Selective expression of a unique glutathione S-transferase Y_{b3} gene in rat brain. J Biol Chem 262:7770–7773.
166. Baltimore D (1981) Gene conversion: Some implications for immunoglobulin genes. Cell 24:592–594.
167. Board PG (1981) Biochemical genetics of glutathione S-transferase in man. Am J Hum Genet 33:36–43.
168. Seidegard J, Guthenberg C, Piro RW, Mannervik B (1987) The trans-stilbene oxide-active glutathione transferase in human mononuclear leukocytes is identical with the hepatic glutathione transferase μ. Biochem J 246:783–785.
169. Board PG, Suzuki T, Shaw DC (1988) Human muscle glutathione S-transferase (GST-4) shows close homology to human liver GST-1. Biochim Biophys Acta 953:214–217.
170. Seidegard J, Pero RW (1985) The hereditary transmission of high glutathione transferase activity towards trans-stilbene oxide in human mononuclear leukocytes. Hum Genet 69:66–68.
171. Seidegard J, Pero RW, Miller DG, Beattle EJ (1986) A glutathione transferase in human leukocytes as a marker for the susceptibility to lung cancer. Carcinogenesis 7:751–753.
172. Seidegard J, Pero RW, Markowitz MM, Roush G, Miller DG, Beattie EJ (1990) Isoenzyme(s) of glutathione transferase (class Mu) as a marker for the susceptibility to lung cancer: A follow up study. Carcinogenesis 11:33–36.
173. DeJong JL, Chang C-M, Whang-Peng J, Knutsen T, Tu C-PD (1988) The human liver glutathione S-transferase gene superfamily: Expression and chromosome mapping of an H_b subunit cDNA. Nucleic Acids Res 16:8541–8554.
174. Singh SV, Kurosky A, Awasthi YC (1987) Human liver glutathione S-transferase ψ. Chemical characterization and secondary-structure comparison with other mammalian glutathione S-transferases. Biochem J 243:61–67.
175. De Jong JL, Mohandas T, Tu C-PD (1991) The human H_b (mu) class glutathione S-ransferases are encoded by a dispersed gene family. Biochem Biophys Res Commun 180:15–22.
176. Vorachek WR, Pearson WR, Rule GS (1991) Cloning, expression and characterization of a class mu glutathione transferase from human muscle, the product of the GST 4 locus. Proc Natl Acad Sci USA 88:4443–4447.
177. Campbell E, Takahashi Y, Abramovitz M, Peretz M, Listowsky I (1990) A distinct human testis and brain class μ glutathione S-transferase: Molecular cloning and characterization of a form present even in individuals lacking hepatic type μ isoenzymes. J Biol Chem 265:9188–9193.
178. Ross VL, Board PG (1993) Molecular cloning and heterologous expression of an alternatively spliced human mu class glutathione S-transferase transcript. Biochem J 294:373–380.
179. Takahashi Y, Campbell EA, Hirata Y, Takayama T, Listowsky I (1993) A basis for differentiating among the multiple human mu-glutathione S-transferases and molecular cloning of brain GSTM5. J Biol Chem 268:8893–8898.
180. Suguoka Y, Kano T, Okuda A, Sakai M, Kitagawa T, Muramatsu M (1985) Cloning and the nucleotide sequence of rat glutathione S-transferase P cDNA. Nucleic Acids Res 13:6049–6057.
181. Pemble SE, Taylor JB, Ketterer B (1986) Tissue distribution of rat glutathione transferase subunit 7, a hepatoma marker. Biochem J 240:885–889.
182. Okuda A, Sakai M, Muramatsu M (1987) The structure of the rat glutathione S-transferase P gene and related pseudogenes. J Biol Chem 262:3858–3863.
183. Kano T, Sakai M, Muramatsu M (1987) Structure and expression of a human π glutathione S-transferase messenger RNA. Cancer Res 47:5626–5630.
184. Cowell LC, Dixon KH, Pemble SE, Ketterer B, Taylor JB (1988) The structure of the human glutathione S-transferase π gene. Biochem J 255:79–83.
185. Morrow CS, Cowan KH, Goldsmith ME (1989) Structure of the human genomic glutathione S-transferase π gene. Gene 75:3–11.
186. Dixon KH, Cowell IG, Xia CL, Pemble SE, Ketterer B, Taylor JB (1989) Control of expression of the human glutathione S-transferase π gene differs from its rat orthologue. Biochem Biophys Res Commun 163:815–822.
187. Morrow CS, Goldsmith ME, Cowan KH (1990) Regulation of human glutathione S-transferase π gene transcription: Influence of 5′-flanking sequences and trans-activating factors which recognize AP-1 binding sites. Gene 88:215–225.
188. De Jong JL, Morgenstern R, Jornvall H, De Pierre JW, Tu C-PD (1988) Gene expression of rat and human microsomal glutathione S-transferases. J Biol Chem 263:8430–8436.
189. De Jong JL, Mohandas T, Tu C-PD (1990) The gene for the microsomal glutathione S-transferase is on human chromosome 12. Genomics 6:379–382.

190. Sakai M, Okuda A, Muramatsu M (1988) Multiple regulatory elements and phorbol 12-O-tetradecanoate 13-acetate responsiveness of the rat placental glutathione transferase gene. Proc Natl Acad Sci USA 85:9456–9460.

191. Okuda A, Imagawa M, Maeda Y, Sakai M, Muramatsu M (1989) Structural and functional analysis of an enhancer GPEI having a phorbol-12-O-tetradecanoate 13-acetate responsive element-like sequence found in the rat glutathione transferase P gene. J Biol Chem 264:16919–16926.

192. Okuda A, Imagawa M, Sakai M, Muramatsu M (1990) Functional cooperativity between two TPA responsive elements in undifferentiated F9 embryonic stem cells. EMBO J 9:1131–1135.

193. Diccianni MB, Imagawa M, Muramatsu M (1992) The dyad palindromic glutathione transferase P enhancer binds multiple factors including AP-1. Nucleic Acids Res 20:5153–5158.

194. Oridate N, Nishi S, Imayama Y, Sakai M (1994) Jun and fos related gene products bind to and modulate the GPE-I, a strong enhancer element of the rat glutathione S-transferase P gene. Biochim Biophys Acta 1219:499–504.

195. Imagawa M, Osada S, Koyama Y, Suzuki T, Hirom PC, Diccianni MB, Morimura S, Muramatsu M (1991) SF-B that binds to a negative element in glutathione transferase P gene is similar or identical to trans-activator LAP/IL-6-DBP. Biochem Biophys Res Commun 179:293–300.

196. Muramatsu M, Okuda A, Imagawa M, Sakai M (1989) Regulation of glutathione transferase P gene during hepatocarcinogenesis of the rat. In: JD Hayes, CB Pickett, MY Mantle, eds. Glutathione S-Transferases and Drug Resistance. London: Taylor and Francis, p 165.

197. Xia CL, Cowell IG, Dixon KH, Pemble SE, Ketterer B, Taylor JB (1991) Glutathione transferase π its minimal promoter and downstream cis-acting element. Biochem Biophys Res Commun 176:233–240.

198. Norris JS, Schwartz DA, MacLeod SL, Fan WM, O'Brien TJ, Harris SE, Trifiletti R, Cornett LE, Cooper TE, Levi WM, Smith RG (1991) Cloning of a mu-class glutathione S-transferase complementary-DNA and characterization of its glucocorticoid inducibility in a smooth-muscle tumor-cell line. Mol Endocrinol 5:979–986.

199. Fan W, Trifiletti R, Cooper R, Norris JS (1992) Cloning of a μ-class glutathione S-transferase gene and identification of the glucocorticoid regulatory domains in its 5′ flanking sequence. Proc Natl Acad Sci USA 89:6104–6108.

200. Paulson EK, Darnell JE, Jr Rushmore TH, Pickett CB (1990) Analysis of the upstream elements of the xenobiotic compound-inducible and positionally regulated glutathione S-transferase Y_a gene. Mol Cell Biol 10:1841–1852.

201. Rushmore TH, King RG, Paulson EK, Pickett CB (1990) Regulation of glutathione S-transferase Y_a subunit gene expression: Identification of a unique xenobiotic-responsive element controlling inducible expression by planar aromatic compounds. Proc Natl Acad Sci USA 87:3826–3830.

202. Rushmore TH, Pickett CB (1990) Transcriptional regulation of the rat glutathione S-transferase Y_a subunit gene. Characterization of a xenobiotic-responsive element controlling inducible expression by phenolic antioxidants. J Biol Chem 265:14648–14653.

203. Whitlock JP, Jr (1987) The regulation of gene expression by 2,3,7,8-tetrachlorodibenzo-p-dioxin. Pharmacol Rev 39:147–161.

204. Denison MS, Fisher JM, Whitlock JP, Jr (1988) The DNA recognition sites for the dioxin-Ah receptor complex: Nucleotide sequence and functional analysis. J Biol Chem 263:17221–17224.

205. Denison MS, Fisher JM, Whitlock JP, Jr (1989) Protein-DNA interactions at recognition sites for the dioxin-Ah receptor complex. J Biol Chem 264:16478–16482.

206. Neuhold LA, Shirayoshi Y, Ozato K, Jones JE, Nebert DW (1989) Regulation of mouse Cyp 1a1 gene expression by dioxin: Requirement of two cis-acting elements during induction. Mol Cell Biol 9:2378–2386.

207. Pimental RA, Liang B, Yee GK, Wilhelmsson A, Poellinger L, Paulson KE (1993) Dioxin receptor and C/EBP regulate the function of the glutathione S-transferase Y_a gene xenobiotic response element. Mol Cell Biol 13:4365–4373.

208. Hapgood J, Cuthill S, Soderkvist A, Wilhelmsson I, Pongratz RH, Tukey RH, Johnson EF, Gustafsson J-A, Poellinger L (1991) Liver cells contain constitutive DNase I-hypersensitive sites at the xenobiotic response elements 1 and 2 (XRE1 and -2) of the rat cytochrome P-450IA1 gene and a constitutive, nuclear XRE-binding factor that is distinct from the dioxin receptor. Mol Cell Biol 11:4314–4323.

209. Paulson KE (1991) Xenobiotic regulation of glutathione S-transferase Y_a gene expression. Mol Toxicol 2:215–235.

210. Prochaska HJ, De Long MJ, Talalay P (1985) On the mechanism of induction of cancer protective enzymes: A unifying proposal. Proc Natl Acad Sci USA 82:8232–8236.

211. De Long MJ, Santamaria AB, Talalay P (1987) Role of cytochrome P_1-450 in the induction of NAD(P)H:quinone reductase in a murine hepatoma cell line and its mutants. Carcinogenesis 8:1549–1553.

212. Prochaska HJ, Talalay P (1988) Regulatory mechanisms of monofunctional and bifunctional anticarcinogenic enzyme inducers in murine liver. Cancer Res 48:4776–4782.

213. Talalay P, De Long MJ, Prochaska HJ (1988) Identification of a common chemical signal regulating the induction of enzymes that protect against chemical carcinogenesis. Proc Natl Acad Sci USA 85:8261–8265.

214. Rushmore TH, Morton MR, Pickett CB (1991) The antioxidant responsive element. Activation by oxidative stress and identification of the DNA consensus sequence required for functional activity. J Biol Chem 266:11632–11639.

215. Nguyen T, Pickett CB (1992) Regulation of rat glutathione S-transferase Y_a subunit gene expression: DNA-protein interaction at the antioxidant responsive element. J Biol Chem 267:13535–13539.

216. Friling RS, Bensimon A, Tichauer Y, Daniel V (1990) Xenobiotic-inducible expression of murine glutathione S-transferase Y_a subunit gene is controlled by an electrophile-responsive element. Proc Natl Acad Sci USA 87:6258–6262.

217. Friling RS, Bergelson S, Daniel V (1992) Two adjacent AP-1-like binding sites form the electrophile-responsive element of the murine glutathione S-transferase Y_a subunit gene. Proc Natl Acad Sci USA 89:668–672.

218. Rushmore TH, Pickett CB (1993) Glutathione S-transferases: Structure, regulation, and therapeutic implications. J Biol Chem 268:11475–11478.

219. Wang B, Williamson G (1994) Detection of a nuclear protein which binds specifically to the antioxidant responsive element (ARE) of the human NAD(P)H:quinone oxidoreductase gene. Biochim Biophys Acta 1219:645–652.

220. Riley RJ, Workman P (1992) DT-diaphorase and cancer chemotherapy. Biochem Pharmacol 43:1657–1669.

221. Favreau LV, Pickett CB (1991) Transcriptional regulation of the rat NAD(P)H:quinone reductase gene: Identification of regulatory elements controlling basal level expression and inducible expression by planar aromatic compounds and phenolic antioxidants. J Biol Chem 266:4556–4561.

222. Jaiswal AK (1991) Human NAD(P)H:quinone oxidoreductase (NQO_1) gene structure and induction by dioxin. Biochemistry 30:10647–10653.

223. Li Y, Jaiswal AK (1992) Regulation of human NAD(P)H:quinone oxidoreductase gene. Role of AP-1 binding site contained within human antioxidant response element. J Biol Chem 267:15097–15104.

224. Xie T, Belinsky M, Xu Y, Jaiswal AK (1995) ARE- and TRE-mediated regulation of gene expression. Response to xenobiotics and antioxidants. J Biol Chem 270:6894–6900.

225. Wattenberg LW (1985) Chemoprevention of cancer. Cancer Res 45:1–8.

226. Talalay P, De Long MJ, Prochaska HJ (1987) Molecular mechanisms in protection against carcinogenesis. In JG Cory, A Szentivanyi, eds. Cancer Biology and Therapeutics. New York: Plenum Press, p 197.

227. Kensler TW, Davidson NE, Groopman JD, Roebuck BD, Prochaska HJ, Talalay P (1993) Chemoprotection by inducers of electrophile detoxication enzymes. Basic Life Sci 61;127–136.

228. Pearson WR, Windle JJ, Morrow JF, Benson AM, Talalay P (1983) Increased synthesis of glutathione S-transferases in response to anticarcinogenic antioxidants. Cloning and measurement of messenger RNA. J Biol Chem 258:2052–2062.

229. Prochaska HJ, Santamaria AB, Talalay P (1992) Rapid detection of inducers of enzymes that protect against carcinogens. Proc Natl Acad Sci USA 89:2394–2398.

230. Zhang Y, Talalay P, Cho C-G, Posner GH (1992) A major inducer of anticarcinogenic protective enzymes from broccoli: Isolation and elucidation of structure. Proc Natl Acad Sci USA 89:2399–2403.

231. Zhang Y, Kensler TW, Cho CG, Posner Talalay P (1994) Anticarcinogenic activities of sulforaphane and structurally related synthetic norbornyl isothiocyanates. Proc Natl Acad Sci USA 91:3147–3150.

232. Zhang Y, Talalay P (1994) Anticarcinogenic activities of organic isothiocyanates: Chemistry and mechanisms. Cancer Res 54(Suppl):1976–1981S.

233. Posner GH, Cho CG, Green JV, Zhang Y, Talalay P (1994) Design and synthesis of bifunctional isothiocyanate analogs of sulforaphane: Correlation between structure and potency as inducers of anticarcinogenic detoxication enzymes. J Med Chem 37:170–176.

234. Egner PA, Kensler TW, Prestera T, Talalay P, Libby AH, Joyner HH, Curphey TJ (1994) Regulation of phase 2 enzyme induction by oltipraz and other dithiolethiones. Carcinogenesis 15:177–181.
235. Spencer SR, Xue L, Klenz EM, Talalay P (1991) The potency of inducers of NAD(P)H: (quinone acceptor) oxidoreductase parallels their efficiency as substrates for glutathione transferases. Structural and electronic correlations. Biochem J 273:711–717.
236. Nakabeppu Y, Ryder K, Nathans D (1988) DNA binding activities of three murine Jun proteins: Stimulation by fos. Cell 55:907–915.
237. Cohen DR, Ferreira PCP, Gentz R, Franza BR, Jr Curran T (1989) The product of a fos-related gene, fra-1, binds cooperatively to the AP-1 site with Jun: Transcription factor AP-1 is comprised of multiple protein complexes. Genes Dev 3:173–184.
238. Hirai S-I, Ryseck R-P, Mechta F, Bravo R, Yaniv M (1989) Characterization of jun-D: A new member of the jun proto-oncogene family. EMBO J 8:1433–1439.
239. Zerial M, Toschi L, Ryseck R-P, Schuermann M, Muller R, Bravo R (1989) The product of a novel growth factor activated gene, fos B, interacts with Jun proteins enhancing their DNA binding activity. EMBO J 8:805–813.
240. Matsui M, Tokuhara M, Konuma Y, Nomura N, Ishizaki R (1990) Isolation of human fos-related genes and their expression during monocyte-macrophage differentiation. Oncogene 5:249–255.
241. Chiu R, Angel P, Karin M (1989) Jun-B differs in its biological properties from, and is a negative regulator of, c-Jun. Cell 59:979–986.
242. Chiu R, Boyle W, Meek J, Smeal T, Hunter T, Karin M (1988) The c-Fos protein interacts with c-Jun/AP-1 to stimulate transcription of AP-1 responsive genes. Cell 54:541–552.
243. Halzonetis TD, Georgopoulos K, Greenberg M, Leder P (1988) c-Jun dimerizes with itself and with c-Fos forming complexes of different DNA binding affinities. Cell 55:917–924.
244. Kouzarides T, Ziff E (1988) The role of the leucine zipper in the fos-jun interaction. Nature 336:646–651.
245. Rauscher F III, Voulalas P, Franza BR, Jr Curran T (1988) Fos and Jun bind cooperatively to the AP-1 site: Reconstitution in vitro. Genes Dev 2:1687–1699.
246. Sassone-Corsi P, Ransone LJ, Lamph WW, Verma IM (1988) Direct interaction between fos and nuclear oncoproteins: Role of the "leucine zipper" domain. Nature 336:692–695.
247. Hirai S-I, Yaniv M (1989) Jun DNA-binding is modulated by mutations between the leucines or by direct interaction of Fos with the TGACTCA sequence. New Biol 1(2):181–191.
248. Ryseck R-P, Hirai SI, Yaniv M, Bravo R (1988) Transcriptional activation of c-jun during the G_0/G_1 transistion in mouse fibroblasts. Nature 334:535–537.
249. Quantin R, Breathnach R (1988) Epidermal growth factor stimulates transcription of the c-jun proto-oncogene in rat fibroblasts. Nature 334:538–539.
250. Greenberg ME, Ziff EB, Greene LA (1986) Stimulation of neuronal acetylcholine receptors induces rapid gene transcription. Science 234:80–83.
251. Sonnenberg JL, Macgregor-Leon PF, Curran T, Morgan JI (1989) Dynamic alterations occur in the levels and composition of transcription factor AP-1 complexes after seizure. Neuron 3:359–365.
252. Bravo R, Burckhardt J, Curran T, Muller R (1985) Stimulation and inhibition of growth by EGF in different A431 cell clones is accompanied by the rapid induction of c-fos and c-myc proto-oncogenes. EMBO J 4:1193–1197.
253. Curran T, Morgan JI (1986) Barium modulates c-fos expression and posttranslational modification. Proc Natl Acad Sci USA 83:8521–8525.
254. Morgan JI, Curran T (1986) Role of ion flux in the control of c-fos expression. Nature 322:552–555.
255. Shibanuma M, Kuroki T, Nose K (1987) Inhibition of proto-oncogene c-fos transcription by inhibitors of protein kinase C and ion transport. Eur J Biochem 164:15–19.
256. Imler JL, Schatz C, Wasylyk C, Chatton B, Wasylyk B (1988) A Harvey-ras responsive transcription element is also responsive to a tumor-promoter and to serum. Nature 332:275–278.
257. Piette J, Hirai SI, Yaniv M (1988) Constitutive synthesis of activator protein-1 transcription factor after viral transformation of mouse fibroblasts. Proc Natl Acad Sci USA 85:3401–3405.
258. Schonthal A, Herrlich P, Rahmsdorf HJ, Ponta H (1988) Requirement for fos gene expression in the transcriptional activation of collagenase by other oncogenes and phorbol esters. Cell 54:325–334.
259. Wasylyk C, Imler JL, Wasylyk B (1988) Transforming but not immortalizing oncogenes activate the transcription factor PEA1. EMBO J 7:2475–2483.
260. Pinkus R, Bergelson S, Daniel V (1993) Phenobarbital induction of AP-1 binding activity mediates

activation of glutathione S-transferase and quinone reductase gene expression. Biochem J 290:637–640.

261. Puga A, Nebert DW, Carrier F (1992) Dioxin induces expression of c-fos and c-jun proto-oncogenes and a large increase in transcription factor AP-1. DNA Cell Biol 11:269–281.

262. Daniel V, Bergelson S, Pinkus R (1993) The role of AP-1 transcription factor in the regulation of glutathione S-transferase Y_a subunit gene expression by chemical agents. In KD Tew, CB Pickett, TJ Mantle, B Mannervik, J Hayes, eds. Structure and Function of Glutathione S-Transferases. Boca Raton, FL: CRC Press, pp 129–136.

263. Vogel K, Bentley P, Platt K-L, Oesch F (1980) Rat liver cytoplasmic dihydrodiol dehydrogenase: Purification to apparent homogeneity and properties. J Biol Chem 255:9621–9625.

264. Penning TM, Mukharji I, Barrows S, Talalay P (1984) Purification and properties of 3α-hydroxysteroid dehydrogenase of rat liver cytosol and its inhibition by anti-inflammatory drugs. Biochem J 222:601–611.

265. Poland A, Knutson JC (1982) 2,3,7,8-Tetrachlorodibenzo-p-dioxin and related halogenated aromatic hydrocarbons: Examination of the mechanism of toxicity. Annu Rev Pharmacol Toxicol 22:517–554.

266. Li GC (1983) Induction of thermotolerance and enhanced heat shock protein synthesis in Chinese hamster fibroblasts by sodium arsenite and by ethanol. J Cell Physiol 115:116–122.

267. Kim Y-J, Shuman J, Sette M, Przybyla A (1983) Arsenate induces stress proteins in cultured rat myoblasts. J Cell Biol 96:393–400.

268. Bortelero F, Pozzi G, Sabbioni E, Saffiotti U (1987) Cellular uptake and metabolic reduction of pentavalent to trivalent arsenic as determinants of cytotoxicity and morphological transformation. Carcinogenesis 8:803–808.

269. Goldstein BD, Rozen MG, Quintavalla JC, Amoruso MA (1979) Decrease in mouse lung and liver glutathione peroxidase activity and potentiation of the lethal effects of ozone and paraquat by the superoxide dismutase inhibitor diethyldithiocarbamate. Biochem Pharmacol 28:27–30.

270. Solanki V, Rana RS, Slaga TJ (1982) Diminution of mouse epidermal superoxide dismutase and catalase activities by tumor promoters. Carcinogenesis 2:1141–1146.

271. Packard BS, Saxton MJ, Bissell MJ, Klein MP (1984) Plasma membranes reorganization induced by tumor promoters in an epithelial cell line. Proc Natl Acad Sci USA 81:449–453.

272. Cerutti PA (1985) Prooxidant states and tumor promotion. Science 227:375–381.

273. Clark JD, Lin L-L, Kriz RW, Ramesha CS, Sultzman LA, Lin AY, Milona N, Knopf JL (1991) A novel arachidonic acid-selective cytosolic PLA_2 contains a Ca^{++}-dependent translocation domain with homology to PKC and GAP. Cell 65:1043–1051.

274. Sharp JD, White DL, Chiou XG, Goodson T, Gambra GC, McClure D, Burgett Haskins J, Skatruid PL, Sportsman JR, Beeker GW, King LH, Roberts EF, Kramer RM (1991) Molecular cloning and expression of human Ca^{++}-sensitive cytosolic phospholipase A_2. J Biol Chem 266:14850–14853.

275. Piper PJ (1984) Formation and actions of leukotrienes. Physiol Rev 64:744–761.

276. Ford-Hutchinson AW (1990) Leukotriene B_4 in inflammation. Crit Rev Immunol 10:1–12.

277. Nicholson DW, Ali A, Klemba NW, Munday NA, Zamboni RJ, Ford-Hutchinson AW (1992) Human leukotriene C_4 synthase expression in dimethyl sulfoxide-differentiated U937 cells. J Biol Chem 267:17849–17857.

278. Nicholson DW, Klemba NW, Rasper DM, Metters KM, Zamboni RJ, Ford-Hutchinson AW (1992) Purification of human leukotriene C_4 synthase from dimethyl sulfoxide-differentiated U937 cells. Eur J Biochem 209:725–734.

279. Frey EA, Nicholson DW, Metters KM (1993) Characterization of the leukotriene D_4 receptor in dimethyl sulphoxide-differentiated U937 cells: Comparison with the leukotriene D_4 receptor in human lung and guinea pig lung. Eur J Pharmacol 244:239–250.

280. Ford-Hutchinson AW (1992) In PJ Barnes, ed. New Drugs for Asthma, Vol. 2 London: IBC Technical Services, pp 94–102.

281. Kouitert L, Barnes NC (1992) In PJ Barnes, ed. New Drugs for Asthma, Vol. 2. London: IBC Technical Services, pp 78–93.

282. Farber E (1984) The biochemistry of preneoplastic liver: A common metabolic pattern in hepatocyte nodules. Can J Biochem Cell Biol 62:486–494.

283. Buchmann A, Kuhlmann W, Schwarz M, Kunz W, Wolf CR, Moll E, Friedberg T, Oesch F (1985) Regulation and expression of four cytochrome P-450 isoenzymes, NADPH-cytochrome P-450 reductase, the glutathione transferases B and C and microsomal epoxide hydrolase in preneoplastic and neoplastic lesions in rat liver. Carcinogenesis 6:513–521.

284. Jensson H, Eriksson LC, Mannervik B (1985) Selective expression of glutathione transferase isoenzymes in chemically induced preneoplastic rat hepatocyte nodules. FEBS Lett 187:115–120.
285. Satoh K, Kitahara A, Soma Y, Inaba Y, Hatayama I, Sato K (1985) Purification, induction, and distribution of placental glutathione transferase: A new marker enzyme for preneoplastic cells in the rat chemical hepatocarcinogenesis. Proc Natl Acad Sci USA 82:3964–3968.
286. Sato K, Satoh K, Hatayama I, Tsuchida S, Soma Y, Shiratori Y, Tateoka N, Inaba Y, Kitahara A (1987) Placental glutathione S-transferase as a marker for (pre)neoplastic tissues. In TJ Mantle, CB Pickett, JD Hayes, eds. Glutathione S-Transferases and Carcinogenesis. London: Taylor and Francis, pp 127–137.
287. Sato K (1988) Glutathione S-transferases and hepatocarcinogenesis. Jpn J Cancer Res 79:556–572.
288. Di Ilio C, Del Boccio G, Aceto A, Federici G (1987) Alteration of glutathione transferase isoenzyme concentrations in human renal carcinoma. Carcinogenesis 8:861–864.
289. Mannervik B, Castro VM, Danielson UH, Kalim TM, Hansson J, Ringborg U (1987) Expression of class Pi glutathione transferase in human malignant melanoma cells. Carcinogenesis 8:1929–1932.
290. Peters WHM, Nagengast FM, Wobbes T (1989) Glutathione S-transferases in normal and cancerous human colon. Carcinogenesis 10:2371–2374.
291. Howie AF, Forrester LM, Glancey MJ, Schlager JJ, Powis G, Beckett GH, Hayes JD, Wolf CR (1990) Glutathione S-transferase and glutathione peroxidase activity in normal and tumour human tissues. Carcinogenesis 11:451–458.
292. Clapper ML, Hoffman SJ, Tew KD (1991) Glutathione S-transferases in normal and malignant human colon tissue. Biochim Biophys Acta 1096:209–216.
293. Adams DJ, Carmichael H, Wolf CR (1986) Glutathione and glutathione transferase levels in response to cytotoxins. Cancer Res 45:1669–1673.
294. Carmichael J, Adams DJ, Ansell J, Wolf CR (1986) Glutathione and glutathione levels in mouse granulocytes following cyclophosphamide administration. Cancer Res 46:735–739.
295. Lee W-H, Morton RA, Epstein JI, Brooks JD, Campbell PA, Bova GS, Hsieh W-S, Isaacs WB, Nelson WG (1994) Cytidine methylation of regulatory sequences near the π-class glutathione S-transferase gene accompanies human prostatic carcinogenesis. Proc Natl Acad Sci USA 91:11733–11777.
296. Castro VM, Soderstrom M, Carlbeg I, Widersten M, Platz A, Mannervik B (1990) Differences among human tumor cell lines in the expression of glutathione transferases and other glutathione-linked enzymes. Carcinogenesis 11:1569–1576.
297. Tew KD, Clapper ML, Greenberg RE, Weese TL, Hoffman SJ, Smith TM (1987) Glutathione S-transferases in human prostate. Biochim Biophys Acta 926:8–15.
298. Peters WHN, Roelofs HMJ (1989) Time-dependent activity and expression of glutathione S-transferases in the human colon adenocarcinoma cell line Caco-2. Biochem J 264:613–616.
299. Awasthi YC, Singh SV, Ahmad H, Moller PC, Gupta V (1988) Expression of glutathione S-transferase isoenzymes in human cell lung cancer cell lines. Carcinogenesis 9:89–93.
300. Schisselbauer JC, Silber R, Papadopoulos E, Abrams K, LaCreta FP, Tew KD (1990) Characterization of glutathione S-transferase expression in lymphocytes from chronic lymphocytic leukemia patients. Cancer Res 50:3562–3568.
301. Lewis AD, Hickson ID, Robson CN, Harris AL, Hayes JD, Griffiths SA, Manson MM, Hall AE, Moss JE, Wolf CR (1988) Amplification and increased expression of alpha class glutathione S-transferase-encoding genes associated with resistance to nitrogen mustards. Proc Natl Acad Sci USA 85:8511–8515.
302. Wang AL, Tew KD (1985) Increased glutathione S-transferase activity in a cell line with acquired resistance to nitrogen mustards. Cancer Treat Rep 69:677–682.
303. Batist G, Tulpule A, Sinha BK, Katki AG, Myers CE, Cowan KH (1986) Overexpression of a novel anionic glutathione transferase in multidrug-resistant human breast cancer cells. J Biol Chem 261:15544–15549.
304. Cowan KH, Batist G, Tulpule A, Sinha BK, Myers CE (1986) Similar biochemical changes associated with multidrug resistance in human breast cancer cells and carcinogen-induced resistance to xenobiotics in rats. Proc Natl Acad Sci USA 83:9328–9332.
305. Buller AM, Clapper ML, Tew KD (1987) Glutathione S-transferases in nitrogen mustard-resistant and -sensitive cell lines. Mol Pharmacol 31:575–578.
306. Evans CG, Bodell WJ, Tokuda K, Doane-Setzer P, Smith MT (1987) Glutathione and related enzymes in rat brain tumor cell resistance to 1,3-bis(2-chloroethyl)-1-nitrosourea and nitrogen mustard. Cancer Res 47:2525–2530.
307. Dahllof B, Martinsson T, Mannervik B, Jensson H, Levan G (1987) Characterization of multidrug

resistance in SEWA mouse tumor cells. Increased glutathione transferase activity and reversal of resistance with verapamil. Anticancer Res 7:65–70.

308. Robson CN, Lewis AD, Wolf CR, Hayes JD, Hall A, Proctor SJ, Harris AL, Hickson ID (1987) Reduced levels of drug-induced DNA cross-linking in nitrogen mustard-resistant Chinese hamster ovary cells expressing elevated glutathione S-transferase activity. Cancer Res 47:6022–6027.

309. Gupta V, Singh SV, Ahmad H, Medh RD, Awasthi YC (1989) Glutathione and glutathione S-transferases in a human plasma cell line resistant to melphalan. Biochem Pharmacol 38:1993–2000.

310. Saburi Y, Nakagawa M, Ono M, Sakai M, Muramatsu M, Kohno K, Kuwano M (1989) Increased expression of glutathione S-transferase gene in cis-diamminedichloro platinum (II)-resistant variants of a Chinese hamster. Cancer Res 49:7020–7025.

311. Schisselbauer JC, Crescimanno M, D'Alessandro N, Clapper M, Tapiero H, Tew KD (1989) Glutathione, glutathione S-transferases, and related redox enzymes in Adriamycin resistant cell lines with a multidrug resistant phenotype. Cancer Commun 1:133–139.

312. Whelan RDH, Hosking LK, Townsend AJ, Cowan KH, Hill BT (1989) Differential increases in glutathione S-transferase activities in a range of multidrug-resistant human tumor cell lines. Cancer Commun 1:359–365.

313. Wolf CR, Wareing CJ, Black SM, Hayes JD (1989) Glutathione S-transferases in resistance to chemotherapeutic drugs. In JD Hayes, CB Pickett, TJ Mantle, eds. Glutathione S-Transferases and Drug Resistance. London: Taylor and Francis, pp 295–307.

314. Clapper ML, Tew KD (1989) Identification of a glutathione S-transferase associated with microsomes of tumor cells resistant to nitrogen mustards. Biochem Pharmacol 35:1915–1921.

315. Clapper ML, Kuzmich S, Seestaller LM, Tew KD (1993) Time course of glutathione S-transferase elevation in Walker mammary carcinoma cells following chlorambucil exposure. Biochem Pharmacol 45:683–690.

316. Hall AG, Matheson E, Hickson ID, Foster SA, Hogarth L (1994) Purification of an α class glutathione S-transferase from melphalan-resistant Chinese hamster ovary cells and demonstration of its ability to catalyze melphalan-glutathione adduct formation. Cancer Res 54:3369–3372.

317. Berhane K, Hao X-Y, Egyhazi S, Hansson J, Ringborg U, Mannervik B (1993) Contribution of glutathione transferase M3-3 to 1,3-bis (2-chloroethyl)-1-nitrosourea resistance in a human non-small cell lung cancer cell line. Cancer Res 53:4257–4261.

318. Mimnaugh EG, Dusre L, Atwell J, Myers CE (1989) Differential oxygen radical susceptibility of Adriamycin-sensitive and -resistant MCF-7 human breast tumor cells. Cancer Res 49:8–15.

319. Burt RK, Garfield S, Johnson K, Thorgeirsson SS (1988) Transformation of rat liver epithelial cells with v-H-ras or v-raf causes expression of MDR-1, glutathione S-transferase-P and increased resistance to cytotoxic chemicals. Carcinogenesis 9:2329–2332.

320. Tew KD (1994) Glutathione-associated enzymes in anticancer drug resistance. Cancer Res 54:4313–4320.

321. Lewis AD, Hayes JD, Wolf CR (1988) Glutathione and glutathione-dependent enzymes in ovarian adenocarcinoma cell lines derived from a patient before and after the onset of drug resistance: Intrinsic differences and cell cycle effects. Carcinogenesis 9:1283–1288.

322. Moscow JA, Townsend AJ, Cowan KH (1989) Elevation of π class glutathione S-transferase activity in human breast cancer cells by transfection of the GST π gene and its effect on sensitivity to toxins. Mol Pharmacol 36:22–28.

323. Black SM, Beggs JD, Hayes JD, Bartoszek A, Muramatsu M, Sakai M, Wolf CR (1990) Expression of human glutathione S-transferases in Saccharomyces cerevisiae confers resistance to the anticancer drugs Adriamycin and chlorambucil. Biochem J 268:309–315.

324. Fairchild CR, Moscow JA, O'Brien EE, Cowan KH (1990) Multidrug resistance in cells transfected with human genes encoding a variant P-glycoprotein and glutathione S-transferase-π. Mol Pharmacol 37:801–809.

325. Miyazaki M, Kohno K, Saburi Y, Matsuo K-I, One M, Kuwano M, Tsuchida S, Sato K, Sakai M, Muramatsu M (1990) Drug resistance to cis-diamminedichloroplatinum (II) in Chinese hamster ovary cell lines transfected with glutathione S-transferase pi gene. Biochem Biophys Res Commun 166:1358–1364.

326. Nakagawa K, Saijo N, Tsuchida S, Sakai M, Tsunokawa Y, Yokota J, Muramatsu M, Sato K, Terada M, Tew KD (1990) Glutathione S-transferase π as a determinant of drug resistance in transfectant cell lines. J Biol Chem 265:4296–4301.

327. Schecter RL, Aloui-Jamali MA, Woo A, Fahl WE, Batist G (1993) Expression of rat glutathione S-transferase complementary DNA in rat mammary carcinoma cells: Impact upon alkylator-induced toxicity. Cancer Res 53:4900–4906.

328. Greenbaum M, Letourneau S, Assar H, Schecter RL, Batist G, Cournoyer D (1994) Retrovirus-mediated gene transfer of rat glutathione S-transferase Y_c confers alkylating drug resistance in NIH 3T3 mouse fibroblasts. Cancer Res 54:4442–4447.

329. Nakagawa K, Saijo N, Tsuchida S, Sakai M, Tsunokawa Y, Yokota J, Muramatsu M, Sato K, Terada M, Tew KD (1990) Glutathione S-transferase π as a determinant of drug resistance in transfectant cell lines. J Biol Chem 265:4296–4301.

330. Fairchild CR, Moscow JA, O'Brien EE, Cowan KH (1990) Multidrug resistance in cells transfected with human genes encoding a variant P-glycoprotein and glutathione S-transferase-π. Mol Pharmacol 37:801–809.

331. Puchalski RB, Fahl WE (1990) Expression of recombinant glutathione S-transferase π, Y_a, or Y_{b1} confers resistance to alkylating agents. Proc Natl Acad Sci USA 87:2443–2447.

332. Giaccia AJ, Lewis AD, Denko NC, Cholon A, Evans JW, Waldren CA, Stamato TD, Brown JM (1991) The hypersensitivity of the Chinese hamster ovary variant BL-10 to bleomycin killing is due to a lack of glutathione S-transferase α activity. Cancer Res 51:4463–4469.

333. Smith MT, Evans CG, Doane-Setzer P, Castro VM, Kalim Tahir M, Mannervik B (1989) Denitrosation of 1,3-bis (2-chloroethyl)-1-nitrosourea by class mu glutathione transferases and its role in cellular resistance in rat brain tumor cells. Cancer Res 49:2621–2625.

334. Jensen DE, Mackay RL (1990) Rat, mouse, and hamster isozyme specificity in the glutathione transferase-mediated denitrosation of nitrosoguanidinium compounds. Cancer Res 50:1440–1448.

335. Dedon PC, Borch RF (1964) Characterization of the reactions of platinum antitumor agents with biologic and nonbiologic sulfur-containing nucleophiles. Biochem Pharmacol 36:1955–1964.

336. Hamilton TC, Winker MA, Louis KG, Batist G, Behrens BC, Tsuruo T, Grotzinger KR, McKoy WM, Young RC, Ozols RF (1985) Augmentation of Adriamycin, melphalan, and cisplatin cytotoxicity in drug-resistant and -sensitive human ovarian carcinoma cell lines by buthionine sulfoximine mediated glutathione depletion. Biochem Pharmacol 34:2583–2586.

337. Ciaccio PJ, Tew KD, LaCreta FP (1990) The spontaneous and glutathione S-transferase-mediated reaction of chlorambucil with glutathione. Cancer Commun 2:279–286.

338. Ciaccio PJ, Tew KD, LaCreta FP (1991) Enzymatic conjugation of chlorambucil with glutathione by human glutathione S-transferase enzymes and inhibition by ethacrynic acid. Biochem Pharmacol 42:1504–1507.

339. Bolton MG, Colvin OM, Hilton J (1991) Specificity of isozymes of murine hepatic glutathione S-transferase for the conjugation of glutathione with L-phenylalanine mustard. Cancer Res 51:2410–2415.

340. Dulik DM, Fenselau C, Hilton J (1986) Characterization of melphalan-glutathione adducts whose formation is catalyzed by glutathione transferases. Biochem Pharmacol 35:3405–3409.

341. Dirven HAAM, Dictus ELJT, Broeders NLHL, van Ommen B, van Bladeren PJ (1995) The role of human glutathione S-transferase isoenzymes in the formation of glutathione conjugates of the alkylating cytostatic drug thiotepa. Cancer Res 55:1701–1706.

342. Berhane K, Mannervik B (1989) Inactivation of the genotoxic aldehyde acrolein by human glutathione transferases of classes alpha, mu, and pi. Mol Pharmacol 37:251–254.

343. Yvan Z-M, Smith PB, Brundrett RB, Colvin M, Fenselau C (1991) Glutathione conjugation with phosphoramide mustard and cyclophosphamide. Drug Metab Dispos 19:625–629.

344. Pallante SL, Lisek CA, Dulik DM, Fenselau C (1986) Glutathione conjugate. Immobilized enzyme synthesis and characterization by fast atom bombardment mass spectrometry. Drug Metab Dispos 14:313–318.

345. Ploemen JHTM, Van Ommen B, Van Bladeren PJ (1990) Inhibition of rat and human glutathione S-transferase isoenzymes by ethacrynic acid and its glutathione conjugate. Biochem Pharmacol 40:1631–1635.

346. Phillips MF, Mantle TJ (1991) The initial-rate kinetics of mouse glutathione S-transferase $Y_f Y_f$. Evidence for an allosteric site for ethacrynic acid. Biochem J 275:703–709.

347. Tew KD, Bomber AM, Hoffman SJ (1988) Ethacrynic acid and piriprost as enhancers of cytotoxicity in drug resistant and sensitive cell lines. Cancer Res 48:3622–3625.

348. Hansson J, Berhane K, Castro VM, Jungnelius U, Mannervik B, Ringborg U (1991) Sensitization of human melanoma cells to the cytotoxic effect of melphalan by the glutathione transferase inhibitor ethacrynic acid. Cancer Res 51:94–98.

349. O'Dwyer PJ, LaCreta F, Nash S, Tinsley PW, Schilder R, Clapper ML, Tew KD, Panting L, Litwin S, Comis RL, Ozols RF (1991) Phase I study of thio-TEPA in combination with the glutathione transferase inhibitor ethacrynic acid. Cancer Res 51:6059–6065.

350. LaCreta FP, Brennan JM (1991) Effects of ethacrynic acid and SKF525A on hepatic thio-TEPA elimination. Proc Am Assoc Cancer Res 32:339.
351. Petrini M, Conte A, Caraccioli F, Sabatini A, Grassi B, Ronca G (1993) Reversing of chlorambucil resistance by ethacrynic acid in a B-CLL patient. Br J Hematol 85:409–410.
352. Kuzmich S, Vanderveer LA, Walsh ES, LaCreta FP, Tew KD (1992) Increased levels of glutathione S-transferase π transcript as a mechanism of resistance to ethacrynic acid. Biochem J 281:219–224.
353. Shen H, Ranganathan S, Kuzmich S, Tew KD (1995) The influence of ethacrynic acid on glutathione S-transferase π transcript and protein half-lives in human colon cancer cells. Biochem Pharmacol 50:1233–1238.
354. Ranganathan S, Kuzmich S, Walsh E, Tew KD (1992) Determination of mRNA and protein half-lives of glutathione S-transferase π (GST π) in ethacrynic acid (EA) sensitive and resistant colon carcinoma cell lines. Proc Am Assoc Cancer Res 33:2963.
355. Ranganathan S, Ciaccio PJ, Tew KD (1993) Principles of drug modulation applied to glutathione S-transferases. In KD Tew, CB Pickett, TJ Mantle, B Mannervik, JD Hayes, eds. Structure and Function of Glutathione Transferases. Boca Raton, FL: CRC Press, pp 249–256.
356. Ciaccio PJ, Stuart JE, Tew KD (1993) Overproduction of a 37.5 kD cytosolic protein structurally related to prostaglandin F synthase in ethacrynic acid resistant human colon cells. Mol Pharmacol 43:845–853.
357. Ciaccio PJ, Jaiswal AK, Tew KD (1994) Regulation of human dihydrodiol dehydrogenase by Michael acceptor xenobiotics. J Biol Chem 269:15558–15562.
358. Flatgaard JE, Bauer KE, Kauvar LM (1993) Isozyme specificity of novel glutathione S-transferase inhibitors. Cancer Chemother Pharmacol 33:63–70.
359. Lyttle MH, Hocker MD, Hui HC, Cladwell CG, Aaron DT, Engqvist-Goldstein A, Flatgaard JE, Bauer K (1994) Isozyme-specific glutathione S-transferase inhibitors: Design and synthesis. J Med Chem 37:189–194.
360. Lyttle MH, Satyam A, Hocker MD, Bauer KE, Cladwell CG, Hui HC, Morgan AS, Mergia A, Kauvar LM (1994) Glutathione S-transferase activates novel alkylating agents. J Med Chem 37:1501–1507.
361. Morgan AS, Ciaccio PJ, Tew KD, Kauvar LM (1996) Isozyme specific glutathione S-transferase inhibitors potentiate drug sensitivity in cultured human tumor cell lines. Cancer Chemother Pharmacol 37:363–370.
362. Ciaccio PJ, Shen H, Jaiswal AK, Lyttle MH, Tew KD (1996) Modulation of detoxification gene expression in human colon HT-29 cells by glutathione S-transferase inhibitors. Mol Pharmacol 48:639–647.
363. Ciaccio PJ, Tew KD (1993) Glutathione S-transferases. In BA Teicher, ed. Drug Resistance in Oncology. Marcel Dekker, Inc., New York, NY, pp 351–374.

5. ROLE OF DNA REPAIR IN RESISTANCE TO DRUGS THAT ALKYLATE O⁶ OF GUANINE

OMER N. KOÇ, WELDON P. PHILLIPS, JR., KEUNMYOUNG LEE, LILI LIU, NASIR H. ZAIDI, JAMES A. ALLAY, AND STANTON L. GERSON

This review focuses on DNA repair as a mechanism of resistance to chemotherapeutic agents that attack at the O^6 position of guanine. This class of agents includes the methylating agents, temozolomide, procarbazine, dacarbazine (DTIC), and steptozotocin, and the chloroethylating agents, carmustine (1,3 bis-chloroethyl 2-nitrosourea, BCNU), lomustine (3-cyclohexyl-1-chloroethyl-nitrosourea, CCNU), (2-chloroethyl)-3-sarcosinamide-1-nitrosourea (SarCNU), and agents used in other countries, including clomosome and 1-(4-amino-2-methyl-5-pyrimidinyl)methyl-3-(2-chlorethyl)-3-nitrosourea (ACNU). Both groups of agents attack at the same site, but their mechanism of cytotoxicity appears to differ. For instance, methylating agents form numerous methyl–DNA adducts, including O^6-methylguanine (O^6-mG). In cells with persistent O^6–mG adducts, over 6,000 lesions are required to induce cell death [1]. In contrast, chloroethylating agents lead to the formation of DNA-interstrand crosslinks, only a few of which are required for cytotoxicity [2].

MISMATCH REPAIR–MEDIATED CYTOTOXICITY DUE TO METHYLATING AGENTS

The formation of O^6mG DNA adducts by methylating agents is not directly cytotoxic. Rather, the presence of O^6mG in DNA appears to initiate a DNA repair process that can result in cytotoxicity. During DNA synthesis, O^6mG adducts are preferentially paired with thymine (T), forming O^6mG:T. Both O^6mG:C and O^6mG:T base pairs have recently been shown to elicit unscheduled long-patch DNA synthesis in the strand of DNA opposite O^6mG. Karran et al. termed this activity *repair synthesis* when the base pair was $O^6mG:C$. In contrast, the $O^6mG:T$ base pairs are recognized by the mismatch repair machinery [3,4]. In the absence of direct repair of O^6mG by O^6-alkylguanine DNA alkyltransferase (AGT) (see later), both "repair synthesis" and the mismatch repair activities appear to be targeted to the strand opposite to O^6mG [5–7].

It is worth noting that O^6mG is a highly mutagenic adduct, inducing predominantly G to A transitions, and repair of O^6mG by alkyltransferase (see later) decreases methylating agent mutagenicity [8]. However, O^6mG's propensity to cause mutations is probably not a critical component of methylating agent cytotoxicity, as highly mutagenic alkylation-tolerant cell lines have been identified [9–11]. In some cell lines, this highly resistant phenotype is now recognized to be due to defects in the mismatch repair machinery [12,13]. In fact, microsatellite instability, seen in a large percentage of tumors from several human cancer types, has recently been associated with mismatch repair defects [14–17].

Current evidence suggests that methylating agent–induced cell death involves an aborted effort at mismatch repair. In many cells, low levels of methylation at the O^6 position of guanine are repaired by the DNA repair protein, O^6-alkylguanine-DNA alkyltransferase (AGT) [18] and, as noted later, there is no sequel to the single-step repair process. However, persistent O^6mG DNA adducts in cells lacking alkyltransferase become the sites of a DNA repair process that is ultimately cytotoxic (Figure 5–1). Paully et al. [19], in bacterial systems, and Karran et al. [4], in mammalian systems, have shown that the replicative DNA polymerase machinery pauses at O^6mG and preferentially inserts a thymine (T) at the site [20,21]. Using a plasmid replication assay, in which a plasmid containing a single O^6mG is transfected into E. coli, Paully et al. [19] found that polymerase pauses sufficiently long to result in preferential synthesis of the complimentary strand not containing O^6mG. Nonetheless, replication continues on both strands, and mutations arising at sites of $O^6mG:C$ are predominantly G to A [20,21], indicating that replication produces a $O^6mG:T$ mismatch.

The $O^6mG:T$ base pair is recognized by the mismatch repair (MMR) system [4]. In human cells, the MMR complex consists of at least five proteins involved in the recognition and repair of mismatch lesions: hMLH1, hMSH2, hPMS1, hPMS2, and GT binding protein (GTBP) [22–24], all of which appear to be homologues of E. coli and yeast MMR proteins. In E. coli, mismatch repair is initiated in the postreplication state by MutS binding the mismatch (a function of MSH2 and GTBP in human cells) and is coupled to a GATC site within the DNA by MutL (human homologue, hMLH1). Incision is directed towards the newly synthesized strand (the strand with the unmethylated A) within GATC by MutH endonuclease, which acts in an ATP-dependent manner [25,26]. How mammalian cell MMR proteins recognize the newly synthesized stand or the transcribed strand is an area of active investigation. Following binding recognition, an endonuclease removes a patch containing both the GATC region and the mismatch, DNA polymerase δ or ϵ fills in the patch, and DNA ligase closes the strand break [26,27]. Curiously, in contrast to other mismatch lesions introduced by errors in replication, the $O^6mG:T$

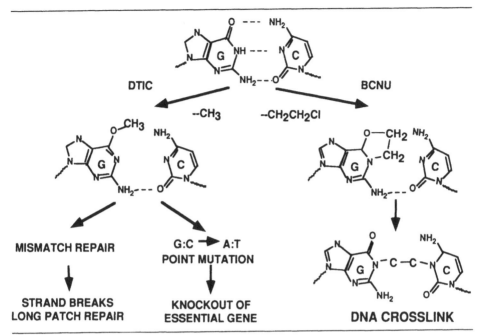

Figure 5–1. Methyl and chloroethyl alkylation of the O⁶ of guanine by nitrosoureas, triazines, and tetrazines. Representative reactions for methylating agents, such as dacarbazine (DTIC), and chloroethylating agents, such as carmustine (BCNU), are shown. The subsequent cytotoxic lesions are thought to involve the crosslink derived from the chloroethylating agents and aberrant repair of the methyl adduct produced by the methylating agents.

mismatch is not successfully repaired by the MMR complex, because the exonuclease appears to preferentially remove the T on the newly synthesized strand [4,26], leaving O⁶mG intact and resulting in reinsertion by the polymerase of T opposite the O⁶mG.

This abortive DNA repair process may repeat itself a number of times and appears, by ill-defined means, to be cytotoxic [4]. Cell death may ensue from extensive chromosomal breakage or energy depletion in response to the enzymatic repair of single strand breaks [28]. Furthermore, cells wild type for MMR arrest DNA replication, again, most likely as a result of strand break recognition, and may be induced into the apoptotic pathway, even after exposure to very low levels of methylating agents [5], a finding that is not observed in mismatch repair mutants. This may involve wild-type p53 but preferentially occurs during the second round of DNA synthesis, suggesting that it is instigated after O⁶mG:T recognition by the MMR pathway.

Human tumor lines that fail to repair base mismatches apparently fail to activate the mismatch repair process in stretches of DNA containing O⁶mG and, even in the face of many adducts, fail to induce a cytotoxic response [12,29]. Thus, defects in components of base mismatch repair complex seem to explain the alkylation-tolerant phenotype.

CROSSLINK-INDUCED CELL DEATH DUE TO CHLOROETHYLATING AGENTS

Chloroethylating agents induce DNA damage primarily by forming chloroethyl-DNA adducts [30]. Of these, the most important appears to be O^6-chloroethylguanine, which may undergo hydrolysis to O^6-hydroxyethylguanine or rearrange to the cyclic intermediate, N^1-O^6-ethanoguanine [31,32]. Nucleophilic attack by N^3 of the opposing strand's cytosine on the cyclic adduct results in the formation of the stable DNA-interstrand crosslink, 1-[N^3-deoxycytidyl]-2-[N^1-deoxyguanosinyl]-ethane, a lesion that may lack repairability (see Figure 5–1) [31,32]. Although the pathway(s) by which DNA-interstrand crosslinks kill cells are not well understood, it is likely to involve a blockage in DNA replication and/or transcription. These crosslinks disrupt DNA synthesis, giving rise to chromosomal aberrations, rearrangements, sister chromatid exchanges (SCEs), and strand breaks, each of which correlates with cytotoxicity [33–35]. Both of the precrosslink lesions, O^6-chloroethylguanine and N^1-O^6-ethanoguanine, as well as O^6-hydroxyethyl-guanine, are susceptible to repair by alkyltransferase, although repair of the cyclic adduct may be the most critical as it directly proceeds crosslink formaiton [36–39]. Of note, repair of N^1-O^6-ethanoguanine leads to a DNA–protein linkage between N^1 postion of guanine and the alkyltransferase, a lesion of unknown consequence [40,41]. Chloroethylating agent–induced O^6-chloroethylguanine forms interstrand DNA crosslinks over a period of 12 hours following formation of the intermediate, O^6-N^1-ethanoguanine [42]. Preventing crosslinks by repairing precrosslink lesions up to 12 hours after BCNU treatment reduces its cytotoxicity [42,43].

In this regard, repair of the interstrand crosslink induced by chloroethylnitro-soureas appears to be a lesser mechanism of resistance than repair of the precrosslink lesion and stands in sharp contrast to the repair of melphalan- or cisplatin-induced crosslinks in which nucleotide excision repair and topoisomerase II activity are important, especially in instances of acquired resistance [44,45]. What separates the nitrogen mustard class of alkylating agents from the chloroethylnitrosoureas is the lack of attack at the O^6 position of guanine attack occurs instead at N^7G, resulting in a guanine–guanine intrastrand crosslink. The precrosslink lesion at N^7G is specifi-cally recognized by the N^7-methylguanine glycosylase, which appears to reduce the cytotoxicity of the nitrogen mustard class of agents. In contrast, repair of the chloroethylnitrosourea-induced precrosslink lesion, because it initiates at the O^6G position, occurs via the alkyltransferase DNA repair protein.

O^6-ALKYLGUANINE DNA ALKYLTRANSFERASE

We and others have extensively studied O^6-alkylguanine DNA alkyltransferase (AGT) as a mediator of resistance to drugs that attack at O^6 of guanine. This protein serves as the stoichiometric acceptor protein for O^6-alkylguanine DNA monoadducts, transferring the alkyl group from DNA to the active site of the protein, hence inactivating the protein and restoring DNA to normal [18,46]. The natural targets for this protein are small alkyl groups, including methyl, ethyl, isopropyl, hydroxyethyl, and chloroethyl adducts. In addition, the O^6 bond of the

O^6N^1 ethanoguanine is a target for the alkyltransferase [42]. Since the crosslink that follows chloroethylation occurs between the N^1 of guanine and the N^3 of cytosine [31], the crosslink is not a substrate for the alkyltransferase protein.

Much of what is known about alkyltransferase has been learned from analysis in *E. coli,* in which two genes encoding for this enzyme have been identified, *ada* [47] and *Ogt* [48]. The product of the *ada* gene is a 39 kDa protein that repairs O^6-alkyl-guanine (O^6-alkyl-G), O^4-methylthymine, and the *s*-stereoisomer of methyl-phosphotriesters. The *ada* alkyltransferase can undergo a host-dependent cleavage to liberate a 19 kDa fragment responsible for the repair of O^6-alkyl-G or O^4-methylthymine, with a methyl group acceptor site at cysteine-321, and a 20 kDa fragment that repairs the methyl-phosphotriesters, with a methyl acceptor site at cysteine-69 in the N-terminal part of the *ada* protein. Replacement of the methyl acceptor cysteine with another amino acid in either fragment abolishes the methyl acceptor activity of the respective part of the protein [8]. The second *E. coli* alkyltransferase gene, *Ogt,* encodes a 19 kDa protein and repairs only O^6-alkyl-G or O^4-methylthymine. The *Ogt* alkyltransferase is expressed constitutively and cannot be induced, in contrast to the *ada* protein [18,49].

In eukaryotes, alkyltransferase activity has been found in all the mammalian species examined [50]. The human alkyltransferase gene MGMT is located on chromosome 10 [51], and the molecular weight of the product protein is approximately 22 kDa. The mammalian alkyltransferase repairs alkyl groups predominantly from the O^6 position of guanine [8,18,52], although recent work has shown its ability to repair O^4-alkylthymine in vitro when excessive amounts of the protein are used [53]. The mammalian alkyltransferase requires no cofactor and has an optimum pH of about 7.5–8.5. Its activity is inhibited by certain divalent metal ions (Zn^{2+}, Cd^{2+}, Hg^{2+}) and aldehydes. The preferred substrate is double-stranded DNA, but it can repair a single-stranded DNA at a slower rate [18,50,54]. There appears to be some DNA sequence preference in the rate of repair, which appears slower when the lesion is located 3′ of another guanine [18].

A variety of mammalian cell strains have been identified that have either a little or no alkyltransferase activity (Mer⁻ or Mex⁻), although the MGMT gene is present and other strains have a measurable alkyltransferase activity (Mer⁺ or Mex⁺ [8,18,50,54,55]. The molecular basis of Mer⁻ cell is not clear; it is suggested that it involves switching off of transcription of the MGMT gene as a result of immortalization of cells or of the culture conditions [8,18,50,54]. Recent studies by Brent and coworkers indicate that expression of alkyltransferase is related to methylation at CpG islands in the promoter region of the gene [56].

The cellular functions and fate of an inactivated molecule of alkyltransferase are partially understood. For example, once alkyltransferase covalently transfers an alkyl group forming *S*-alkyl-cysteine, it is not regenerated to an active protein [57]. Thus, the repair capacity of a cell is limited to the number of alkyltransferase molecules present in the nucleus at the time of DNA damage or synthesized soon after the damage. Recently a ubiquitin-mediated protein degradation system was shown to be involved in the turnover of inactivated alkyltransferase proteins, yet it remains unclear what molecular signal triggers this pathway [58]. Selective ubiquitination of human alkyltransferase in HT-29 colon carcinoma or CEM leukermic cells after exposure to O^6-bG or BCNU was demonstrated by utilizing antibodies to both ubiquitin and alkyltransferase [58]. In addition, small levels of ubiquinated alkyltransferase observed in untreated control cells, suggesting the presence of endogenously inactivated alkyltransferase proteins. These results make it attractive to hypothesize that a molecule of alkyltransferase, once inactivated, can selectively signal for its own degradation. It is also possible that conjugation of ubiquitin to active molecules of alkyltransferase takes place, suggesting a regulatory role for the ubiquitin degradation system in alkyltransferase expression and turnover.

Role of alkyltransferase in drug resistance

Over a decade ago, a series of papers by Day and colleagues demonstrated that the sensitivity of human cell lines to methylating agents was related to their ability to reactivate MNNG treated adenovirus (Mer⁺), and that the Mer⁻ phenotype corresponded with the inability to repair O^6mG in DNA [59–61]. The role of alkyltransferase in human tumor cell resistance to methylating agents was further solidified by studies demonstrating a direct correlation between alkyltransferase expression and resistance to both procarbazine and temozolomide [62,63]. Since the bulk of alkyltransferase-mediated repair occurs within minutes of DNA damage, alkyltransferase appears to be the first line of defense against methylating agents.

Erickson was the first to demonstrate that expression of alkyltransferase corresponded with resistance to DNA crosslink formation and cell death in human tumor cells treated with chloroethylating agents [2]. Since then, correlations between alkyltransferase activity and resistance to BCNU, CCNU, and ACNU in cell culture have been reported in separate studies in 54 tumor cell lines [62,64,65]. A strong correlation is indicated for chloroethylating agent responsiveness in vivo as well as in vitro. For example, the therapeutic responsiveness of human rhabdosarcoma and colon cancer xenografts to 1-(2-chloroethyl)-3-(trans-4-methylcyclohexyl)-1-nitrosourea (methyl-CCNU) and BCNU, respectively, correlates with alkyltransferase expression in the xenograft [66; Gerson, unpublished]. Cell lines lacking alkyltransferase activity are typically quite sensitive to chloroethylating agents when grown in cell culture or as a xenograft [2,66–68]. Transfection of those lines with alkyltransferase encoding genes imparts significant resistance to chloroethylating agents, demonstrating that the aforementioned sensitivity was due to insufficient alkyltransferase-mediated DNA repair [67]. Thus, the predominant role of alkyltransferase in tumor cell resistance to chloroethylating agents seems clear, further solidifying the contention that the DNA-interstrand crosslink formation is the major cytotoxic lesion.

Alkyltransferase structure and function

The function of AGT has been conserved in evolution since bacteria, and there is striking amino acid sequence homology between species, suggesting that this protein

Putative DNA Binding Domain

```
Human    94 FTRQVLWKLLKVVKFGEVISYQQLAALAGNPKAARAVGGAMR  135
E. coli 270 AFQQQVWQALRTIPCGETVSYQQLANAIGKPKAVRAVASACA  311
```

Active Site Domain

```
Human   136 GNPVPILIPCHRVVCSSGAVGNYSGGLAVKEWLLAHEGHRLGK  178
E. coli 312 ANKLAIIIPCHRVVRGDGTLSGYRWGVSRKAQLLRREAENEER  354
```

Figure 5–2. O⁶-alkylguanine-DNA alkyltransferases of human (from Phe94 to Lys178) and *E. coli* (*ada*, from Ala270 to Arg354) are compared by sequence alignment of the conserved amino acids. Both AGTs have a putative DNA binding domain followed by an active site domain. Three α-helixes in the DNA binding domain are shaded. In the active site domain, amino acids involved in the H-bonded network are in bold face and the stretch of amino acids that allows swivel of the C-terminal α-helix is in a box. The C-terminal α-helix is shaded.

has a fundamental role in maintaining the integrity of DNA. The crystallographic structure of the *E. coli ada* gene *C*-terminal fragment, a biologically active 19 kDa alkyltransferase, reveals a putative DNA-binding domain as well as a hydrogen (H)-bonded network within an active site domain [69]. This H-bonded network involves two ordered water molecules, Asn¹³⁷, Cys¹⁴⁵, His¹⁴⁶, Tyr¹⁵⁸ and Glu¹⁷² (numbered from the amino terminus of the human alkyltransferase), which are absolutely conserved among all alkyltransferase proteins (Figure 5–2). Eighteen other residues are 100% conserved among all alkyltransferase proteins, 12 of which reside within the putative DNA-binding domain. Sequences within this domain are well conserved in both prokaryotic and eukaryotic proteins, and it is speculated that the three α-helices within this region represent a variant helix-turn-helix DNA binding motif. It will be interesting to see how mutations within this region affect both DNA-binding and alkyltransferase function in both prokaryotic and eukaryotic proteins.

The rate-determining step in O⁶-alkylguanine repair by human alkyltransferase is DNA binding [70]. A swivel about the loop domain corresponding to Val¹⁴⁹-Ser¹⁵⁹ in the human repair protein should simultaneously expose the putative DNA-binding domain and render duplex DNA accessible to Cys¹⁴⁵ [69]. Thus, a conformational change is predicted for DNA binding by alkyltransferase proteins, a prediction that is corroborated by fluorescence and circular dichroism studies with alkyltransferase proteins [70,71]. Molecular modeling by Moore et al. predicts the bacterial protein will lie within the major groove covering about eight base pairs, which again agrees with experimental results with the *ada*-encoded and human alkyltransferase [69–71]. This conformation change would disrupt the active-site H-bonded network and may initiate events leading to the generation of a reactive cysteine-derived thiolate anion. Serine proteases as well as lipases utilize acid-histidine stereochemistry in the generation of a nucleophile, suggesting that aklyltransferases may utilize a similar mechanism involving the H-bonded residues His¹⁴⁶ and Glu¹⁷² [72]. In support of this fact, alkyltransferase proteins with mutations at either amino acid site have very little or no activity [73–75].

Differences in substrate specificity of alkyltransferases amongst species reveal more clues in the structure–function relationship of the protein. Mammalian alkyltransferases recognize the pseudosubstrate O^6-benzylguanine (O^6bG) and are inactivated in vitro and in vivo by O^6bG treatment, whereas the *ada*-encoded alkyltransferase is inert to O^6bG [76,77]. These differences in substrate specificity and sensitivity to O^6bG stem from conformational differences of the H-bonded network. A stretch of amino acids from Val^{148} to Ser^{159} within the human alkyl-transferase swivels the C-terminal α-helix amino acids from Leu^{162} to His^{171} upon substrate binding to the active site, facilitating the alkyl group transfer to the sulfur side chain of Cys^{145}. Glycine-156 is located in this stretch, and if mutated to alanine it may cause subtle conformational changes in the H-bonded network. This point mutation does not significantly affect alkyltransferase removal of either the methyl or chloroethyl adduct from DNA, but reduces its ability to react with O^6bG, resulting in alkyltransferase (AGT-Gly156Ala) resistance to O^6bG [78].

Heterogeneity of alkyltransferase expression

Alkyltransferase levels vary in different species, strains, and also in various tissues of the same animal. In mouse liver, alkyltransferase activity is lower in preweaning and old mice compared with young adults [79]. Human tissues contain considerably higher alkyltransferase levels compared with rodents [18,54,79,80]. In many species the levels of alkyltransferase are relatively higher in liver and spleen than those in brain and mammary gland. When alkyltransferase activity was measured in normal and malignant human tissue, there was a marked interindividual variation, with a range of greater than 10-fold [18,50,81–84]. Some laboratories reported the complete absence of alkyltransferase activity in a proportion of tumors, especially brain tumors [83,85].

In addition, studies have reported that alkyltransferase levels also vary among different cells from the same tissue. Alkyltransferase was higher in rat hepatocytes compared with nonparenchymal cells [86,87]. Belinsky and coworkers [88] reported that alkyltransferase was two times higher in the macrophages and type II cells compared with that in the alveolar small cells and Clara cells in the lung of rats.

Recent studies utilizing in situ hybridization and immunohistochemistry have confirmed the heterogeneity of alkyltransferase expression within different cells of the same organ [89]. In human liver, alkyltransferase is located in hepatocytes and bile duct cells, while the periportal region is deficient [90]. In human colon, alkyltransferase is dominantly located in the mucosal epithelial cells, while the submucosal tissue is deficient [84]. In human breast, alkyltransferase is dominantly expressed in connective tissue and myoepithelial cells, while the ductal epithelial cells are relatively deficient [91].

There is also heterogenous expression of alkyltransferase among cells that comprise a variety of human tumors, including melanoma, Hodgkin's disease, and ovarian, breast, and colon cancer. Alkyltransferase levels are generally higher in the malignant parenchymal cells, while the stoma is relatively deficient [84,92; Gerson, unpublished]. Availability of human alkyltransferase-specific monoclonal antibodies that can be used for immunohistochemistry with an image analysis system will soon be providing better histological localization of alkyltransferase in human tumors [84,93].

BIOCHEMICAL MODULATION OF DRUG RESISTANCE BY INHIBITION OF ALKYLTRANSFERASE

From these observations, we can conclude that for many human tumors, alkyltransferase is a major source of resistance to the nitrosourea class of alkylating agents. To overcome this form of resistance, two methods have been employed to inhibit alkyltransferase. The first, described by Erickson and coworkers [94,95], involves using a methylating agent, such as streptozotocin or dacarbazine, to form O^6-methylguanine DNA adducts, which in turn deplete the enzyme through the repair process, while the second method involves the use of direct inhibitors of the enzyme, as outlined later [96,97].

Taking advantage of different toxicity profiles of streptozotocin and BCNU, combination treatment has been studied in a series of phase I trials using the maximally tolerated dose (MTD) of each drug. Streptozotocin significantly enhanced the myelotoxicity of the BCNU but failed to improve its antitumor effect [98]. In a series of phase I clinical trials of streptozotocin as a modulator of alkyltransferase-directed DNA repair, the MTD of BCNU decreased from 200 mg/m² to 100–150 mg/m², with dose-limiting myelosuppression and hepatic toxicity [99–101]. These studies showed that it is possible to inhibit alkyltransferase in peripheral blood mononuclear cells by a total dose of 2,000 mg/m² streptozotocin given as a single bolus or over 4 days [46]. When we administered streptozotocin as a single iv dose, it led to a 78% (range 69–89%) decrease in the alkyltransferase levels in metastatic colon cancer samples obtained 5 hours after the drug infusion and a comparable drop in the alkyltransferase activity of peripheral blood mononuclear cells. No clinical responses were observed with 130 mg/m² BCNU, given 6 hours following streptozotocin [101]. It may be that the poor modulatory effect of the streptozotocin resulted in residual alkyltransferase activity in tumor cells that was sufficient to maintain BCNU resistance. Micetich et al. [99] noted responses in patients with carcinoid syndrome. Dose-limiting toxicity of the combination appears to be myelosuppression observed at doses of BCNU of between 100 and 125 mg/m². We are now engaged in clinical studies to evaluate other combinations of steptozotocin temozolomide and/or hydroxyurea in combination with BCNU in an effort to define synergistic effects clinically.

Of interest, while the blood samples were a good predictor of the biochemical modulation that took place in the target tumor, there was no correlation with tumor and biopsies from the same patient after streptozotocin treatment. For this reason, we are cautious about suggesting that there will be a correlation between the two, indicating that the blood cells are not a "surrogate" maker for the activity in tumor samples. In addition, relying on the lymphocyte to estimate the duration of modulaton may be ill advised because the resting lymphocyte regenerates alkyltransferase quite slowly after depletion [102,103], whereas tumor cells may regenerate activity much more quickly.

In a study recently reported by Willson, et al., sequential CT-guided 14 g cutting needle tumor biopsies were used to measure changes in tumor alkyltransferase 6 hours after infusion of 2,000 mg/m^2 streptozotocin. Tumor samples had a greater than 80% decrease in alkyltransferase activity [101]. There were no complications of the sequential biopsies, and in most instances biopsies contained viable tumor so that paired analysis of tumor alkyltransferase could be made. While tumors showed evidence of biochemical modulation, all tumors continued to express alkyltransferase activity after streptozotocin. The inability to completely deplete the alkyltransferase in the tumor may have decreased the likelihood that therapeutic responses would be seen. Nonetheless, this study indicates that it is technically feasible to monitor biochemical changes within the tumor to guide phase I trials and to correlate biochemical modulation with clinical response.

O⁶-BENZYLGUANINE

The most selective and potent direct inhibitor of alkyltransferase is O^6-benzylguanine (O^{6}bG), one of a large series of related compounds synthesized by Moschel [97]. While each of these compounds has a slightly different inhibitory profile, and has different pKa and solubility, they are all very potent inhibitors of the alkyltransferase. Earlier studies evaluated O^6-methylguanine as a potential inhibitor of the protein [96], but the results with O^{6}bG are far superior and most investigators are pursuing research on this agent.

O^6-benzylguanine acts as a pseudo-substrate for alkyltransferase: The benzyl group is transferred to the active site of alkyltransferase, causing its irreversible inactivation by the same mechanism employed in DNA repair (Figure 5-3). O^6-benzylguanine is a potent inhibitor of alkyltransferase, with an ED$_{50}$ of approximately 0.2 μM [104]. In cells expressing alkyltransferase, O^6-benzylguanine inactivates the protein in a dose- and time-dependent manner [105]. Maximal inhibition is reached within 4 hours, but at higher concentrations inhibition can occur much sooner. In animal studies, intraperitoneal injection of O^6-benzylguanine results in rapid depletion of alkyltransferase in both animal tissues and in human xenograft tumors expressing high levels of the protein [105]. The compound is relatively nontoxic, with an IC$_{50}$ of 30–60 μM, well above the concentrations required to achieve biochemical modulation of the protein, 0.5–5 μM, [67,105].

O^6-benzylguanine markedly potentiates the cytotoxicity of chloroethylnitrosoureas in a number of human tumor cell lines, including colon cancer, breast cancer, lung cancer, medulloblastoma, and glioblastoma [67,96,105–107]. When cells are preincubated in O^6-benzylguanine to deplete alkyltransferase and then are treated with cytotoxic agents, there is increased tumor cell cytotoxicity. The best enhancement is seen when the inhibitor remains in the culture medium after drug exposure to prevent regeneration of the alkyltransferase [103,108]. In most instances, a dose-modification factor, that is, a reduction in the IC$_{50}$, of 2.5- to 10-

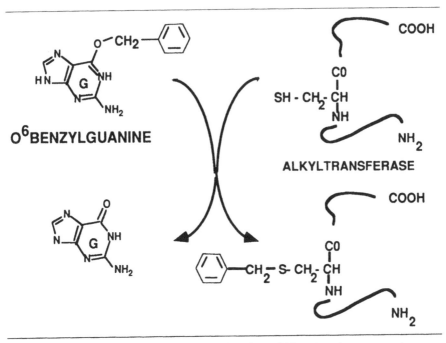

Figure 5–3. O⁶-benzylguanine inactivation of alkyltransferase. O⁶-benzylguanine acts as a substrate for the alkyltransferase, resulting in the transfer of the benzyl group to the active site of the alkyltransferase, causing its irreversible inactivation. The alkyltransferase protein is shown schematically on the right.

fold, has been observed and a significant synergistic effect has been noted [67,105,109,110].

Human colon cancer, medulloblastoma, glioma, and lung cancer xenografts, tumors that express high levels of alkyltransferase and are partially or completely resistant to maximally tolerated doses of BCNU, can be markedly sensitized to BCNU by O⁶bG [67,106,107,110–112]. A single dose of 30 mg/kg O⁶bG formulated in PEG-400 (40% PEG-400, 60% PBS) appears sufficient to deplete tumor alkyltransferase 16–>24 hours [67,108,114]. This is sufficient time to allow the BCNU-induced pre-crosslink N¹O⁶-ethanoguanine intermediate to complete the crosslink reaction and may increase the efficacy of the combination, presumably because, as noted earlier, prolonged depletion of the protein for at least 12 hours prevents repair of pre-crosslink lesions in the tumor. Even in BCNU-resistant tumors, the animal studies indicate that the combination of O⁶bG and BCNU results in substantial tumor growth delays and, in some instances, tumor regressions.

The xenograft studies also identified increased toxicity of the combination with a reduction in the MTD of the chloroethylnitorourea of approximately twofold [67,111,114]. There is little evidence of selectivity in the rate of depletion or regeneration of alkyltransferase activity in different tissues or between tumor and normal tissues in the murine models [67,115], predicting for increased toxicity to normal tissues, in particular, the bone marrow, by the combination of O⁶bG and nitrosoureas. This raises the possibility that there may be a much more narrow therapeutic index observed in human clinical trials of the combination than was observed in the xenograft studies. Nonetheless, the xenograft studies show a promising degree of efficacy in tumors that are resistant to BCNU alone.

POTENTIAL FOR TOXICITY IN TRIALS COMBINING ALKYLTRANSFERASE DEPLETION WITH A NITROSOUREA OR RELATED COMPOUND

While an increased level of tumor alkyltransferase activity is the major resistance mechanism against nitrosoureas, the level of the alkyltransferase in normal host tissues determines the toxicity profile of these drugs. There is a wide variation in alkyltransferase activity in normal human tissues. The highest activity is observed in liver (55.4 ± 25.8 fmol/μg DNA), closely followed by the intestine, lung, brain, and lymphocytes. Myeloid precursors in the human bone marrow consistently reveal low activity (3 ± 1.6 fmol/μg DNA), which explains the dose-limiting myelotoxicity of the nitrosoureas [86]. Alkyltransferase activity does not seem to vary as myeloid cells differentiate from the immature CD34+ cell to the myeloblast through the myelocyte stage [116; Gerson, unpublished]. These laboratory observations correlate well with the clinically observed myelotoxicity of the nitrosoureas, in which delayed recovery of the neutrophil count and cumulative toxicity of repeated exposures are observed, indicating a cytotoxic effect on very early progenitor cells. This is in contrast to the relative resistance of early progenitors to cyclophosphamide, due to increased levels of aldehyde dehydrogenase, and to anthracyclines, due to increased expression of the MDR gene.

In addition to myelotoxicity, transient abnormalities in liver and renal function have been reported in 10–30% of patients in phase I–II studies of BCNU [117]. Although the pathogenesis is not well defined, pulmonary toxicity in the form of interstitial fibrosis occurs in 15–30% of the patients treated with high cumulative doses of BCNU [118]. When BCNU was used in the setting of autologous bone marrow transplantation, significant dose escalation could be achieved, with the dose-limiting toxicity of fatal interstitial pneumonitis and hepatic necrosis at 1,200 mg/m² [119]. In contrast to the chloroethylating nitrosoureas, streptozotocin has minimal myelotoxicity but induces dose-limiting renal tubular toxicity in the form of proteinuria and a reduction in creatinine clearance [120]. Despite its toxicity toward pancreatic islets and its diabetogenic action on laboratory animals, streptozotocin has not resulted in diabetes in clinical studies.

Nitrosoureas are also potent carcinogens and mutagens, and bone marrow once again is the most vulnerable target due to its low alkyltransferase activity. This effect was clinically recognized in a trial evaluating adjuvant use of methyl-CCNU in colon cancer patients when a high incidence of secondary leukemias was noted [121]. In another review, use of CCNU in 269 patients with Hodgkin's disease was associated with15 cases of acute leukemia over 15 years of follow-up, resulting in a cumulative risk of over 10% [122]. Of interest, a similar secondary leukemia is observed in mice and rats following exposure to methylnitrosourea. In a transgenic animal model, the leukemogenic effect of methylnitrosourea was prevented by overexpression of the human MGMT gene, which resulted in high levels of human alkyltransferase in the target cell and rapid removal of the mutagenic O^6-methylguanine DNA adduct [123].

None of the available alkyltransferase inhibitors, including O^6-benzylguanine, are selective for tumor alkyltransferase activity, and in animal studies they potentiate host tissue toxicity when given in combination with nitrosoureas. The degree of potentiation correlates with the alkyltransferase activity of the cell. Similar to tumor cell lines with high levels of alkyltransferase and marked resistance to nitrosoureas, normal tissues with high alkyltransferase activity can be rendered sensitive by O^6-benzylguanine pretreatment [103,112]. This implies that clinical toxicity of the O^6-benzylguanine/nitrosourea combination should shift to include tissues with high alkyltransferase activity, but would also exacerbate renal, hepatic, and pulmonary toxicity. Increased toxicity toward hematopoietic stem cells with BCNU has been observed following depletion of the alkyltransferase by O^6-methylguanine [104] and O^6-benzylguanine [124]. Thus, myelosuppression may remain dose limiting. In preclinical toxicology studies involving mice and beagle dogs, O^6-benzylguanine resulted in marked potentiation of BCNU-induced myelosuppression [125]. Xenograft studies in mice have shown that pretreatment with O^6-benzylguanine reduced the MTD of BCNU by twofold when assessed by animal weight loss and survival [68].

In addition, recent data revealed that in cell-free systems, the ED_{50} for O^6-benzylguanine depletion of the mouse alkyltransferase was threefold greater than for the human protein [77]. Our group has recently confirmed that in isogenic cell lines expressing either mouse or human MGMT, and in MGMT transgenic mice, the mouse alkyltransferase protein is more resistant to inhibition by O^6-benzylguanine compared with human alkyltransferase protein [126]. This suggests that there may be increased toxicity of the combination in human trials than predicted based on the trials in xenograft-bearing mice. Interspecies differences in alkyltransferase activity and its sensitivity to O^6-benzylguanine mandates careful design of phase I human clinical trials.

Although O^6-benzylguanine is predicted to potentiate clinical nitrosourea toxicity by two- to threefold, xenograft and in vitro studies suggest a reduction in IC_{50} of BCNU in human tumor cell lines of between 2.5- and 10-fold. If this degree of antitumor effect can be achieved clinically, it would significantly improve the therapeutic index of nitrosoureas. Since the modulation would be greater in tumors with high alkyltransferase activity, tumor alkyltransferase levels could be utilized as an indicator of the therapeutic index for nitrosoureas. Pretreatment analysis of tumor alkyltransferase activity could define whether a particular partient would benefit from combination therapy or only experience toxicity without enhancement of antitumor effect.

CLINICAL TRIALS OF O^6-BENZYLGUANINE AND BCNU COMBINATION

The ability of O^6-benzylguanine to overcome nitrosourea resistance of tumor cell lines in vitro and in xenograft models stimulated rapid completion of preclinical testing of the combination in large animal models under the auspices of the NCI

Decision Network, followed by approval of this agents for phase I clinical trials. Such a trial was designed at our institution to address questions pertaining to both biochemical and clinical endpoints. In Table 5–1, a schematic outline of the strategy that will be pursued is presented. The initial objective is to establish a dose of O^6-benzylguanine required to deplete the tumor alkyltransferase activity to undetectable levels for a sufficient duration to allow cytotoxic crosslinks to form after subsequent BCNU administration. Since the optimal duration of sustained alkyltransferase inhibition for cytotoxicity is thought to be between 12 and 18 hours [42], tumor alkyltransferase depletion at 18 hours is the target. In order to minimize the number of tumor biopsies, we plan to use peripheral blood mononuclear cell (PBMC) alkyltransferase activity to perform the initial dose escalation to achieve 90% or greater alkyltransferase inhibition in these cells. The duration of this inhibition can be easily followed in PBMCs, but the correlation with tumor alkyltransferase activity at later time points is expected to be poor due to anticipated differences in alkyltransferase regeneration rates of different tissues. Once PBMC depletion is noted, tumor biopsies will be performed. Patients are scheduled to undergo tumor biopsies 2 and 18 hours after the 1-hour O^6-benzylguanine infusion. Tumor samples will be obtained by a 14 G cutting needle, and will be processed for histology, immunohistochemistry, and alkyltransferase measurments. If the single-dose O^6-benzylguanine schedule fails to produce more than 90% depletion in tumor samples at 18 hours, an alternative dose schedule aimed at achieving the same biochemical endpoint will be developed.

Table 5–1. Phase I trial of sequential O^6-benzylguanine and BCNU in adults with metastatic solid tumors at CWRU (principal investigator, James K.V. Willson, MD)

Process	Time (hours)							
	−24	0	1	2	6	18	24	Wkly
O^6BG^a		X-----------						
BCNU[b] (day 21)				X------				
PBM AGT[c]	X	X-----------		X	X	X	X	X
Tumor AGT[d]	X			[X]		[X]		
Pharm[e]		X	X---	X---	X---	X---	X—	

[a] O^6-benzylguanine (O^6-BG) is administered on day 1 and day 21 over 1 hour at a starting dose of 10 mg/m^2 and is escalated first to the biochemical modulatory dose (BMD) in peripheral blood mononuclear cells (PBM) at 2 hours, and then to the BMD at 2 hours in the tumor and finally to achieve the BMD in the tumor at 18 hours. The BMD of O^6BG is defined as the dose required to deplete the alkyltransferase (AGT) to undetectable levels.

[b] BCNU is administered on day 21 at a starting does of 13 mg/m^2 and subsequently escalated after the BMD in the tumor at 18 hours is determined. The drug combination is repeated every 6 weeks.

[c] The AGT in peripheral blood mononucolear cells is measured at multiple time points to determine the kinetics of AGT inactivation and regeneration.

[d] Tumor biopsies will be obtained prior to and after the first dose of O^6BG, either at 2 or 18 hours after O^6BG treatment to define the doses required to deplete the tumor AGT.

[e] Pharmacology (Pharm) measurements of O^6BG and metabolites will be determined after each administration of O^6BG and will be correlated with the depletion of AGT in both PBM and tumor samples.

Once the biochemical modulatory dose of O^6-benzylguanine is established, BCNU dose escalation can be undertaken until MTD is reached. Patients will be given a 60 minute iv infusion of BCNU, 1 hour following the completion of O^6-benzylguanine, at a starting dose of $13 \, mg/m^2$, which is 10% of the MTD in dogs when given in combination. BCNU dose will be escalated until grade 2 nonhematologic and grade 3 or worse hematologic toxicity is observed in at least 2 out of 6 patients. Based on the preclinical toxicity studies, we anticipate a three- to eightfold reduction in the MTD of BCNU from $200 \, mg/m^2$ to $25–60 \, mg/m^2$. While myelosuppression is expected to be the dose-limiting toxicity, other organ toxicities will be monitored closely.

GENE THERAPY WITH MGMT

Since myelosuppression is dose limiting for nitrosoureas and is likely to be dose limiting for their combination with modulatory agents such as O^6-benzylguanine, there is research interest in enhancing bone marrow resistance by increasing its alkyltransferase activity. Since there is currently no known inducer of MGMT [127], efforts have been concentrated on the transfer and expression of the MGMT gene into hematopoietic progenitors [128,129]. Besides simply overexpressing MGMT, gene transfer technology would allow transfer of a mutant MGMT gene that is markedly resistant to inhibition by O^6-benzylguanine, as recently described by Crone and Pegg [78]. The inhibitory dose 50 (ID_{50}) of O^6-benzylguanine against such mutant alkyltransferase proteins varies from 60 to $>300 \, \mu M$, as opposed to $0.25 \, \mu M$ for wild-type protein [97]. If successful, such an approach would further increase the therapeutic index of the O^6-benzylguanine/nitrosourea combination by ameliorating myelosuppression and also reducing the incidence of secondary leukemias related to these agents.

Hematopoietic cell gene therapy designed for treatment of single gene disorders [130–133] or reduction of chemotherapy-induced myelosuppression [134–137] has shown potential both in vitro and in animal models. Currently replication-defective retroviruses provide the most developed methodology in terms of safety, gene integration and expression, and efficacy to deliver new genetic material to hematopoietic cells. For instance, retroviral-mediated gene transfer of the MDR-1 gene encoding the p-glycoprotein transmembrane pump has reduced cytotoxicity in murine and human hematopoietic progenitors in vitro to Taxol. Following murine bone marrow transplantation, MDR-1–transduced hematopoietic progenitors maintain their increased drug resistance and reduce the myelosuppression associated with systemic drug treatment [134,136,137].

Increased alkyltransferase expression in hematopoietic cells by retroviral-mediated gene transduction has been shown to reduce the cytotoxic potential of nitrosoureas, particularly BCNU. Successful transduction of the human alkyltransferase cDNA, MGMT [128,129], or the *E. coli ada* gene [138] into murine bone marrow progenitors has been achieved. Transduction efficiencies of clonogenic cells has ranged from 20–30% [129] to greater than 75% [128]. In vitro expression of the transduced gene has been noted in all cases, and in the case of MGMT transduction has significantly increased the resistance of hematopoietic progenitors to BCNU [128,129]. Transduction of *ada*, which, unlike the mammalian alkyltransferase protein is resistant to the potent inhibitor O^6-benzylguanine, required prior treatment of progenitors with O^6-benzylguanine in order to provide enhanced BCNU survival [138]. This treatment resulted in an increased IC_{50} from 15 µM BCNU for control transduced progenitors (transduction with a vector lacking *ada*) to 18 µM for *ada*-transduced progenitors. O^6-benzylguanine + BCNU treatment also resulted in selection of *ada*-expressing progenitors.

Murine bone marrow transplantation models have allowed the examination of the efficacy of increased hematopoietic alkyltransferase expression. In one model designed to mimic the delayed myelotoxicity associated with nitrosourea therapy, Moritz et al. [129] used weekly BCNU treatments combined with biweekly infusion of marrow progenitors. Animals receiving mock-transduced cells suffered from severe pancytopenia, whereas animals receiving bone marrow progenitors transduced with MGMT had significantly higher hematocrits, leukocyte counts, and platelet counts.

Models employing conventional transplantation of transduced hematopoietic progenitors following lethal irradiation of the recipient have shown multilineage reconstitution and maintenance of MGMT-transduced cells in primary and secondary transplant mice. Primary transplant mice showed increases in mean alkyltransferase levels of 40-fold in bone marrow, 10-fold in spleen, and 14-fold in thymus. High alkyltransferase expression led to increased BCNU resistance of bone marrow-derived colony forming progenitors (Figure 5–4) [128] and high proliferative potential-colony forming cells from MGMT-transplanted mice [129].

Reduction in BCNU-induced myelosuppression has been described for mice having increased hematopoietic alkyltransferase expression. Mice transplanted with MGMT transduced marrow progenitors that were treated weekly for 5 weeks with 40 mg/kg ip BCNU showed significantly higher peripheral blood counts, with platelet and hematocrits at normal levels, and a greater than fivefold increase in bone marrow and spleen cellularity relative to mice transplanted with control transduced marrow progenitors [129]. A similar effect in platelets, hematocrits, and red blood cells was noted in mice transplanted with *ada*-transduced marrow progenitors that were treated twice, 6 weeks apart, with the combination of 30 mg/kg O^6-benzylguanine + 12.5 mg/kg BCNU. Increased survival of *ada*-transplanted mice compared with control transplanted mice was also noted [138].

These studies show the feasibility of decreasing myelosuppression and increasing nitrosourea resistance of hematopoietic progenitors by increasing alkyltransferase expression. It is anticipated that MGMT transduction of human hematopoietic progenitors will lead to similar results in vitro. Anticipated clinical trials may show a benefit of increased nitrosourea resistance in bone marrow cells by enhancing their tolerance to this class of chemotherapy agents. Increased alkyltransferase expression in cells of the hematopoietic lineage may also allow dose escalation, especially for agents without other organ toxicity, such as temozolomide, and may limit the late

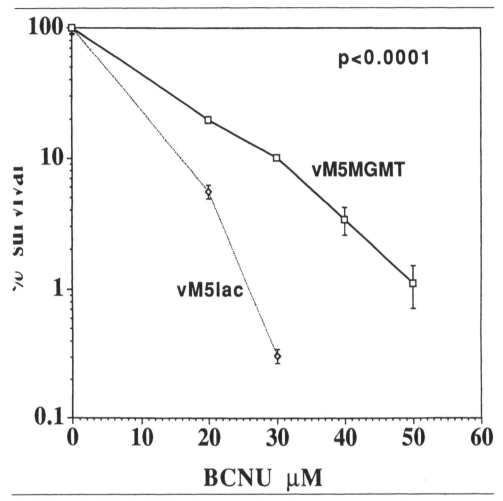

Figure 5–4. BCNU resistance in murine hematopoietic progenitors. Mice transplanted with vM5MGMT- or vM5lac-transduced bone marrow cells were treated with BCNU 2 weeks and 10 weeks after transplantation and were sacrificed after 18 weeks. Bone marrow from these animals was analyzed for BCNU resistance p < 0.0001 for all BCNU concentrations examined.

toxicity associated with chemotherapeutic agents that induce bone marrow failure and secondary leukemia.

SUMMARY

The mechanism of cytotoxicity of a number of chemotherapeutic agents involves alkylation at the O^6 position of guanine, a site that strongly influences cytotoxicity. Repair of these lesions by the alkyltransferase protects from cytotoxicity and is a major mechanism of resistance to these agents. O^6-benzylguanine inhibition of alkyltransferase sensitizes tumor cells, and clinical trials are underway to determine its efficacy. The use of gene therapy to enhance the expression of alkyltransferase in hematopoietic cells may prevent dose-limiting myelosuppression and may enhance the utility of this class of chemotherapeutic agents.

REFERENCES

1. Rasouli-Nia A, Sibghat U, Mirzayans R, Paterson MC, Day R III (1994) On the quantitative relationship between O^6-methylguanine residues in genomic DNA and production of sister-chromatid exchanges, mutations and lethal events in a Mer-human tumor cell line. Mutat Res 314:99–113.
2. Erickson LC, Laurent G, Sharkey NA, Kohn KW (1980) DNA cross-linking and monoadduct repair in nitrosourea-treated human tumour cells. Nature 288:727–729.
3. Griffin S, Xu Y-Z, Karran P (1994) DNA mismatch binding and incision at modified guanine bases by extracts of mammalian cells: Implications for tolerance to DNA methylation damage. Biochemistry 33:4787–4793.
4. Karran P, Macpherson P, Ceccotti S, Dogliotti E, Griffin S, Bignami M (1993) O^6-methylguanine residues elicit DNA repair synthesis by human cell extracts. J Biol Chem 286:15878–15886.
5. Zhukovskaya N, Branch P, Aquilina G, Karran P (1994) DNA replication arrest and tolerance to DNA methylation damage. Carcinogenesis 15:2189–2194.
6. Samson L, Derfler B, Waldstein EA (1986) Suppresion of human DNA alkylation-repair defects by Escherichia coli DNA repair gene. Proc Natl Acad Sci USA 83:5607–5610.
7. Bignami M, Terlizzese M, Zijno A, Calcagnite A, Abbondondolo A, Dogliotti E (1987) Cytotoxicity, mutations and SCEs induced by methylating agents are reduced in CHO cells expressing an active mammalian O^6-methylguanine-DNA methyltransferase gene. Carcinogenesis 8:1417–1421.
8. Lindahl T, Sedgwick B, Sekiguchi M, Nakabeppu Y (1988) Regulation and expression of the adaptive response to alkylating agents. Ann Rev Biochem 57:133–157.
9. Goldmacher VS, Cuzick RA Jr, Thilly WG (1986) Isolation and partial characterization of human cell mutants differing in sensitivity to killing and mutation by methylnitrosourea and N-methyl-N'-nitro-N-nitrosoguanidine. J Biol Chem 261:12462–12471.
10. Green MHL, Lowe JE, Petit-Frere C, Karran P, Hall J, Kataoka H (1989) Propeties of N-methylnitrosourea-resistant mex- derivatives of an SV-40-immortalized human fibroblast cell line. Carcinogenesis 10:893–898.
11. Aquilina G, Giammarioli AM, Zijno A, Di Muccio A, Dogliotti E, Bignami M (1990) Tolerance to O^6-methylguanine and 6-thioguanine cytotoxic effects: A cross-resistant phenotype in N-methylnitrosourea-resistant Chinese hamster ovary cells. Cancer Res 50:4248–4253.
12. Kat A, Thilly WG, Fang W (1993) N alkylation tolerant mutant human cell line is deficient in strand specific mismatch repair. Proc Natl Acad Sci USA 90:6434–6428.
13. Papadopoulos N, Nicolaides N, Liu B, Parsons R, Lengauer C, Palombo F, D'Arrigo A, Markowitz S, Willson J, Kinzler K (1995) Mutations of GTBP in genetically unstable cells. Science 268:1915–1917.
14. Thibodeau S, Bren G, Schaid D (1993) Microsatellite instability in cancer of the proximal colon. Science 260:816–819.
15. Risinger J, Berchuck A, Kohler M, Watson P, Lynch H, Boyd J (1993) Genetic instability of microsatellites in endometrial carcinoma. Cancer Res 53:5100–5103.
16. Han H-J, Yanagisawa A, Kato Y, Park J-G, Nakamura Y (1993) Genetic instability in pancreatic cancer and poorly differentiated type of gastric cancer. Cancer Res 53:5087–5089.
17. Branch P, Hampson R, Karran P (1995) DNA mismatch binding defects, DNA damage tolerance, and mutator phenotypes in human colorectal carcinoma cell lines. Cancer Res 55:2304–2309.
18. Pegg AE (1990) Mammalian O^6-alkylguanine-DNA alkyltransferase: Regulation and importance in response to alkylating carcinogenic and therapeutic agents. Cancer Res 50:6119–6129.
19. Pauly GT, Highes SH, Moschel RC (1994) Response of repair-competent and repair-deficient Escherichia coli to three O^6-substituted guanines and involvement of methyl-directed mismatch repair in the processing of O^6-methylguanine residues. Biochemistry 33:9169–9177.
20. Snow E, Foote R, Mitra S (1984) Base-pairing properties of O^6-methylguanine in template NA during in vitro DNA replication. J Biol Chem 259:8095–8100.
21. Singer B, Chavez F, Goodman M, Essigmann J, Dosanjh M (1989) Effect of 3'flanking neighbors

on kinetics of pairing of dCTP or dTTP opposite O^6-methylguanine in a defined primed oligonucleotide when *E. coli* DNA polymerase I is used. Proc Natl Acad Sci USA 86:8271–8274.

22. Prolla TA, Christie D-M, Lisskay RM (1994) Dual requirement in yeast DNA mismatch repair for MLH1 and PMS1, two homologs of the bacterial *mutL* gene. Mol Cell Biol 14:407–415.

23. Prolla TA, Pang Q, Alani E, Kolodner RD, Liskay RM (1994) MLH1, PMS1, and MSH2 interactions during the initiation of DNA mismatch repair in yeast. Science 265:1091–1095.

24. Horii A, Han H-J, Sasaki S, Shimada M, Nakamura Y (1994) Cloning, characterization and chromosomal assignment of the human genes homologous to yeast *PMS1*, a member of mismatch repair genes. Biochem Biophys Res Commun 204:1257–1263.

25. Modrich P (1994) Mismatch repair, genomic stability and cancer. Science 266:1959–1960.

26. Au K, Welsh K, Modrich P (1992) Initiation of methyl-directed mismatch repair. J Biol Chem 267:12142–12148.

27. Grilley M, Griffith J, Modrich P (1993) Bidirectional excision in methyl-directed mismatch repair. J Biol Chem 268:11830–11837.

28. Chatterjee S, Berger NA (1994) Growth-phase-dependent response to DNA damage in poly(ADP-ribose) polymerase deficient cell lines: Basis for a new hypothesis describing the role of poly(ADP-ribose) polymerase in DNA replication and repair. Mol Cell Biochem 138:61–69.

29. Parsons R, Li G, Longley M, Fang W, Papadopoulus N, Jen J, de la Chapelle A, Kinzler KW, Vogelstein B, Modrich P (1994). Hypermutability and mismatch repair defficiency in RER+ tumor cells. Cell 75:1227–1236.

30. Ludlum D (1990) DNA alkylation by the haloethyl nitrosoureas: Nature of modifications produced and their enzymatic repair or removal. Mutat Res 233:117–126.

31. Tong WP, Kirk MC, Ludlum DB (1982) Formation of the cross-link 1-[N^3-deoxycyctidyl],2-[N^1-deoxyguanosinyl]-ethan in DNA treated with N,N^1-bis(2-chloroethyl)-N-nitrosourea. Cancer Res 42:3102–3105.

32. Tong W, Kohn K, Ludlum D (1982) Modifications of DNA by different haloethylnitrosoureas. Cancer Res 42:4460–4464.

33. Srivenugopal KD (1992) Formation and disappearance of DNA interstrand cross-links in human colon tumor cell lines with different levels of resistance to chlorozotocin. Biochemi Pharmacol 433:1159–1163.

34. Trey JE, Gerson SL (1989) The role of O^6-alkylguanine DNA alkyltransferase in limiting nitrosourea-induced sister chromatid exchanges in proliferating human lymphocytes. Cancer Res 49:1899–1903.

35. Wiencke JK, Bodell WJ (1985) N-methyl-N-nitrosourea potentiation of cytogenetic damage induced by 1,3-bis(2-chloroethyl)-1-nitrosourea in normal human lymphocytes. Cancer Res 45:4798–4803.

36. Brent T, Lestrud S, Smith D, Remack JS (1987) Formation of DNA interstrand cross-links by the novel chloroethylating agent 2-chloroethyl(methylsulfonyl)-methanesulfonate: Suppression by O^6-alkylguanine-DNA alkyltransferase purified from human leukemic lymphoblasts. Cancer Res 47:3384–3387.

37. Brent T (1984) Suppression of cross-link formation in chloroethylnitrosourea-treated DNA by an activity in extracts of human leukemic lymphoblasts. Cancer Res 44:1887–1892.

38. Ewig R, Kohn K (1978) DNA-protein cross-linking and DNA interstrand cross-linking by haloethylnitrosoureas in L1210 cells. Cancer Res 38:3197–3203.

39. Ludlum DB, Mehta JR, Tong WP (1986) Prevention of 1-(3-deoxycytidyl),2-(1-deoxyguanosinyl)ethane cross-link formation in DNA by rat liver O^6-alkylguanine-DNA alkyltransferase. Cancer Res 46:3353–3357.

40. Brent T, Remack J, Smith D (1987) Characterization of a novel reaction by human O^6-alkylguanine-DNA-alkyltransferase with 1,3-bis(2-chloroethyl)-1-nitrosourea-treated DNA. Cancer Res 47:6185–6188.

41. Gonzaga PE, Potter PM, Niu TQ, Yu D, Ludlum DB, Rafferty JA, Margison GP, Brent TP (1992) Identification of the cross-link between human O^6-methylguanine-DNA methyltransferase and chloroethylnitrosourea-treated DNA. Cancer Res 52:6052–6058.

42. Brent TP, Smith DG, Remack JS (1987) Evidence that O^6-alkylguanine-DNA alkyltransferase becomes covalently bound to DNA containing 1,3-bis(2-chloroethyl)-1-nitrosourea-induced precursors of interstrand cross-links. Biochem Biophys Res Commun 142:341–347.

43. Brent TP, Remack JS (1988) Formation of covalent complexes between human O^6-alkylguanine-DNA alkyltransferase and BCNU-treated defined length synthetic oligodeoxynucleotides. Nucleic Acids Res 16:6779–6788.

44. Zdziencka M, Roza L, Westerveld A, Boostsma D, Simons J (1987) Biologicial and biochemical consequences of the human ERCC-1 repair gene after transfection into a repair deficient CHO cell line. Mutat Res 183:69–74.

45. Yang LY, Li L, Li MJ, Keating MJ, Plunkett W (1995) Fludarabine tri phosphate suppresses nucleotide excision repair of cisplatin-induced lesions by blocking incision and repair synthesis. Proc Am Assoc Cancer Res 37:363.

46. Gerson SL, Miller K, Berger NA (1985) O^6 alkylguanine-DNA alkyltransferase activity in human myeloid cells. J Clin Invest 76:2106–2114.

47. Sedgwick B (1983) Molecular cloning of a gene which regulates the adaptive response to alkylating agentts in E. coli. Mol Gen Genet 191:466–472.

48. Potter P, Wilkinson M, Fitton F, Brennand J, Cooper D, Marginson G (1987) Characterization and nucleotide sequence of Ogt, the O^6-alkylguanine-DNA alkyltransferase gene of E. coli. Nucleic Acids Res 15:9177–9193.

49. Margison G, O'Connor PJ, Cooper DP, Davies R, Hall CN, Redmond SMS, Buser K, Cerny T, Citti L, D'Incalci M (1990) O^6-alkylgunine-DNA alkyltransferase: Significance, methods of measurement and some human tumour and normal tissue levels. In Giraldi T ed. Triazenes. New York: Plenum Press, pp 195–206.

50. Pegg AE, Byers TL (1992) Repair of DNA containing O^6-alkylguanine. FASEB J 6:2302–2310.

51. Natarajan AT, Vermeulen S, Darroudi F, Valentine MB, Brent TP, Mitra S, Tano K (1992) Chromosomal localization of human O^6-methylguanine-DNA methyltransferase (MGMT) gene by in situ hybridization. Mutagenesis 7:83–85.

52. Brent T, Dolan ME, Fraenkel-Conrat H, Hall J, Karran P, Laval F, Margison GP, Montesano R, Pegg AE, Potter PM, Singer B, Swenberg JA, Yavosh DB (1988) Repair of O-alkylpyrimidines in mammalian cells: A present consensus. Proc Natl Acad Sci USA 85:1759–1762.

53. Sassanfar M, Dosanjh MK, Essigmann JM, Samson L (1991) Relative efficiencies of the bacterial, yeast, and human DNA methyltransferases for the repair of O^6-methylguanine and O^4-methylthymine. Suggestive evidence for O^4-methylthymine repair by eukaryotic methyltransferases. J Biol Chem 266:2767–2771.

54. Yarosh DB (1985) The role of O^6-methylguanine-DNA methyltransferase in cell survival, mutagenesis and carcinogenesis. Mutat Res 145:1–16.

55. Arita I, Fujimori A, Takebe H, Tatsumi K (1990) Evidence for spontaneous conversion of Mex− to Mex+ in human lymphoblastoid cells. Carcinogenesis 11:1733–1738.

56. Harris LC, Remack JS, Brent TP (1994) In vitro methylation of the human O^6-methylguanine-DNA methyltransferase promoter reduces transcription. Biochim Biophys Acta 1217:141–146.

57. Demple B, Karran P (1983) Death of an enzyme: Suicide repair of DNA. Trends Biol Sci 8:137–139.

58. Srivenugopal K, Yuan X, Ali-Osman F (1995) Ubiquitination of O^6-alkylguanine-DNA-alkyltransferase in human tumor cells following inactivation with O^6-benzylguanine and 1,3 bis(2-chloroethyl)-1-nitrosourea. Proc Am Assoc Cancer Res 36:508.

59. Scudiero DA, Meyer SA, Clatterbuch BE, Mattern MR, Ziolkowski CHJ, Day RS III (1984) Sensitivity of human cell strains having different abilities to repair O^6-methylguanine in DNA to inactivation by alkylating agents including chloroethylnitrosoureas. Cancer Res 44:2467–2474.

60. Day RSI, Ziolkowski CHJ, Scudiero DA, Meyer SA, Mattern MR (1980) Human tumor cell strains defective in the repair of alkylation damage. Carcinogenesis 1:21–32.

61. Day R III, Ziolkowski C, Scudiero D, Meyer S, Lubiniecki A, Girardi A, Galloway S, Bynum G (1980) Defective repair of alkylated DNA by human tumour and SV40-transformed human cell strains. Nature 288:724–727.

62. Baer JC, Freeman AA, Newlands ES, Watson AJ, Rafferty JA, Margison GP (1993) Depletion of O^6-alkylguanine-DNA alkyltransferase correlates with potentiation of temozolomide and CCNU toxicity in human tumour cells. Br J Cancer 67:1299–1302.

63. Schold SJ, Brent TP, von Hofe E, Friedman HS, Mitra S, Bigner DD, Swenberg JA, Kleihves P (1989) O^6 alkylguanine-DNA alkyltransferase and sensitivity to procarbazine in human brain-tumor xenografts. Neurosurgery 70:573–577.

64. Gerson S, Willson J (1995) O^6-alkylguanine-DNA-alkyltransferase: A target for the modulation of drug resistance. Hematol/Oncol Clin North Am 9:431–449.

65. Tsujimura T, Zhang Y-P, Fujio C, Chang H-R, Watatani M, Ishizaki K, Kitamura H, Ikenaga M (1987) O^6-methylguanine methyltransferase activity and sensitivity of Japanese tumor cell strains to 1-(4-amino-2-methyl-5pyrimidinyl)methyl-3-(2-chloroethyl)-3-nitrosourea hydrochloride. Jpn J Cancer Res 78:1207–1215.

66. Brent TP, Houghton PJ, Houghton JA (1985) O⁶alkylguanine-DNA alkyltransferase activity correlates with the therapeutic response of human rhabdomyosarcoma xenografts to 1-(2-chloroethyl)-3-(trans-4-methyl-cyclohexyl)-1-nitrosourea. Proc Natl Acad Sci USA 82:2985–2989.
67. Gerson S, Markowitz SD, Willson JKV (1993) Induction of BCNU resistance in a sensitive colon cancer xenograft by transfection of alkyltransferase MGMT: A model for tumor drug resistance heterogeneity. Proc Am Assoc Cancer Res 34:271.
68. Gerson SL, Berger NA, Arce C, Petzold SJ, Willson JK (1992) Modulation of nitrosourea resistance in human colon cancer by O⁶-methylguanine. Biochem Pharmacol 43:1101–1107.
69. Moore MH, Gulbis JM, Dodson EJ, Demple B, Moody PC (1994) Crystal structure of a suicidal DNA repair protein: The Ada O⁶-methylguanine-DNA methyltransferase from E. coli. EMBO J 13:1495–1501.
70. Chan CL, Wu Z, Ciardelli T, Eastman A, Bresnick E (1993) Kinetic and DNA-binding properties of recombinant human O⁶-methylguanine-DNA methyltransferase. Arch Biochem Biophys 300:193–200.
71. Takahashi M, Sakumi K, Sekiguchi M (1990) Interaction of ada protein with DNA examined fluorescence anisotropy of the protein. Biochemistry 29:3431–3436.
72. Blow D, Hartley B (1969) Role of a buried acid group in the mechanism of action of chymotrypsin. Nature 221:337–340.
73. Ihara K, Kawate H, Chueh LL, Hayakawa H, Sekiguchi M (1994) Requirement of the Pro-Cys-His-Arg sequence for O⁶-methylguanine-DNA methyltransferase activity revealed by saturation mutagenesis with negative and positive screening. Mol Gen Genet 243:379–389.
74. Ling-Ling C, Nakamura T, Nakatsu Y, Sakumi K, Hayakawa H, Sekiguchi M (1992) Specific amino acid sequences required for O⁶-methyguanine-DNA methyltransferase acttivity: Analysis of three residues at or near the methyl acceptor site. Carcinogenesis 13:837–843.
75. Rafferty JA, Tumelty J, Skorvaga M, Elder RH, Margison GP, Douglas KT (1994) Site-directed mutagenesis of glutamic acid 172 to glutamine completely inactivated human O⁶-alkylguanine-DNA-alkyltransferase. Biochem Biophys Res Commun 199:285–291.
76. Dolan ME, Pegg AE, Dumenco LL, Moschel RC, Gerson SL (1991) Comparison of the inactivation of mammalian and bacterial O⁶-alkylguanine-DNA alkyltransferases by O⁶-benzylguanine and O⁶-methylguanine. Carcinogenesis 12:2305–2309.
77. Elder RH, Margison GP, Rafferty JA (1994) Differential inactivation of mammalian and Escherichia coli O6-alkylguanine-DNA alkyltransferases by O⁶-benzylguanine. Biochem J 298:231–235.
78. Crone TM, Pegg AE (1993) A single amino acid change in human O⁶-alkylguanine-DNA alkyltransferase decreasing sensitivity to inactivation by O⁶-benzylguanine. Cancer Res 53:4750–4753.
79. Nakatsuru Y, Aoki K, Ishikawa T (1989) Age and strain dependence of O⁶-methylguanine DNA methyltransferase activity in mice. Mutat Res 219:51–56.
80. Gerson SL, Trey JE, Miller K, Berger NA (1986) Comparison of O⁶-alkylguanine-DNA alkyltransferase activity based on cellular DNA content in human, rat and mouse tissues. Carcinogenesis 7:745–749.
81. Dyke GW, Craven JL, Hall R, Garner RC (1993) O⁶-alkyltransferase activity in normal and abnormal gastric mucosa. Cancer Lett 68:169–176.
82. Gerson S, Allay E, Vitantonio K, Dumenco L (1995) Determinants of O⁶-alkylguanine-DNA alkyltransferase activity in human colon cancer. Clin Cancer Res 1:525–534.
83. Silber JR, Mueller BA, Ewers TG, Berger MS (1993) Comparison of O⁶-methylguanine-DNA methyltransferase activity in brain tumors and adjacent normal brain. Cancer Res 53:3416–3420.
84. Zaidi N, Liu L, Gerson S (1995) Cell-type and tissue heterogeneity of O⁶-alkylguanine-DNA alkyltransferase expression in normal and malignant human colon. Proc Am Assoc Cancer Res 36:356.
85. Citron M, Decker R, Chen S, Schneider S, Graver M, Kleynerman L, Kahn LB, White A, Schoenhaus M, Yarosh D (1991) O⁶-methylguanine-DNA methyltransferase in human normal and tumor tissue from brain, lung and ovary. Cancer Res 51:4131–4134.
86. O'Connor P, Fan C, Zaidi SNH, Cooper D (1990) Selective alkylation of cells in rat tissue after treatment with N-nitroso compuunds: Immunohistochemical detection of potential target cells. In Garner RC, Farmer PB, Steel GT, Wright AS, eds. Human Carcinogen Exposure: Biomonitoring and Risk Assessment. Oxford University Press: Oxford, pp 355–362.
87. Swengerg J, Bedell M, Billing K, Umbenhaur D, Pegg A (1982) Cell specific differences in O⁶-alkylguanine repair during continous carcinogen exposure. Proc Natl Acad Sci USA 79:5499–5502.
88. Belinsky SA, Dolan ME, White CM, Maronpot RR, Pegg AE, Anderson MW (1988) Cell specific

differences in O⁶-methylguanine-DNA methyltransferase activity and removal of O⁶-methylguanine in rat pulmonary cells. Carcinogenesis 9:2053–2058.

89. Wani G, Wani AA, D'Ambrosio SM (1992) In situ hybridization of human kidney tissue reveals cell-type-specific expression of the O⁶-methylguanine-DNA methyltransferase gene. Carcinogenesis 13:463–468.

90. Lee SM, Rafferty JA, Elder RH, Fan CY, Bromley M, Harris M, Thatcher N, Potter PM, Altermatt HJ, Perinat-Frey T (1992) Immunohistological examination of the inter- and intracellular distribution of O⁶-alkylguanine DNA-alkyltransferase in human liver and melanoma. Br J Cancer 66:355–360.

91. Wani G, D'Ambrosio S (1995) Differential expression of O⁶-alkylguanine-DNA alkyltransferase gene in normal human breast and skin tissue: In situ mapping of cell specific expression. Mol Carcinogen. 12:177–184.

92. Lee SM, Harris M, Rennison J, McGown A, Bromley M, Elder RH, Rafferty JA, Crowther D, Margison GP (1993) Expression of O⁶-alkylguanine-DNA-alkyltransferase in situ in ovarian and Hodgkin's tumours. Eur J Cancer 9:1306–1312.

93. Belanich M, Ayi T, Li B, Kibitel J, Grob D, Randall T, Citron M, Yarosh D (1994) Analysis of O⁶-methylguanine-DNA methyltransferase in individual human cells by quantitative immunofluorescence microscopy. Oncol Res 6:128–137.

94. Gibson NW, Hartley JA, Barnes D, Erickson LC (1986) Combined effects of streptozotocin and mitozolomide against four human cell lines of the Mer+ phenotype. Cancer Res 46:4995–4998.

95. Zlotogorski C, Erickson LC (1983) Pretreatment of normal human fibroblasts and human colon carcinoma cells with MNNG allows chloroethylnitrosourea to produce DNA interstrand crosslinks not observed in cells treated with chloroethylnitrosourea alone. Carcinogenesis 4:759–763.

96. Dolan ME, Morimoto K, Pegg AE (1985) Reduction of O⁶-alkylguanine-DNA alkyltransferase activity in HeLa cells treated with O⁶-alkylguanines. Cancer Res 45:6413–6417.

97. Dolan ME, Moschel RC, Pegg AE (1990) Depletion of mammalian O⁶-alkylguanine-DNA alkyltransferase activity by O⁶-benzylguanine provides a means to evaluate the role of this protein in protection against carcinogenic and therapeutic alkylating agents. Proc Natl Acad Sci USA 87:5368–5372.

98. Lodich J, Chawla PL, Frei E (1975) 1,3 Bis-(2 chloroethyl)-1-nitrosourea and streptozotocin chemotherapy. Clin Pharmacol Ther 17:374–378.

99. Micetich K, Futscher B, Koch D, Fisher RI, Erickson LC (1992) Phase I study of streptozocin- and carmustine-sequenced administration in patients with advanced cancer. J Natl Cancer Inst 84:256–262.

100. Panella TJ, Smith DC, Schold SC, Rogers MP, Winer EP, Fine RL, Crawford J, Herndon JE2d. Trump DL (1992) Modulation of O⁶-alkylguanine-DNA alkyltransferase-mediated carmustine resistance using streptozotocin: A phase I trial. Cancer Res 52:2456–2459.

101. Willson J, Gerson S, Haaga J, Berger S, Berger N (1992) Biochemical modulation of drug resistance in colon cancers. Am Assoc Cancer Res 33:326.

102. Lee SM, Thatcher N, Margison GP (1991) O⁶-alkylguanine-DNA alkyltransferase depletion and regeneration in human peripheral lymphocytes following dacarbazine and fotemustine. Cancer Res 51:619–623.

103. Gerson S, Zborowska E, Norton K, Gordon N, Willson JKV (1993) Synergistic efficacy of O⁶benzylguanine and BCNU in human colon cancer xenografts completely resistant to BCNU alone. Biochem Pharmacol 46:483–491.

104. Moschel RC, Dolan ME, Stine L, Pegg AE (1992) Structural features of substituted purine derivatives compatible with depletion of human O⁶-alkylguanine-DNA alkyltransferase. J Med Chem 23:4486–4491.

105. Dolan ME, Mitchell RB, Mummert C, Moschel RC, Pegg AE (1991) Effect of O⁶-benzylguanine analogues on sensitivity of human tumor cells to the cytotoxic effects of alkylating agents. Cancer Res 51:3367–3372.

106. Felker GM, Friedman HS, Dolan ME, Moschel RC, Schold C (1993) Treatment of subcutaneous and intracranial brain tumor xenografts with O⁶-benzylguanine and 1,3 bis-chloroethyl 2-nitrosourea, BCNU. Cancer Chemother Pharmacol 32:471–476.

107. Dolan ME, Stine L, Mitchell RB, Moschel RC, Pegg AE (1990) Modulation of mammalian O⁶-alkylguanine-DNA alkyltransferase in vivo by O⁶-benzylguanine and its effect on the sensitivity of a human glioma tumor to 1-(2-chloroethyl)-3-(4-methylcyclohexyl)-1-nitrosourea. Cancer Commun 2:371–377.

108. Marathi UK, Kroes RA, Dolan ME, Erickson LC (1993) Prolonged depletion of O⁶-methylguanine DNA methyltransferase activity following exposure to O⁶-benzylguanine with or without

streptozotocin enhances 1,3-bis(2-chloroethyl)-1-nitrosourea sensitivity in vitro. Cancer Res 53:4281–4286.

109. Gerson SL, Trey JE, Miller K (1988) Potentiation of nitrosourea cytotoxicity in human leukemic cells by inactivation of O⁶-alkylguanine-DNA alkyltransferase. Cancer Res 48:1521–1527.

110. Chen JM, Zhang YP, Wang C, Sun Y, Fujimoto J, Ikenaga M (1992) O⁶-methylguanine-DNA methyltransferase activity in human tumors. Carcinogenesis 13:1503–1507.

111. Dolan ME, Pegg AE, Moschel RC, Grindey GB (1993) Effect of O⁶-benzylguanine on the sensitivity of human colon tumor xenografts to 1,3-bis(2-chloroethyl)-1-nitrosourea (BCNU). Biochem Pharmacol 46:285–290.

112. Dolan ME, Pegg AE, Biser ND, Moschel RC, English HF (1993) Effect of O⁶-benzylguanine on the response to 1,3-bis(2-chloroethyl)-1-nitrosourea in the Dunning R3327G model of prostatic cancer. Cancer Chemother Pharmacol 32:221–225.

113. Mitchell RB, Dolan ME (1993) Effect of temozolomide and dacarbazine on O⁶-alkylguanine-DNA alkyltransferase activity and sensitivity of human tumor cells and xenografts to 1,3-bis(2-chloroethyl)-1-nitrosourea. Cancer Chemother Pharmacol 32:59–63.

114. Friedman HS, Dolan ME, Moschel RC, Pegg AE, Felker GM, Rich J, Bigner DD, Schold S Jr (1992) Enhancement of nitrosourea activity in medulloblastoma and glioblastoma multiforme. J Natl Cancer Inst 84:1926–1931.

115. Mitchell R, Moschel RC, Dolan ME (1992) Effect of O⁶-benzylguanine on the sensitivity of human tumor xenografts to 1,3-bis(2-chloroethyl)-1-nitrosourea and on DNA interstrand cross-link formation. Cancer Res 52:1171–1175.

116. Gerson SL, Trey JE (1988) Modulation of nitrosourea resistance in myeloid leukemias. Blood 71:1487–1494.

117. De Vita V, Carbone P, Owens AH Jr, Gold G, Krant M, Edmonson J (1965) Clinical trials with 1,3-bis(2-chloroethyl)-1-nitrosourea, NSC-409962. Cancer Res 25:1876–1881.

118. Weiss R, Poster D, Penta J (1981) The nitrosoureas and pulmonary toxicity. Cancer Treat Rev 8:111–125.

119. Phillips GL, Fay JW, Herzig GP, Herzig RH, Weiner RS, Wolff SN, Lazarus HM, Karanes C, Ross W, Kramer B (1983) Intensive 1,3-bis(2-chloroethyl)-1-nitrosourea (BCNU), NSC #436650 and cryopreserved autologous marrow transplantation for refractory cancer: A phase I–II study. Cancer 52:1792–1802.

120. Schein P, O'Connell M, Blom J, Hubbard S, Magrath I, Bergevin P, Wiernik P, JL Z, De Vita V (1974) Clinical antitumor activity and toxicity of streptozotocin (NSC-85998). Cancer 34:993–1000.

121. Boice JJ, Greene MH, Killen JY Jr (1983) Leukemia and preleukemia after adjuvant treatment of gastrointestinal cancer with semustine (methylCCNU). N Engl J Med 309:1079–1084.

122. Devereux S, Selassie TG, Hudson GV, Hudson BV, Linch DC (1990) Leukemia complicating treatment for Hodgkin's disease: The experience of the British National Lymphoma Investigation. Bri Med J 301:1077–1080.

123. Dumenco LL, Allay E, Norton K, Gerson SL (1993) The prevention of thymic lymphomas in transgenic mice by human O⁶-alkylguanine-DNA alkyltransferase. Science 259:219–222.

124. Fairbairn L, Watson A, Rafferty J, Elder RH, Margison GP (1994) O⁶-benzylguanine increases the sensitivity of human primary bone marrow cells to the cytotoxic effects of temozolomide. Proc Am Assoc Cancer Res 35:323.

125. Page J, Giles HD, Phillips W, Gerson SL, Smith AC, Tomaszewski JE (1994) Preclinical toxicology study of O⁶-benzylguanine (NSC-637037) and BCNU (Carmustine, NSC-409962) in male and female beagle dogs. Proc Am Assoc Cancer Res 35:328.

126. Liu L, Lee K, Wasan E (1996) Differential Sensitivity of human and mouse alkyltransferase to O⁶-benzylguanine using a transgenic model. Cancer Res 56:1880–1885.

127. Gerson S (1988) Regeneration of O⁶alkylguanine-DNA alkyltransferase in human lymphocytes after nitrosourea exposure. Cancer Res 48:5368–5373.

128. Allay J, Dumenco L, Koc O, Liu L, Gerson S (1995) Retroviral transduction and expression of the human alkyltransferase cDNA provides nitrosourea resistance to hematopoietic cells. Blood 85:3342–3351.

129. Moritz T, Mackay W, Glassner B, Williams D, Samson L (1995) Retrovirus-mediated expression of a DNA repair protein in bone marrow protects hematopoietic cells from nitrosourea-induced toxicity in vitro and in vivo. Cancer Res 55:2608–2614.

130. Cournoyer D, Scarpa M, Mitani K, Moore KA, Markowitz D, Bank A, Belmont JW, Caskey CT (1991) Gene transfer of adenosine deaminase into primitive human hematopoietic progenitor cells. Hum Gene Ther 2:203–213.

131. Karlsson S (1991) Treatment of genetic defects in hematopoietic cll function by gene transfer. Blood 78:2481.
132. Kantoff PW, Gillo AP, MacLachlin JR, Bordignon C, Eglitis MA, Kernan NA, Moen RC, Kohn DB, Yu SF, Karson E (1987) Expression of human adenosine deaminase in nonhuman primates after retrovirus-mediated gene transfer. J Exp Med 166:219.
133. Nienhuis AW, McDonagh KT, Bodine DM (1991) Gene transfer into hematopoietic stem cells. Cancer 67:2700–2704.
134. Hanania EG, Deisseroth AB (1994) Serial transplantation shows that early hematopoietic precursor cells are transduced by MDR-1 retroviral vector in a mouse gene therapy model. Cancer Gene Ther 1:21–25.
135. McLachlin JR, Eglitis MA, Ueda K, Kantoff PW, Pastan IH, Anderson WF, Gottesman MM (1990) Expression of a human complementary DNA for the multidrug resistance gene in murine hematopoietic precursor cells with the use of retroviral gene transfer. Natl Cancer Inst 82:1260–1263.
136. Podda S, Ward M, Himelstein A, Richardson C, de la Flor-Weiss E, Smith L, Gottesman M, Pastan I, Bank A (1992) Transfer and expression of the human multiple drug resistance gene into live mice. Proc Natl Acad Sci USA 89:9676.
137. Sorrentino B, Brandt S, Bodine D, Gottesman M, Pastan I, Cline A, Nienhuis A (1992) Selection of drug-resistant bone marrow cells in-vivo after retroviral transfer of human MDR1. Science 257:99–103.
138. Harris L, Marathi U, Edwards C, Houghton P, Vanin E, Sorrentino B, Brent T (1995) Retroviral transfer of a bacterial alkyltransferase gene into murine bone marrow protects agains nitrosourea cytotoxicity. Proc Am Assoc Cancer Res 36:419.

III. RESISTANCE TO MICROTUBULE ACTIVE DRUGS

6. PACLITAXEL (TAXOL®) MECHANISMS OF RESISTANCE*

ANNA M. CASAZZA AND CRAIG R. FAIRCHILD

INTRODUCTION

Paclitaxel (Taxol #®) is one of the most promising new anticancer agents developed in recent years [1]. Taxol® has been approved for the treatment of refractory ovarian [2,3] and breast cancer [4] in several countries, and has shown activity against after human malignancies, such as lung cancer head and neck cancer, esophageal cancer, hematological malignances, and melanomas. However, even in patients with responding tumors, response rates have not been superior to 50%, and relapses have always been the case, indicating that (1) even among the sensitive tumor types, there are examples of cancers that are naturally resistant to Taxol therapy (and these tumors are defined as having *intrinsic resistance or insensitivity to Taxol*, and (2) treatment with Taxol inexorably leads to development of resistance to paclitaxel (and these tumors are defined as having *acquired resistance to Taxol*). An understanding of the mechanisms of intrinsic or acquired resistance of cancer cells to paclitaxel can result in (1) design of better therapeutic modalities (drug combinations, sequences, schedule of treatment) for the treatment of cancer patients; (2) development of appropriate experimental models that represent as closely as possible the clinical cause of paclitaxel insensitivity or resistance; and (3) identification of novel anticancer drugs, and in particular paclitaxel analogs, active against paclitaxel-resistant cancer cells. An agent active against such tumor cells in vitro and in vivo would, in fact, be an important candidate for clinical development.

*TAXOL® is a registered trademark of Bristol-Myers Squibb Company. The approved generic name for the drug is paclitaxel.
This review is dedicated to the memory of Matt Suffness.

The interest in understanding the mechanisms of insensitivity or resistance of cancer cells to paclitaxel also stems from the fact that some preclinical observations have not been predictive of the clinical findings. For example, one attractive feature of Taxol is its clinical activity in patients resistant to treatment with other agents, such as doxorubicin and cisplatin. However, in experimental models the lack of crossresistance of paclitaxel has been confirmed only with platinum agents (cisplatin, carboplatin) and not with anthracyclines, such as doxorubicin. In addition, one of the most important mechanisms of drug resistance, multiple drug resistance (MDR), has been demonstrated to have a definite role in paclitaxel resistance in experimental models. However, recent observations do not support a firm association of the MDR phenotype and P-gp expression with anticancer drug resistance in the patient. This renders the picture of paclitaxel resistance even more confusing, and its elucidation more challenging.

In this chapter we review the mechanisms of resistance to paclitaxel that have been described so far and discuss their possible clinical relevance, as well as the predictivity of preclinical models and preclinical results for the clinical outcome.

MULTIPLE DRUG RESISTANCE

The first mechanism of paclitaxel resistance to be identified involves the MDR phenotype. This well-studied form of resistance occurs when cells selected for resistance to one of a variety of hydrophobic natural product anticancer agents display a group of common characteristics, such as crossresistance to structurally unrelated drugs, reduced drug accumulation, overexpression of a high molecular weight membrane glycoprotein, and genetic alterations, including gene amplification and overexpression [5,6]. This membrane glycoprotein, called *P-glycoprotein* (P-gp), is energy dependent and acts as a drug efflux pump, which increases the efflux of cytotoxic drugs from the cell, thereby reducing their cytotoxic potency. P-gp is encoded by a small family of *mdr* genes in mammalian cells. Most natural product anticancer agents are affected by this mechanism, such as anthracyclines (doxorubicin and daunorubicin), epipodophyllotoxins (etoposide and teniposide), *Vinca* alkaloids (vincristine and vinblastine), actinomycin D, and several others.

Cells selected for resistance to paclitaxel have been shown to express the MDR phenotype. In early studies by Gupta and Cabral, Chinese hamster ovary (CHO) cells were selected for resistance to paclitaxel in a single-step selection that included mutagenesis, leading to the isolation of cells that were 3- to 10-fold more resistant to paclitaxel and expressed the MDR phenotype [7–9]. These resistant cell lines were termed *permeability mutants*, because of reduced ^{3}H-daunorubicin intracellular accumulation, and were crossresistant to a number of MDR drugs, including vinblastine, doxorubicin, and etoposide. Similar results were obtained in mouse cell lines. When mouse macrophage J774.2 cells were selected for paclitaxel resistance in stepwise increasing concentrations of paclitaxel, the result was a cell line that was highly resistant to paclitaxel (833-fold) [10] and expressed an MDR phenotype, as shown by the crossresistance to doxorubicin, vinblastine, colchicine, and actinomycin D. ^{3}H-paclitaxel accumulation in this resistant cell line was reduced to only 12% of that seen in the parental cell line. A phosphoglycoprotein was found to be highly expressed on the plasma membrane and was later shown by western blotting to be P-gp [11]. The elevated expression of the protein was attributed to overexpression of mRNA for P-gp.

Cell lines that have *not* been selected directly for paclitaxel resistance, but rather for resistance to other MDR anticancer agents, are also crossresistant to paclitaxel. Indeed, oftentimes it has been observed that cells are more resistant to paclitaxel than to the selecting drug. For example, a colon carcinoma cell line, HCT116(VM)46, originally selected for resistance to VM-26 and expressing the MDR phenotype, is 125-fold resistant to paclitaxel, yet is only 10-fold resistant to the selecting agent [12,13]. The reason for particular patterns of crossresistance in cells is unclear. In some instances genetic mutations in the P-gp have been implicated. In a colchicine-selected series of MDR KB cells, preferential resistance to colchicine was observed that resulted from spontaneous mutations in the *mdr*1 gene that produced a single amino acid change at position 185 (glycine to valine) in the human P-gp [14]. Those KB cells that expressed the mutant valine amino acid at position 185 demonstrated increased resistance to colchicine and decreased resistance to vinblastine compared with cells that expressed wild-type P-gp with a glycine at the same position. Subsequently, patterns of drug resistance were compared in transfected KB or NIH3T3 cells that expressed either wild-type or mutant P-gp. Those cells that expressed the wild-type protein were preferentially resistant to vinblastine and paclitaxel, and less resistant to colchicine and etoposide [15,16].

Paclitaxel has been shown to bind to P-gp using a technique based on displacement of photoaffinity analogs such as ^{3}H-azidopine. In MDR J774.2 cells selected for paclitaxel resistance, paclitaxel at a 1,000-fold molar excess reduced ^{3}H-azidopine labeling of P-gp by up to 60%, which was nearly as much as vinblastine and better than colchicine [17]. Although structural conformations of the putative drug binding site on P-gp in the membrane have been postulated, the exact binding site(s) for paclitaxel and other hydrophobic molecules on P-gp remain to be determined. It has also been suggested that mutations at position 185 do not affect the initial binding of drugs to P-gp but may instead affect the release of P-gp–bound drugs to the other side of the membrane [15]. In addition, binding to P-gp may not be the only requirement for transport. In fact, progesterone is able to inhibit the binding to ^{3}H-azidopine to P-gp, but it does not appear to be transported [18,19]. A better understanding of how paclitaxel interacts with P-gp would certainly be useful in designing paclitaxel analogs that would not be transported by this efflux pump.

MDR is one of the possible mechanisms, but not the only mechanism, for resistance to paclitaxel, as described later in this chapter. Of particular relevance are the mechanisms of resistance to paclitaxel that involve tubulin, which is the target of paclitaxel activity. How common is the occurrence of MDR relative to other resistance mechanisms, such as those related to tubulin, in cells selected in vitro for paclitaxel resistance? Several studies have addressed this question directly using single-step selection and clonal isolation of resistant cells. In CHO cells, after single-step selection with paclitaxel, only 10% of the resistant cell lines were permeability (MDR) mutants [9]. These results contrast with those obtained when selecting for resistance using microtubule-disrupting drugs, such as colchicine or maytansine. In this case, permeability mutants with crossresistance to the MDR drug puromycin were the primary type of mutant isolated (70–88%) [20,21]. Therefore, the predominant form of resistance may depend on the type of selecting drug that is used. However, the results of more recent studies using the human sarcoma cell line MES-SA suggest that as many as 40% of the resistant clones isolated from a single-step paclitaxel selection expressed the MDR phenotype [22]. In these single-step selection studies, the non-MDR clones had alterations in tubulin. These results suggest that, even though paclitaxel is quite susceptible to resistance mediated by P-gp, overexpression of P-gp may not be the principal mechanism of resistance for paclitaxel when a single-step selection is used. The situation may be different during longer term stepwise selection for paclitaxel resistance. In this case, indirect evidence suggests that P-gp overexpression is a dominant mechanism of resistance, so much so that when an MDR-reversing agent, such as verapamil, SDZ PSC 833, or Cremophor® EL, was added to the selection regimen, mechanisms of resistance to paclitaxel other than P-gp–mediated MDR were induced [23–25]. These results are discussed in more detail later.

The resistance of MDR tumor cells to paclitaxel has also been observed in in-vivo models. When a panel of resistant P388 leukemia sublines was tested for sensitivity to paclitaxel in vivo, paclitaxel was clearly crossresistant with amsacrine, and marginally crossresistant with doxorubicin, actinomycin D, and mitoxantrone [26]. Therefore, the different pattern of crossresistance between MDR drugs and paclitaxel that was found in vitro was also observed in vivo. Other studies have shown that treatment of tumor cells in vivo with paclitaxel can select for resistant cells that show the MDR phenotype. In mouse M109 lung carcinoma tumors, exposure to paclitaxel in vivo over the course of months resulted in cells that were resistant to paclitaxel both in vivo and in vitro. These cells were shown to overexpress P-gp mRNA and to be crossresistant to vinblastine both in vitro and in vivo, and their paclitaxel resistance was reversed by verapamil in vitro [27]. These resistant M109 cells are discussed in more detail in a later section.

Finally, it is likely that P-gp–mediated resistance to paclitaxel can be exploited. Recent studies have demonstrated that in vivo expression of *mdr*1, transferred by retroviral vector into mouse bone marrow cells, conferred a selective advantage of the cells after treatment of the mice with paclitaxel [28,29]. The results from these experiments suggest a possible new approach for the production of paclitaxel-resistant bone marrow in cancer patients undergoing bone marrow transplantation.

MECHANISMS RELATED TO TUBULIN

As mentioned earlier, in addition to sharing being affected by MDR with other cytotoxic agents, paclitaxel can elicit or be affected by mechanisms of cell resistance that are related to its primary biochemical target, tubulin. One of the biochemical effects of paclitaxel on tumor cells is the induction of tubulin bundles, which can be easily observed after treatment of the cells with paclitaxel, followed by exposure to antibodies to tubulin and to fluorescent double staining. As soon as the clinical activity of Taxol was recognized, studies were conducted to identify biochemical markers that could help select patients who were sensitive to this new drug. One such pioneering study, carried out on four human leukemia cell lines [30], showed that the induction of persistent microtubules bundles in vitro correlated with the cytotoxic effect of paclitaxel. It is important to note that the *persistence* of the bundles, and not the quantitative amount of microtubules organized in bundles, was the differentiating factor between cells with low sensitivity and cells with high sensitivity to paclitaxel.

Cabral carried out extensive studies on paclitaxel resistance by selecting CHO cells for their ability to grow in this drug in a single-step procedure after first mutagenizing the cells. He initially isolated a number of paclitaxel-resistant mutants (with two- to threefold resistance), one of which had an electrophoretic variant of α-tubulin [31]. This suggested that an alteration in α-tubulin could produce resistance to paclitaxel. Indeed, revertants of the mutant cell line simultaneously lost their resistance to paclitaxel and the electrophoretic variant α-tubulin.

In later work, mutants were identified that required paclitaxel to survive [32,33]. These resistant cells, which demonstrated increased sensitivity to colcemid, became rounder, flatter, and multinucleated when deprived of paclitaxel. Furthermore, they accumulated in G2 + M, but leaked through the block, an event that resulted in cells with DNA content increased beyond the tetraploid amount. These observations suggested that the cells were unable to process the increased amount of DNA/chromosomes. It was subsequently demonstrated that the resistant cells were defective in spindle, but not cytoplasmic microtubule, assembly, which suggested an alteration in a spindle-specific tubulin. Indeed, this was the case, as defects in both α and β tubulin were shown to occur in these paclitaxel-dependent cell lines [9].

Taking into account the results of these studies, a model was proposed to explain the properties observed in these resistant cells [34]. The model postulates that mutations in tubulin that lead to resistance to paclitaxel change the conformation of tubulin so that hyperlabile microtubules are produced. These microtubules are able to tolerate a higher concentration of microtubule-stabilizing agent, but they should be more sensitive to microtubule-disrupting agents, such as colchicine or colcemid. On the other hand, mutations that produce colchicine resistance would result in tubulin that is hyperstable and cells that are hypersensitive to paclitaxel. In the paclitaxel-dependent cells, the mutation has resulted in microtubules that are so hyperlabile that they cannot perform their necessary cellular functions. Therefore, the addition of small amounts of paclitaxel is required to stabilize the microtubules enough to rescue the cells. Too much paclitaxel, however, can still be toxic to the cells. Evidence for this model was obtained by direct measurement of the amount of tubulin in the assembled or polymerized state in wild-type CHO cells (ca. 40%) and mutants. Results demonstrated that paclitaxel-resistant cell lines maintained less tubulin in the polymerized form (ca. 28%) and colcemid-resistant cell lines maintain more assembled tubulin (ca. 50%) [35]. The levels of total tubulin and actin were unchanged in the mutant cell lines relative to the parental cell lines. This suggests that the resistance involves alterations in tubulin that affect the assembly properties of the protein in the absence of changes in the total amount of tubulin. The possibility of predicting the sensitivity of a cell to paclitaxel on the basis of the proportion of polymerized tubulin warrants further investigation.

Following these original observations, several cell lines have been reported that are resistant to paclitaxel and show tubulin alterations. The properties of these cell lines are summarized in Table 1. The murine macrophage cell line J7.T1-50, selected for resistance to paclitaxel in vitro, in addition to the P-gp mechanism and MDR phenotype previously described, also shows a twofold increase in the amount of α- and β-tubulin and their corresponding mRNAs in comparison with the parent line J774.2 [36]. Similar to the CHO cell lines described earlier, this cell line is partially dependent on paclitaxel for its growth. To better characterize the tubulin

Table 6–1. Tumor cell lines resistant to paclitaxel that present tubulin alterations

Tumor type	Cell line	MDR	Tubulin	Ref.
Chinese hamster ovary (CHO)	Tax-1 Tax-18 (paclitaxel dependent) Selected in vitro	No	Altered α- and β-tubulin	31, 32
Murine macrophage-like (J774.2)	J7.T1-50 Selected in vitro	Yes	Increased α- and β-tubulin, and MAP-4	36
Human lung carcinoma (H69)	H69/Txl Selected in vitro	No	3rd more acidic α-tubulin species Increase of tubulin acetylation	38
Human bladder carcinoma (J82)	J82-NVB Selected with navelbine	No	Decreased stability of microtubules	40
Human colon carcinoma (HCT116)	HCT116/TX15CR Selected in vitro in presence of Cremophor EL	No	Tubulin less sensitive to polymerization; total tubulin levels are equivalent	25
Human ovarian carcinoma (A 2780)	A2780/PTX Selected in vitro in presence of verapamil	No	Tubulin is decreased or unchanged, but less sensitive to polymerization by paclitaxel	23, 42
Human leukemia (K562)	K562 Selected in vitro in presence of SDZ PSC 833	No	Overexpression of 5β and β2 tubulin isotypes	24, 43
Mouse lung carcinoma (M109)	M109/TXLR1 Selected in vivo	No	Increased tubulin mRNA levels	27
Human sarcoma (MES-SA)	MES-SA Selected in vitro in presence of SDZ PSC 833	No	Overexpression of tubulin isotype 5β	22

isotypes that were found to be increased, additional J774.2 sublines selected in vitro for resistance to paclitaxel or docetaxel were investigated using a polymerase chain reaction (PCR)–based technology [37]. It was found that Mβ5 was increased in all the resistant lines, and Mβ2 was specifically increased in the cell line most resistant to paclitaxel.

Tubulin-related mechanisms of paclitaxel resistance have also been described for the human lung carcinoma cell line H69/Tx that was generated by exposing the parent cells to increasing stepwise paclitaxel concentrations in vitro [38]. The H69/Tx cell line was fourfold resistant to paclitaxel, did not show any difference from the parent line in terms of intracellular paclitaxel amounts nor in amounts of total and polymerized tubulin content, did not express mdr1 mRNA, and was not crossresistant to other MDR agents. Actually, this cell line was hypersensitive to the *Vinca* alkaloids. The only differences from the parent line were that (1) in addition to the two isoforms of α-tubulin that were present in the parent line, the resistant cell line contained one third more acidic α-tubulin species; and (2) there was an increase of tubulin acetylation. Consistent with the finding reported earlier, the H69/Tx cell line was also partially dependent on paclitaxel for its growth.

Another example of resistance to paclitaxel related to changes in tubulin is exemplified by the bladder carcinoma cell line J82-NVB. This cell line was selected for resistance to the *Vinca* alkaloid navelbine [39], did not show the full MDR phenotype, but was crossresistant to *Vinca* alkaloids and taxanes [40]. Analysis of assembly and disassembly of microtubules using immunofluorescence showed that resistant cells had the ability to reassemble their microtubule network after disassembly had been induced by navelbine, suggesting that the mechanism of resistance was related to changes in the microtubules. In this cell line, it was the *stability* of the microtubules that was affected, and not the mass of polymerized microtubules. This important observation is consistent with the observations described earlier for leukemia cell lines [30] and recent information on the mechanism of action of paclitaxel. In fact, according to Jordan et al. [41], at the lowest effective concentrations paclitaxel appears to block mitosis by kinetically stabilizing spindle microtubules, and not by changing the mass of the polymerized microtubules.

In order to avoid the onset of P-gp overexpression and MDR in cells exposed in vitro to paclitaxel, some researchers have combined paclitaxel treatment with an MDR-reversing agent. This approach was first used by Schibler and others [44] using verapamil and paclitaxel in a single-step procedure. These authors found no evidence of altered membrane permeability (based on MDR drug crossresistance patterns), but the resistant clones had well-defined alterations in α- and β-tubulin. Using this approach, a group of non-MDR paclitaxel-resistant cell lines was generated from the human ovarian carcinoma A2780 by treatment in vitro with paclitaxel and verapamil [23,42]. These resistant cells lines were originally reported to have *decreased* tubulin levels [23], but were later found to have unchanged tubulin levels and similar levels of soluble and polymerized tubulin when examined in the absence of paclitaxel [42]. In addition, the three β-tubulin isotypes (M40, β2, 5β) were expressed at comparable levels in sensitive and resistant cells. More importantly, however, it was shown that tubulin in resistant cells was less sensitive to the polymerizing activity of paclitaxel than in sensitive cells [23,42]. It is possible that tubulin in these resistant cells is somewhat unstable, so that increased levels of paclitaxel could be tolerated. This would explain why these cells have increased sensitivity to *Vinca* alkaloids, which destabilize microtubules.

Another set of resistant cell lines was obtained from the K562 erythroleukemia cells through double selection in vitro in the presence of paclitaxel (or vinblastine), and the MDR-reversing agent SDZ PSC 833 [45]. The resistant lines did not exhibit the MDR phenotype and did not overexpress P-gp, but showed overexpression of the β-tubulin isotypes 5β [24]. Recently, these investigators established two additional paclitaxel-resistant cell lines by exposure of the parent human MES-SA sarcoma cell line in vitro to paclitaxel alone, or to paclitaxel in combination with SDZ PSC 833 [43]. Only the cell line selected in the presence of paclitaxel alone was positive for mdr1 mRNA, whereas the line selected with the combined treatment showed alterations in the β-tubulin isotypes 5β and β2.

Another cell line resistant to paclitaxel by non-MDR mechanisms has been obtained in vitro by selection with paclitaxel in combination with Cremophor EL [25]. This cell line, derived from the HCT116 human colon carcinoma cell line, did not overexpress P-gp, was not resistant to *Vinca* alkaloids, did not show reduced ^{3}H-paclitaxel accumulation, and its resistance was not reversed by verapamil. Sensitive and resistant cell lines had the same levels of total tubulin, although tubulin was refractory to polymerization by paclitaxel, an observation that suggests the presence of an altered tubulin.

In an attempt to reproduce in the laboratory the conditions that induce the emergence of resistant cell clones in cell populations treated with Taxol in the clinic, some investigators have chosen to generate tumor lines in which the resistance to paclitaxel is induced by in vivo treatment. With this aim, mice bearing the M109 lung carcinoma, which is sensitive to paclitaxel treatment, were serially treated with paclitaxel [27]. Two paclitaxel-resistant cell lines were generated during two different stages of paclitaxel selection. The first line, M109/TXLR1, generated after treatment with paclitaxel (in Cremophor EL-ethanol) at its maximal tolerated dose of 36 mg/kg/treatment, was resistant to paclitaxel in vivo but not in vitro, did not present any change in mdr1 mRNA expression, nor did it exhibit the MDR phenotype, but showed a 5.5-fold increased levels of tubulin mRNA. The second cell line, M109/TXLR2, was obtained after further treatment with frankly toxic doses of paclitaxel. This line was resistant to paclitaxel in vivo *and* in vitro, and showed the MDR phenotype in terms of crossresistance to other MDR agents, overexpression of P-gp mRNA, and reversal of resistance by verapamil.

The results of these experiments suggest that the presence of Cremophor EL in the Taxol formulation may favor the selection in patients of non-MDR paclitaxel-resistant tumor cells, which probably have mechanisms of resistance related to tubulin alterations. The importance of these findings in view of a rationale use of Taxol in the clinc will be addressed later in this chapter when discussing the utility (or lack of utility) of combining MDR-reversing agents with Taxol treatment.

Changes in tubulin levels can also cause increased sensitivity (collateral sensitivity) to paclitaxel. The human ovarian carcinoma cell subline 2008/C13 * 5.25 is 11-fold resistant to cisplatin and is crossresistant to colchicine, but is hypersensitive to paclitaxel [46,47]. Interestingly, this cell line showed a 45% decrease in the amount of membrane-associated β-tubulin, as compared with the parent line, whereas the levels of α-tubulin were unchanged. Similarly, the cisplatin-resistant cell line KB-CP20 showed changes in cytoskeletal distribution and dynamics, in particular a decrease in tubulin levels [48]. In another pair of cisplatin-sensitive and -resistant cell lines, no paclitaxel hypersensitivity and no change in β-tubulin content were observed, indicating that cisplatin-resistant and paclitaxel-hypersensitive phenotypes do not segregate together, but that paclitaxel hypersensitivity could be related to the decrease in β-tubulin content. An intriguing finding was that paclitaxel efflux was slower, and paclitaxel seemed to be more extensively bound to the cell in the paclitaxel-hypersensitive 2008/C13 * 5.25 cell line than in the parent 2008 cell line.

Together, these data indicate that the activity of paclitaxel can be modulated by the amount of tubulin in the cell. In general, non-MDR paclitaxel-resistant cell lines showed increased levels of tubulin, and cell lines with decreased levels of tubulin had increased sensitivity to paclitaxel. Cisplatin treatment seems to decrease the levels of intracellular tubulin. This could explain why tumors resistant to cisplatin have high sensitivity to paclitaxel.

Is there a correlation between drug efflux and tubulin-related mechanisms of resistance to paclitaxel? The murine macrophage cell line described earlier [36], which shows both tubulin modifications as well as P-gp overexpression and enhanced paclitaxel efflux, can be more than an isolated case. Recent observations seem to suggest a relation between membrane alterations related to drug efflux and tubulin alterations. The gastric carcinoma cell line EPG85-257NOV was obtained from the parent line by continuous incubation in vitro in the presence of stepwise increasing concentrations of mitoxantrone [49]. This cell line did not show the biochemical and phenotypic properties of MDR cell lines but was crossresistant to doxorubicin, daunorubicin, and paclitaxel (but not to other MDR drugs). The following structural changes were found to be associated with the emergence of drug resistance [49,50]: intensive formation of surface vesicles that contained the resistance-inducing drug, and appeared to be expelled from the cell, suggesting an increase in vesicular transport [49]; differences in the distribution of microtubules, with a denser network in resistant than in sensitive cells; and the presence of cell surface elements not present on sensitive cells (such as microvillous-like processes and cup-shaped protrusions) [50].

These findings show that drug efflux from resistant tumor cells can be mediated by intracellular vesicular transport and that changes in this form of transport can be associated with tubulin changes, suggesting a role of microtubule function in drug transport. However, not all paclitaxel-resistant cell lines with altered tubulin have reduced paclitaxel accumulation. Accumulation studies were performed using the non-MDR A2780/Tax22 cells described earlier [42], which have tubulin that is refractory to polymerization by paclitaxel. Drug accumulation studies using these cells and the parental A2780 cell line demonstrated that ^{3}H-paclitaxel accumulated to levels that were about 50% *higher* in the resistant cell line than in the sensitive cell line after 1 hour of drug incubation (C. Fairchild, unpublished observation). In the paclitaxel-resistant, non-MDR cell line HCT116/Tax15CR [25], the resistant and parental HCT116 cells had equivalent levels of ^{3}H-paclitaxel accumulation after 1 hour exposure to the drug.

In other studies it has been found that tumor cells made resistant to estramustine, a drug that acts by stabilizing polymerized tubulin, are drug uptake and/or efflux mutants. The change in intracellular drug concentration is not associated with P-gp changes, but rather with microtubular associated protein (MAP) overexpression [51]. These cells are not crossresistant to paclitaxel, but are cited here as an example of drug-resistant cells that show decreased intracellular drug concentrations independent of the classic MDR phenotype.

Modulation of tubulin constitutes a mechanism of resistance to another class of compounds that act on tubulin—colchicine and its derivatives. Tubulin mutations have been reported in CHO cells resistant to colchicine or colcemid [52,53], and reduced tubulin levels have been reported in cells treated with colchicine or nocodazole, another tubulin-interacting compound [54]. The reduction of tubulin levels was attributed to feedback inhibition of tubulin synthesis by unpolymerized tubulin accumulating in cells treated with the above-mentioned compounds, which, in contrast to paclitaxel, inhibit tubulin polymerization. Therefore, one is tempted to speculate that in cells treated with paclitaxel, the decreased levels of unpolymerized tubulin found in paclitaxel-resistant cells could cause an increase in tubulin synthesis.

Whatever the mechanism of paclitaxel resistance, either tubulin alterations or MDR or both, one important question that arises is whether the molecular changes occur due to spontaneous mutation or to induction by the chemotherapeutic treatment. As reported earlier, results of an in vitro study in MES-SA human sarcoma cells support a mechanism of spontaneous mutation rather than induction [22].

OTHER MECHANISMS

GSH

The possible role of glutathione in tumor cell resistance to paclitaxel is still controversial, and conflicting experimental data have so far emerged on this subject. It has been reported that depletion of cellular GSH (glutathione) by L-BSO (L-buthionine sulfoximine) results in resistance to paclitaxel in two human carcinoma cell lines. This effect was accompanied by an increase in the S-phase fraction in paclitaxel-treated cells, whereas no variation in the intracellular paclitaxel concentration was observed [55]. GSH works, in general, as a detoxification molecule, and increased levels of intracellular GSH are often associated with resistance to several anticancer drugs, such as anthracyclines and especially platinum-containing compounds. The observation that paclitaxel is more active when cells have high levels of GSH is therefore of great interest and could explain the clinical effect of paclitaxel in patients resistant to most other anticancer drugs. However, a contradictory observation has been reported [56]. A human ovarian carcinoma cell line selected in vitro for cisplatin resistance showed increased intracellular levels of glutathione. This line was crossresistant to several anticancer agents, including paclitaxel.

In addition to those related to GSH, other biochemical mechanisms may be the basis for the increased sensitivity to paclitaxel by cisplatin-resistant cells. For example, a human ovarian carcinoma cell line selected for resistance in vitro to cisplatin (41M/cisR) showed collateral sensitivity to both paclitaxel and docetaxel in vitro [57]. This cell line is reported to be resistant to cisplatin because of reduced cisplatin uptake.

Oncogenes and tumor suppressor genes

A very important area of investigation in the field of anticancer drug sensitivity and cell transformation is related to the role of apoptosis (see Chapter 14). The p53 and bcl-2 genes have been shown to regulate apoptosis and, in turn, to directly affect the sensitivity of cells to anticancer agents, including paclitaxel. The protein encoded by the p53 gene is a member of a larger family of so-called tumor suppressors, because of their ability to arrest cell growth, and consequently tumor development, when the cell or its DNA has been damaged. The arrest in cell growth allows the cell time to repair the damage; however, should the cells be unable to repair the DNA, the result would be progression to apoptotic cell death. Thus it is likely that the p53 tumor suppressor gene plays an important role in apoptosis, and the absence of normal p53 expression can lead to resistance to anticancer drugs, such as VP-16 and doxorubicin, that act by induction of apoptosis [58,59]. Because p53 is often mutated in human cancer, this may be an important factor in response to therapy.

Recent investigations on the influence of p53 status on the sensitivity of cells to paclitaxel portray a different picture. The results from these studies suggest that, in contrast to DNA-damaging agents, increased sensitivity to paclitaxel occurs with loss of p53 function. Fibroblasts from transgenic mice with homozygous p53 deletion were more sensitive to paclitaxel in vitro than the matched wild-type counterparts and normal mouse embryo fibroblasts [60]. In addition, when normal fibroblasts were depleted of functional p53 by expression of either SV40 (which complexes with p53) or human papilloma virus type 16 E6 (which targets p53 for degradation), the cells became six- to eightfold more sensitive to paclitaxel than untransfected cells [61]. Fibroblasts with diminished p53 function arrested in G2 and underwent apoptosis, in contrast to resistant fibroblasts with intact p53, which progressed through mitosis and arrested in the subsequent G1. The implication is that, in addition to surveillance for DNA damage, p53 may be involved in protection from microtubule disorganization and, as has recently been shown [62], could initiate a protective mitotic checkpoint control.

If confirmed in vivo, these results are of extreme importance and suggest that activity against p53-null or p53-mutated cells can be another mechanism by which Taxol exerts its activity in cancer patients who have developed resistance to other chemotherapeutic agents. These results also suggest that p53 may operate in vivo to protect normal cells from the cytotoxic action of paclitaxel, and may explain why in some studies paclitaxel was found to be much more cytotoxic in vitro for tumor cells than for normal (fibroblast) cells. However, this observation does not seem to apply to all experimental models. When the in vitro sensitivity of primary human mammary epithelial cells to paclitaxel was compared with that of MCF-7 breast carcinoma cells, the sensitivity of each of these cells was equivalent (Fairchild, unpublished observation). Additional studies, and in particular in vivo studies, are needed to better understand the relationship between the status of the p53 suppressor gene and sensitivity to paclitaxel (see Chapter 14).

The Bcl-2 protein has been demonstrated, in some systems, to be able to block apoptotic cell death through p53-dependent and p53-independent pathways and, in other systems, to block apoptosis mediated by chemotherapy [63]. Bcl-x is a member of the Bcl-2 family of genes, and one of its alternately spliced forms, Bcl-x_s, acts as a dominant inhibitor of Bcl-2. When MCF-7 cells were transfected with Bcl-x_s in order to decrease Bcl-2 levels, the MCF-7 cells became 5- to 10-fold more sensitive to apoptosis and cytotoxicity induced by VP-16 or paclitaxel than cells transfected with a control plasmid [64]. These studies suggest that Bcl-2 could also play a role in determining the sensitivity of tumor cells to paclitaxel.

An interesting correlation between expression of c-*myc* and sensitivity to paclitaxel in vitro has been recently reported [65]. In this study, sublines of the Chinese hamster lung fibroblasts cell line DC-3F resistant to 9-OH-ellipticine or to actinomycin D were less tumorigenic than the parent line and showed reduced levels of c-*myc* amplification and overexpression in comparison with those of the parent line. When one of the resistant sublines was transfected with the plasmid pSV-c-myc, the level of c-*myc* expression was again increased, but tumorigenicity was not restored. However, resistance to MDR drugs, including paclitaxel, was reversed, roughly in proportion to the expression of the transfected myc. These results suggest that there can be a correlation between c-*myc* expression and paclitaxel resistance, independent of the effect that c-*myc* expression can have with regard to cell transformation.

WHAT IS THE CAUSE OF CLINICAL RESISTANCE TO PACLITAXEL?

The role of MDR in the clinical resistance to anticancer agents has recently been the subject of animated and interesting debates, and this topic was the subject of a special session at the annual meeting of the American Association for Cancer Research (April 10–13, 1994). In particular, contrasting data have been obtained that can support or negate the importance of this mechanism in the clinical resistance or insensitivity to Taxol. We will briefly summarize these studies.

Paclitaxel is active in tumor populations resistant to treatment with anticancer compounds that are often associated with P-gp–mediated MDR. In particular, lack of clinical crossresistance of Taxol with anthracyclines has been reported in breast carcinoma patients [66]. In this study, responses were at least as frequent in anthracycline-resistant (30%) as in anthracycline-sensitive (19%) patients. Recently these authors have reported on an even more extensive experience [4]. A large group of breast cancer patients previously treated with anthracyclines, and either resistant or refractory to this therapy, were given high-dose Taxol together with granulocyte colony-stimulating factor. Fifty-two patients received Taxol at 200 mg/m^2, and 25 patients received Taxol at 250 mg/m^2. A major objective response was observed in 33% of patients, independent of the outcome of previous anthracycline treatment. In another study, Taxol administered by a 96 hour infusion at a dose of 140 mg/m^2, without concomitant granulocyte colony-stimulating factor administration, was active in breast cancer patients refractory to doxorubicin or mitoxantrone, with a response rate of 48% [67]. In this study, *mdr*1 expression was evaluated in accessible biopsies from 12 patients by detecting total mRNA by PCR. There was no correlation between *mdr*1 level and response to Taxol. These authors attributed the success of the treatment to the long infusion time. However, Taxol can be very effective also when given in a short-term infusion. For example, in another study, Taxol administered at 175 mg/m^2 by a 3 hour infusion produced a 47% response rate in a group of 15 advanced breast cancer patients resistant to anthracyclines [68]. The clinical activity of Taxol in breast cancer patients resistant to anthracyclines has therefore been demonstrated in several studies.

Is the clinical activity supported by biochemical/mechanistic findings on cancer cells from resistant patients?

This question has received the attention of several investigators, and numerous studies are presently in progress whose results will contribute to a better understanding of the mechanisms underlying Taxol resistance in the clinic. The preliminary results reported thus far in the literature (mainly in the form of meeting abstracts) do not provide a clear answer to this question.

In an in vitro study on 20 ovarian cancer specimens from predominantly untreated patients, it was found that 5 of 20 specimens were *mdr*1 or P-gp positive, and were less sensitive to paclitaxel treatment than the negative specimens, supporting a role of MDR in patient insensitivity to paclitaxel [69]. Similarly, the response to Taxol correlated with low levels of *mdr*1 gene expression in a group of patients with metastatic breast cancer treated with Taxol at dose of 135 mg/m^2 administered as a 24 hour infusion, in which an overall 23% response rate was observed [70]. In a recent study, Taxol had limited activity (17% partial responses) in relapsed non-Hodgkin's lymphoma patients who had detectable, albeit low, levels of the *mdr*1 gene, suggesting that low levels of P-gp could cause resistance to Taxol [71].

However, contrasting results were reported by other investigators. Expression of *mdr*1, as determined by quantitative PCR, was low in 20 patients tumor samples obtained before Taxol treatment, and did *not* correlate with response [72]. When the tumors from seven anthracycline-resistant breast cancer patients were examined for *mdr*1 gene expression, little or no immunoreactivity with antibodies to P-gp was found, indicating that overexpression of P-gp may not have played a role in anthracycline resistance. However, these patients did not respond to Taxol treatment, and P-gp immunoreactivity increased in 2 of 2 patients who progressed during Taxol treatment [73].

In this regard, it must be recalled that other biochemical mechanisms can be present at the same time in a cell population and in the same cells that express the MDR phenotype. For example, resistance to anthracyclines and epipodophyllotoxins can be due to so-called atypical MDR, which is sustained by reduced intracellular levels of topoisomerase II, without overexpression of P-gp. We have previously described an HCT116 human colon carcinoma subline [12] that is resistant to doxorubicin and etoposide because of low levels of topoisomerase II, and does not express the MDR phenotype. This cell line showed no resistance to paclitaxel treatment in vitro [13] or in vivo (W. Rose, personal communication). A similar result has been reported with docetaxel, which was found to maintain its activity against cell lines resistant to other chemotherapeutic agents because of modified activities of topoisomerase I and II [74]. This result shows that activity against atypical-MDR tumors is a property common to other taxanes, besides paclitaxel.

Another biochemical mechanism that can make tumor cells resistant to chemo-therapeutic agents is related to MRP. The gene for this membrane-associated protein, when transfected into human carcinoma cell lines, was able to confer resistance to several compounds that are also affected by the MDR mechanism, such as anthracyclines, epipodophyllotoxins, and tubulin-binding agents, such as vincristine and colchicine, but not (or only at a very low level) to paclitaxel [75,76]. This extremely interesting result again demonstrates that the pattern of cross-resistance between paclitaxel and the above-mentioned agents, in particular anthracyclines, is not complete.

Not only may anthracycline-resistant tumor cells be sensitive to paclitaxel, but they may even have increased sensitivity to the latter. In fact, increased levels of GSH, probably due to increased levels of the detoxification enzymes GSH peroxidase and GSH S-transferase [77], can confer resistance to anthracyclines and could actually increase the sensitivity to paclitaxel, as reported earlier [55].

In agreement with the hypothesis that P-gp–mediated MDR is not the only mechanism that confers anthracycline resistance in patients, low levels of P-gp were detected before Taxol treatment was initiated in a group of seven anthracycline-resistant patients with advanced breast cancer [70]. However, P-gp levels increased in 2 of 2 patients who ultimately progressed on Taxol, suggesting that P-gp may have not played a role in anthracyclines resistance but could be easily induced by Taxol treatment in patients.

Efforts to use laboratory techniques to predict the sensitivity of ovarian carcinoma to treatment with Taxol have been reported. In a study of 1,500 ovarian tumor specimens, 23% of the untreated tumors exhibited extreme drug resistance to paclitaxel in a thymidine incorporation assay in soft agar [78]. This percentage increased to 33% when the tumor was taken from the patient after chemotherapy with various agents, including MDR drugs. These observations suggest that induction of P-gp by previous treatment could be responsible for Taxol-induced resistance, but only in a small percentage of patients [78]. In order to evaluate the role of P-gp in drug resistance, a subset of tumors was characterized for increased P-gp expression and was correlated with intrinsic and acquired resistance. The percentage of P-gp–positive tumors increased from 19% in previously untreated patients to 29% in previously treated patients, suggesting that P-gp–mediated MDR can play a role in both intrinsic and acquired resistance to paclitaxel. However, the percent inhibition in vitro by paclitaxel at 1 μg/ml was approximately 45% in P-gp–positive tumor specimens and was approximately 65% in P-gp–negative tumor specimens. The fact that growth inhibition by paclitaxel of P-gp–positive and P-gp–negative patient tumors differs only slightly suggests that the level of MDR-related resistance to paclitaxel in clinical tumor specimens is low.

In order to define the pattern of chemosensitivity of cells from ovarian carcinoma patients who were insensitive or developed resistance to Taxol, human ovarian carcinoma xenografts (HOCs) directly derived from Taxol-treated patients were established in the peritoneal cavity of nude mice [79]. In general, paclitaxel administered intravenously is very active against intraperitoneal HOCs derived from paclitaxel-naive patient tumors, and is able to cure or induce complete responses in a high percentage of the animals at the maximal tolerated dose of 34.5 mg/kg/ treatment, and also at the lower dose of 20 mg/kg/treatment if treatment is initiated early after tumor transplant [80]. The HOCs derived from Taxol-resistant or -insensitive patients seems to maintain sensitivity to paclitaxel treatment in the animal, but the sensitivity was somewhat reduced: one of the HOCs investigated, HOC 79, was sensitive to the highest paclitaxel dose of 34.5 mg/kg/treatment but was much less sensitive to the lower dose of 20 mg/kg/treatment. Additional tumors are presently being investigated. If confirmed, these results again suggest that tumors from Taxol-resistant patients have a low level of resistance, which can be very difficult to maintain and to characterize biochemically in experimental systems, and that Taxol-resistant patients could be sensitive to treatment with higher doses of Taxol. It is interesting to see that a clinical approach that takes into consideration these observations is now being implemented [81].

It has been reported that Taxol has an impressive anticancer effect in the clinic when administered as a long-term infusion. Whether this approach can also increase the activity to a level that would make this drug effective against resistant tumors is not yet clear. Clearly, the activity of taxanes in preclinical models is both time and concentration dependent. This has been well demonstrated in studies in vitro with docetaxel [82] and paclitaxel [83], and in vivo with paclitaxel [84–86]. In addition, longer exposure to paclitaxel partially reversed drug resistance in an MDR breast carcinoma cell line in vitro [87]. In one study, results from in vitro investigation on the activity of paclitaxel in a panel of tumor cell lines that were either established or freshly derived from a patient led to the suggestion that the ratio of paclitaxel exposure time to the culture doubling time was a major factor in cytotoxicity [88]. Additional clinical trials are presently in progress to verify the hypothesis that the activity of Taxol can be modulated by the duration of exposure.

RESISTANCE REVERSAL

Several classes of compounds have been shown to be effective in reversing MDR by blocking the efflux of MDR agents. These compounds include calcium channel blockers (verapamil), phenothiazine calmodulin (thoridazine), indole alkaloids (reserpine), bisbenzylisoquinoline alkaloids (chloroquine), and cyclosporins [5]. Many reversing agents inhibit the binding of photoaffinity labels to P-gp, and in particular verapamil has been shown to bind to P-gp. Indeed, verapamil, cyclosporin A, and its derivative SDZ PSC 833, the semisynthetic cyclopeptolide SDZ 280-446, and transflupenthixol have been shown to substantially reverse paclitaxel resistance in cells that overexpress P-gp [89–91]. These compounds appear to restore sensitivity by maintaining intracellular drug accumulation, suggesting a direct interaction with P-gp [15,92]. However, the possibility that these agents act through P-gp–independent mechanisms, such as through alterations of cell membrane fluidity, that cause increased permeability has been raised [93].

Clinical studies are in progress to evaluate the possible advantages of associating an MDR-reversing agent with Taxol. Preliminary results are not very encouraging. In a phase I study, no remissions were observed in a group of 19 Taxol-resistant patients treated with Taxol in combination with cyclosporin [94]. As discussed earlier, mechanisms of resistance to MDR agents are not limited to P-gp overexpression, and this could explain why MDR-reversing agents have not yet been very successful in clinical trials.

Interestingly, Cremophor EL, which is included in the Taxol formulation as a solubilizing agent, is able to reverse paclitaxel resistance mediated by P-gp in cells in culture and may account for the pattern of resistance that emerges following clinical treatment (see earlier). Cremophor EL is a polyoxyethylated castor oil, reported to have low toxicity in several animals but to evoke a profound clinical syndrome in dogs that is similar the pharmacological effects of histamine [95]. Similar to other surfactants, Cremophor EL was able to reverse the MDR phenotype in vitro, and this effect was associated with increased intracellular drug concentrations [96]. In particular, Cremophor EL has been reported to reverse paclitaxel resistance in murine C1300 multidrug-resistant neuroblastoma cells in vitro [97,98] and in two MDR human breast carcinoma cell lines [99]. The effect was seen at concentrations of 0.003–0.1%, and was reported to be maximal at the subtoxic concentration of 0.03% [97]. At this concentration, Cremophor EL increased the intracellular paclitaxel concentration in the resistant cells by 61%; however, drug efflux did not seem to be affected.

Paired sensitive and resistant human tumor cell lines (derived from the same parental line) offer the advantage of providing reproducible experimental models and allow a better characterization of the biochemical mechanism of resistance. The effect of Cremophor EL was therefore recently investigated in an MDR HCT116 human colon carcinoma cell line, HCT116(VM)46 [100]. This resistant cell line shows more than 100-fold resistance to paclitaxel [12]. The IC_{50} of Cremophor EL in this cell line was 0.077%. Cremophor EL was able to reverse the resistance to paclitaxel in the HCT116(VM)46 cells from 125-fold to 4-fold at a nontoxic concentration of 0.03%. At lower concentrations of Cremophor EL, the resistance reversal was reduced. The results obtained in this study show that Cremophor EL is able to substantially, but only partially, overcome MDR in vitro.

It has been reported that the plasma concentrations of Cremophor EL immediately after 3 hours infusion of Taxol doses of 135 mg/m^2 or 175 mg/m^2 were sufficient to inhibit the activity of the P-gp drug efflux pump associated with the MDR phenotype [101]. This suggests that enough Cremophor EL may be present to affect P-gp–mediated paclitaxel efflux in patient tumors. However, the degree to which these plasma levels would reverse resistance, what quantities of Cremophor EL might be present in the tumors, and the pharmacokinetics of Cremophor EL relative to Taxol remain to be determined.

Some experimental data have been reported suggesting that Cremophor EL, which is cytotoxic by itself, could increase the cytotoxicity of paclitaxel not only against the MDR tumor cells, but also against "sensitive" tumor cells [102]. However, others have reported the opposite effect, that is, Cremophor EL at a concentration of 0.135% was able to antagonize the cytotoxic effect of paclitaxel in vitro against two human carcinoma cell lines in a clonogenic assay [84,103]. In fact, Cremophor EL at the concentration of 0.135% was able to block cells in G1, preventing the entry of the cells into mitosis, and therefore antagonizing the cytotoxicity of paclitaxel, which is more active against dividing than against resting cells [104]. In our experiments, Cremophor EL was not able to potentiate the effect of paclitaxel in vitro against sensitive cell lines when used at a nontoxic concentration of 0.03%, and the activity of paclitaxel in Cremophor EL or in DMSO was similar [100].

Only limited in vivo studies have been so far reported in which the effect of paclitaxel against MDR tumor models was tested in the presence or absence of Cremophor EL. It has been reported that paclitaxel in DMSO is less active than in Cremophor EL-ethanol against a P388 mouse leukemia cell line resistant to vincristine. However, the addition of Cremophor EL to the paclitaxel formulation did not completely overcome the resistance, and no effect was seen in a similar doxorubicin-resistant cell line [105].

At Bristol-Myers Squibb (BMS), paclitaxel in the Cremophor EL-ethanol-saline (12.5/12.5/75) was not active against two sublines of P388, one resistant to doxorubicin (a classic MDR subline) and another resistant to mitomycin C by an undetermined mechanism [106]. In addition, paclitaxel in the Cremophor EL-ethanol-saline vehicle was not active against the HCT116(VM)46 tumor line transplanted subcutaneously into nude mice (W. Rose, personal communication). Therefore, the presence of Cremophor EL was not able to allow paclitaxel to become active in these tumor models. It is possible that a slight increase in paclitaxel accumulation (61% in the MDR neuroblastoma cells described earlier above [97]) can produce partial reversal of paclitaxel resistance in MDR cells in vitro, but not in an in vivo model. However, it should be noted that these tumor models are characterized by a very high level of drug resistance, which is much higher than the level most likely to be present in the clinic.

With regard to the possible role of Cremophor EL in the antitumor activity of paclitaxel against "sensitive" tumors, in studies done at BMS, comparable activity in the intraperitoneal P388 and in the subcutaneous M109 model was observed following treatment with paclitaxel solubilized in ethanol plus Tween 80 or ethanol plus Cremophor EL, or using paclitaxel administered intravenously in 5% or 12.5% Cremophor EL plus matching percent ethanol solutions [106]. In addition, data generated at the National Cancer Institute demonstrated that suspensions of paclitaxel were just as effective as paclitaxel solutions in Cremophor EL-ethanol against intraperitoneal P388 [102]. In vitro, Tween 80 was also able to reverse MDR in HCT116(VM)46 cells to a degree comparable with Cremophor EL [100].

On the basis of these experimental results, we conclude that the possibility, advanced by some authors [107], that Cremophor EL has a role in the antitumor activity of paclitaxel, in particular against resistant tumor cells, is very low.

CONCLUSIONS

Taxol is an extremely interesting and novel anticancer agent. It has a unique mechanism of action and shows activity in patients affected by carcinomas resistant or refractory to other therapies. The reason for the clinical success of Taxol could reside, in part, in the following two properties: (1) its mechanism and (2) its activity against resistant forms of cancer, which are possibly related.

The major mechanisms of resistance to paclitaxel thus far identified have been described in this chapter. Among the first mechanisms of resistance to paclitaxel to be identified was the overexpression of P-gp, which results in the MDR phenotype. However, it seems that this mechanism is favored in experimental models in which resistance occurs after repeated exposure to paclitaxel in the absence of Cremophor EL (which is an important component of the clinical vehicle) or at very high and toxic paclitaxel doses. When clinical conditions were mimicked in experimental models, the mechanism of resistance to paclitaxel that emerged first was related to tubulin changes, as shown by in vivo studies on the M109 lung carcinoma. In addition, tumor cells from cancer patients resistant or insensitive to paclitaxel have a low level of resistance when transplanted in vivo in nude mice. These observations suggest that in the clinic resistance or insensitivity to paclitaxel is related to tubulin changes rather than to selection or induction of the MDR phenotype. Indeed, investigations done on tumor samples from treated patients seem to favor this hypothesis, and cotreatment with MDR-reversing agents has not yet been very successful.

If clinical resistance to Taxol occurs at a low level, it may be overcome by increasing the dose of the drug. Clinical studies are in progress, or are being planned, in which Taxol is administered in conjunction with therapies aimed at protection of the bone marrow (which is the major target organ for Taxol), either with colony stimulating factors or with transfection of bone marrow cells with genes conferring the MDR phenotype. These approaches seem very promising and have the potential to result in an increase in the therapeutic activity of Taxol.

REFERENCES

1. Suffness M, Wall M (1995) Discovery and Development of Taxol. In Taxol, Science and Application. Boca Raton, FL: Ed. by M. Suffness CRC Press, pp 3–26.

2. Caldas C, McGuire WP (1993) Paclitaxel (Taxol) therapy in ovarian carcinoma. Semin Oncol 20:50–55.
3. Ozols RF (1994) Treatment of ovarian cancer: Current status. Semin Oncol 21:1–9.
4. Seidman AD, Reichman BS, Crown JPA, Yao T-J, Currie V, Hakes TB, Hudis CA, Gilewski TA, Baselga J, Forsythe P, Lepore J, Marks L, Fain K, Souhrada M, Onetto N, Arbuck S, Norton L (1995) Paclitaxel as second and subsequent therapy for metastatic breast cancer: Activity independent of prior anthracycline response. J Clin Oncol 13:1152–1159.
5. Gottesman MM, Pastan I (1993) Biochemistry of multidrug resistance mediated by the multidrug transporter. Annu Rev Biochem 62:385–427.
6. Childs S, Ling V (1994) The MDR superfamily of genes and its biological implications. In VT DeVita, S Hellman, SA Rosenberg, eds. Important Advances in Oncology. Philadelphia: JB Lippincot, pp 21–36.
7. Gupta RS (1983) Taxol resistant mutants of Chinese hamster ovary cells genetic biochemical and cross resistance studies. J Cell Physiol 114:137–144.
8. Gupta RS (1985) Cross-resistant of vinblastine and taxol-resistant mutants of Chinese hamster ovary cells to other anticancer drugs. Cancer Treat Rep 69:515–522.
9. Schibler MJ, Cabral F (1986) Taxol-dependent mutants of Chinese hamster ovary cells with alterations in α and β-tubulin. J Cell Biol 102:1522–1531.
10. Roy SN, Horwitz SB (1985) A phosphoglycoprotein associated with taxol resistance in J774.2 cells. Cancer Res 45:3856–3863.
11. Greenberg LM, Lothstein L, Williams SS, Horwitz S (1988) Distinct P-glycoprotein precursors are overproduced in independently isolated drug-resistant cells lines. Proc Natl Acad Sci USA 85:3762–3766.
12. Long B, Wang L, Lorico A, Wang RCC, Brattain MG, Casazza AM (1991) Mechanisms of resistance to etoposide and teniposide in acquired resistant human colon and lung carcinoma cell lines. Cancer Res 51:5275–5284.
13. Fairchild C (1992) Taxol in vitro cytotoxicity studies performed at Bristol-Myers Squibb. Bristol-Myers Squibb Internal Report 50323.
14. Choi K, Chen CJ, Kriegler M, Roninson IB (1988) An altered pattern of cross-resistance in multidrug-resistant cells results from spontaneous mutations in the mdr1 P-gp gene. Cell 53:519–529.
15. Safa AR, Stern RK, Choi K, Agresti M, Tamai I, Mehta ND, Roninson IB, Zhan Z, Kang Y-K, Giannakakov P, Villalba L, Walendowski E, Poruchynski M, Wilsom W, Bates S, Fojo T (1990) Molecular basis of preferential resistance to colchicine in multidrug-resistant human cells conferred by Gly-185 to Val-185 substitution in P-glycoprotein. Proc Natl Acad Sci USA 87:7225–7229.
16. Cardarelli CO, Akesntijevich I, Pastan I, Gottesman MM (1995) Differential effects of P-glycoprotein inhibitors on NIHSTS cells transfected with wild type (G185) or mutant (V185) multidrug transporters. Cancer Res 55:1086–1091.
17. Yang CPH, Mellado W, Horwitz SB (1988) Azidopine photoaffinity labeling of multidrug resistance-associated glycoproteins. Biochem Pharmacol 37:1417–1421.
18. Yang CPH, DePinho SG, Greenberger LM, Arceci RJ, Horwitz SB (1989) Progesterone interacts with p-glycoprotein in multidrug-resistant cells and in the endometrium of gravid uterus. J Biol Chem 264:782–788.
19. Ueda K, Okamura N, Hirai M, Tanigawara Y, Saeki T, Kioka N, Komano T, Hori R (1992) Human p-glycoprotein transports cortisol, aldosterone, and dexamethasone, but not progesterone. J Biol Chem 267:24248–24252.
20. Cabral F, Sobel M, Gottesman M (1980) CHO mutants resistant to colchicine, colcemid or griseofulvine have an altered b-tubulin. Cell 20:29–36.
21. Schibler M, Cabral F (1985) Maytansine-resistant mutants of Chinese hamster ovary cells with an alteration in alpha-tubulin. Can J Biochem Cell Biol 63:503–510.
22. Dumontet CM, Duran GE, Sikic BI (1995) Mechanisms of resistance to paclitaxel (Taxol, TAX) in human sarcoma mutants derived by single-step selection. Proc Am Assoc Cancer Res 36:320.
23. Zhan Z, Kang Y-K, Giannakakou P, et al. (1994) Tubulin expression and polymerization in normal tissues, human tumors and paclitaxel (PTX) selected ovarian and breast carcinoma cells. Proc Am Assoc Cancer Res 35:390.
24. Dumontet C, Jaffrezou J-P, Duran G, Jordan MA, Wilson L, Sikic B (1994) Resistance to paclitaxel (Taxol-R) in KPTA5 variants of K562 cells is associated with the overexpression of 5-beta isotype of tubulin. Blood 84:603A.
25. Cornell L, Peterson R, Johnston KA, Fairchild CR (1995) Selection and characterization of a

paclitaxel resistant cell line which has a non-P-glycoprotein mediated mechanism of resistance. Proc Am Assoc Cancer Res 36:320.

26. Waud WR, Gilbert KS, Harrison Jr SD, Griswold Jr DP (1992) Cross-resistance of drug-resistant murine P388 leukemias to taxol in vivo. Cancer Chemother Pharmacol 31:255–257.

27. Lee FYF, Fager K, Fairchild C, Carboni J (1995) In vivo resistance to paclitaxel in the murine Madison 109 lung carcinoma is acquired in two mechanistically distinct stages. Proc Am Assoc Cancer Res 36:319.

28. Pastan I, Willingham MC, Gottesman M (1991) Molecular manipulations of the multidrug transporter: A new role for transgenic mice. FASEB J 5:2523–2528.

29. Sorrentino BP, Brandt SJ, Bodine D, Gottesman M, Pastan I, Cline A, Nienhuis AW (1992) Selection of drug-resistant bone marrow cells in vivo after retroviral transfer of human MDR1. Science 257:99–103.

30. Rowinsky EK, Donehower RC, Jones RJ, Tucker RW (1988) Microtubule changes and cytotoxicity in leukemic cell lines treated with Taxol. Cancer Res 48:4093–4100.

31. Cabral F, Abraham I, Gottesman MM (1981) Isolation of a taxol resistant Chinese hamster ovary cell mutant that has an alteration in alpha tubulin. Proc Natl Acad Sci USA 78:4388–4391.

32. Cabral FR (1983) Isolation of Chines hamster ovary cell mutants requiring the continuous presence of taxol for cell division. J Cell Biol 97:22–29.

33. Cabral F, Wible L, Brenner S, Brinkley BR (1983) Taxol-requiring mutant of Chinese hamster ovary cells with inpaired mitotic spindle assembly. J Cell Biol 97:30–39.

34. Cabral F, Brady RC, Schibler MJ (1986) A mechanism of cellular resistance to drugs that interfere with microtubule assembly. Ann NY Acad Sci 466:745–756.

35. Minotti AM, Barlow SB, Cabral F (1991) Resistance to antimitotic drugs in Chinese hamster ovary cells correlates with changes in the level of polymerized tubulin. J Biol Chem 266:3987–3994.

36. Rao S, Horwitz SB (1992) A multidrug resistance murine cell line is partially dependent on taxol for growth and has an increased tubulin content. Proc Am Assoc Cancer Res 33:461.

37. Haber M, Burkhart CA, Regl D, Madafiglio J, Norris MD, Horwitz SB (1995) Taxol resistance in murine J774.2 cells is associated with altered expression of specific beta-tubulin isotypes. Proc Am Assoc Cancer Res 36:318.

38. Ohta S, Nishio K, Kubuta N, Ohmori T, Funayama Y, Ohira T, Nakajima H, Adachi M, Saijo N (1994) Characterization of a Taxol-resistant human small-cell lung cancer cell line. Jpn J Cancer Res 85:290–297.

39. Potier P (1989) The synthesis of navelbine prototype of a new series of vinblastine derivatives. Semin Oncol 16:2–4.

40. Debal V, Allam N, Morjani H, Millot JM, Bragver D, Breillout F, Manfait M (1994) Characterization of a navelbine-resistant bladder carcinoma cell line cross-resistant to taxoids. Br J Cancer 70:1118–1125.

41. Jordan M, Toso R, Thrower D, Wilson L (1993) Mechanism of mitotic block and inhibition of cell proliferation by taxol at low concentrations. Proc Natl Acad Sci USA 90:9552–9556.

42. Giannakakou P, Sackett D, Mickley L, Kang Y-K, Fojo AT (1995) Characterization of non-Pgp paclitaxel (PTX) resistance in the human ovarian cancer cell line A2780. Proc Am Assoc Cancer Res 36:456.

43. Mallarino MC, Duran GE, Dumontet CM, Sikic BI (1995) Mechanisms of resistance in a human sarcoma cell line continuously selected with paclitaxel (Taxol, TAX) and SDZ PSC 833. Proc Am Assoc Cancer Res 36:320.

44. Schibler MJ, Barlow SB, Cabral F (1989) Elimination of permeability mutants from selections for drug resistance in mammalian cells. FASEB J 3:163–168.

45. Jaffrezou J-P, Jordan M, Tsuchiya E, Wilson L, Sikic BI (1994) Novel drug resistance in human leukemic cell lines double-selected with SDZ PSC 833 and vinblastine or taxol. Proc Am Assoc Cancer Res 35:342.

46. Christen RD, Jekunen AP, Jones JA, Thiebaut FB, Shalinsky DR, Howell SB (1992) Modulation of cisplatin accumulation in human ovarian carcinoma cells by pharmacological alteration of microtubule function. Proc Am Assoc Cancer Res 33:535.

47. Jekunen AP, Christen R, Shalinsky D, Howell S (1994) Synergistic interaction between cisplatin and taxol in human ovarian carcinoma cells in vitro. Br J Cancer 69:299–306.

48. Rixe O, Alvarez M, Miskley L, Ly H, Parker R, Tsokos M, Reed E, Fojo T (1993) Cisplatin (CP) resistance is multifactorial and includes changes in cytoskeletal distribution and dynamics. Proc Am Assoc Cancer Res 34:406.

49. Dietel M, Arps H, Lage H, Niendorf A (1990) Membrane vesicle formation due to aquired

mitoxantrone resistance in human gastric carcinoma cell line EPG85-257. Cancer Res 50:6100–6106.

50. Seidel A, Nickelsen M, Brandt I, Heinemann G, Dietel M (1991) Pathology and morphology of vesicular transport in drug-resistant tumor cells. J Cancer Res Clin Oncol 117(Suppl III):S90.

51. Speicher LA, Sheridan VR, Tew KD (1991) Human prostatic carcinoma cell (DU 145) resistance to antimitotic drugs. Proc Am Assoc Cancer Res 32:330.

52. Cabral F, Sobel M, Gottesman M (1980) CHO mutants resistant to colchicine, colcemid or griseofulvine have an altered b-tubulin. Cell 20:29–36.

53. Keates R, Sarangi F, Ling V (1981) Structural and functional alterations in microtubule protein from Chinese hamster ovary cell mutants. Proc Natl Acad Sci USA 78:5638–5642.

54. Cleveland D, Lopata M, Sherline P, Kirschner M (1981) Unpolymerized tubulin modulates the level of tubulin mRNAs. Cell 25:537–546.

55. Liebmann JE, Hahn SM, Cook JA, Lipschultz C, Mitchell JB, Kaufman DC (1993) Glutathione depletion by L-butathione sulfoximine antagonizes taxol cytotoxicity. Cancer Res 53:2066–2070.

56. Hamaguchi K, Godwin AK, Chapman JD, Yakushiji M, Hamilton TC (1993) The multidrug-resistance phenotype of ovarian cancer cells with high primary cisplatin resistance correlates with elevated glutathione levels. Proc Am Assoc Cancer Res 34:306.

57. Kelland LR, Abel G (1992) Circumvention of cisplatin (acquired) resistance in an in vitro panel of human ovarian carcinoma cell lines by Taxotere (RP56976). Br J Cancer 65(Suppl 16):20.

58. Lowe SC, Ruley HE, Jacks T, Housman DE (1993) p53-dependent apoptosis modulates the cytotoxicity of anticancer agents. Cell 74:957–967.

59. Rouby Se, Thomas A, Costin D, Rosenberg CR, Potmesil M (1993) p53 gene mutation in B-cell chronic lymphocytic leukemia is associated with drug resistance and is independent of MDR1/MDR3 gene expression. Blood 82:3452–3459.

60. Lee F, Fairchild C, Long B (1994) Chemosensitivity to paclitaxel as a function of the p53 phenotype. Proc Am Assoc Cancer Res 35:419.

61. Wahl A, Donaldson K, Fairchild C, Lee F, Foster S, Galloway D, Demers G (1996) Loss of normal p53 functions confers sensitization to Taxol by increasing GZ/M arrest and apoptosis. Nature Medicine 2:72–79.

62. Cross SA, Sanchez CA, Morgan CA, Schimke MK, Ramel S, Idzerda RL, Raskind WH, Reid BJ (1995) A p53-dependent mouse spindle checkpoint. Science 267:1353–1356.

63. Dole M, Nuñez G, Merchant AK, Maybaum J, Rode CK, Bloch CA, Castle VP (1994) Bcl-2 inhibits chemotherapy-induced apoptosis in neuroblastoma. Cancer Res 54:3253–3259.

64. Sumantran V, Ealovega M, Nuñez G, Clarke M, Wicha M (1995) Overexpression of Bcl-x$_L$ sensitizes MCF-7 cells to chemotherapy-induced apoptosis. Cancer Res 55:2507–2510.

65. Delaprote C, Larsen AK, Dautry F, Jacquemin-Sablon A (1991) Influence of myc overexpression of the phenotypic properties of chinese hamster lung cells resistant to antitumor agents. Exp Cell Res 197:176–182.

66. Seidman A, Crown J, Reichman B (1993) Lack of clinical cross-resistance of Taxol (T) with anthracycline (A) in the treatment of metastatic breast cancer (MBC). Proc Am Soc Clin Oncol 12:53.

67. Wilson WH, Berg SL, Bryant G, Wittes RE, Bates S, Fojo A, Steinberg SM, Goldspiel BR, Herdf J, O'shaughnessy J, Balis FM, Chabner BA (1994) Paclitaxel in doxorubicin-refractory or mitoxantrone-refractory breast cancer: A phase I/II trial of 96-hour infusion. J Clin Oncol 12:1621–1629.

68. Gianni L, Capri G, Munzone E, Straneo M (1994) Paclitaxel (Taxol) efficacy in patients with advanced breast cancer resistant to anthracyclines. Semin Oncol 21(Suppl 8):29–33.

69. Eck L, Pavich D, Fruehauf JP (1993) MDR-1 expression by human ovarian tumors is associated with taxol resistance. Proc Am Assoc Cancer Res 34:232.

70. Uziely B, Delaflor-Weiss E, Lenz H, Groshan S, Jeffers S, Watkins K, Danenberg K, Russell C, Leichman G, Muggia F, Press M (1994) Paclitaxel (Taxol) in refractory breast cancer: Response correlates with low levels of MDR1 gene expression. Proc Am Soc Clin Oncol 13:75.

71. Wilson WH, Chabner BA, Bryant G, Bates S, Fojo A, Regis J, Jatte ES, Steinberg SM, Goldspiel BR, Cheson BD (1995) Phase II study of paclitaxel in relapsed non-Hodgkin's lymphomas. J Clin Oncol 13:381–386.

72. Wilson WH, Berg S, Kang YK (1993) Phase I–II study of Taxol 96-hr infusion in refractory lymphoma and breast cancer: Pharmacodynamics and analysis of multi-drug resistance (mdr-1). Proc Am Soc Clin Oncol 12:335.

73. Linn SC, Kuiper CM, Liefting AJ, Vermorken J, Pinedo H, Giaccone G (1993) MDR1 gene

expression in anthracycline-resistant advanced breast cancer patients undergoing high dose Taxol treatment. Proc Am Soc Clin Oncol 12:87.

74. Riou J-F, Naudin A, Lavelle F (1992) Effects of taxotere on murine and human tumor cell lines. Biochem Biophys Res Comm 187:164–170.

75. Cole SPC, Sparks KE, Fraser K, Loe DW, Grant CE, Wilson GM, Deeley RG (1994) Pharmacological characterization of multidrug resistant MRP-transfected human tumor cells. Cancer Res 54:5902–5910.

76. Zaman GHR, Flens MJ, Leusden MRV, De Haas M, Mulder HS, Lankelma J, Pinedo HM, Scheper RJ, Baas F, Broxterman HJ, Borst P (1994) The human multidrug resistance-associated protein MRP is a plasma membrane drug-efflux pump. Proc Natl Acad Sci USA 91:8822–8826.

77. Lee F, Sciandra J, Siemann D (1989) A study of the mechanism of resistance to Adriamicin in vivo. Glutathione metabolism, p-glycoprotein expression, and drug transport. Biochem Pharmacol 38:3697–3705.

78. Fruehauf JP, Manetta A (1994) Use of the extreme drug resistance assay to evaluate mechanisms of resistance in ovarian cancer: Taxol resistance and MDR-1 expression. Contrib Gynecol Obstet 19:39–52.

79. Nicoletti M, Onorati L, Belotti D, Mangioni C, Casazza A, Giavazzi R (1995) Human ovarian carcinoma xenografts derived from paclitaxel (TAXOL)-treated patients. Proc Am Assoc Cancer Res 36:453.

80. Nicoletti M, Lucchini V, Massazza G, Abbott B, D'Incalci M, Giavazzi R (1993) Antitumor activity of taxol (NSC-125973) in human ovarian carcinomas growing in the peritoneal cavity of nude mice. Ann Oncol 4:151–155.

81. O'Shaugnessy JA, Cowan KH, Nienhuis AW, McDonash KT, Sorrentino BP, Dunbar CE, Chiang Y, Wilson W, Goldspiel B, Kohler D (1994) Retroviral mediated transfer of the human multidrug resistance gene (MDR-1) into hematopoietic stem cells during autologous transplantation after intensive chemotherapy for metastatic breast cancer. Hum Gene Ther 5:891–911.

82. Hill BT, Whelan RD, Shellard SA, McClean S, Hosking LK (1994) Differential cytotoxic effects of docetaxol in a range of mammalian tumor cell lines and certain drug resistant sublines in vitro. Invest New Drugs 12:169–82.

83. Georgiadis M, Russell E, Johnson B (1994) Prolonging the exposure of human lung cancer cell lines to paclitaxel improves the cytotoxicity. Proc Am Assoc Cancer Res 35:341.

84. Liebmann JE, Cook JA, Lipschulta C, Teague D, Fisher J, Mitchell JB (1993) Cytotoxic studies of paclitaxel (Taxol) in human tumor cell lines. Br J Cancer 68:1104–1109.

85. Rose WC (1993) Taxol-based combination chemotherapy and other in vivo preclinical antitumor studies. J Natl Cancer Inst Monogr 15:47–53.

86. Fujimoto S (1994) Schedule dependency of IV-paclitaxel against sc-M 109 mouse lung cancer. Jpn J Cancer Chemother 21:671–677.

87. Zahn Z, Kang Y-K, Regis J, Shives B, Byrant G, Wilson W, Fojo AT, Bates S (1995) Taxol resistance: in vitro and in viro studies in breast cancer lymphoma. Proc Am Assoc Cancer Res 34:215.

88. Baguley BC, Marshall ES, Whittaker JR, Dotchin MC, Nixon J, McCrystal MR, Finlay GJ, Matthews JH, Holdaway KM, van Zijl P (1995) Resistance mechanisms determining the in vitro sensitivity to paclitaxel of tumour cells cultured from patients with ovarian cancer. Eur J Cancer 31A:230–237.

89. Racker E, Wu L-T, Westcott D (1986) Use of slow calcium channel blockers to enhance inhibition by taxol of growth of drug-sensitive and drug-resistant Chinese hamster ovary cells. Cancer Treat Rep 70:275–278.

90. Jachez B, Nordmann R, Loor F (1993) Restoration of taxol sensitivity of multidrug-resistant cells by the cyclosporin SDZ PSC 833 and the cyclopeptolide SDZ 280-446. J Natl Cancer Inst 85:478–483.

91. Yang JM, Sommers S, Hait WN (1994) Reversal of Taxol resistance in vitro and in vivo by transflupenthixol and cyclosporin A. Proc Am Assoc Cancer Res 35:355.

92. Husain HR, Rahman A (1994) Mechanism of interaction of Taxol with P-glycoprotein in multidrug resistant cells. Proc Am Assoc Cancer Res 35:357.

93. Drori S, Eytan G, Assaraf Y (1995) Potentiation of anticancer-drug cytotoxicity by multidrug-resistance chemosensitizers involves alterations in membrane fluidity leading to increased membrane permeability. Eur J Biochem 228:1020–1029.

94. Fisher GA, Bartlett NL, Lum BL, Brophy NA, Duran GE, Ehsan MN (1994) Phase I trial of taxol

(T) with high dose cyclosporine (CsA) as a modulator of multidrug resistance (MDR). Proc Am Soc Clin Oncol 13:144.

95. Lorenz W (1977) Histamine release in dogs by Cremophor EL and its derivatives: Oxethylated oleic acid is the most effective constituent. Agents Action 7:63–67.

96. Woodcock D, Jefferson S, Linsenmeyer M (1990) Reversal of the multidrug resistance phenotype with Cremophor EL, a common vehicle for water-insoluble vitamins and drugs. Cancer Res 50:4199–4203.

97. Chervinsky D, Brecher ML, Hoelcle MJ (1992) Cremophor-EL reverses taxol cross-resistance in murine C1300 multidrug resistant neuroblastoma cells. Proc Am Assoc Cancer Res 33:477.

98. Chervinsky D, Brecher M, Hoelcle M (1993) Cremophor-EL enhances taxol efficacy in a multidrug resistant C-1300 neuroblastoma cell type. Anticancer Res 13:93–96.

99. Fjallskog M-L, Frii L, Bergh J (1994) Paclitaxel-induced cytotoxicity. The effects of cremophor EL (castor oil) on two human breast cancer cell lines with acquired multidrug resistant phenotype and induced expression of the permeability glycoprotein. Eur J Cancer 30:687–690.

100. Fairchild CR (1993) Reversal of taxol resistance in a multidrug resistant human colon carcinoma cell line in vitro by cremophor EL and Tween 80. Bristol Myers Squibb Internal Report 910028780.

101. Webster L, Linsenmeyer M, Millward M, Morton C, Bishop J, Woodcock D (1993) Measurement of Cremophor EL following taxol: Plasma levels sufficient to reverse drug exclusion mediated by the multidrug-resistant phenotype. J Natl Cancer Inst 85:1685–1690.

102. Nygren P, Csoka K, Jonsson B, Fridborg H, Bergh J, Hagberg H, Glimelius B, Brodin D, Tholander B, Krueger A, Lonnerholm G, Jakobsson A, Olsen L, Kristensen J, Larsson R (1995) The cytotoxic activity of Taxol in primary cultures of tumour cells from patients is partly mediated by Cremophor EL. Br J Cancer 71:478–81.

103. Liebmann JE, Cook JA, Mitchell JB (1993) Cremophor EL, solvent for paclitaxel, and toxicity. Lancet 342:1428.

104. Liebmann J, Cook JA, Lipschultz C, Teague D, Fisher J, Mitchell JB (1994) The influence of Cremophor EL on the cell cycle effects of paclitaxel (Taxol®) in human tumor cell lines. Cancer Chemother Pharmacol 33:331–339.

105. Fujimoto S (1994) Study for modifying activity of solvents on antitumor activity of paclitaxel. Jpn J Cancer Chemother 21:665–670.

106. Rose WC (1992) Taxol: A review of its preclinical in vivo antitumor activity. Anti-Cancer Drugs 3:311–321.

107. Fjallskog M-L, Frii L, Bergh J (1993) Is Cremophor EL, solvent for paclitaxel, cytotoxic? Lancet 342:873.

IV. RESISTANCE TO ANTIMETABOLITES

7. MECHANISMS OF CLINICAL RESISTANCE TO 5-FLUOROURACIL CHEMOTHERAPY

EDWARD CHU AND CARMEN J. ALLEGRA

In the late 1950s, the era of fluoropyrimidine antimetabolite chemotherapy was ushered in with the synthesis of 5-fluorouracil (5-FU) by Heidelberger and colleagues [1]. The rationale for the development of this class of compounds arose from studies that showed preferential utilization of the nucleobase uracil for nucleic acid biosynthesis by rat hepatoma cells when compared with normal rat intestinal mucosa [2]. In view of this finding and the fact that profound biological effects had been observed upon substitution of fluorine for hydrogen in several classes of compounds, it was postulated that fluorine-substituted pyrimidine analogs might display selective antitumor activity.

The fluoropyrimidine 5-FU has shown clinical efficacy in the treatment of a wide variety of solid tumors, including breast, head and neck, ovary, and gastrointestinal malignancies. To date, it remains the single most active agent for the treatment of patients with colorectal cancer, with an overall response rate in the range of 10–15% [3,4]. Unfortunately, the responses are partial in nature with virtually no associated complete remissions. For this reason, it is not surprising that therapy with single-agent 5-FU has not translated into an improvement in overall patient survival. Given the rather dismal response rate to single-agent 5-FU, significant efforts have focused on enhancing the cytotoxic effects of 5-FU through modulation with either biochemical agents or with biological response modifiers. Studies performed in both the preclinical and clinical settings have demonstrated significant enhancement of 5-FU cytotoxicity when it is used in combination with other agents, such as leucovorin, methotrexate (MTX), PALA, and the interferons (IFNs), in particular, alpha-IFN [5–14]. Given these promising studies, significant efforts continue to be placed on designing clinical protocols that incorporate each of these modulatory agents, either alone or in combination with 5-FU–based therapies.

It is clear that a more complete understanding of the mechanisms by which the class of fluoropyrimidines exert their cytotoxic action is central to the design and development of more effective treatment strategies. In order to exert their cytotoxic effects, the fluoropyrimidines must first be metabolized within the cell to their active nucleotide metabolites. The cytotoxic mechanisms of 5-FU have been well characterized, and they include [3,15–17]: (1) inhibition of the target enzyme thymidylate synthase (TS) by the 5-FU metabolite 5-fluoro-2'-deoxyuridine-5'-monophosphate (FdUMP), with resultant inhibition of thymidylate and DNA biosynthesis; (2) incorporation of the 5-FU metabolite 5-fluorouridine-5'-triphosphate (FUTP) into RNA, resulting in interference with RNA processing and translation; and (3) incorporation of the 5-FU metabolite 5-fluoro-2'-deoxyuridine-5'-triphosphate (FdUTP) into DNA, resulting in inhibition of DNA synthesis and subsequent DNA fragmentation. However, despite over 30 years of study, the relative contribution of each of these mechanisms in mediating the clinical activity of 5-FU remains unclear. In part, this may be attributed to alterations in the pattern and level of intracellular metabolism of 5-FU, which may show interpatient and intrapatient variation, and which may vary amongst different tumor types and normal host tissues. As suggested by Bertino et al. [18], another factor that must also be considered relates to the schedule of fluoropyrimidine drug administration, which may impact on the final pathway by which 5-FU exerts its cytotoxicity.

One of the principal obstacles to the clinical efficacy of fluoropyrimidine chemotherapy has been the rapid emergence of cellular resistance. Given the multiple sites of 5-FU action, it is not surprising that various resistance mechanisms have been identified in a host of in vitro and in vivo experimental model systems. These mechanisms are presented in Table 7–1 and include [19–31] increased levels of the target enzyme, TS; alterations in binding affinity of TS for the 5-FU metabolite, FdUMP; decreased incorporation of 5-FU into cellular RNA; decreased incorporation of 5-FU into cellular DNA; decreased intracellular pools of the reduced folate substrate, 5,10-methylenetetrahydrofolate; increased levels of dUTPase, preventing

Table 7–1. Mechanisms of resistance to 5-FU[a]

1. Increased level of expression of TS
2. Altered binding affinity of TS for FdUMP
3. Decreased incorporation of 5-FU into RNA
4. Decreased incorporation of 5-FU into DNA
5. Decreased pools of the reduced folate 5,10-methylenetetrahydrofolate
6. Increased level of expression of dUTPase
7. Decreased level of anabolic enzymes
8. Increased activity of catabolic enzymes, acid, and alkaline phosphatase

[a]5-FU = 5-fluorouracil; TS = thymidylate synthase; FdUMP = 5-fluoro-2'-deoxyuridine-5'-monophosphate; dUTPase = deoxy uridine triphosphatase.

accumulation of dUTP and FdUTP into cellular DNA; decreased levels of anabolic enzymes, resulting in decreased formation of active 5-FU metabolites; and increased activity of catabolic enzymes, such as acid and alkaline phosphatases, leading to decreased formation of active 5-FU metabolites. Recent work also suggest that the schedule of drug administration may play a critical role in determining the ultimate mechanism of 5-FU resistance. Using human colon cancer HCT-116 cells, Bertino et al. [18] observed that exposure to high-dose (1 mM) 5-FU for 4 hours led to drug resistance that was mediated by decreased incorporation of 5-FU metabolites into cellular RNA [15]. In contrast, when these same cells were continuously exposed to low concentrations (15 μM) of 5-FU for 7 days, sublines were selected that were resistant to 5-FU on the basis of a TS-directed, DNA-dependent process.

While each of these mechanisms of 5-FU resistance have been documented in both in vitro and in vivo model systems, their relative contribution in mediating clinical drug resistance remains uncertain. However, there is a growing body of evidence to suggest that malignant cells develop resistance to the cytotoxic effects of the fluoropyrimidines through a TS-mediated process. Specifically, two mechanisms have been identified that appear to have particular clinical relevance, and they include (1) a relative deficiency in intracellular folates, resulting in decreased inhibition of TS, and/or (2) increased expression of TS.

Given that the catalytic conversion of dUMP to thymidylate by TS is an ordered and sequential biochemical process [32,33], considerable attention has focused on strategies to enhance the formation of the ternary complex composed of TS enzyme, FdUMP, and the reduced folate substrate 5,10-methylenetetrahydrofolate. Various investigators have shown that the ternary complex is significantly more stable in the presence of increasing concentrations of the polyglutamated reduced folate substrate. These cell-free studies were subsequently extended to the intact cell setting, where it was observed that 5-FU cytotoxicity in a host of human malignant cell lines was enhanced upon addition of the reduced folate leucovorin [34–37]. The biochemical modulatory effects of leucovorin were especially marked in those cell lines whose endogenous levels of reduced folate, specifically 5,10-methylenetetra hydrofolate, were relatively low and, therefore, suboptimal for ternary complex formation.

With this preclinical information in hand, the combination of 5-FU and leucovorin was brought into the clinical setting for the treatment of patients with a variety of malignancies, including advanced colorectal, breast, and head and neck cancer. Specifically, with regard to the treatment of patients with advanced colorectal cancer, the collective results from several randomized clinical trials have demonstrated that the overall response rate to the combination of 5-FU and leucovorin is superior (25–35%) to treatment with single-agent 5-FU (10–15%) [6–9]. Of note, in one study reported from the North Central Oncology group and the Mayo Clinic, a small but significant improvement in overall patient survival continues to be observed in those patients treated with the 5-FU/leucovorin combination [7]. These studies, taken together, suggest that a relative depletion of critical intracellular reduce folates represents an important mechanism by which malignant cells develop resistance to the fluoropyrimidines in the clinical setting. Moreover, they lend support to the view that TS is a clinically relevant chemotherapeutic target.

The role of gene amplification in mediating drug resistance is well established. The initial studies by Schimke and colleagues identified marked amplification of the DHFR gene in Chinese hamster ovary cells made resistant to MTX, and this observation was subsequently extended to MTX-resistant murine and human leukemic cell lines [38]. In addition to being observed in the laboratory setting, there is evidence that amplification of the DHFR gene has clinical relevance in that it was identified in clinical specimens taken directly from patients treated with MTX [39,40]. With regard to TS, amplification of the TS gene has been observed in cultured malignant cells treated with either 5-FU [41], FdUrd [42,43], or with the specific antifolate TS inhibitor 10-propargyl-5,8-dideazafolate (CB3717) [44]. In each of these studies, a strong association between the level of intracellular expression of TS and relative fluoropyrimidine and/or antifolate sensitivity has been observed. Consequently, malignant cell lines and tumors with higher levels of TS enzyme activity and TS protein are relatively more resistant to the cytotoxic effects of the fluoropyridines. To date, there is little evidence in the literature to directly link TS gene amplification as a relevant mechanism of clinical resistance to the fluoropyrimidines. However, Clark et al. [26] reported a four- to six-fold increased in the TS gene copy number in a tumor sample obtained from a patient with progressive colon cancer following treatment with 5-FU and leucovorin chemotherapy. Although a pretreatment biopsy sample was not obtained to determine the baseline tumor TS gene copy number, this clinical study does provide suggestive evidence that the process of TS gene amplification may play a clinically important role in the acquisition of resistance following fluoropyrimidine therapy.

While amplification of the TS gene is a well-documented mechanism for the increased expression of TS, other mechanisms have been described that involve both transcriptional and post-transcriptional regulatory events. Studies by Scanlon and colleagues [45] demonstrated that selection of human ovarian cancer cells in cisplatin led to the development of cross-resistance to 5-FU. They found that cisplatin-resistant cells expressed three- to four-fold higher levels of TS when compared with wild-type parental cells. Moreover, the increased level of expression of TS was not associated with TS gene amplification but rather was the direct result of an increased transcriptional rate. A series of Adriamycin-resistant human breast cancer MCF-7 and human colon cancer DLD-1 cells were found to be cross-resistant to both 5-FU and FdUrd [46]. Of note, these resistant cell lines had not previously been exposed to either of the fluoropyrimidines.

Further evaluation revealed that the development of fluoropyrimidine resistance was directly associated with increased expression of TS protein. Moreover, maintenance of the selective pressure of Adriamycin within the growth medium of these cells was essential in establishing the enhanced expression of TS and consequent crossresistance to 5-FU. As in the case of the cisplatin-resistant human ovarian cancer cell line described by Scanlon and colleagues [45], the increased expression of TS was not the result of gene amplifacation of the TS gene but rather was directly regulated at the transcriptional lelvel. While the precise molecular mechanism(s) by which this occurs remains to be characterized, these two studies suggest that the ability to increase the expression of TS in response to chronic exposure to cytotoxic agents other than fluoropyrimidines serves as an important adaptive response mechanism for malignant cells to circumvent the effects of various cytotoxic stresses and thereby to maintain cellular synthetic function.

Using both in vitro and in vivo experimental model systems, a number of groups have described acute elevations in TS enzyme levels following short-term (12–24 hours) exposure to 5-FU [47–52]. Based on these earlier observations, it was proposed that the increase in TS enzyme activity in response to fluoropyrimidine exposure might represent one mechanism by which malignant cells rapidly developed cellular resistance to drug. A group from the National Cancer Institute determined the effect of fluoropyrimidine treatment on the levels of TS enzyme in direct patient tumor specimens. To do so, Swain et al. [53] measured TS enzyme levels in the cutaneous tumor specimens of female patients with advanced breast cancer pretreatment and 24 hours post-treatment with 5-FU and leucovorin. they observed an approximately threefold increase in total levels of TS enzyme in those tumor samples taken 24 hours post 5-FU exposure when compared with pretreatment levels. Moreover, patients with unresponsive disease had a significantly lower fraction of TS enzyme bound in the ternary complex when compared with those patients with responsive disease. Thus, given that exposure to 5-FU resulted in the acute elevation of TS enzyme levels in clinical tumor samples, this finding suggested that the acute induction of TS enzyme may represent a mechanism of fluoropyrimidine resistance with biological and clinical relevance.

Significant efforts have focused, over the past few years, on elucidating the critical biochemical and molecular events that underlie the 5-FU–mediated acute induction of TS. Using a human colon cancer H630 cell line [54], it was shown that exposure to 5-FU resulted in the acute induction of both TS enzyme activity and TS protein. Although Western immunoblot analysis revealed that the majority of the increased level of TS protein was in the form of TS protein complexed with the 5-FU metabolite FdUMP, there was also an approximately 30–40% increase in the levels of free, uncomplexed TS protein [55]. This small increase in free TS as determined by Western immunoblot analysis was consistent with the nearly 40% increase in free levels of TS enzyme activity, as determined by the radioenzymatic FdUMP binding assay [54]. Thus, the induction of TS in response to 5-FU exposure would allow for free TS to remain at a level 40% above baseline, thereby allowing for thymidylate and subsequent DNA biosynthesis to be maintained in the face of the cytotoxic stress of 5-FU.

Further studies revealed that the use of gamma-IFN, at noncytotoxic concentrations, effectively repressed the 5-FU–associated induction of TS, maintaining TS at levels observed in control, non–drug-treated cells. As evidence for the biological effect of the repression of gamma-IFN on TS expression, cytotoxicity studies demonstrated that simultaneous treatment with gamma-IFN resulted in a nearly 20-fold enhancement in the sensitivity of the human colon cancer H630 cells to 5-FU.

These findings thus provided the first direct evidence that the acute induction of TS represented an important mechanism for malignant cells to rapidly develop resistance to 5-FU.

Further work demonstrated that the increased level of expression of TS following exposure to 5-FU was not accompanied by a corresponding increase in the level of expression of TS mRNA [55]. Investigations measuring both the synthetic rate and stability of TS in human colon cancer cells treated with 5-FU demonstrated that the increased intracellular synthesis of TS was directly mediated by an enhanced translational efficiency of TS mRNA. Thus, the acute induction of TS in human colon cancer cells following 5-FU exposure was regulated at the translational level.

The possibility of translational control with regard to expression of the *Escherichia coli* TS thyA gene was first postulated by Belfort et al. [56]. Shortly thereafter, Kisliuk et al. [57,58] reported that TS isolated from an MTX-resistant *Streptococcus faecium* species was bound to a poly G tetraribonucleotide sequence. While the nature of this RNA–protein interaction was not further characterized, these investigators postulated that this short RNA sequence might, by itself, affect TS enzyme activity or that it might be part of a longer RNA sequence with potential regulatory activities. In their initial analysis of the human TS cDNA, Takeishi et al. [59] also suggested the possibility of translational control, given the theoretical potential of three interconvertible secondary structures, each containing a stem-loop structure in the 5'-untranslated region (5'-UTR) of the TS cDNA. In a follow-up study, Kaneda et al. [60] showed that deletion of these tandem repeat sequences significantly altered TS mRNA translational efficiency in vivo.

Recent work by Keyomarsi et al. [61] suggests that the changes in the levels of TS enzyme activity in both normal mammary epithelial cells and human breast cancer MCF-7 cells as they go through the cell cycle may also be controlled by a translational regulatory event. They also showed that exposure of human breast cancer MCF-7 cells to the antifolate analog ZD1694, a specific inhibitor of TS, resulted in a 10- to 40-fold increase in TS protein levels, while TS mRNA levels remained unchanged. These findings, taken together, provide further evidence for the critical role of translational regulatory mechanisms in determining the expression of TS. Furthermore, the ability to regulate the expression of TS at the translational level in the setting of an acute cellular stress may represent (1) a critical mechanism for normal cells to rapidly maintain their cellular synthetic function and (2) an important defense mechanism for malignant cells to protect themselves against the cytotoxic effects of various antineoplastic agents.

Within the past few years, there has been a heightened interest in elucidating the role of translational control mechanisms in the regulation of cellular gene expression [62–64]. There now is a growing list of eukaryotic genes for which translational regulation of mRNA has been described. The regulated synthesis of the storage protein ferritin by the intracellular levels of iron represents one of the best-characterized examples of translational regulation [65,66]. Detailed studies have identified a specific iron-responsive element (IRE) within the 5'-untranslated region (5'-UTR) of the ferritin mRNA to which a 90kDa cytosolic protein binds, the iron-responsive factor (IRF). The binding affinity of IRF for this target RNA sequence is principally determined by the iron status within the cell. Recent investigations have shown that, in addition to binding to and repressing the translation of ferritin, IRF can bind with high affinity to the IRE contained within the 5'-UTR of erythroid 5-aminolevulinate synthase mRNA and thereby repress synthesis of this protein that catalyzes the rate-limiting step in hemolobin biosynthesis [64].

Since the expression of TS in response to cytotoxic agents was controlled at the translational level, studies were subsequently undertaken to more directly characterize the regulation of TS mRNA translation. Using a rabbit reticulocyte lysate in vitro translation system, Chu et al. [67] observed that the addition of exogenous pure human recombinant TS protein repressed the translation of human TS mRNA in a dose-dependent manner. This inhibitory effect was specific in that the translational efficiencies of a host of unrelated mRNA transcripts, such as human chromogranin A, human folate receptor, human pre-placenental lactogen, yeast, and brome mosaic virus, remained unaffected by human recombinant TS protein. Moreover, the addition of a different folate-dependent enzyme, such as dihydrofolate reductase (DHFR), was unable to repress translation of the human TS mRNA. This initial set of studies suggested that translation of human TS mRNA was regulated by its own protein product via an autoregulatory mechanism. While this form of regulation has been well described for a number of bacteriophage T4 proteins and various *E. coli* ribosomal proteins [62,68–71], this autoregulatory process has not been previously described in a eukaryotic system.

The rabbit lysate experimental system employed only rabbit lysate, pure human TS protein, and in vitro transcribed TS mRNA. As a result, these initial studies suggested a direct interaction between TS protein and its own TS mRNA. To directly address this issue, an RNA electrophoretic gel mobility shift assay system was used to show a specific interaction between human recombinant TS protein and its corresponding TS mRNA [68,72]. Moreover, no other cofactor or protein was required for TS to directly bind to its TS mRNA, given that RNA binding activity was preserved in different preparations of human recombinant TS that varied in their level of enzyme purity.

A working model for the TS protein–TS mRNA interaction and the translational autoregulatory control of TS is presented in Figure 7–1. Two different regions on TS mRNA have been identified that bind with high affinity, on the order of 1–2nM to TS [72]. The first site is located within the first 188 nucleotides and includes the translational start site, while the second site is contained within a 100-nt sequence in the protein-coding region. In many of the studies described to date, the 5'-UTR has been identified as an important *cis*-acting element involved in repression of translation initiation of a number of genes [65–67]. For this reason, significant efforts were made to define the 5'-upstream binding site on TS mRNA. A Zuker RNA fold analysis of this binding site predicted for a stable stem-loop secondary structure with the translational AUG start site contained within the loop aspect.

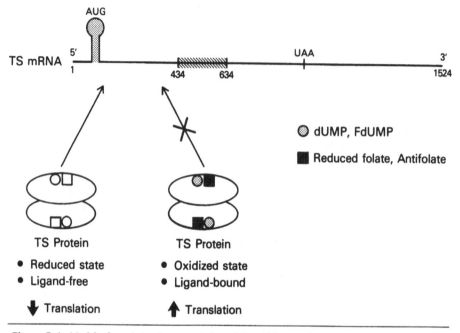

Figure 7–1. Model of translational autoregulation of thymidylate synthase.

Using both mutant and deletion RNA sequences, Chu et al. [72] reported that a hexanucleotide GCCAUG sequence contained within the loop aspect of this putative stem-loop structure was critical for protein recognition. Further studies using a combinatorial approach are currently in progress to identify the optimal nucleotide sequences required for this 5′-upstream binding site. In addition, further studies are required to more precisely characterize the sequence and structure determinants for protein recognition of the second binding site located within the protein-coding region. Initial comparison of the nucleotide sequence for both binding sites, however, has failed to reveal any apparent consensus sequence. Moreover, a preliminary secondary structure analysis suggests that the downstream binding site can form a pseudoknot structure, which is significantly different from the stem-loop structure observed for the 5′-site.

Significant efforts have focused on defining the essential molecular factors that determine RNA–protein interactions. The R17 bacteriophage coat protein [73,74] and aminoacyl-tRNA synthetase [75,76] represent two particularly well-studied examples of RNA binding proteins. In an elegant series of experiments, Starzyk et al. [76] conclusively demonstrated that the C-6 position of uridine 8 in aminoacyl-tRNA was subject to direct nucleophilic attack by a cysteine sulfhydryl group within the aminoacyl-tRNA synthase protein. This interaction resulted in formation of a transient covalent bond, referred to as the *Michael adduct*. The interaction between the R17 replicase protein and its target mRNA was also shown by Uhlenbeck and colleagues to be mediated by a cysteine sulfhydryl group [74].

Both TS catalytic activity and TS enzyme-ternary complex formation with FdUMP and 5,10-methylenetetrahydrofolate require the highly conserved cysteine sulfhydryl positioned in the nucleotide active site of TS to be in a fully reduced state [77–79]. During the catalytic reaction, the C-6 on the uracil ring of dUMP undergoes nucleophilic attack by the active site cysteine to form a Michael adduct. Since Michael addition of a protein nucleophile represents the critical step in the TS enzyme-catalyzed reaction and appears to be an important process underlying RNA–protein interactions, the potential role of the redox state in determining the interaction between TS protein and its target TS mRNA was examined. Chu et al. [80] demonstrated that the RNA binding activity of human recombinant TS was markedly sensitive to the presence of reducing agents and required the presence of at least one free sulfhydryl group. In the presence of either 2-mercaptoethanol (2-ME) or dithiothreitol, the RNA binding activity of TS was significantly enhanced. In contrast, treatment of TS with an oxidizing agent such as diamide effectively inhibited RNA binding in a dose-dependent manner. However, this inhibitory effect was readily reversible in that the simulaneous presence of the reducing agent fully restored RNA binding activity. In addition, the catalytic activity of this human TS protein was significantly enhanced in the presence of 2-ME, a finding that suggested the potential for a single common redox site on TS to simultaneously control RNA binding and catalysis by switching TS from inactive to active forms. However, a detailed mathematical analysis demonstrated that the reduced form of TS engaged in RNA binding and enzyme catalysis was not mediated by a single common redox site but suggested that RNA binding was a complex process, potentially involving multiple redox sites.

Although the precise mechanism(s) by which the cysteine sulfhydryl group(s) on TS mediates RNA binding remains to be more precisely defined, alternative possibilities to explain its central role include: (1) direct formation of a covalent Michael adduct between the active site sulfhydryl and the C-6 position of a uracil ring on TS mRNA occurs, (2) occupation of the active site cysteine alters RNA binding via a steric hindrance mechanism, and/or (3) the cysteine sulfhydryl groups in their maximally reduced state maintain TS protein in a certain conformation that allows for optimal RNA binding elsewhere on the protein.

In addition to the role of the redox state of the TS protein, the state of occupancy of the protein is critical in determining its RNA binding function. Specifically, when TS was ligand-free, maximal RNA binding activity was maintained, thereby resulting in complete translational inhibition of TS mRNA. In contrast, when TS was bound by either of its physiologic substrates dUMP or 5,10-methylenetetrahydrofolate, or was bound by the 5-FU nucleotide metabolite FdUMP, TS was no longer able to bind to its target mRNA. The end result of this decreased RNA binding activity was to relieve translational repression, resulting in an increased synthesis of new TS protein. Such a condition would exist in cells exposed to either 5-FU or to inhibitors of TS. Thus, this model provides a rational mechanism for the acute induction of TS that arises in response to exposure to 5-FU and antifolate analogs that target TS (see later).

Several investigators have proposed that modulation of the critical folate-dependent enzyme dihydrofolate reductase (DHFR) by the antifolate analogs methotrexate (MTX) and trimetrexate (TMQ) is mediated by post-transcriptional events [81–83]. There is now experimental evidence to suggest that the expression of DHFR is, in part, regulated at the translational level. Using an in vitro translation system, Chu et al. [84] demonstrated that the expression of DHFR was controlled by a negative autoregulatory mechanism in which human recombinant DHFR binds to its own mRNA, resulting in repression of new DHFR protein synthesis. In vitro experiments revealed that dihydrofolate and MTX can each interact with DHFR to disallow binding of the protein to its corresponding DHFR mRNA, thereby resulting in enhanced translation of DHFR mRNA.

Recent molecular modeling studies have identified ligand-induced conformational changes for both *E. coli* and human DHFR [85,86]. These findings would then support the possibility that MTX and dihydrofolate might prevent DHFR from exerting its normal autoregulatory function by either altlering enzyme conformation or by directly occupying the protein–mRNA binding site. The regulated expression of thymidine kinase during the cell cycle and periods of stimulated growth has also been shown to be controlled at the translational level [87–89]. In contrast to TS and DHFR, however, further studies are required to more precisely define the specific *cis*- and *trans*-acting elements involved in the translational regulation of thymidine kinase. It is intriguing to note that the expression of three different enzymes that catalyze reaction pathways critical for DNA biosynthesis, namely, TS, DHFR, and thymidine kinase, is controlled at the translational level. Thus, the ability to control the expression of each of these genes by translational regulatory events would appear to provide further evidence that this process represents a biologically important response mechanism that allows for cellular synthetic function to be maintained in the face of an acute cellular stress.

A more refined characterization of the molecular elements underlying the interaction between TS protein and its own TS mRNA should provide the rational basis for the future design and development of novel therapeutic approaches. Several potential strategies that may arise from these molecular-based studies are presented in Figure 2. For example, identification of the specific RNA binding domain may lead to the development of new inhibitors of TS enzymatic activity that would still allow for formation of the TS protein–TS mRNA interaction. A stable ternary complex composed of inhibitor, TS protein, and TS mRNA would then result in effective inhibition of synthesis of new TS protein. As an alternative approach, identification of the RNA binding domain may lead to the development of a small peptide that would then be used to bind to the target TS mRNA and to inhibit new TS protein synthesis. Moreover, molecular modeling techniques may help identify a small "designer" molecule that would mimic the structural features of the peptide.

NEW CONSIDERATIONS FOR THYMIDYLATE SYNTHASE INHIBITION

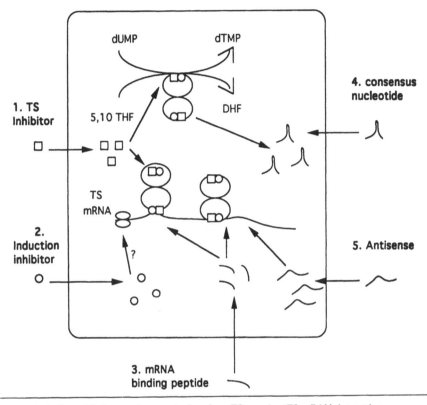

Figure 7–2. Potential therapeutic strategies based on TS protein–/TS mRNA interaction.

The theoretical advantage of this kind of molecular modeling analysis would be that novel organic molecules with enhanced spatial and biophysical characteristics could be designed.

Such an approach is presently be taken in anti-HIV drug development, where small basic Rev and Tat peptides that mimic the function of their corresponding native proteins are being tested to inhibit HIV viral replication. Identification of the consensus nucleotide sequence and/or secondary structure containing the high-affinity protein binding site may lead to the design and development of an RNA oligonucleotide that can then be used to sequester and/or inhibit TS enzymatic function. One potential drawback to this approach, however, is the inherent difficulty in efficiently and specifically delivering nucleic acids into cells. To circumvent this problem, molecular modeling programs may be applied to design small organic molecules that closely resemble the consensus RNA sequence/structure. In contrast to nucleic acids, such compounds might then be delivered with far greater efficiency and at relatively high concentrations into malignant cells.

A consensus nucleotide sequence/structure might also serve as the target for either antisense- or ribozyme-based strategies, with consequent inhibition of steady-state levels of TS. Finally, previous studies had shown that gamma-IFN effectively repressed the 5-FU–mediated induction of TS expression. A more detailed characterization of the mechanism(s) by which gamma-IFN downregulates TS expression may lead to the development of "small molecules" that mimic the structure and function of gamma-IFN and that would be used to bind to the cis-acting sites on TS mRNA, thereby leading to repression of new TS protein synthesis.

While the future clinical development of new therapeutic strategies incorporating potentially novel "small organic molecules" awaits further molecular studies examining the TS protein–TS mRNA interaction, considerable focus continues to be placed on the development of new inhibitors of TS. Since thymidylate synthase binds both a nucleotide and a reduced folate, recent efforts have been directed toward identifying antifolate compounds that potently inhibit the activity of the enzyme. Several such compounds have been developed and are currently in various phases of preclinical and clinical development. While they each appear to specifically inhibit the TS enzymatic reaction, they vary in a number of other characteristics that may be important determinants of their cellular pharmacology and pharmacokinetic disposition in patients (Table 7–2).

N-10-propargyl-5,8-dideazafolate (CB3717) was the first pure antifolate inhibitor of thymidylate synthase to be developed and ultimately tested in patients [90–92]. This compound requires intracellular metabolism to the polyglutamate form for its potent inhibitory activity and requires the reduced folate carrier for cellular entry [93]. While evidence of clinical activity was demonstrated in early phase I testing, this compound was withdrawn from further testing due to unpredictable nephrotoxicity, presumably resulting from precipitation of the poorly soluble parent compound in the acidic pH of the urine [94–96].

Table 7–2. Selected characteristics of thymidylate synthase inhibitors

Inhibitor	Transport	Polyglutamation	Potency (nM)
CB3717	? RFC[a]	+	2.7 (monoglutamate)
			0.04 (pentaglutamate)
ZD1694	RFC	+++	60 (monoglutamate)
			1.0 (tetraglutamate)
LY231514	RFC	+++	340 (monoglutamate)
			3.4 (pentaglutamate)
ZD9331	RFC	−	0.4
BW1843U89	RFC	+ (only diglutamate)	0.09 (mono or di glutamate)
AG331	Diffusion	−	2
AG337	Diffusion	−	15

[a]RFC = reduced folate carrier.

ZD1694 (Tomudex) was developed as a more water-soluble analog of CB3717 [97–99]. It was found to be devoid of nephrotoxicity in animal models yet retained a potent ability to inhibit thymidylate synthase [98]. Like the index compound, ZD1694 utilizes the reduced folate carrier for cellular transport and is one of the most avidly polyglutamated antifolate compounds to enter clinical investigation, being a 100-fold better substrate for the folyl polyglutamate synthetase enzyme (FPGS) when compared with CB3717. Polyglutamation of ZD1694 results in an approximately 60-fold increase in the potency of thymidylate synthase inhibition. In addition to enhancing enzymatic inhibition, polyglutamation of ZD1694 and CB3717 results in a prolonged intracellular half-life of these compounds in much the same fashion as polyglutamation of the physiologic folates and methotrexate results in their prolonged intracellular retention.

The prolonged intracellular half-life of ZD1694 was demonstrated by Aherne and colleagues in a murine model wherein these investigators noted tissue to plasma ratios of up to 1,000 in the liver of mice 1–2 weeks following ZD1694 injections [100]. These investigators further demonstrated that polyglutamates accounted for 75% of the retained drug 24 hours following drug administration [101]. The importance of polyglutamation has been underscored by recent investigations from several groups illustrating that deficient polyglutamation is a critical mechanism by which malignant cells become resistant to the cytotoxic effects of ZD1694 [102–104]. Preclinical investigations suggest that ZD1694 may be used in combination with 5-fluorouracil with greater than additive effects, since the polyglutamates of ZD1694 stabilize ternary complex formation with fluorodeoxyuridine monophosphate and thymidylate synthase [105]. In addition, alteration of thymidine triphosphate pools resulting from thymidylate synthase inhibition by ZD1694 may promote the incorporation of 5-fluorouracil into nucleic acids [106].

Two independent phase I trials of ZD1694 have been conducted by the National Cancer Institute and a group from the United Kingdom [107,108]. Both groups employed a 15 minute infusion given every 3 weeks, reasoning that the avid polyglutamation of ZD1694 could be used to selective advantage between normal and malignant cells, which have a greater propensity for polyglutamation. The major toxicities observed in these studies included an anorexia/fatigue syndrome, GI toxicity, principally in the form of diarrhea, and myelotoxicity. While transaminasemia was noted, it appeared to be reversible in all cases, and no long-term hepatic or renal toxicities were observed. The recommended dose for phase II investigations was 3–4 mg/m2. Phase II investigations have now been completed in patients with advanced colorectal, pancreas, non–small cell lung, breast, and ovarian cancers [109–113]. The overall response rates in preliminary reports of patients with advanced breast cancer (45 patients) and pancreas cancer (22 patients) were 25% and 14%, respectively. Response rates in 31 patients with advanced ovarian cancer and in 21 patients with non–small cell lung cancer were less than 10%.

The largest experience, to date, has been for first-line treatment of patients with advanced colorectal carcinoma. A recent update of 176 evaluable patients demonstrated an overall response rate of 26%, with an average response duration of 6 months [113]. The major toxicities observed in this trial using 3 mg/m2 intravenously every 3 weeks included WHO grade III or IV diarrhea in 10%, leukopenia in 6%, asthenia in 12%, and reversible transaminasemia in 14%. The overall median survival of patients on study was 42 weeks. Phase III trials are currently underway to compare the efficacy of ZD1694 with the combination of 5-fluorouracil and leucovorin for the treatment of patients with advanced colorectal carcinoma.

LY231514 is another antifolate thymidylate synthase inhibitor requiring polyglutamation for potent inhibitory effects [114]. This compound has undergone phase I testing with several schedules, including a single intravenous dose given over 10 minutes every 21 days [115–117]. This schedule has been chosen for a phase II study in patients with advanced colorectal carcinoma using a dose of 60 mg/m^2. The major toxicities noted with LY231514 include neutropenia, an anorexia/fatigue syndrome, gastrointestinal toxicity, and reversible transaminasemia [117].

Since alterations in the ability of malignant cells to polyglutamate appears to be an important mechanism of resistance to agents requiring polyglutamation for their activity, several new compounds have been developed that do not require polyglutamation but still retain a potent ability to inhibit thymidylate synthase. This group of compounds includes 1843U89 [118], ZD9331 [119–121], and two lipophilic compounds, namely, AG331 and AG337 [122,123]. While polyglutamation of 1843U89 is not required for potent enzymatic inhibition, the compound is metabolized rapidly to the diglutamate form by folyl polyglutamate synthetase. Polyglutamation to the diglutamate level appears to be important for optimal activity of 1843U89, presumably by enhancing intracellular retention [124,125]. This compound is currently undergoing phase I testing. While requiring the reduced folate carrier for cellular entry, ZD9331 does not require polyglutamation for its inhibitory effects and is not a substrate for folyl polyglutamate synthetase. Unfortunately, the lack of polyglutamation necessitates administration of the drug by prolonged infusion schedules for activity in vivo. Using infusional schedules in mice, ZD9331 appears to be principally associated with hematologic toxicity and demonstrates a broad spectrum of activity against a variety of human tumor xenografts [121]. This compound has yet to enter clinical investigations.

An interesting approach has been taken in the development of AG331 and AG337, two novel analogs that were designed based on knowledge of the x-ray crystal structure of the active site of thymidylate synthase [122]. These two compounds represent the first to enter clinical investigations based on such a molecular modeling analysis. Both compounds are less potent inhibitors of thymidylate synthase when compared with the aforementioned antifolate analogs, but they do not rely on polyglutamation for their cytotoxic activity [122,123,126,127]. Moreover, they enter the cell via passive diffusion rather than using the reduced folate carrier for transmembrane transport. Due to the rapid intracellular half-life observed in early phase I testing, prolonged infusion schedules have been explored. Recent investigations have focused on the use of a 5 day continuous infusion of AG337 and AG331 given every 3 weeks. Toxicities observed with this schedule include myelosuppression, mucositis, nausea, vomiting, rash, fatigue, and transient transaminasemia. The recommend dose for phase II testing is $1,000 \, mg/m^2/day$ for AG337 [128–130].

The antifolate inhibitors of thymidylate synthase have clearly demonstrated antineoplastic activity, particularly in patients with advanced colorectal and breast carcinomas. It remains to be determined which of the various characteristics of the compounds under current clinical investigations will ultimately prove to be critical for clinical antineoplastic activity. Since polyglutamation differences between normal and malignant tissues provides selective advantage to those compounds requiring polyglutamation for their activity, it remains to be seen if selectivity with respect to normal tissues will be retained by antifolate analogs that do not require polyglutamation for their inhibitory activity. Hopefully, the respective roles of polyglutamation, transmembrane transport, and enzyme inhibitory potency will be more clearly defined by future investigations examining these various compounds.

REFERENCES

1. Heidelberger C, Chaudhuri NK, Danenberg P, Mooren D, Griesbach L, Duschinsky R, Schnitzer RJ, Pleven E, Scheiner J (1957) Fluorinated pyrimidines, a new class of tumour-inhibitory compounds. Nature 179:663–666.
2. Rutman RJ, Cantarow A, Paschkis KE (1954) Studies on 2-acetylaminofluorene carcinogenesis: II. The utilization of uracil-2-C^{14} by preneoplastic rat liver. Cancer Res 14:199–126.
3. Pinedo HM, Peters GFJ (1988) Fluorouracil: Biochemistry and pharmacology. J Clin Oncol 6:1653–1664.
4. Moertel CG (1994) Chemotherapy for colorectal cancer. N Engl J Med 330:1136–1142.
5. Petrelli N, Douglass HI, Herrera L, Russell D, Stablein DM, Bruckner HW, Mayer RJ, Schinella R, Green MD, Muggia FM, Megibow A, Greenwald ES, Bukowski RM, Harris J, Levin B, Gaynor E, Loutfi A, Kaiser MH, Barkin JS, Benedetto P, Woolley PV, Nauta R, Weaver DW, Leichman LP (1989) The modulation of fluorouracil with leucovorin in metastatic colorectal carcinoma: A prospective randomized phase III trial. J Clin Oncol 7:1419–1426.
6. Erlichman C, Fine S, Wong A, Elhakim T (1988) A randomized trial of fluorouracil and folinic acid in patients with metastatic colorectal carcinoma. J Clin Oncol 6:469–475.
7. Poon MA, O'Connell MJ, Moertel CG, Wieand HS, Cullinan SA, Everson LK, Krook JE, Mailliard JA, Laurie JA, Tschetter LK, Wiesenfeld M (1989) Biochemical modulation of fluorouracil: Evidence of significant improvement of survival and quality of life in patients with advanced colorectal carcinoma. J Clin Oncol 7:1407–1417.
8. Doroshow JH, Multhauf P, Leong L, Margolin K, Kitchfield T, Akman S, Carr B, Mertrand M, Goldberg D, Blayney D, Odujinrin O, DeLap R, Shuster J, Newman E (1990) Prospective randomized comparison of fluorouracil versus fluorouracil and high-dose continuous infusion leucovorin calcium for the treatment of advanced measurable colorectal cancer in patients previously unexposed to chemotherapy. J Clin Oncol 8:491–501.
9. Poon MA, O'Connell MJ, Wieand HS, Krook JE, Gerstner JB, Tschetter LK, Levitt R, Kardinal CG, Mailliard JA (1991) Biochemical modulation of fluorouracil with leucovorin: Confirmatory evidence of improved therapeutic efficacy in advanced colorectal cancer. J Clin Oncol 9:1967–1972.
10. Sotos GA, Grogan LM, Allegra CJ (1994) Preclinical and clinical aspects of biomodulation of 5-fluorouracil. Cancer Treat Rev 20:11–49.
11. Wadler S, Schwartz EL (1990) Antineoplastic activity of the combination of interferon and cytotoxic agents against experimental and human malignancies: A review. Cancer Res 50:3473–3486.
12. Grem JL, McAtee N, Murphy RF, Balis FM, Steinberg SM, Hamilton JM, Sorensen JM, Sartor I, Kramer BS, Goldstein LJ, Gay LM, Caubo KM, Goldspiel B, Allegra CJ (1991) A pilot study of interferon alfa-2a in combination with 5-fluorouracil plus high-dose leucovorin in metastatic gastrointestinal carcinoma. J Clin Oncol 9:1811–1820.
13. Grem JL, Jordan E, Robson ME, Binder RA, Hamilton JM, Steinberg SM, Arbuck SG, Beveridge

RA, Kales AN, Miller JA, Weiss RB, McAtee N, Chen A, Brewster L, Goldspiel B, Sover E, Bastian A, Allegra CJ (1993) Phase II study of 5-fluorouracil, leucovorin and interferon alfa-2a in metastatic colorectal carcinoma. J Clin Oncol 11:1737–1745.

14. Kohne-Wompner C-H, Schmoll H-J, Harstrick A, Rustum YM (1992) Chemotherapeutic strategies in metastatic colorectal cancer: An overview of current clinical trials. Semin Oncol 19:105–125.

15. Heidelberger C (1975) Fluorinated pyrimidines and their nucleosides. In A Sartorelli, D Johns, eds. Antineoplastic and Immunosuppressive Agents. New York: Springer, pp 193–231.

16. Heidelberger C, Danenberg PV, Moran RG (1989) Fluorinated pyrimidines and their nucleosides. Adv Enzymol Relat Areas Mol Biol 54:57–119.

17. Santi DV, McHenry CS, Sommer H (1974) Mechanism of interaction of thymidine synthetase with 5-fluorodeoxyuridylate. Biochemistry 13:471–481.

18. Aschele C, Sobrero A, Faderan MA, Bertino JR (1992) Novel mechanisms of resistance to 5-fluorouracil in human colon cancer (HCT-8) sublines following expsoure to two different clinically relevant dose schedules. Cancer Res 52:1855–1864.

19. Ardalan B, Cooney DA, Jayaram HN, Carrico CK, Glazar RI, Macdonald J, Schein PS (1980) Mechanisms of sensitivity and resistance of murine tumors to 5-fluorouracil. Cancer Res 40:1431–1437.

20. Spiegelman S, Sawyer R, Nayak R, Ritzi E, Stolfi R, Martin D (1980) Improving the antitumor activity of 5-fluorouracil by increasing its incorporation into RNA via metabolic modulation. Proc Natl Acad Sci USA 77:4966–4970.

21. Houghton JA, Maroda SJ, Phillips JO, Houghton PJ (1981) Biochemical determinants of responsiveness to 5-fluorouracil and its derivatives in xenografts of human colorectal adenocarcinomas in mice. Cancer Res 41:144–149.

22. Mulkins MA, Heidelberger C (1982) Biochemical characterization of fluoropyrimidine-resistant murine leukemic cell lines. Cancer Res 42:965–973.

23. Yin MB, Zakrzewski SF, Hakala MT (1983) Relationship of cellular folate cofactor pools to the activity of 5-fluorouracil. Mol Pharmacol 23:190–197.

24. Fernandes DJ, Crawford SK (1985) Resistance to CCRF-CEM cloned sublines to 5-fluorodeoxyuridine associated with enhanced phosphatased activities. Biochem Pharmacol 34:125–132.

25. Berger SH, Jenh C-H, Johnson LF, Berger F (1985) Thymidylate synthase overproduction and gene amplification in fluorodeoxyuridine-resistant human cells. Mol Pharmacol 28:461–467.

26. Clark JL, Berger SH, Mittleman A, Berger F (1987) Thymidylate synthase gene amplification in a colon tumor resistant to fluoropyrimidine chemotherapy. Cancer Treat Rep 71:261–265.

27. Berger SH, Barbour KW, Berger F (1988) A naturally occurring variation in thymidylate synthase structure is associated with a reduced response to 5-fluoro-2'-deoxyuridine in a human colon tumor cell line. Mol Pharmacol 34:480–484.

28. Kessel D, Hall TC, Wodinsky I (1966) Nucleotide formation as a determinant of 5-fluorouracil response in mouse leukemia. Science 154:911–913.

29. Chu E, Lai G-M, Zinn S, Allegra CJ (1990) Resistance of a human ovarian cancer line to 5-fluorouracil associated with decreased levels of 5-fluorouracil in DNA. Mol Pharmacol 38:410–417.

30. Canman CE, Tang H-Y, Normolle DP, Lawrence TS, Maybaum J (1992) Variations in patterns of DNA damage induced in human colorectal tumor cells by 5-fluorodeoxyuridine: Implications for mechanisms of resistance and cytotoxicity. Proc Natl Acad Sci USA 89:10474–10478.

31. Canman CE, Radany EH, Parsels LA, Davis MA, Lawrence TS, Maybaum J (1994) Induction of resistance to fluorodeoxyuridine cytotoxicity and DNA damage in human tumor cells by expression of Escherichia coli deoxyuridinetriphosphatase. Cancer Res 54:2296–2298.

32. Danenberg KD, Danenberg PV (1979) Evidence for a sequential interaction of the subunits of thymidylate synthetase. J Biol Chem 254:4345–4348.

33. Danenberg PV, Lockshin A (1982) Tight-binding complexes of thymidylate synthetase, folate analogs, and deoxyribonucleotides. Adv Enzyme Regul 20:99–101.

34. Keyomarsi K, Moran RG (1986) Folinic acid augmentation of the effects of fluoropyrimidines on murine and human leukemic cells. Cancer Res 46:5229–5235.

35. Radparvar S, Houghton PJ, Houghton JA (1989) Effect of polyglutamylation of 5,10-methylenetetrahydrofolate on the binding of 5-fluoro-2'-deoxyuridylate to thymidylate synthase purified from a human colon adenocarcinoma xenograft. Biochem Pharmacol 38:335–342.

36. Mini E, Mazzei T, Coronnello M, Criscuoli L, Gualtieri M, Periti P, Bertino JR (1987) Effects of 5-methyltetrahydrofolate on the activity of fluoropyrimidines against human leukemia (CCRF-CEM) cells. Biochem Pharmacol 36:2905–2911.

37. Houghton JA, Williams LG, de Graaf SSN, Cheshire PJ, Rodman JH, Maneval DC, Wainer IW, Jadaud P, Houghton PJ (1990) Relationship between dose rate of [6RS] leucovorin administration, plasma concentrations of reduced folates, and pools of 5,10-methylenetetrahydrofolates and tetrahydrofolates in human colon adenocarcinoma xenografts. Cancer Res 50:3493–3502.
38. Schimke RT (1984) Gene amplification in cultured animal cells. Cell 37:705–713.
39. Carman MD, Schornagel JH, Rivest RS, Srimatkandada S, Portlock CS, Duffy T, Bertino JR (1984) Resistance to methotrexate due to gene amplification in a patient with acute leukemia. J Clin Oncol 2:16–20.
40. Horns CR Jr, Dower WJ, Schimke RT (1984) Gene amplification in a leukemic patient treated with methotrexate. J Clin Oncol 2:2–7.
41. Lesuffleur T, Kornowski A, Luccioni C, Muleris M, Barbat A, Beaumatin J, Dussaulx E, Dutrillaux B, Zweibaum A (1991) Adaptation to 5-fluorouracil of the heterogeneous human colon tumor cell line HT-29 results in the selection of cells committed to differentiation. Int J Cancer 49:721–730.
42. Jenh C-H, Geyer PK, Baskin F, Johnson LF (1985) Thymidylate synthase gene amplification in fluorodeoxyuridine-resistant mouse cell lines. Mol Pharmacol 28:80–85.
43. Imam AMA, Crossley PH, Kackman AL, Little PFR (1987) Analysis of thymidylate synthase gene amplification and of mRNA levels in the cell cycle. J Biol Chem 262:7268–7373.
44. Danenberg KD, Danenberg PV (1989) Activity of thymidylate synthetase and its inhibition by 5-fluorouracil in highly enzyme-overproducing cells resistant to 10-propargyl-5,8-dideazafolate. Mol Pharmacol 36:219–223.
45. Scanlon KJ, Kashani-Saabet M (1988) Elevated expression of thymidylate synthase cycle genes in cisplatin-resistant human ovarian carcinoma A2780 cells. Proc Natl Acad Sci USA 85:650–653.
46. Chu E, Drake JC, Koeller DM, Zinn S, Jamis-Dow CA, Yeh GC, Allegra CJ (1991) Induction of thymidylate synthase associated with multidrug resistance in human breast and colon cancer cell lines. Mol Pharmacol 39:136–143.
47. Spears CP, Shahinian AH, Moran RG, Heidelberger C, Corbett TH (1982) In vivo kinetics of thymidylate synthetase inhibition in 5-fluoro-uracil sensitive and resistant murine colon adenocarcinomas. Cancer Res 42:450–456.
48. Washtein WL (1984) Increased levels of thymidylate synthetase in cells exposed to 5-fluorouracil. Mol Pharmacol 25:171–177.
49. Berne MHO, Gustavsson BG, Almersjo O, Spears PC, Frosing R (1986) Sequential methotrexate/5-FU: FdUMP formation and TS inhibition in a transplantable rodent colon adenocarcinoma. Cancer Chemother Pharmacol 16:237–242.
50. Berne M, Gustavsson B, Almersjo I, Spears CP, Waldenstrom J (1987) Concurrent allopurinol and 5-fluorouracil: 5-Fluoro-2'-deoxyuridylate formation and thymidylate synthase inhibition in rat colon carcinoma and in regenerating rat liver. Cancer Chemother Pharmacol 20:193–197.
51. Keyomarsi K, Moran RG (1988) Mechanism of the cytotoxic synergism of fluoropyrimidines and folinic acid in mouse leukemic cells. J Biol Chem 263:14402–14409.
52. Van der Wilt CL, Pinedo HM, Smit K, Peters GJ (1992) Elevation of thymidylate synthase following 5-fluorouracil treatment is prevented by the addition of leucovorin in murine colon tumors. Cancer Res 52:4922–4928.
53. Swain SM, Lippman ME, Egan EF, Drake JC, Steinberg SM, Allegra CJ (1989) 5-Fluorouracil and high-dose leucovorin in previously treated patients with metastatic breast cancer. J Clin Oncol 7:890–899.
54. Chu E, Zinn S, Boarman D, Allegra CJ (1990) Interaction of gamma interferon and 5-fluorouracil in the H630 human colon carcinoma cell line. Cancer Res 50:5834–5840.
55. Chu E, Koeller DM, Johnston PG, Zinn S, Allegra CJ (1993) Regulation of thymidylate synthase in human colon cancer cells treated with 5-fluorouracil and interferon-gamma. Mol Pharmacol 43:527–533.
56. Belfort M, Maley G, Pedersen-Lane J, Maley F (1983) Primary structure of the *Escherichia coli* thyA gene and its thymidylate synthase product. Proc Natl Acad Sci USA 80:4914–4918.
57. Rao KN, Kisliuk RL (1983) Association of RNA with thymidylate synthase from methotrexate-resistant *Streptococcus faecium*. Proc Natl Acad Sci USA 80:916–920.
58. Thorndike J, Kisliuk RL (1986) Identification of poly G bound to thymidylate synthase. Biochem Biophys Res Commun 139:461–465.
59. Takeishi K, Kaneda S, Ayusawa D, Shimizu K, Gotoh O, Seno T (1985) Nucleotide sequence of a functional cDNA for human thymidylate synthase. Nucleic Acids Res 13:2035–2043.
60. Kaneda S, Takeishi K, Ayusawa D, Shimizu K, Seno T, Altman S (1987) Role in translation of a

triple tandemly repeated seqduence in the 5'-untranslated region of human thymidylate synthase mRNA. Nucleic Acids Res 15:1259–1270.

61. Keyomarsi K, Samet J, Molnar G, Pardee AB (1993) The thymidylate synthase inhibitor, ICI D1694, overcomes translational detainment of the enzyme. J Biol Chem 268:15142–15149.

62. Gold L (1988) Posttranscriptional regulatory mechanisms in *Escherichia coli*. Ann Rev Biochem 57:199–233.

63. Hershey JWB (1991) Translational control in mammalian cells. Annu Rev Biochem 60:717–755.

64. Melefors O, Hentze MW (1993) Translational regulation by mRNA/protein interactions in eukaryotic cells: Ferritin and beyond. Bioessays 15:85–90.

65. Theil EC (1990) Regulation of ferritin and transferrin receptor mRNAs. J Biol Chem 265:4771–4774.

66. Klausner RD, Rouault TA, Harford JB (1993) Regulating the fate of mRNA: The control of cellular iron metabolism. Cell 72:19–28.

67. Chu E, Koeller DM, Casey JL, Drake JC, Chabner BA, Elwood PC, Zinn S, Allegra CJ (1991) Autoregulation of human thymidylate synthase messenger RNA translation by thymidylate synthase. Proc Natl Acad Sci USA 88:8977–8981.

68. Yates JL, Arfsten AE, Nomura M (1980) In vitro expression of *Escherichia coli* ribosomal protein genes: Autogenous inhibition of translation. Proc Natl Acad Sci USA 77:1837–1841.

69. Winter RB, Morrissey L, Gauss P, Gold L, Hsu T, Karam J (1987) Bacteriophage T4 regA protein binds to mRNAs and prevents translation initiation. Proc Natl Acad Sci USA 84:7822–7826.

70. Andrake M, Guild N, Hsu T, Gold L, Tuerk C, Karam J (1988) DNA polymerase of bacteriophage T4 is an autogenous translational repressor. Proc Natl Acad Sci USA 85:7942–7946.

71. Bernardi A, Spahr P-F (1972) Nucleotide sequence at the binding site for coat protein on RNA of bacteriophage R17. Proc Natl Acad Sci USA 69:3033–3037.

72. Chu E, Voeller D, Koeller DM, Drake JC, Takimoto CH, Maley GF, Maley F, Allegra CJ (1993) Identification of an RNA binding site for human thymidylate synthase. Proc Natl Acad Sci USA 90:517–521.

73. Carey J, Cameron V, de Haseth PL, Uhlenbeck OC (1983) Sequence-specific interaction of R17 coat protein with its ribonucleic acid binding site. Biochemistry 22:2601–2610.

74. Romaniuk PJ, Uhlenbeck OC (1985) Nucleoside and nucleotide inactivation of the R-17 coat protein: Evidence for a transient covalent RNA-protein bond. Biochemistry 24:4239–4244.

75. Koontz SW, Schimmel PR (1979) Aminoacyl-tRNA synthetase-catalyzed cleavage of the glycosidic bond of 5-halogenated uridines. J Biol Chem 254:12277–12280.

76. Starzyk RM, Koontz SW, Schimmel P (1982) A covalent adduct between the uracil ring and the active site of an aminoacyl tRNA synthetase. Nature 298:136–140.

77. Leary RP, Beaudette N, Kisliuk RL (1975) Interaction of deoxyuridylate with thymidylate synthetase. J Biol Chem 250:4864–4868.

78. Plese PC, Dunlap RB (1977) Sulfhydryl group modification of thymidylate synthetase and its effect on activity and ternary complex formation. J Biol Chem 252:6139–6144.

79. Danenberg PV (1977) Thymidylate synthase: A target enzyme in cancer chemotherapy. Biochem Biophys Acta 473:73–97.

80. Chu E, Voeller DM, Morrison PF, Jones KL, Takechi T, Maley GF, Maley F, Allegra CJ (1994) The effect of reducing reagents on binding of thymidylate synthase protein to thymidylate synthase messenger RNA. J Biol Chem 269:20289–20293.

81. Bastow KF, Prabhu R, Cheng YC (1984) The intracellular content of dihydrofolate reductase: Possibilities for control and implications for chemotherapy. Adv Enzyme Regul 22:15–26.

82. Domin BA, Grill SP, Bastow KF, Cheng YC (1982) Effect of methotrexate on dihydrofolate reductase activity in methotrexate-resistant human KB cells. Mol Pharmacol 21:478–482.

83. Cowan KH, Goldsmith ME, Ricciardone MD, Levine R, Rubalcaba E, Jolivet J (1986) Regulation of dihydrofolate reductase in human breast cancer cells and in mutant hamster cells transfected with a human dihydrofolate reductase minigene. Mol Pharmacol 30:69–76.

84. Chu E, Takimoto CH, Voeller D, Grem JL, Allegra CJ (1993) Specific binding of human dihydrofolate reductase protein to dihydrofolate reductase messenger RNA in vitro. Biochemistry 32:4756–4760.

85. Davies JF II, Delcamp TJ, Prendergast NJ, Ashford VA, Freisheim JH, Kraut J (1990) Crystal structures of recombinant human dihydrofolate reductase complexed with folate and 5-deazafolate. Biochemistry 29:9467–9479.

86. Bystroff C, Kraut J (1991) Crystal structure of unliganded *Escherichia coli* dihydrofolate reductase ligand-induced conformational changes and cooperativity in binding. Biochemistry 30:2227–2239.
87. Sherley JL, Kelly TJ (1988) Regulation of human thymidine kinase during the cell cycle. J Biol Chem 263:8350–8358.
88. Ito M, Conrad SE (1990) Independent regulation of thymidine kinase mRNA and enzyme levels in serum-stimulated cells. J Biol Chem 265:6954–6960.
89. Knofler M, Waltner C, Wintersberger E, Mullner EW (1993) Translational repression of endogenous thymidine kinase mRNA in differentiating and arresting mouse cells. J Biol Chem 268:11409–11416.
90. Jones TR, Calvert AH, Jackman AL, Brown SJ, Jones M, Harrap KR (1981) A potent antitumor quinazoline inhibitor of thymidylate synthetase: Synthesis, biological properties and therapeutic results in mice. Eur J Cancer 17:11–19.
91. Jackson RC, Jackman AL, Calvert AH (1983) Biochemical effects of a quinazoline inhibitor of thymidylate synthetase N-(4-(N-((2-amino-4-hydroxy-6-quinazolinyl)methyl) prop-2-ynylamino)-benzyol)-L-glutamic acid (CB3717), on human lymphoblastoid cells. Biochem Pharmacol 32:3783–3790.
92. Jackman AL, Taylor GA, Calvert AH, Harrap KR (1984) Modulation of anti-metabolite effects: Effects of thymidine on the efficacy of the quinazoline-based thymidylate synthetase inhibitor, CB3717. Biochem Pharmacol 33:3269–3275.
93. Jansen G, Schornagel JH, Westerhof GR, Rijksen G, Newell DR, Jackman AL (1990) Multiple membrane transport systems for the uptake of folate-based thymidylate synthase inhibitors. Cancer Res 50:7544–7548.
94. Alison DL, Newell DR, Sessa C, Harland SJ, Hart LI, Harrap KR, Calvert AH (1985) The clinical pharmacokinetics of the novel antifolate N^{10}-propargyl-5,8-dideazafolic acid (CB3717). Cancer Chemother Pharmacol 14:265–271.
95. Calvert AH, Harland SJ, Robinson BA, Jackman AL, Jones TR, Newell DR, Siddik ZH, Wiltshaw E, McElwain TJ, Smith IE, Harrap KR (1986) A phase I evaluation of the quinazoline antifolate thymidylate synthase inhibitor N^{10}-propargyl-5,8-dideazafolic acid, CB3717. Clin Oncol 4:1245–1252.
96. Cantwell BMJ, MaCaulay V, Harris AL, Kaye SB, Smith IE, Milsted RAV, Calvert AH (1988) Phase II study of the antifolate N^{10}-propargyl-5,8-dideazafolic acid (CB 3717) in advanced breast cancer. Eur J Cancer Clin Oncol 24:733–736.
97. Jones TR, Thornton TJ, Flinn A, Jackman AL, Newell DR, Calvert AH (1989) Quinazoline antifolates inhibiting thymidylate synthase: 2-Desamino derivatives with enhanced solubility and potency. J Med Chem 32:847–852.
98. Jackman AL, Taylor GA, Gibson W, Kimbell R, Brown M, Calvert AH, Judson IR, Hughes LR (1991) ICI D1694, a quinazoline antifolate thymidylate synthase inhibitor that is a potent inhibitor of L1210 tumor cell growth in vitro and in vivo: A new agent for clinical study. Cancer Res 51:5579–5586.
99. Harrap KR, Jackman AL, Newell DR, Taylor GA, Hughes LR, Calvert AH (1989) Thymidylate synthase: A target for anticancer drug design. Adv Enzyme Regul 29:161–179.
100. Aherne GW, Farrugia DC, Ward E, Sutcliffe F, Jackman AL (1995) ZD1694 (Tomudex) and polyglutamate levels in mouse plasma and tissues measured by radioimmunoassay (RIA) and the effect of leucovorin (LV) Proc Am Assoc Cancer Res 36:2243.
101. Jackman AL, Gibson W (1995) Polyglutamation of the thymidylate synthase (TS) inhibitor, ZD1694 (Tomudex), in normal mouse tissues. Proc Am Assoc Cancer Res 36:2245.
102. Drake JC, Allegra CJ, Moran RG, Johnston PG (1995) The development and characterization of Tomudex (ZD1694) resistant human breast and colon carcinoma cell lines. Proc Am Assoc Cancer Res 36:2271.
103. Lu K, McGuire JJ, Rustum YM (1995) Characterization of a folylpolyglutamate synthetase deficient, ZD1694-resistant/methotrexate-sensitive HCT-8 human ileocecal adenocarcinoma subline. Proc Am Assoc Cancer Res 36:1895.
104. Takemura Y, Walton MI, Gibson W, Kimbell R, Miyachi H, Kobayashi H, Jackman AL (1995) The influence of drug exposure manner on the development of ZD1694-resistance in cultured human leukemia cells. Proc Am Assoc Cancer Res 36:1890.
105. Van der Wilt CL, Pinedo HM, Kuiper CM, Smid K, Peters GJ (1995) Biochemical basis for the combined antiproliferative effect of AG337 or ZD1694 and 5-fluorouracil. Proc Am Assoc Cancer Res 36:2260.

106. Izzo J, Zielinski Z, Chang YM, Bertino JR (1995) Molecular mechanisms of the synergistic sequential administration of D1694 (Tomudex) followed by Fura in colon carcinoma cells. Proc Am Assoc Cancer Res 36:2272.

107. Clarke SJ, Ward J, de Boer M, Planting A, Verweij J, Sutcliffe F, Azab M, Judson IR (1994) Phase I study of the new thymidylate synthase inhibitor Tomudex (ZD1694) in patients with advanced malignancy. Ann Oncol 5:240.

108. Sorensen JM, Jordan E, Grem JL, Arbuck SG, Chen AP, Hamilton JM, Johnston P, Kohler DR, Goldspiel BR, Allegra CJ (1994) Phase I trial of ZD1694 (Tomudex), a direct inhibitor of thymidylate synthase. Ann Oncol 5:241.

109. Smith IE, Speilmann M, Bonneterre J, Namer M, Green M, Wandar HE, Toussaint C, Azab M (1994) Tomudex (ZD1694), a new thymidylate synthase inhibitor with antitumour activity in breast cancer. Ann Oncol 5:242.

110. Burris III H, Von Hoff D, Bowen K, Heaven R, Rinaldi D, Eckardt J, Fields S, Campbell L, Robert F, Patton S, Kennealey G (1994) A phase II trial of ZD1694, a novel thymidylate synthase inhibitor, in patients with advanced non-small cell lung cancer. Ann Oncol 5:244.

111. Gore M, Earl H, Cassidy J, Tattersal M, Mansi J, Azab M (1994) Phase II study of Tomudex (ZD1694) in refractory ovarian cancer. Ann Oncol 5:245.

112. Pazdur R, Casper ES, Meropol NJ, Fuchs C, Kennealey GT (1995) Phase II trial of Tomudex (ZD1694), a thymidylate synthase inhibitor, in advanced pancreatic cancer. Proc Am Soc Clin Oncol 13:613.

113. Zalcberg J, Cunningham D, Francois E, van Cutsem E, Schornagel J, Adenis A, Green M, Seymour L, Azab M (1995) The final results of a large phase II study of the potent thymidylate synthase (TS) inhibitor "Tomudex" (ZD1694) in advanced colorectal cancer. Proc Am Soc Clin Oncol 13:494.

114. Taylor EC, Kuhnt D, Shih C, Rinzel SM, Grindey GB, Barredo J, Jannatipour M, Moran RG (1992) A dideazatetrahydrofolate analogue lacking a chiral center at C-6,N-[4-[2-(2-amino-3,4-dihydro-4-oxo-7H-pyrolo[2,3-d]pyrimidin-5-yl)ethyl]benzoyal]-L-glutamic acid, is an inhibitor of thymidylate synthase. J Med Chem 35:4450–4454.

115. Rinaldi DA, Burris HA, Dorr FA, Nelson J, Fields SM, Kuhn JG, Eckardt JR, Lu P, Woodworth JR, Corso SW, Von Hoff DD (1994) A phase I evaluation of the novel thymidylate synthase inhibitor, LY231514, in patients with advanced solid tumors. Proc Am Soc Clin Oncol 13:430.

116. Vasey PA, Calvert AH, Kaye SB, Cassidy J (1994) Clinical phase I study of LY231514 (an inhibitor of thymidylate synthase) using a daily ×5 q21 schedule. Ann Oncol 5:237.

117. Rinaldi D, Burris H, Dorr F, Eckardt J, Fields S, Langley C, Clark G, Von Hoff D (1995) A phase I evaluation of LY231514 administered every 21 days, utilizing the modified continual reassessment method for dose escalation. Proc Am Soc Clin Oncol 14:1539.

118. Duch DS, Banks S, Dev IK, Dickerson SH, Ferone R, Health LS, Humphreys J, Knick V, Pendergast W, Singer S, Smith GK, Waters K, Wilson HR (1993) Biochemical and cellular pharmacology of 1843U89, a novel benzoquinazoline inhibitor of thymidylate synthase. Cancer Res 53:810–818.

119. Walton MI, Gibson W, Aherne GW, Lawrence N, Stephens T, Smith M, Jackman AL (1994) Pharmacokinetics of the potent, non-polyglutamatable thymidylate synthase inhibitors CB 30900 and ZD9331 in mice. Proc Am Assoc Cancer Res 35:1793.

120. Boyle FT, Wardleworth JM, Hennequin LF, Kimbell R, Marsham PR, Stephens TC, Jackman AL (1994) ZD9331-Design of a novel non-polyglutamatable quinazoline-based inhibitor of thymidylate synthase (TS). Proc Am Assoc Cancer Res 35:1817.

121. Jackman AL, Aherne GW, Kimbell R, Brunton L, Hardcastle A, Wardleworth JW, Stephens TC, Boyle FT (1994) ZD9331, a non-polyglutamatable quinazoline thymidylate synthase (TS) inhibitor. Proc Am Assoc Cancer Res 35:1791.

122. Webber SE, Bleckman TM, Attard J, Deal JG, Kathardekar V, Welsch KM, Webber S, Janson CA, Mattews DA, Smith WW, Freer ST, Jordan SR, Bacquet RJ, Howland EF, Booth CLJ, Ward RW, Hermann SM, White J, Morse CA, Hilliard JA, Bartlett CA (1993) Design of thymidylate synthase inhibitors using protein crystal structures: The synthesis and biological evaluation of a novel class of 5-substituted quinazolinones. Med Chem 36:733–746.

123. Johnston AL, Sherry BV, Webber S, Welsch KM (1992) Experimental antitumor activity of AG-331, a novel lipophilic thymidylate synthase inhibitor. 7th NCI-EORTC Symposium on New Drugs in Cancer Therapy, Amsterdam, p 131.

124. Ferone R, Hanlon MH, Waters KA, Dev IK (1993) Influence of intracellular polyglutamation on the cytotoxicity of the thymidylate synthase inhibitor 1843U89. Proc Am Assoc Cancer Res 34:1630.

125. Humphreys J, Smith G, Waters K, Duch D (1993) Antitumor activity of the novel thymidylate synthase inhibitor 1843U89. Proc Am Assoc Cancer Res 34:1625.
126. Mitrovski B, Johnston PG, Erlichman C (1994) Cytotoxic and biochemical effects of a lipophilic (AG-331) and a non-lipophilic (D1694) thymidylate synthase inhibitor in MHG-U1 cells. Proc Am Assoc Cancer Res 35:1787.
127. Calvete JA, Balmanno K, Taylor GA, Rafi I, Newell DR, Lind MJ, Calvert AH (1994) Pre-clinical and clinical studies of prolonged administration of the novel thymidylate synthase inhibitor, AG337. Proc Am Assoc Cancer Res 35:1821.
128. Clendeninn NJ, Peterkin JJ, Webber S, Shetty BV, Koda RT, Leichman L, Leichman CG, Jeffers S, Muggia FM, O'Dwyer PJ (1994) AG-331, a "non-classical," lipophilic thymidylate synthase inhibitor for the treatment of solid tumors. Ann Oncol 5:246.
129. Rafi I, Taylor GA, Calvete JA, Balmanno K, Boddy AV, Bailey NB, Lind MJ, Newell D, Calvert AH (1995) A phase I clinical study of the novel antifolate AG337 given by a 5 day continuous infusion. Proc Am Assoc Cancer Res 36:1433.
130. Giantonio B, Qian M, Gallo J, DiMaria D, Legerton K, Johnston AL, Clendeninn NJ, O'Dwyer PJ (1995) Phase I trial of AG-331 as a 5-day continuous infusion. Proc Am Soc Clin Oncol 14:1562.

8. ANTIFOLATES: CURRENT DEVELOPMENTS

ELIZABETH A. RAYL AND GIUSEPPE PIZZORNO

This group of chemotherapic agents represents the first class of antimetabolites synthesized and successfully proven to have antitumor activity. The concept of antimetabolite was conceived in 1940 when Woods and Fildes described the activity of sulfonamides on bacteria and suggested that the antimicrobial effect was related to some sort of competition with the normal utilization of p-aminobenzoic acid, a fundamental metabolite for bacteria [1,2]. Following the characterization and synthesis of folic acid in 1946, a number of analogues were synthesized and tested [3]. The first derivative was x-methyl-folic acid, which produced changes in blood counts, particularly granulocytes, and bone marrow in rats [4]. However, this antagonist had no activity in humans.

Almost simultaneously, Farber had described an acceleration phenomenon in the leukemic process of children affected by acute lymphoblastic leukemia treated with the folic acid conjugates pteroyl-di- and pteroyl-tri-glutamic acid (diopterin and teropterin), suggesting the possible merits of folic acid antagonists in the treatment of these patients [5].

A new series of folic acid antagonists, in which the hydroxy group in the pteridine ring was replaced by an amino group, proved to be deadly poisons in mice [6]. As expected, the toxic effects were reversed by folic acid. The first antifolate in this series, 4-amino-pteroyl glutamic acid (aminopterin), was introduced in the clinic at the end of 1947 by Farber and was shown to produce temporary remission in 10 out of 16 children terminally ill with acute leukemia [7]. Despite the initial success, the severe side effects associated with aminopterin, mostly stomatitis, hindered further clinical development. A second antifolate in this series, methotrexate, in which the N^{10} proton was replaced by a methyl group, proved to be equally effective but had a slightly better therapeutic index [8].

METHOTREXATE

Methotrexate (MTX) has been the most widely studied and clinically utilized folate agonist. Since the inception of its use in the early 1950s, methotrexate has been used clinically to treat a wide variety of cancers, including leukemia, choriocarcinoma, and solid tumors of the head, neck, and breast. While MTX has proven to be effective against certain cancers either as the sole agent or in combination therapies, one major obstacle to its use has been the development of drug resistance. A considerable effort has been undertaken over the past 40 years to investigate the biochemistry of MTX metabolism and pharmacology, as well as the mechanisms of MTX resistance.

Methotrexate is a classical antifolate and therefore is a structural analogue of folic acid, comprised of three main substituents: a substituted pteridine ring, para-aminobenzoate, and a terminal glutamate. The hydroxyl group at the C_4 position of the pteridine ring of folate has been replaced with an amino group in MTX. In addition, the N^{10} proton of folate has been substituted with a methyl group (Figure 8-1). The disodium salt of this molecule is water soluble and is readily transported across eukaryotic cell membranes.

Transport and accumulation of methotrexate

Folates and antifolates are transported into cells via two distinct transport systems, the low-affinity reduced-folate carrier or the high-affinity folate receptor. While MTX may be transported by either of these two mechanisms, the primary route of intracellular uptake is via the reduced-folate carrier. Methotrexate competes for uptake with physiological concentrations of folic acid, N^5-methyltetrahydrofolate (5-methyl FH_4), and N^5-formyltetrahydrofolate (5-formyl FH_4) [9–12].

Upon entry into cells, MTX is polyglutamylated via folylpolyglutamate synthase (FPGS). Mammalian FPGS adds glutamate residues in gamma-carboxyl linkage to folate coenzymes as well as folate antagonists, such as MTX [13–20]. As many as two to seven glutamate residues may be added by FPGS. Polyglutamylation of MTX, like other folate coenzymes, is important for intracellular accumulation of the drug within cells. Polyanionic forms of MTX result in drug retention at levels that are much higher than would be expected based on simple diffusion.

The effectiveness of MTX as a chemotherapeutic agent is directly related to the retention of the drug within cells and consequently the level of polyglutamylation by the cytosolic FPGS. Intracellular retention of MTX is proportional to the number of glutamate residues added. Unlike the case with other antifolates, polyglutamylation does not significantly increase the inhibitory effect of MTX for dihydrofolate reductase (DHFR) [21–26]. Furthermore, the level of polyglutamylation may vary between cell types. Although MTX monoglutamates

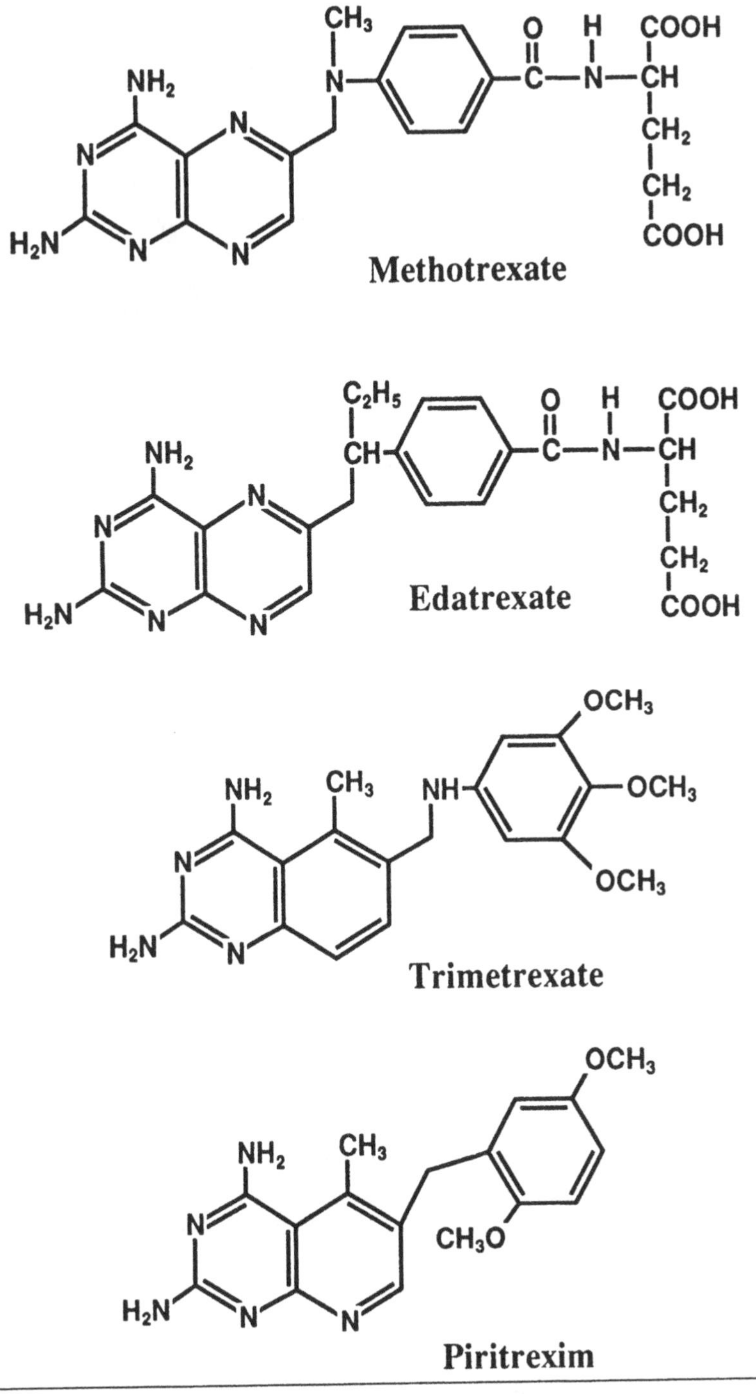

Figure 8–1. Dihydrofolate reductase inhibitors.

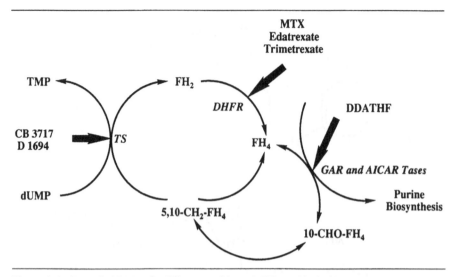

Figure 8–2. Sites of inhibition for different antifolates. *DHFR* = dihydrofolate reductase; *TS* = thymidylate synthase; *GAR Tase* = glycinamide ribonucleotide transformylase; *AICAR Tase* = aminoimidazole carboxamide ribonucleotide transformylase; FH_4 = tetrahydrofolate; FH_2 = dihydrofolate; $5,10\text{-}CH_2\text{-}FH_4$ = $N^{5,10}$-methylene tetrahydrofolate; $10\text{-}CHO\text{-}FH_4$ = 10-formyl tetrahydrofolate; dUMP = deoxyuridine monophosphate; TMP = thymidine monophosphate.

are good substrates for FPGS, diglutamate derivatives are poor substrates. In some tissues, including rat and beef liver, rat hepatocyte primary cultures, and a human leukemia cell line, the predominant species of MTX is either the diglutamate or the triglutamate [21,25,27,28]. In other tissues and cultured mammalian cells, longer length derivatives of MTX glutamate have been observed [19,21,25,29,30]. It has been suggested that these differences in polyglutamate chain length may be a consequence of differential efflux rates of short-chain MTX polyglutamates from the different cell types or may result from differences in the specificity of the folylpolyglutamate synthase from each of the different cell types [19,21,25].

Metabolic action of methotrexate

Dihydrofolate reductase is an essential enzyme required for the maintenance of intracellular folate pools. Dihydrofolate reductase reduces dihydrofolate to tetrahydrofolate in the presence of NADPH (Figure 8–2). Tetrahydrofolate is subsequently converted to a variety of other reduced-folate coenzymes. There are 18 folate-dependent enzymes in mammalian cells. These enzymes carry out single-carbon transfer reactions involved in DNA, RNA, and protein biosynthesis. Each of these enzymes play pivotal roles in metabolic processes in neoplastic as well as normal mammalian cells.

The primary cytotoxic effect of MTX is competitive inhibition of DHFR [31]. Methotrexate is a tight-binding inhibitor of DHFR, with its dissociation constants being measured in the range of 10^{-9}M, and binds in a stoichiometric ratio to DHFR at pH 6.0 [32,33]. At physiological pH levels, MTX binds less tightly and displays reversible competitive kinetics with the substrate dihydrofolate. Unlike the natural folate substrates, polyglutamylation of MTX does not enhance the inhibitory effect of MTX for DHFR.

Polyglutamates of MTX have been demonstrated to be potent inhibitors of glycinamide ribonucleotide transformylase (GARTF), aminoimidazole carboxamide ribonucleotide transformylase (AICARTF), as well thymidylate synthase (TS) [34]. GARTF and AICARTF both utilize the coenzyme N^{10}-formyltetrahydrofolate (10-formyl-FH$_4$) and are required for *de novo* purine biosynthesis. The latter is required for thymidine biosynthesis. In addition, secondary inhibitory effects are observed as a result of DHFR inhibition. As dihydrofolates accumulate within cells, they serve as substrates for FPGS. These polyglutamylated forms of dihydrofolate have demonstrated to be effective inhibitors of TS, glycinamide ribonucleotide transformylase, and aminoimidazole carboxamide ribonucleotide transformylase [34,35].

Methotrexate displays similar binding affinities for DHFR from either normal or neoplastic tissues. Therefore, selectivity of MTX depends upon a variety of other physiological factors. Such factors include differential transport, polyglutamylation, gamma-glutamyl hydrolase activity, as well as differential interactions with DHFR.

Resistance of methotrexate

Problems associated with any chemotherapeutic agent include the development of resistance as well as toxicity. Intrinsic drug resistance results from naturally occurring polymorphisms in the absence of selective pressure. However, more commonly, resistance due to chemotherapeutic drugs is acquired. The documented forms of acquired resistance to methotrexate include: defective transport of MTX, polyglutamylation defects, elevation in the level of gamma-glutamyl hydrolase activity, mutations in DHFR, and gene amplification of DHFR. Acquired resistance often results from either one or a combination of several forms of resistance.

One of the most common forms of resistance to MTX is due to defects in the transport mechanisms. Several mammalian cell lines have been determined to be resistant to MTX as a result of alterations in the expression or structural alterations of the reduced-folate carrier [36–39]. These cells are also defective for transport of 5-methyl FH$_4$ and 5-formyl FH$_4$. The low-affinity, reduced-folate carrier cDNA has been cloned from a mouse L1210 leukemia cell line. Transfection of this cDNA into human breast tumor cells, MTX-ZR-75-1, which are resistant to MTX due to transport defects, renders the cells sensitive to MTX [40]. Possible mutant forms of the reduced-folate carriers have yet to be identified or characterized.

Two isoforms of the high-affinity folate carrier receptor have been identified in humans. The two 28 kDa proteins are approximately 70% identical based upon the deduced amino acid sequence of the cDNAs. Despite these similarities, these two folate carrier receptors demonstrated different stereospecificities for reduced folate coenzymes [41]. Expression of the folate receptor has been implicated in MTX transport. Dixon *et al.* transfected wild-type as well as MTX-resistant cells, ZR-75-1 and MTX-ZR-75-1, respectively, with an expression recombinant harboring a human high-affinity folate receptor cDNA. Stably transfected cells sustained growth in low-folate medium and displayed enhanced intracellular concentrations of MTX as well as 5-formyl FH$_4$ and folic acid. Furthermore, accumulated intracellular concentrations of MTX and folates were similar between the wild-type and MTX-resistant transfectants [11]. Other studies have suggested that folate receptor mRNA expression may be regulated by the stability of the mRNA itself [42].

Transport defects in several MTX-resistant cell lines have been described. However, resistance in these cells is often accompanied by a combination of mechanisms. Decreased FPGS activity has been described as a mechanism of resistance to MTX [43–48]. Conversely, cells expressing very high levels of FPGS have demonstrated increased sensitivity to MTX [49].

In addition to FPGS, the interconversion and regulation of cellular polyglutamtes is dependent upon the function of another intracellular enzyme, gamma-glutamyl hydrolase. This enzyme removes glutamate residues from polyglutamylated forms of folates and antifolates. A variety of folate-requiring enzymes demonstrate differential specificity for folate substrates based, in part, upon the numbers of attached glutamate residues. Increased gamma-glutamyl hydrolase activity in human H35 hepatoma cells contributes to MTX resistance [50]. The nature of increased gamma-glutamyl hydrolase activity in these cells has not been elucidated but may serve as an alternate target in overcoming resistance.

Several MTX-resistant tumor cell lines have been attributed to mutations in DHFR [51–58]. More commonly, amplification of the DHFR gene appears to be a mechanism of MTX resistance [59–63]. Some patients treated with MTX have demonstrated resistance due to gene amplification of DHFR [64–67]. Reversible resistance due to gene amplification is associated with the presence of double-minute chromosomes [68–70]. DHFR gene amplification associated with chromosomes displaying homogeneous staining regions (HSR) is a stably maintained form of MTX resistance [71–76]. While the mechanisms of gene amplification in mammalian cells are not well understood, gene amplification occurs at a higher frequency in transformed cells than in normal cells [77–79].

Overexpression in the absence of DHFR gene amplification has been documented [80,81]. Studies indicate that translation of DHFR mRNA is reduced by DHFR binding *in vitro*. Furthermore, addition of MTX stimulated translation of the DHFR mRNA, probably by binding with DHFR and interrupting the DHFR/mRNA interaction [81].

Clinical use

Since the early 1950s, MTX has been utilized against acute lymphoblastic leukemia (ALL) in children as a single agent. Methotrexate is an important drug currently used in combination protocols to treat acute leukemia as well as certain other leukemias and lymphomas. Methotrexate is used in combination with leucovorin, L-asparaginase, or 6-mercaptopurine in the treatment of ALL [82–87].

Methotrexate administered in a high-dose/aggressive regimen in the treatment of choriocarcinoma has been highly successful, with response rates up to 50% [88]. The reason for the exquisite MTX sensitivity of this neoplasm is unclear. However, accumulation of MTX long-chain polyglutamates in choriocarcinoma cells may allow for intracellular retention and subsequently increased sensitivity [35].

Other neoplasms, such as breast cancer and tumors of the head and neck, have been successfully treated with combination therapies that include MTX. Sequential use of MTX with 5-fluorouracil and cyclophosphamide has demonstrated response rates up to 50% for breast cancer [89]. Methotrexate is often used in combination with cisplatin for the treatment of advanced head and neck neoplasms. Methotrexate treatment followed by leucovorin rescue has been shown to improve response rates from 30% to 50%. However, long-term survival rates remain unchanged [90]. Methotrexate has also been utilized in the treatment of several non-neoplastic disorders, such as psoriasis, systemic lupus erythematous, and rheumatoid arthritis [91–93]. Treatment of these disorders is usually with oral, low-dose administration of MTX.

Despite successful therapy with MTX, either alone or in combination with other drugs, drug resistance remains a major obstacle. While combination therapy response rates for patients with ALL or with acute non-lymphocytic leukemia (ANLL), are 90% and 70%, respectively, the 5-year survival rates of these patients are 50% and 15%, respectively [94]. Subsequent treatment with the same drugs has been demonstrated to be less effective. This is indicative of acquired drug resistance. High-dose therapy may overcome MTX resistance due to transport defects. However, resistance due to ineffective polyglutamylation, defects in DHFR, or amplification of DHFR may not readily be overcome by high-dose regimens with MTX.

Toxicity

Common toxic effects of MTX include mucositis, neutropenia, renal tubule damage, hepatic fibrosis, and frank cirrhosis. These toxic side effects often occur together. Hematologic and gastrointestinal toxicity is most often observed because these cells are rapidly dividing and are consequently more susceptible to MTX. Administration of MTX in high doses may result in renal toxicity, especially in adults. Adjustment of the urine pH to alkaline values, as well as extensive hydration, increase the solubility of MTX, thereby reducing this form of toxicity. Liver damage may result from long-term, low-dose treatment with MTX. While this is a rare problem in the treatment of cancers, this is a potential toxic threat in the treatment of non-neoplastic disorders.

In order to find better DHFR inhibitors with improved tumor selectivity and to overcome drug resistance mechanisms that could preclude the antitumor activity of classical antifolates, a number of DHFR inhibitors have been developed during the past 30 years. Because of their different structural charcteristics, we will mainly focus on two inhibitors that have shown to be superior to MTX at the preclinical level and have recently received thorough clinical testing.

EDATREXATE

Edatrexate (10-ethyl-10-deazaaminopterin) is a classical antifolate DHFR inhibitor lacking a nitrogen in position 10 with an alkyl substitutent in the same location (see

Figure 8–1). These modifications result in an increased tumor selectivity in both murine and human xenograft *in vivo* tumor models [96–98]. This antifolate has several improved properties over MTX. It has increased membrane transport via the reduced folate carrier as well as better affinity for FPGS. Subsequently polyglutamates accumulate more efficiently intracellularly [99,100]. However, the enhanced tumor selectivity of edatrexate may be primarily due to differences in kinetic parameters between tumor and normal cells [101]. Transport studies in L1210, S180, and Manca tumor cells versus murine small intestine epithelial cells have shown lower Km and higher Vmax values for both influx and efflux in normal cells. Furthermore, *in vivo* studies of polyglutamation revealed that only a small percentage of edatrexate is present as polyglutamates in the small intestine (~8%). In contrast, the majority of the drug (~60%) was polyglutamated in tumor cells [102]. In these studies, edatrexate showed a substantial advantage in selectivity for the tumor cells over methotrexate and aminopterin, and consequently resulted in a better therapeutic index for this new antifolate. In several *in vivo* experiments against murine tumors and human xenografts, edatrexate was far superior to MTX in terms of antitumor activity, even in tumors refractory to other classical antifolates, producing not only a reduction in tumor burden but also a cure in some of the tumor models [97,98].

Phase I clinical trials have been conducted in patients with advanced solid tumors receiving weekly iv doses ranging from 5 to 120 mg/m². The dose-limiting toxicity was mucositis in 20–30% of the patients accompanied by myelosuppression, mostly leukopenia and thrombocytopenia. Other side effects that were not dose dependent included nausea, vomiting, fatigue, macular rash, and mild hepatic toxicity. Some activity was observed in patients with breast cancer and non–small cell lung cancer [103].

A series of phase II trials was conducted in patients with lung, breast, head and neck, and colon cancers, and non-Hodgkin's lymphoma. An average of 32% of patients enrolled in non–small cell lung cancer trials experienced some objective responses, with tolerable toxicities at the dose of 80 mg/m² weekly for 5 weeks [104,105]. An equally interesting feature was that the antitumor activity of edatrexate in patients with metastatic breast cancer resulted in a response rate of 41% [106]. A randomized phase II trial comparing edatrexate with MTX in patients with head and neck cancer showed a small advantage of edatrexate over MTX (27% vs. 21% response rate) [107]. In patients with metastatic colon carcinoma [108] as well as in patients with small cell lung cancer [109], edatrexate did not show significant activity.

Because the preclinical data demonstrated synergistic effects of edatrexate in combination with other anticancer agents, such as 5-FU, cyclophosphamide, cisplatin, and melphalan [110,111], several clinical trials were conducted to explore the activity of combination regimens containing this new antifolate for the treatment of non–small cell lung cancer. A 60% response rate was observed in previously untreated patients who received the combination edatrexate, vinblastine, and mitomycin [112]. A similar set of patients was treated with edatrexate combined with cisplatin and cyclophosphamide [113]. In the first group of patients who received the full dose of chemotherapy, a 47% response rate was observed. Since serious toxicities were experienced by the first group of patients, the second group received a reduced dose. Only 27% of individuals in the second group experienced a major response. Despite a 12.5% reduction of the starting dose of each drug, stomatitis remained the major dose-limiting toxicity [113]. To alleviate the side effects of edatrexate, low doses of leucovorin (15 mg every 6 hours for 4 doses) were added, 24 hours after each administration of the antifolate to the full-dose regimen. Compared to the patients who received the reduced-dose combination, the addition of leucovorin had a protective effect against stomatitis without affecting the response rate, which remained above 40% [114]. Several studies that combine leucovorin with edatrexate- and edatrexate-containing regimens are now in progress.

LIPOPHILIC DIHYDROFOLATE REDUCTASE INHIBITORS

A number of quinazoline and pyrimidine antifolate analogs have been synthesized over the past 30 years and have been shown to be potent inhibitors of DHFR. Because of the emergence of drug resistance to methotrexate, several groups concentrated their efforts on the development of nonclassical antifolates that possess lipophilic characteristics. This class of lipophilic antifolates lacks the glutamic acid portion present in the first generation DHFR inhibitors [115], such as MTX and aminopterin, and was designed with the intent of overcoming MTX resistance related to (1) reduced-folate transport and (2) intracellular retention and accumulation. Since these antifolates lack a terminal glutamate, they do not form polyglutamates. Therefore, activation and retention of these molecules is not dependent on an active FPGS.

Among the many lipophilic antifolates synthesized, trimetrexate (see Figure 8–1) proved to be a potent inhibitor of DHFR, with an affinity for the enzyme similar to that of MTX. Moreover, it was shown to be a potent inhibitor of cell growth in different *in vitro* and *in vivo* tumor models [115–118], including L1210 leukemia cells resistant to methotrexate [119]. These resistant L1210 cells have a rapid intracellular accumulation of the drug despite impaired MTX transport [119]. A specific carrier involved in the transport of trimetrexate had not been described, suggesting that passive diffusion was the main mechanism of uptake, but it probably was not the only one. Several investigators had shown cross-resistance of this lipophilic antifolate in cells expressing the MDR phenotype, indicating some specificity of this structure for the aforementioned mechanism of efflux [120–123].

Preclinical studies have indicated the superiority of trimetrexate over MTX in a number of murine tumor models. However, as with MTX, this nonclassical antifolate was not effective against several human xenograft tumors [124]. Due to the broad spectrum of antitumor activity and its ability to overcome MTX-related drug resistance in certain tumor models, trimetrexate was clinically evaluated in phase I trials during the mid-1980's. The main administration of the drug was by infusion over a 60 minute period with doses of 10–200 mg/m² every 2 weeks. The dose-limiting toxicity was hematological, mostly leukopenia. Thrombocytopenia was modest. Nonhematological toxicities were sporadic and mild. Responses were observed in patients with colon, head and neck, breast, and non–small cell lung cancer [125–130].

Several phase II clinical trials had been conducted in a number of diseases previously shown to be sensitive to methotrexate. The results have been somewhat disappointing. Trimetrexate has demonstrated considerable activity in non–small cell lung cancer, with a response rate of approximately 20% [131–133]. A 26% objective response rate was observed in patients with head and neck cancer [134]. Minor antineoplastic activity was also observed in breast cancer [135,136]. No significant activity was observed in esophageal and renal cancer [137–140], melanoma [141,142], mesothelioma [143], soft tissue sarcoma [144,145], and gastric, pancreatic, and uterine cancer [146–149]. Furthermore, trimetrexate failed to show any antitumor activity in recurrent childhood ALL.

Recently, trimetrexate has received FDA approval for the treatment of moderate to severe *Pneumocystis carinii* pneumonia in immunosuppressed patients whose disease was refractory to co-trimoxazole treatment [150]. Trimetrexate was shown to be a potent inhibitor of the protozoan DHFR. Despite the myelosuppressive activity of this antifolate, the lack of a folate transport system in the *Pneumocystis* had provided the possibility of a differential rescue of the host tissues by the concurrent administration of leucovorin without interfering with the antiprotozoan effect [151]. Trimetrexate is administered iv as a 60 minute infusion once daily at a dose of $45 \, mg/m^2$ concomitant with or followed by $20 \, mg/m^2$ of leucovorin every 6 hours [150].

Piritrexim (see Figure 8–1) is another lipophilic DHFR inhibitor tested as an anticancer agent in clinical trials. This compound, like trimetrexate, does not require an active transport mechanism, is not a substate for FPGS, and is ineffective in tumor cells expressing the MDR phenotype [152,153]. Piritrexim has shown minimal activity in non–small cell lung cancer, melanoma, sarcoma, colon cancer, and head and neck cancer [154].

It is difficult to identify the reasons for the lack of success of these two lipophilic DHFR inhibitors. However, a few critical points should be kept in mind during the development of the next generations of lipophilic antifolates. (1) Because of the lack of polyglutamylation of these compounds and subsequent limited intracellular retention of these drugs, schedules involving continuous infusion of the drug rather than bolus administrations should be tested. (2) Since these lipophilic antifolates were mainly developed for overcoming drug resistance to MTX, besides classical phase II trials, where the drug is administered to previously untreated patients, additional phase II trials should select patients with tumors that are resistant to methotrexate. The mechanisms of resistance may subsequently be evaluated using the current available assays in order to correlate the clinical outcome.

THYMIDYLATE SYNTHASE INHIBITORS

Methotrexate, besides its primary inhibitory activity on DHFR and following its intracellular convertion to polyglutamates, has been shown to inhibit other folate-dependent enzymes, such as thymidylate synthase and AICAR transformylase [34,35]. The contribution of these secondary inhibitory activities to the mechanism of action of MTX and the need to overcome MTX resistance due to amplified or altered DHFR led to the development in the past decade of a new series of folate analogs having the ability to inhibit other folate-dependent enzymes.

Thymidylate synthase (TS), the enzyme that catalyzes the methylation of dUMP to dTMP using 5,10-methylenetetrahydrofolate as a methyl donor, has been an important target for cancer chemotherapy. 5-Fluorouracil, once metabolized to FdUMP, forms a ternary complex with TS in the presence of 5,10-methylene tetrahydrofolate [156]. The formation of the ternary complex with FdUMP results in the inhibition of dTMP formation, therefore causing a block of DNA synthesis [157,158]. 5-FU is also converted to ribonucleotides and incorporated into RNA, resulting in an increased cytotoxic effect [159,160]. A folate analog inhibitor directed against TS might have a better therapeutic advantage over a pyrimidine derivative since it would more likely affect a single target, TS, and inhibition could not be overcome by dUMP accumulated as a result of the enzymatic blockage [161,162].

2-Amino-4-hydroxy quinazoline analogs of folic acid were shown in the past to have not only inhibitory activity against TS but also better affinity for TS over DHFR [163]. Jones and collegues developed a series of 5,8-dideaza analogues substituted at the N^{10} position, and the corresponding propargyl derivative (CB 3717) (Figure 8–3) was selected for further development because of its potent TS inhibition and antiproliferative activity [164] (Figure 8–2).

N^{10}-propargyl-5,8-dideazafolic acid as a monoglutamate is a tight binding inhibitor of TS with a Ki value of ~4nM. Its mechanism of inhibition is mixed noncompetitive with the natural enzyme substrate, 5,10-methylenetetrahydrofolate [165,166]. *In vitro* experiments on different cell lines have shown that the antiproliferative activity of CB 3717 can be reversed by the addition of thymidine, thus indicating the specificity of this quinazoline analog for TS [164]. Furthermore, cell lines that developed resistance to this antifolate by continous exposure possessed an amplification of the TS gene [167,168].

CB 3717 is transported into the cells through two main mechanisms: (1) the reduced-folate transport system, which is also utilized by MTX and other classical antifolates, and has not demonstrated to be a very effective carrier for this substrate; (2) the membrane folate binding protein system, also referred to as the high-affinity folate receptor [169]. The folate binding protein has high affinity for CB 3717 and other TS inhibitors. Only folic acid has a threefold advantage over these series of compounds. However, the membrane carrier system demonstrated a low affinity for the classical DHFR inhibitors, MTX and edatrexate. Despite the high affinity of TS inhibitors for this second transport system, the process of internalization of the drug by the folate binding protein, probably through a receptor-mediated endocytosis, is not very efficient and its role in the cytotoxicity of the drug is still unclear.

Following the uptake process, CB 3717 has been shown both *in vitro* and *in vivo* to be converted to polyglutamate forms [170,171]. These metabolites, particularly

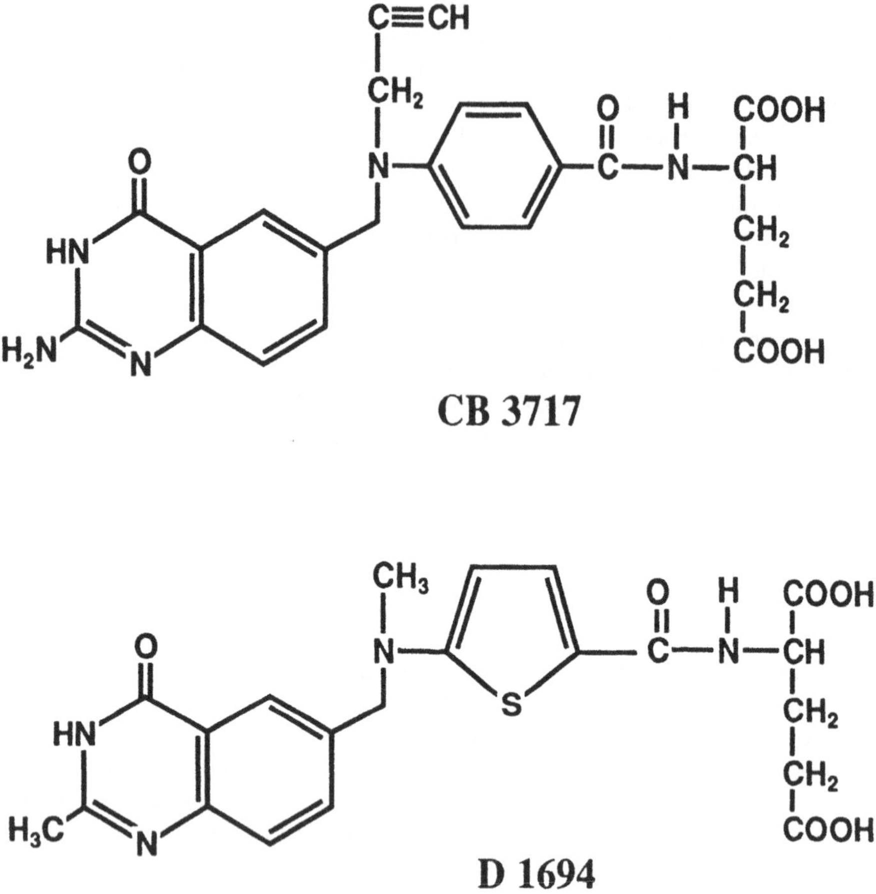

CB 3717

D 1694

Figure 8–3. Thymidylate synthase inhibitors.

tetra- and penta-glutamates, are at least 100-fold more effective inhibitors of TS than the parent compound, and appear to contribute significantly to the anti-proliferative effect of CB 3717 [172].

Clinically, CB 3717 was tested in a phase I trial with a starting dose of 140 mg/m^2 infused over 1 hour period every 3 weeks. The dose-limiting toxicity was found to be mainly renal at a dose of 450 mg/m^2. Other relevant toxicities were liver function abnormalities, mostly elevation of alanine aminotransferase, and fatigue, anorexia, and lethargy. Surprisingly, myelosuppression was mild and mucositis was limited to very few patients [173]. CB 3717 had a modest antitumor activity against ovarian, breast, colon, and non–small cell lung cancer [173–175]. Phase II trials were conducted at a dose of 400 mg/m^2, and a number of responders were again seen in breast, ovarian, and hepatocellular carcinomas. Toxicities were similar to those encountered during the phase I evaluation [176–179].

The cause of nephrotoxicity was found to be related to the physical properties of the drug and not to the inhibitory effect on TS [180,181]. The limited aqueous solubility of CB 3717 at acidic pH in the urine caused crystallization and accumulation in the kidneys of mice; alkalinization of the urine to pH 9 increased the solubility up to 100-fold [182].

In order to circumvent the insolubility of CB 3717, 2-desamino CB 3717 was the first derivative of the parent compound synthesized with reduced intermolecular hydrogen-bonding capability. This new antifolate proved to be soluble at physiological pH and maintained TS inhibition [183]. Further structural modifications led to the synthesis of a N^{10}-methylthiophene derivative, D1694 [184] (see Figure 8–3). D1694 was a weaker TS inhibitor than CB 3717 (20-fold less effective) but was 500-fold more cytotoxic than the parent compound [185]. As in the case of CB 3717, the inhibition is mixed noncompetitive with respect to 5,10-methylene tetrahydrofolate. D1694 is rapidly internalized through the reduced-folate carrier, in contrast with CB 3717, and maintains high affinity for the membrane folate binding protein [185]. This second-generation TS inhibitor has high affinity for FPGS, and the polyglutamates are rapidly accumulated in the cells. As seen for other TS inhibitors, the polyglutamate forms are better inhibitors of TS with at least a two log advantage over the monoglutamate [185]. The parent compound, D1694, as well its polyglutamates, are highly specific for TS, with a 100-fold greater affinity over DHFR. Despite a lower affinity for the target enzyme, the more efficient uptake and the rapid accumulation of polyglutamates make D1694 a better cytotoxic agent than CB 3717.

D1694 demonstrated its antitumor activity in several *in vivo* murine models, such as L1210 leukemia, L5178Y lymphoma, and human xenograft tumors, with high cure rates and no hepatic or renal toxicities [185,186]. Studies in dogs identified gastrointestinal and hematological toxicities [187].

Phase I clinical trials of D1694 were conducted administering the drug as a 15 minute iv infusion every 3 weeks [188–190]. The maximum tolerated dose recommended for further phase II trials was 3 mg/m^2 [191]. Mild hepatic toxicity was encountered at 1.6 mg/m^2, with an increase in alanine aminotransferase, which returned to normal after the treatment [191,192]. At higher doses, gastrointestinal and hematological limiting toxicities were observed. Nausea, vomiting, and severe diarrhea occurred at 3.0 and 3.5 mg/m^2, as well as myelosuppression, leukopenia, and granulocytopenia [191,192]. Few responses have been reported in breast, ovarian, and nasopharyngeal cancers [191]. Phase II clinical trials indicated that D1694 had activity in advanced colorectal cancer (25% objective responses) and pancreatic cancer (14% response), with an acceptable safety profile at 3.0 mg/m^2 [193–195].

LIPOPHILIC THYMIDYLATE SYNTHASE INHIBITORS

Similar to the goal expressed for the development of the lipophilic DHFR inhibitors, a number of lipophilic TS inhibitors have been synthesized with the intention of creating compounds that would diffuse passively into the cells, thereby overcoming possible resistance due to an impaired active transport system and not requiring polyglutamylation for their activation and intracellular retention, as needed by CB 3717 and D1694.

Two of these new generation TS inhibitors have reached the clinic. Both were developed utilizing information obtained from a high-resolution crystal structure of the *E. coli* protein and molecular modeling techniques. N6-[4-(N-morpholinosulfonyl)-benzyl]-N6-methyl-2,6-diamino-benz[c,d]indole   (AG-331) [196]   and   2-amino-3,4,-dihydro-6-methyl-4-oxo-5-(4-pyridylthio)-quinazoline (AG-337) [197] represent two new classes of TS inhibitors structurally unrelated to previously known TS inhibitors (Figure 8–4).

AG-337 is a potent inhibitor of human TS with a Ki of 10 nM and an anti-proliferative effect against several murine and human tumor cell lines, with ID_{50} values of approximately 1 μM. *In vivo* studies of AG-337 in murine and human xenograft models have shown cure rates of 100% in two thymidine kinase–deficient tumors. This lipophilic TS inhibitor was also active against L5178Y (TK−) lymphoma when administered orally [198].

Phase I clinical studies of AG-337, administered as a 5-day continous infusion every 3 weeks, determined a maximum tolerated dose of 1,130 mg/m², with myelosuppression as the dose-limiting toxicity and transient mucositis. No organ toxicity was observed. A partial response has been registered in a patient with colorectal cancer previously treated with 5-FU [199]. Phase II clinical trials at a dose of 1,000 mg/m² are currently being conducted to evaluate the efficacy of AG-337 against colon, lung, liver, pancreas, prostate, and head/neck cancers. A current phase I clinical trial using an oral formulation has shown a rapid absorption of the drug and a bioavailability of 80% [200].

AG-331, a benzindole derivative [196], is a more potent inhibitor of the human enzyme (Ki 2 nM) and has ID_{50} values for growth inhibition in the range of 0.4–5 μM against several tumor cell lines [201,202]. This lipophilic TS inhibitor is currently in phase I trials as well, being administered as a 5-day infusion. At doses above 400 mg/m², acute elevation of bilirubin and other liver enzymes was observed. Other side effects were mild fatigue, nausea, vomiting, and diarrhea [203].

DE NOVO PURINE SYNTHESIS INHIBITORS

As mentioned earlier, reduced folates are essential for several critical one-carbon transfer reactions. There are at least 18 enzymes that require folates as cofactors for their enzymatic activity, including those involved in the formation of thymidine and in *de novo* purine biosynthesis. The 5,10-dideazafolates were designed according to the principle of critical bond blocking [204]. The substitution of nitrogens in positions 5 and 10, atoms essential for one-carbon transfer reactions, with less reactive carbon atoms precludes this new molecule from serving as a substrate for the enzymes involved in these reactions. Furthermore, the 2-amino-4-hydroxy substituents in this tetrahydrofolate-like design make this molecule a poor inhibitor for DHFR [204,205].

5,10-Dideazatetrahydrofolic acid (DDATHF) (Figure 8–5) has been shown to be a potent antiproliferative agent in L1210 and CCRF-CEM leukemia cell lines at

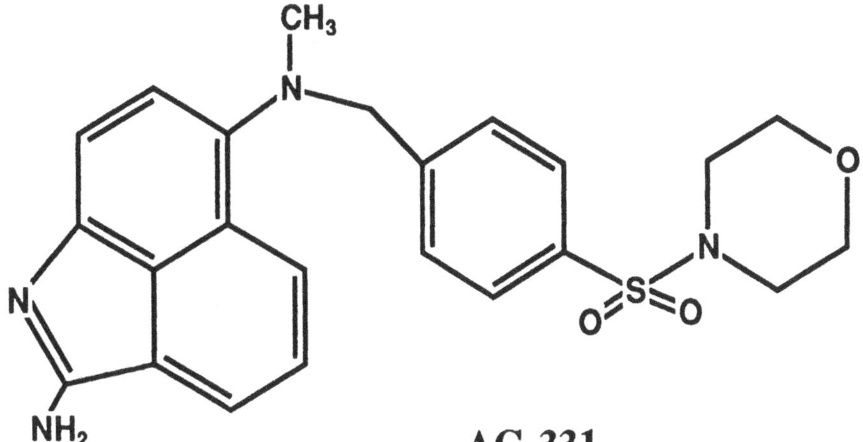

AG-331

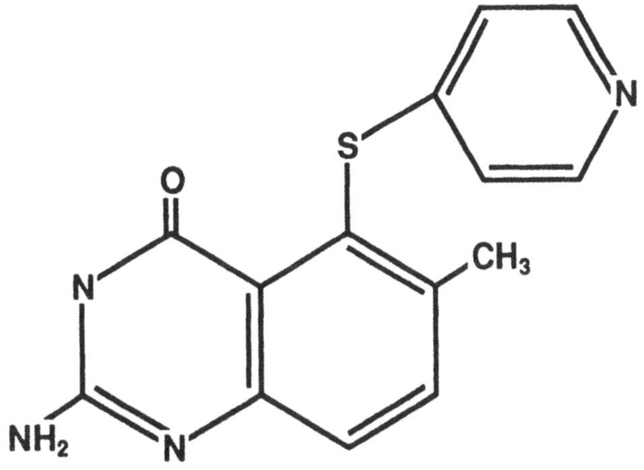

AG-337

Figure 8–4. Lipophilic thymidylate synthase inhibitors.

nanomolar concentrations. Its inhibitory activity is reversed by hypoxanthine and aminoimidazole carboxamide, indicating its specific inhibition of *de novo* purine biosynthesis. As the original study suggests, glycinamide ribonucleotide trans-formylase (GARTF) was found to be the primary target for DDATHF, but higher concentrations of the drug were also able to inhibit the second folate-dependent enzyme in *de novo* purine biosynthesis, aminoimidazole carboxamide ribonucleotide

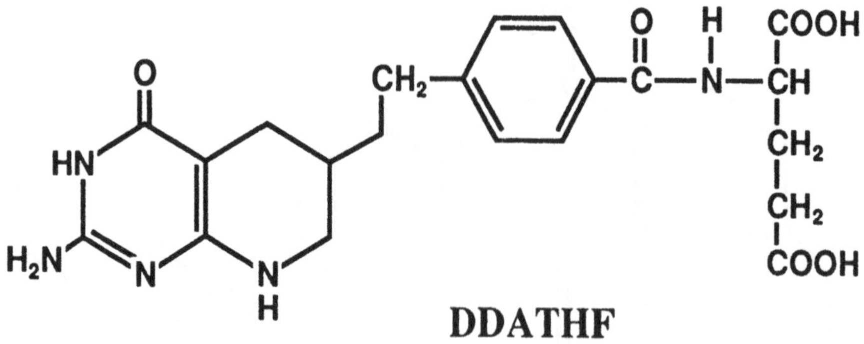

Figure 8–5. De novo purine biosynthesis inhibitor. 5,10-Dideazatetrahydro folic acid.

transformylase (AICARTF) [205]. The antitumor activity of DDATHF is also seen in murine and human xenograft tumor models, showing a wider spectrum of activity than the classical DHFR inhibitor, MTX [206].

DDATHF is a substrate for FPGS *in vitro* [207] and has been found to be metabolized to long-chain polyglutamates *in vivo* [208]. As in the case of CB 3717 with thymidylate synthase, the polyglutamates of DDATHF are 100-fold better inhibitors of both GAR and AICAR transformylases [209]. In a cell line with an impaired mechanism of polyglutamation, the activity of DDATHF was greatly diminished after either short- or long-term exposure to the drug, suggesting the importance of this step in the activations of the deazafolate [210].

Cell lines selected after exposure to increasing concentrations of this antifolate developed resistance to the drug. This resistance was primarily associated with reduction in the accumulation of polyglutamate forms due to diminished FPGS activity. In addition, highly resistant cell lines had increased activity of gamma-glutamyl hydrolase, the enzyme that regulates the intracellular catabolism of folate polyglutamates [211]. Also common to many resistant cell lines was an increased intracellular elevation of reduced folate pools, particularly 10-formyl-tetrahydrofolate, the natural substrate for both GAR and AICAR transformylases [211,212]. DDATHF is efficiently transported intracellularly by the reduced-folate carrier, with an affinity that is fivefold higher than MTX [213]. Studies in MA104 cells revealed that DDATHF has a high affinity for the folate receptor, with a value similar to 5-methyltetrahydrofolate, and is rapidly internalized via a receptor-coupled process, even at low nanomolar concentrations [213].

A number of clinical trials conducted with one of the two DDATHF diasteromers, (6R)DDATHF (lometrexol), using different schedules of administration, indicated the potency of this antifolate purine inhibitor. DDATHF toxicity is observed upon administration of doses lower than those of other antifolates. The most common side effects were thrombocytopenia and stomatitis, with a tendency to become more severe during later cycles of therapy [214–218]. The high affinity of DDATHF for FPGS and the efficient uptake at low nanomolar concentrations may explain this cumulative toxicity. The toxic effects of DDATHF were rapidly reversed by the administration of leucovorin. However, leucovorin has been shown to prevent the antitumor effect of DDATHF [219]. Clinical studies conducted with folic acid as a modulator of DDATHF toxicity have been inconclusive [219,220].

SUMMARY

In summary, the problem of MTX resistance has been approached in a mechanistic fashion, based on the wealth of information generated over the years. To date, these strategies have produced several new classes of anticancer drugs, with a variety of anticipated and unanticipated mechanisms of action. Several of these have shown promising preclinical activity, and these are moving into more stringent testing in the clinic.

ACKNOWLEDGMENTS

This work was partially supported by a NIH research grant CA-16359.

REFERENCES

1. Woods DD (1940) The relation of p-aminobenzoic acid to the mechanism of the action of sulphanilamide. Br J Exp Pathol 21:74–90.
2. Fildes P, Camb MB (1940) A rational approach to research in chemotherapy. Lancet 5:955–957.
3. Angier RB, Boothe JH, Hutchings BL, Mowat JH, Semb J, Stokstad ELR, Subbarow Y, Waller CW (1946) The structure and synthesis of the liver L. Casei factor. Science 103:667–669.
4. Franklin AL, Stokstad ELR, Belt M, Jukes TH (1947) Biochemical experiments with a synthetic preparation having an action antagonistic to that of pteroylglutamic acid. J Biol Chem 169:427–435.
5. Farber S, Culter EC, Hawkins JW, Harrison JH, Peirce EC, Lenz GG (1947) The action of pteroylglutamic conjugates on man. Science 106:619–621.
6. Seeger DR, Smith JM, Hultquist ME (1947) Antagonist for pteroylglutamic acid. Am J Chem Soc 69:2567.
7. Farber S, Diamond LK, Mercer RD, Sylvester RF, Wolff JA (1948) Temporary remissions in acute leukemia in children produced by folic acid antagonist, 4-aminopteroyl-glutamic acid (aminopterin). N Engl J Med 238:788–793.
8. Schoenbach EB, Colsky J, Greenspan EM (1952) Observations on the effects of the folic acid antagonists, aminopterin and amethopterin, in patients with advanced neoplasms. Cancer 5:1210–1220.
9. Goldman ID, Lichtenstein NS, Oliverio VT (1968) Carrier-mediated transport of the folic acid analogue, methotrexate, in the L1210 leukemia cell. Biol Chem 243:5007–5017.
10. Schilsky RL, Bailey BD, Chabner BA (1981) Characteristics of membrane transport of methotrexate by cultured human breast cancer cells. Biochem Pharm 30:1537–1542.
11. Dixon KH, Mulligan T, Chung K-N, Elwood PC, Cowan KH (1992) Effects of folate receptor expression following stable transfection into wild type and methotrexate transport-deficient ZR-75-1 human breast cancer cells. J Biol Chem 267:24140–24147.
12. Henderson GB, Strauss BP (1990) Characteristics of a novel transport system for folate compounds in wild-type and methotrexate-resistant L1210 cells. Cancer Res 50:1709–1714.
13. McGuire JJ, Hsieh P, Coward JK, Bertino JR (1980) Enzymatic synthesis of folylpolyglutamates. J Biol Chem 255:5776–5788.
14. Kim JS, Lowe KE, Shane B (1993) Regulation of folate and one-carbon metabolism in mammalian cells. J Biol Chem 268:21680–21685.
15. Garrow TA, Admon A, Shane B (1992) Expression cloning of a human cDNA encoding folylpoly-(gamma-glutamate) synthetase and determination of its primary structure. Proc Natl Acad Sci USA 89:9151–9155.

16. Cichowicz DJ, Shane B (1987) Mammalian folylpoly-gamma-glutamate synthetase. 1. Purification and general properties of the hog liver enzyme. Biochemistry 26:504–512.

17. Cichowicz DJ, Shane B (1987) Mammalian folylpoly-gamma-glutamate synthetase. 2. Substrate specificity and kinetic properties. Biochemistry 26:513–521.

18. Clarke L, Waxman DJ (1987) Human liver folylopolyglutamate synthetase: Biochemical characterization and interactions with folates and folate antagonists. Arch Biochem Biophys 256:585–596.

19. Cook JD, Cichowicz DJ, George S, Lawler A, Shane B (1987) Mammalian folylpoly-gamma-glutamate synthetase. 4. In vitro and in vivo metabolism of folates and analogues and regulation of folate homeostasis. Biochemistry 26:530–539.

20. Moran RG, Colman PD (1984) Mammalian folyl polyglutamate synthetase: Partial purification and properties of the mouse liver enzyme. Biochemistry 23:4580–4589.

21. Samuels LL, Moccio DM, Sirotnak FM (1985) Similar differential for total polyglutamylation and cytotoxicity among various folate analogues in human and murine tumor cells in vitro. Cancer Res 45:1488–1495.

22. Fabre I, Fabre G, Goldman ID (1984) Polyglutamylation, an important element in methotrexate cytotoxicity and selectivity in tumor versus murine granulocytic progenitor cells in vitro. Cancer Res 44:3190–3195.

23. Samuels LL, Goutas LJ, Priest DG, Piper JR, Sirotnak FM (1986) Hydrolytic cleavage of methotrexate gamma-polyglutamates by folylpolyglutamyl hydrolase derived from various tumors and normal tissues of the mouse. Cancer Res 46:2230–2235.

24. Johnson TB, Nair MG, Galivan J (1988) Role of folylpolyglutamate synthetase in the regulation of methotrexate polyglutamate formation in H35 hepatoma cells. Cancer Res 48:2426–2431.

25. McGuire JJ, Mini E, Hsieh P, Bertino JR (1985) Role of methotrexate polyglutamates in methotrexate- and sequential methotrexate-5-fluorouracil-mediated cell kill. Cancer Res 45:6395–6400.

26. Osborne CB, Lowe KE, Shane B (1993) Regulation of folate and one-carbon metabolism in mammalian cells. J Biol Chem 268:21657–21664.

27. Schoo MMJ, Pristupa ZB, Vickers PJ, Scrimgeour KG (1985) Folate analogues as substrates of mammalian folylpolyglutamate synthetase. Cancer Res 45:3034–3041.

28. Rhee MS, Galivan J (1986) Conversion of methotrexate to 7-hydroxymethotrexate and 7-hydroxymethotrexate polyglutamates in cultured rat hepatic cells. Cancer Res 46:3793–3797.

29. Jolivet J, Schilsky RL, Bailey BD, Drake JC, Chabner BA (1982) Synthesis, retention, and biological activity of methotrexate polyglutamates in cultured human breast cancer cells. J Clin Invest 70:351–360.

30. Fabre G, Fabre I, Matherly LH, Cano JP, Goldman ID (1984) Synthesis and properties of 7-hydroxymethotrexate polyglutamyl derivatives in Ehrlich ascites tumor cells in vitro. J Biol Chem 259:5066–5072.

31. Osborn MJ, Freeman M, Huennekens FM (1958) Inhibition of dihydrofolic reductase by aminopterin and amethopterin. Proc Soc Exp Biol Med 97:429–435.

32. Werkheiser WC (1961) Specific binding of 4-amino folic acid analogues by folic acid reductase. J Biol Chem 236:888–893.

33. Bertino JR, Booth BA, Bieber AL, Cashmore A, Sartorelli AC (1964) Studies on the inhibition of dihydrofolate reductase by the folate antagonists. J Biol Chem 239:479–485.

34. Allegra CJ, Drake JC, Jolivet J, Chabner BA (1985) Inhibition of phosphoribosylaminoimidazolecarboxamide transformylase by methotrexate and dihydrofolic acid polyglutamates. Biochemistry 82:4881–4885.

35. Allegra CJ (1990) Antifolates. In BA Chabner, JM Collins, eds. Cancer Chemotherapy: Principles and Practice. Philadelphia: JB Lippincott, pp 110–153.

36. Fisher GA (1967) Defective transport of amethopterin (methotrexate) as a mechanism of resistance to the antimetabolite in L5178Y leukemic cells. Biochem Pharmacol 11:1233–1237.

37. Kamen BA, Cashmore AR, Dreyer RN, Moroson BA, Hsieh P, Bertino JR (1980) Effect of [³H]methotrexate impurities on apparent transport of methotrexate by a sensitive and resistant L1210 cell line. J Biol Chem 255:3254–3257.

38. Hakala MT (1965) On the role of drug penetration in amethopterin resistance of sarcoma-180 cells in vitro. Biochem Biophys Acta 102:198–209.

39. Sirotnak FM, Moccio DM, Kelleher LE, Goutas LJ (1981) Relative frequency and kinetic properties of transport-defective phenotypes among methotrexate-resistant L1210 clonal cell lines derived in vivo. Cancer Res 41:4447–4452.

40. Dixon KH, Lanpher BC, Chiu J, Kelley K, Cowan KH (1993) A novel cDNA restores reduced folate carrier activity and methotrexate sensitivity to transport deficient cells. J Biol Chem 269:17–20.

41. Wang X, Shen F, Freisheim JH, Gentry LE, Ratnam M (1992) Differential stereospecificities and affinities of folate receptor isoforms for folate compounds and antifolates. Biochem Pharmacol 44:1898–1901.

42. Hsueh C-T, Dolnick BJ (1993) Altered folate-binding protein and mRNA stability in KB cells grown in folate-deficient medium. Biochem Pharmacol 45:2537–2545.

43. Pizzorno G, Mini E, Coronnelo M, McGuire JJ, Moroson BA, Cashmore AR, Dreyer RN, Lin JT, Mazzei T, Periti P, Bertino JR (1988) Impaired polyglutamylation of methotrexate as a cause of resistance in CCRF-CEM cells after short-term, high-dose treatment with this drug. Cancer Res 48:2149–2155.

44. McCloskey DE, McGuire JJ, Russell CA, Rowan BG, Bertino JR, Pizzorno G, Mini E (1991) Decreased folylpolyglutamate synthetase activity as a mechanism of methotrexate resistance in CCRF-CEM Human Leukemia Sublines. J Biol Chem 266:6181–6187.

45. Cowan KH, Jolivet J (1984) A methotrexate-resistant human breast cancer cell line with multiple defects, including diminished formation of methotrexate polyglutamates. J Biol Chem 259:10793–10800.

46. Pizzorno G, Chang YM, McGuire JJ, Bertino JR (1989) Inherent resistance of human squamous carcinoma cell lines to methotrexate as a result of decreased polyglutamylation of this drug. Cancer Res 49:5275–5280.

47. Li WW, Lin JT, Tang WP, Trippett TM, Brennan MF, Bertino JR (1992) Mechanisms of natural resistance to antifolates in human soft tissue sarcomas. Cancer Res 52:1434–1436.

48. Li WW, Lin JT, Schweitzer BI, Tong WP, Niedzwiecki D, Bertino JR (1992) Intrinsic resistance to methotrexate in human soft tissue sarcoma cell lines. Cancer Res 52:3908–3913.

49. Barredo J, Moran RG (1992) Determinants of antifolate cytotoxicity: Folylpolyglutamate synthetase activity during cellular proliferation and development. Mol Pharmacol 42:687–694.

50. Rhee MS, Wang Y, Nair MG, Galivan J (1993) Acquisition of resistance to antifolates caused by enhanced gamma-glutamyl hydrolase activity. Cancer Res 53:2227–2230.

51. Dicker AP, Waltham MC, Volkenandt M, Schweitzer BI, Otter GM, Schmid FA, Sirotnak FM, Bertino JR (1993) Methotrexate resistance in an in vivo mouse tumor due to a non-active-site dihydrofolate reductase mutation. Biochemistry 30:11797–11801.

52. Jackson RC, Niethammer D (1977) Acquired methotrexate resistance in lymphoblasts resulting from altered kinetic properties of dihydrofoltate reductase. Eur J Cancer 13:567–575.

53. Goldie JH, Krystal G, Hartley D, Gudauskas G, Dedhar S (1980) A methotrexate insensitive variant of folate reductase present in two lines of methotrexate-resistant L5178Y cells. Eur J Cancer 16:1539–1546.

54. Hanggi UJ, Littlefield JW (1974) Isolation and characterization of the multiple forms of dihydrofolate reductase from methotrexate-resistant hamster cells. J Biol Chem 249:1390–1397.

55. Haber DA, Beverley SM, Kiely ML, Schimke RT (1981) Properties of an altered dihydrofolate reductase encoded by amplified genes in cultured mouse fibroblasts. J Biol Chem 256:9501–9510.

56. Flintoff WF, Essani K (1980) Methotrexate-resistant Chinese hamster ovary cells contain a dihydrofolate reductase with an altered affinity for methotrexate. Biochemistry 19:4321–4327.

57. Simonsen CC, Levinson AD (1983) Isolation and expression of an altered mouse dihydrofolate reductase cDNA. Proc Natl Acad Sci USA 80:2495–2499.

58. Srimatkandada S, Schweitzer BI, Moroson BA, Dube S, Bertino JR (1989) Amplification of a polymorphic reductase gene expressing an enzyme with decreased binding to methotrexate in a human colon carcinoma cell line, HCT-8R4, resistant to this drug. J Biol Chem 264:3524–3528.

59. Srimatkandada S, Medina WD, Cashmore AR, Whyte W, Engel D, Moroson BA, Franco CT, Dube SK, Bertino JR (1983) Amplification and organization of dihydrofolate reductase genes in a human leukemic cell line, K-562, resistant to methotrexate. Biochemistry 22:5781–5789.

60. Alt FW, Kellems RE, Bertino JR, Schimke RT (1978) Selective multiplication of dihydrofolate reductase genes in methotrexate-resistant variants of cultured murine cells. J Biol Chem 253:1357–1370.

61. Tyler-Smith C, Alderson T (1981) Gene amplification in methotrexate-resistant mouse cells I. DNA rearrangement accompanies dihydrofolate reductase gene amplification in a T-cell lymphoma. J Mol Biol 153:203–218.

62. Dolnick BJ, Berenson RJ, Bertino JR, Kaufman RJ, Nunberg JH, Schimke RT (1979) Correlation of dihydrofolate reductase elevation with gene amplification in a homogeneously staining chromosomal region in L5178Y cells. J Cell Biol 83:394–402.
63. Melera PW, Lewis JA, Biedler JL, Hession C (1980) Antifolate-resistant Chinese hamster cells evidence for dihydrofolate reductase gene amplification among independently derived sublines overproducing different dihydrofolate reductases. J Biol Chem 255:7024–7028.
64. Trent JM, Buick RN, Olson S, Horns RC, Schimke RT (1984) Cytologic evidence for gene amplification in methotrexate-resistant cells obtained from a patient with ovarian adenocarcinoma. J Clin Oncol 2:8–15.
65. Horns RC, Dower WJ, Schimke RT (1984) Gene amplfication in a leukemic patient treated with methotrexate. J Clin Oncol 2:2–7.
66. Carman MD, Schornagel JH, Rivest RS, Srimatkandada S, Portlock CS, Duffy T, Bertino JR (1984) Resistance to methotrexate due to gene amplification in a patient with acute leukemia. J Clin Oncol 2:16–21.
67. Curt GA, Carney DN, Cowan KH, Jolivet J, Bailey BD, Drake JC, Kao-Shan CS, Minna JD, Chabner BA (1983) Unstable methotrexate resistance in human small-cell carcinoma associated with double minute chromosomes. N Engl J Med 308:199–202.
68. Schimke RT, Kung AL, Rush DF, Sherwood SW (1991) Differences in mitotic control among mammalian cells. Cold Spring Harb Symp Quant Biol 56:417–423.
69. Schimke RT (1984) Gene amplification in cultured animal cells. Cell 37:705–713.
70. Brown PC, Beverley SM, Schimke RT (1981) Relationship of amplified dihydrofolate reductase genes to double minute chromosomes in unstably resistant mouse fibroblast cell lines. Mol Cell Biol 1:1077–1083.
71. Biedler JL, Spengler BA (1976) Metaphase chromosome anomaly: Association with drug resistance and cell-specific products. Science 191:185–187.
72. Bostock CJ, Tyler-Smith C (1981) Gene amplification in methotrexate-resistant mouse cells II. Rearrangement and amplification of non-dihydrofolate reductase gene sequences accompany chromosomal changes. J Mol Biol 153:219–236.
73. Tyler-Smith C, Bostock CJ (1981) Gene amplification in methotrexate-resistant mouse cells III. Interrelationships between chromosome changes and DNA sequence amplification or loss. J Mol Biol 153:237–256.
74. Kaufman RJ, Schimke RT (1981) Amplification and loss of dihydrofolate reductase genes in a chinese hamster ovary cell line. Mol Cell Biol 1:1069–1076.
75. Kaufman RJ, Brown PC, Schimke RT (1981) Loss and stabilization of amplified dihydrofolate reductase genes in mouse sarcoma S-180 cell lines. Mol Cell Biol 1:1084–1093.
76. Kaufman RJ, Bertino JR, Schimke RT (1978) Quantitation of dihydrofolate reductase in individual parental and methotrexate-resistant murine cells. J Biol Chem 253:5852–5860.
77. Wright JA, Smith HS, Watt FM, Hancock MC, Hudson DL, Stark GR (1990) DNA amplification is rare in normal human cells. Proc Natl Acad Sci USA 87:1791–1795.
78. Tlsty TD, Margolin BH, Lum K (1989) Differences in the rates of gene amplification in nontumorigenic and tumorigenic cell lines as measured by Lauria-Delbruck fluctuation analysis. Proc Natl Acad Sci USA 86:9441–9445.
79. Stark GR, Debatisse M, Giulotto E, Wahl GM (1989) Recent progress in understanding mechanisms of mammalian DNA amplification. Cell 57:901–908.
80. Eastman HB, Swick AG, Schmitt MC, Azizkhan JC (1991) Stimulation of dihydrofolate reductase promoter activity by antimetabolic drugs. Proc Natl Acad Sci USA 88:8572–8576.
81. Chu E, Takimoto CH, Voeller D, Grem JL, Allegra CJ (1993) Specific binding of human dihydrofolate reductase protein to dihydrofolate reductase messenger RNA in vitro. Biochemistry 32:4756–4760.
82. Freeman AI, Weinberg V, Brecher ML, Jones B, Glickman AS, Sinks LF, Weihl M, Pleuss H, Hananian J, Burgert EO, Gilchrist GS, Necheles T, Harris M, Kung F, Patterson RB, Maurer H, Leventhal B, Chevaliers L, Forman E, Holland JF (1983) Comparison of intermediate dose methotrexate with cranial irradiation for the post-induction treatment of acute lympocytic leukemia in children. N Engl J Med 308:477–480.
83. Moe PJ, Seip M, Finne PH, Kolsmannskog S (1986) Methotrexate infusions in poor prognosis acute lymphoblastic leukemia in children: I. The Norwegian methotrexate study in acute lymphoblastic leukemia in childhood. Eur Pediatr Haematol Oncol 1:113–117.
84. Hudson MM, Dahl GV, Kalwinsky DK, Pui CH (1990) Methotrexate plus L-asparaginase an active combination for children with acute nonlymphocytic leukemia. Cancer 65:2615–2618.

85. Lobel JS, O'Brien RT, McIntosh S, Aspnes GT, Capizzi RL (1979) Methotrexate and asparaginase combination chemotherapy in refractory acute lymphoblastic leukemia of childhood. Cancer 43:1089–1094.

86. Camitta B, Leventhal B, Lauer S, Shuster JJ, Adair S, Casper J, Civin C, Graham M, Mahoney D, Munoz L, Kiefer G, Kamen B (1989) Intermediate-dose intravenous methotrexate and mercaptopurine therapy for non-T, non-B acute lymphocytic leukemia of childhood: A Pediatric Oncology Group study. J Clin Oncol 7:1539–1544.

87. Bokkerink JPM, Bakker MAH, Hulscher TW, DeAbreu RA, Schretlen EDAN (1988) Purine de novo synthesis as the basis of synergism of methotrexate and 6-mercaptopurine in human malignant lymphoblasts of different lineages. Biochem Pharmacol 37:2321–2327.

88. Hertz R, Lewis J, Lipsett MB (1961) Five years' experience with the chemotherapy of metastatic choriocarcinoma and related trophoblastic tumors in women. Am J Obstet Gynecol 82:631–640.

89. Fisher B, Redmond C, Dimitrov NV, Bowman D, Legault-Poisson S, Wickerham L, Wolmark N, Fisher ER, Margolese R, Sutherland C, Glass A, Foster R, Caplan R (1989) A randomized clinical trial evaluating sequential methotrexate and fluorouracil in the treatment of patients with node-negative breast cancer who have estrogen-receptor-negative tumors. N Engl J Med 320:473–478.

90. Browman GP, Levine MN, Goodyear MD, Russell R, Archibald SD, Jackson BS, Young JEM, Basrur V, Johanson C (1988) Methotrexate/fluorouracil scheduling influences normal tissue toxicity but not antitumor effects in patients with squamous cell head and neck cancer: Results from a randomized trial. J Clin Oncol 6:963–968.

91. Rees RB, Bennett JH, Maibach HI, Arnold HL (1967) Methotrexate for psoriasis. Arch Dermatol 95:2–11.

92. Hoffmeister RT (1983) Methotrexate therapy in rheumatoid arthritis: 15 years experience. Am J Med 30:69–73.

93. Storb R, Deeg J, Fisher L, Appelbaum R, Buckner CD, Bensinger W, Clift R, Doney K, Irie C, McGuffin R (1988) Cyclosporine vs methotrexate for graft-vs-host disease prevention in patients given marrow grafts for leukemia: Long-term follow-up of three controlled trials. Blood 71:293–298.

94. Poplack DG (1989) Acute lymphoblastic leukemia. In PA Pizzo, DG Poplack, eds. Principles and Practice of Pediatric Oncology. Philadelphia: JB Lippincott, pp 323–366.

95. DeGraw JI, Brown VH, Tagawa H, et al. (1982) Synthesis and antitumor activity of 10-alkyl, 10-deazaaminopterins. A convenient synthesis of 10-deazaaminopterin. J Med Chem 25:1227–1230.

96. Sirotnak FM, DeGraw JI, Chello PL (1982) Biochemical and pharmacologic properties of a new folate analog, 10-deazaaminopterin, in mice. Cancer Treat Rep 66:351–358.

97. Sirotnak FM, DeGraw JI, Schmid FA, et al. (1984) New folate analogs of the 10-deaza-aminopterin series. Further evidence for markedly increased antitumor efficacy compared with methotrexate in ascitic and solid murine tumor models. Cancer Chemother Pharmacol 12:26–30.

98. Schmid FA, Sirotnak FM, Otter GM, et al. (1985) New folate analogs of the 10-deaza-aminopterin series: Markedly increased antitumor activity of the 10-ethyl analog compared to the parent compound and methotrexate against some human tumor xenografts in nude mice. Cancer Treat Rep 69:551–553.

99. Samuels LL, Moccio DM, Sirotnak FM (1985) Similar differential for total polyglutamylation and cytotoxicity among various folate analogs in human and murine tumor cells in vitro. Cancer Res 45:1488–1495.

100. Rumberger BG, Barrueco JR, Sirotnak FM (1990) Differing specificities for 4-aminofolate analogs of folylpolyglutamyl synthetase from tumors and proliferating intestinal epithelium of the mouse with significance for selective antitumor action. Cancer Res 50:4639–4643.

101. Sirotnak FM, Schmid, FA, Samuels LL, DeGraw JI (1987) 10-Ethyl-10-deaza-aminopterin: Structural design and biochemical, pharmacologic, and antitumor properties. NCI Monogr 5:127–131.

102. Sirotnak FM, DeGraw JI, Moccio DM, Samuels LL, Goutas LJ (1984) New folate analogues of the 10-deaza-aminopterin series. Basis for structural design and biochemical and pharmacologic properties. Cancer Chemother Pharmacol 12:18–25.

103. Kris MG, Kinahan JJ, Gralla RJ et al. (1988) Phase I trial and clinical pharmacological evaluation of 10-ethyl-10-deaza-aminopterin in adult patients with advanced cancer. Cancer Res 48:5573–5579.

104. Shum KY, Kris MG, Gralla RJ, et al. (1988) Phase II study of 10-ethyl-10-deaza-aminopterin in patients with stage III and IV non-small cell lung cancer. J Clin Oncol 6:446–450.

105. Less JS, Libshitz HI, Murphy WK et al. (1990) Phase II study of 10-ethyl-10-deaza-aminopterin

(10-EdAM: CGP 30 694) for stage IIIB or IV non-small cell lung cancer. Invest New Drugs 8:299–304.

106. Vandenberg TA, Pritchard KI, Eisenhauer EA, Trudeau ME, Norris BD, Lopez P, Verma SS, Buckman RA, Muldal A (1993) Phase II study of weekly edatrexate as first-line chemotherapy for metastatic breast cancer: A National Cancer Institute of Canada Clinical Trials Group Study. J Clin Oncol 11:1241–1244.

107. Schornagel JH, Cappelaere P, Cognetti F, et al. (1989) A randomized phase II trial of 10-ethyl-10-deaza-aminopterin and methotrexate in advanced head and neck squamous cell cancer (AHNC), an EORTC study. Proc Am Soc Clin Oncol 8:174.

108. Kemeny N, Israel K, O'Hehir M (1990) Phase II trial of 10-Edam in patients with advanced colorectal carcinoma. J Clin Oncol 13:42–44.

109. Souhami R, Hartley J, Allen R, Rudd R, Harper P, Spiro S (1991) 10-EdAM (10-ethyl-10-deaza-aminopterin in untreated advanced non-small cell lung cancer (NSCLC). Lung Cancer 7:A500.

110. Schmid FA, Sirotnak FM, Otter GM, et al. (1987) Combination chemotherapy with a new folate analog: Activity of 10-ethyl-10-deaza-aminopterin compared to methotrexate with 5-fluorouracil and alkylating agents against advanced metastatic disease in murine tumor models. Cancer Treat Rep 71:727–732.

111. Sirotnak FM, Schmid FA, DeGraw JI (1989) Intracavitary therapy of murine ovarian cancer with cis-diamminedichloroplatinum (II) and 10-ethyl-10-deazaaminopterin incorporating system leucovorin protection. Cancer Res 49:2890–2893.

112. Kris MG, Gralla RJ, Potanovich LM, et al. (1990) Assessment of pretreatment symptoms and improvement after edam + mitomycin + vinblastine (EMV) in patients with inoperable non-small cell lung cancer (NSCLC). Proc Am Soc Clin Oncol 9:229.

113. Lee JS, Libshitz HI, Fossela FV, Murphy WK, Pang A, Lippman SM, Shin DM, Dimery IW, Glisson BS, Hong WK (1991) Edatrexate improves the antitumor effects of cyclophosphamide and cisplatin against non-small cell lung cancer. Cancer 68:959–964.

114. Lee JS, Murphy WK, Shirinian MH, Pang A, Hong WK (1991) Alleviation by leucovorin of the dose-limiting toxicity of edatrexate: Potential for improved therapeutic efficacy. Cancer Chemother Pharmacol 28:199–204.

115. Bertino JR, Sawicki WL (1977) Potent inhibitory activity of trimethoxyquine (TMQ), "nonclassical" 2,4-diaminoquinazoline, on mammalian DNA synthesis. Proc Am Assoc Cancer Res 18:168.

116. Jackson RC, Fry DW, Boritzki TJ, Besserer JA, Leopold WR, Sloan BJ, Elslager EF (1984) Biochemical pharmacology of the lipophilic antifolate, trimetrexate. Adv Enzyme Regul 22:187–206.

117. Bertino JR, Sawicki WL, Moroson BA, Cashmore AR, Elslager EF (1979) 2,41-Diamino-5-methyl-6-[(3,4,5-trimethoxyanilino)methyl]quinazoline (TMQ). A potent non-classical folate antagonist inhibitor. Biochem Pharmacol 28:1983–1987.

118. O'Dwyer JP, Shoemaker DD, Plowman J, Cradock J, Grillo-Lopez A, Leyland-Jones B (1985) Trimetrexate: A new antifol entering clinical trials. Invest New Drugs 3:71–75.

119. Kamen BA, Eibl B, Cashmore AR, Bertino JR (1984) Uptake and efficacy of trimetrexate (TMQ, 2,4-diamino-5-methyl-6-[(3,4,5-trimethoxy-anilino)methyl]quinazoline), a non-classical antifolate in methotrexate-resistent leukemia cells in vitro. Biochem Pharmacol 33:1697–1699.

120. Klohs WD, Steinkampf RW, Besserer JA, Fry DW (1986) Cross resistance of pleiotropically drug resistant P338 leukemia cells to the lipophilic antifolates trimetrexate and BW 301U. Cancer Lett 31:253–260.

121. Klohs WD, Steinkampf RW (1988) Possible link between the intrinsic drug resistance of colon tumors and a detoxification mechanism of intestinal cells. Cancer Res 48:3025–3030.

122. Zamora JM, Pearce HL, Beck WT (1988) Physical-chemical properties shared by compounds that modulate multidrug resistance in human leukemic cells. Mol Pharmacol 33:454–462.

123. Ramu N, Ramu A (1989) Circumvention of adriamycin resistance by dipyridamole analogues: A structure-activity relationship study. Int J Cancer 43:487–491.

124. Jackson RC, Leopold WR, Hamelehle KL, Fry DW (1988) Preclinical studies with trimetrexate: A review of conclusions and unanswered questions. Semin Oncol 15:1–7.

125. Donehower RC, Graham ML, Thompson GE, Dole GB, Ettinger DS (1985) Phase I and pharmacokinetic study of trimetrexate (TMTX) in patients with advanced cancer. Proc Am Soc Clin Oncol 4:32.

126. Legha S, Tenney D, Ho DH, Krakoff I (1985) Phase I clinical and pharmacology study of trimetrexate (TMQ). Proc Am Soc Clin Oncol 4:48.

127. Stewart JA, McCormack JJ, Tong W, DeLap RJ, Grillo-Lopez AJ (1985) A Phase I study of trimetrexate. Proc Am Assoc Cancer Res 26:159.
128. Fanucchi M, Fleisher M, Vidal P, Williams L, Bauer T, Cassidy C, Chou T-C, Young C (1985) Phase I and pharmacologic study of trimetrexate (TMTX). Proc Am Assoc Cancer Res 26:179.
129. Lin JT, Cashmore AR, Baker M, Dreyer RN, Ernstoff M, Marsh JC, Bertino JR, Whitfield LR, Delap R, Grillo-Lopez A (1987) Phase I studies with trimetrexate: Clinical pharmacology, analytical methodology, and pharmacokinetics. Cancer Res 47:609–616.
130. Lin JT, Bertino JR (1987) Trimetrexate: A second generation folate antagonist in clinical trial. J Clin Oncol 5:2032–2040.
131. Mauron J (1988) Clinical response to trimetrexates as sole therapy for nonsmall cell lung cancer. Semin Oncol 15(Suppl 2):17–21.
132. Kris MG, D'Acquisto RW, Gralla RJ, et al. (1989) Phase II trial of trimetrexate in patients with stage III and IV non-small-cell lung cancer. J Clin Oncol 12:24–26.
133. Fosella FV, Winn RJ, Holoye PY (1992) Phase II trial of trimetrexate for unresectable or metastatic non-small cell bronchogenic carcinoma. Invest New Drugs 10:331–335.
134. Robert F (1988) Trimetrexate as a single agent in patients with advanced head and neck cancer. Semin Oncol 15(Suppl 2):22–26.
135. Dawson NA, Costanza ME, Korzun AH, et al. (1991) Trimetrexate in untreated and prevously treated patients with metastatic breast cancer: A Cancer and Leukemia Group B study. Med Pediatr Oncol 19:283–288.
136. Leiby JM (1988) Trimetrexate: A phase II study in previously treated patients with metastatic breast cancer. Semin Oncol 15(Suppl 2):27–31.
137. Alberts AS, Falkson G, Badat M, et al. (1988) Trimetrexate in advanced carcinoma of the esophagus. Invest New Drugs 6:319–321.
138. Falkson G, Ryan LM, Haller DG (1992) Phase II trial for the evaluation of trimetrexate in patients with inoperable squamous carcinoma of the esophagus. J Clin Oncol 15:433–435.
139. Sternberg CN, Yagoda A, Scher H, et al. (1989) Phase II trial of trimetrexate in patients with advanced renal cell carcinoma. Eur J Cancer Clin Oncol 25:753–754.
140. Wittes RS, Elson P, Bryan GT, et al. (1992) Trimetrexate in advanced renal cell carcinoma. Invest New Drugs 10:51–54.
141. Odujinrin O, Goldberg D, Doroshow J, et al. (1990) Treatment of metastatic malignant melanoma with trimetrexate. A phase II study. Med Pediatr Oncol 18:49–52.
142. Iscoe NA, Eisenhauer EA, Bodurtha AJ (1990) Phase II study of trimetrexate in malignant melanoma: A National Cancer Institute of Canada clinical trials group study. Invest New Drugs 8:121–123.
143. Vogelzang NJ, Weissman LB, Herndon JE 2nd, Antman KH, Cooper MR, Corson JM, Green MR (1994) Trimetrexate in malignant mesothelioma: A Cancer and Leukemia Group B Phase II study. J Clin Oncol 12:1436–1442.
144. Licht JD, Gonin R, Antman KH (1991) Phase II trial of trimetrexate in patients with advanced soft-tissue sarcoma. Cancer Chemother Pharmacol 28:223–225.
145. Eisenhauer EA, Wierzbicki R, Knowling M, et al. (1991) Phase II trials of trimetrexate in advanced adult soft tissue sarcoma. Ann Oncol 2:689–690.
146. Hantel A, Tangen CM, Macdonald JS, Richman SP, Pugh RP, Pollock T (1994) Phase II trial of trimetrexate in untreated advanced gastric carcinoma. A Southwest Oncology Group study. Invest New Drugs 12:155–157.
147. Carlson RW, Doroshow JH, Odjuinrin OO, et al. (1990) Trimetrexate in locally advanced or metastatic adenocarcinoma of the pancreas. Invest New Drugs 8:387–389.
148. Weiss GR, Liu PY, O'Sullivan J, et al. (1992) A randomized phase II trial of trimetrexate or didemnin B for the treatment of metastatic or recurrent squamous carcinoma of the uterine cervix. A Southwest Oncology Group trial. Gynecol Oncol 45:303–306.
149. Pappo A, Dubowy R, Ravindranath Y, et al. (1990) Phase II trial of trimetrexate in the treatment of recurrent childhood acute lymphoblastic leukemia. A Pediatric Oncology Group study. J Natl Cancer Inst 82:1641–1642.
150. Hussar DA (1994) New drugs. Nursing 24:48–56.
151. Allegra CJ, Chabner BA, Tuazon CU, Ogata-Arakaki D, Baird B, Drake JC, Simmons JT, Lack EE, Shelhamer JH, Balis F, Walker R, Kovacs JA, Lane HC, Masur H (1987) Trimetrexate for the treeatment of *Pneumocystis carinii* pneumonia in patients with the acquired immunodeficiency syndrome. N Engl J Med 317:978–985.

152. Duch DS, Edelstein MP, Bowers SW, Nichol CA (1982) Biochemical and chemotherapeutic studies on 2,4-diamino-6-(2,5-dimethoxybenzyl)-5-methylypyrido (2,3-d) pyrimidine (BW301), a novel lipid soluble inhibitor of dihydrofolate reductase. Cancer Res 42:3987–3994.
153. Sedwick WD, Hamrell M, Brown OE, Laszlo J (1982) Metabolic inhibition by a new antifolate, 2,4-diamino-6-(2,5-dimethoxybenzyl)-5-methyl-pyrido[2,3-d]pyrimidine (BW301U), and effective inhibitor of human lymphoid and dihydrofolate reductase-overproducing mouse cell lines. Mol Pharmacol 22:766–770.
154. Laszlo J, Brenckman WD Jr, Morgan E, Clendeninn NJ, Williams T, Currie V, Young C (1987) Initial clinical studies of piritrexim. NCI Monogr 5:121–125.
155. Duschinsky R, Pleven E, Heidelberger C (1957) The synthesis of 5-fluoropyrimidines. J Am Chem Soc 79:4559–4560.
156. Santi DV, McHenry CS, Sommer H (1974) Mechanism of interaction of thymidylate synthetase with 5-fluorodeoxyuridylate. Biochemistry 13:471–481.
157. Cohen SS, Flaks JG, Barner HD, Loeb MR, Lichtenstein J (1958) The mode of action of 5-fluorouracil and its derivatives. Proc Natl Acad Sci USA 44:1004–1012.
158. Hartmann KU, Heidelberger C (1961) Studies on fluorinated pyrimidines. VIII. Inhibition of thymidylate synthetase. J Biol Chem 236:3006–3013.
159. Glazer RI, Lloyd LS (1982) Association of cell lethality with incorporation of 5-fluorouracil and 5-fluorouridine into nuclear RNA in human colon carcinoma cells in culture. Mol Pharmacol 21:468–473.
160. Kufe DW, Major PP (1981) 5-Fluorouracil incorporation into human breast carcinoma RNA correlates with cytotoxicity. J Biol Chem 256:9802–9808.
161. Berger SH, Hakala MT (1984) Relationship of dUMP and FdUMP pools to inhibition to thymidylate synthase by 5-fluorouracil. Mol Pharmacol 25:303–309.
162. Houghton JA, Weiss KD, Williams LG, Torrance PM, Houghton PJ (1986) Relationship between 5-fluoro-2'-deoxyuridylate, 2'-deoxyuridylate, and thymidylate synthase activity subsequent to 5-fluorouracil administration in xenografts of human colon adenocarcinomas. Biochem Pharmacol 35:1351–1358.
163. Bird OD, Vaitkus JW, Clarke J (1970) 2-Amino-4-hydroxyquinazolines as inhibitors of thyumidylate synthetase. Mol Pharmacol 6:573–575.
164. Jones TR, Calvert AH, Jackman AL, Brown SJ, Jones M, Harrap KR (1981) A potent antitumour quinazoline inhibitor of thymidylate synthetase: Synthesis, biological properties and therapeutic results in mice. Eur J Cancer 17:11–19.
165. Jackman RC, Jackman AL, Calvert AH (1983) Biochemical effects of a quinazoline inhibitor of thymidylate synthetase, CB3717, on human lymphoblastoid cells. Biochem Pharmacol 32:3782–3790.
166. Jackman AL, Calvert AH, Hart LI, Harrap KR (1984) Inhibition of thymidylate synthetase by the new quinazoline antifolate CB3717: Enzyme purification and kinetics. In CHMM DeBruyn, HA Simmonds, M Muller, eds. Purine Metabolism in Man—IV, Vol. 165B. New York: Plenum Press, pp 375–378.
167. Jackman AL, Alison DL, Calvert AH, Harrap KR (1986) Increased thymidylate synthase in L1210 cells possessing acquired resistance to N^{10}-propargyl-5,8-dideazafolic acid (CB3717): Development, characterization and cross-resistance studies. Cancer Res 46:2810–2815.
168. Iman AM, Crossley PH, Jackman AL, Little PFR (1987) Analysis of thymidylate synthase gene amplification and of mRNA levels in the cell cycle. J Biol Chem 262:7368–7373.
169. Jansen G, Schornagel JH, Westerhof GR, Rijkson GR, Newell DR, Jackman AL (1990) Multiple membrane transport systems for the uptake of folate-based thymidylate synthase inhibitors. Cancer Res 50:7422–7548.
170. Sikora E, Jackson AL, Newell DR, Calvert AH (1988) Formation and retention and biological activity of N^{10}-propargyl-5,8-dideazafolic acid (CB3717) polyglutamates in L1210 cells in vitro. Biochem Pharmacol 37:4047–4054.
171. Manteuffel-Cymborowski M, Sikora E, Grzelakowski-Sztabert B (1986) Polyglutamation of the antifolate anticancer drug, N^{10}-propargyl-5,8-dideazafolic acid (CB3717) in the mouse. Anticancer Res 6:807–812.
172. Sikora E, Jackman AL, Newell DR, Harrap KR, Calvert AH, Jones TR, Pawelczak K, Rzesozotarska B (1986) N^{10}-propargyl-5,8-dideazafolic acid polyglutamates as inhibitors of thymidylate synthase and their intracellular formation. In: BA Cooper, VM Whitehead, eds. Chemistry and Biology of Pteridines. Berlin: Walter de Gruyter, pp 675–679.
173. Calvert AH, Alison DL, Harland SJ, Robinson BA, Jackman AL, Jones TR, Newell DR, Siddik

HZ, Wiltshaw E, McElwain TJ, Smith IE, Harrap KR (1986) A phase I evaluation of the quinazoline antifolate thymidylate synthase inhibitor, N^{10}-propargyl-5,8-dideazafolic acid, CB3717. J Clin Oncol 4:1245–1252.

174. Vest S, Bork E, Hansen HH (1988) A phase I evaluation of N^{10}-propargyl-5,8-dideazfolic acid. Eur J Cancer Clin Oncol 24:201–204.

175. Sessa C, Zucchetti M, Ginier M, Willems Y, D'Incalci M, Cavalli F (1988) Phase I study of the antifolate N^{10}-propargyl-5,8-dideazafolic acid, CB3717. Eur J Cancer Clin Oncol 24:769–775.

176. Cantwell BMJ, Earnshaw M, Harris AL (1986) Phase II study of a novel antifolate, N^{10}-propargyl-5,8-dideazafolic acid (CB3717), in malignant mesothelioma. Cancer Treat Rep 70:1335–1336.

177. Cantwell BMJ, Macaulay V, Harris AL, Kay SB, Smith IE, Milsted RAV, Calvert AH (1988) Phase II study of the antifolate N^{10}-propargyl-5,8-dideazafolic acid (CB3717) in advanced breast cancer. Eur J Cancer Clin Oncol 24:733–736.

178. Harding MJ, Cantwell BMJ, Milstead RAV, Harris AL, Kaye SB (1988) Phase II study of the thymidylate synthetase inhibitor CB3717 (N^{10}-propargyl-5,8-dideazafolic acid) in colorectal cancer. Br J Cancer 57:628–629.

179. Bassendine MF, Curtin NJ, Loose H, Harris AL, James OFW (1987) Induction of remission in hepatocellular carcinoma with a new thymidylate synthase inhibitor, CB3717. J Hepatol 4:349–356.

180. Alison DL, Newell RD, Sessa C, Harland SJ, Hart LI, Harrap KR, Calvert AH (1985) The clinical pharmacokinetics of the novel antifolate N^{10}-propargyl-5,8-dideazafolic acid (CB3717). Cancer Chemother Pharmacol 14:265–271.

181. Jodrell DI, Newell DR, Morgan SE, Clinton S, Bensted JPM, Hughes LR, Calvert AH (1991) The renal effects of N^{10}-propargyl-5,8-dideazafolic acid (CB3717) and a non-nephrotoxic analogue ICI D1694, in mice. Br J Cancer 64:833–838.

182. Newell DR, Alison DL, Calvert AH, Harrap KR, Jarman M, Jones TR, Manteuffel-Cymborowska M, O'Connor P (1986) Pharmacokinetics of the thymidylate synthase inhibitor N^{10}-propargyl-5,8-dideazafolic acid (CB3717) in the mouse. Cancer Treat Rep 70:971–979.

183. Jones TR, Thornton TJ, Flinn A, Jackman AL, Newell DR, Calvert AH (1989) Quinazoline antifolates inhibiting thymidylate synthase: 2-Desamino derivatives with enhanced solubility and potency. J Med Chem 32:847–852.

184. Marsham PR, Hughes LR, Jackman AL, Hayter AJ, Oldfield J, Wardleworth JM, Bishop JA, O'Connor BM, Calvert AH (1991) Quinazoline antifolate thymidylate synthase inhibitors: Heterocyclic benzol; ring modifications. J Med Chem 34:1594–1605.

185. Jackman AL, Taylor GA, Gibson W, Kimbell R, Brown M, Calvert AH, Judson IR, Hughes LR (1991) ICI D1694, a quinazoline antifolate thymidylate synthase inhibitor that is a potent inhibitor of L1210 tumor cell growth in vitro and in vivo; a new agent for clinical study. Cancer Res 51:5579–5586.

186. Stephens TC, Valcaccia BE, Sheader ML, Hughes JR, Jackman AL (1991) The thymidylate synthase (TS) inhibitor ICI D1694 is superior to CB3717, 5-fluorouracil (5-FU) and methotrexate (MTX) against a panel of human tumor xenografts. Proc Am Assoc Cancer Res 32:328.

187. Jackman AL, Jodrell DI, Gibson W, Stephens TC (1991) ICI D1694 an inhibitor of thymidylate synthase for clinical study. In RA Harkness, G Elion, N Zollner, eds. Purine and Pyrimidine Metabolism in Man VII. New York: Plenum Press, pp 19–23.

188. Clarkes S, Ward J, Planting A, Spiers J, Smith R, Verweij J, Judson I (1992) Phase I trial of ICI D1694. A novel thymidylate synthase inhibitor. Proc Am Assoc Cancer Res 33:A2426.

189. Judson I, Clarke S, Ward J, Planting A, Verweij J, Spiers J, Smith R, Sutcliffe F (1992) A phase I trial of the thymidylate synthase (TS) inhibitor ICI D1694. Br J Cancer 65(Suppl 16):12.

190. Sorensen JM, Jordan E, Grem JL, Hamilton JM, Arbuck SG, Johnston P, Kohler DR, Goldspiel BR, Allegra CJ (1993) Phase I trial of D1694, a pure thymidylate synthase inhibitor. Proc Am Soc Clin Oncol 12:A432.

191. Clarke SJ, Jackman AL, Judson IR (1993) The history of the development and clinical use of CB3717 and ICI D1694. Adv Exp Med Biol 339:277–287.

192. Clarke SJ, Jackman AL, Judson IR (1993) The toxicity of ICI D1694 in man and mouse. Adv Exp Med Biol 338:601–604.

193. Cunningham D, Zalcberg J, Francois E, Van Cutsem E, Schornagel JH, Adenis A, Green M, Starkhammer H, Hanrahan A, Ellis P, Azab M (1994) Tomudex (ZD1694) A new thymidylate synthase inhibitor with good antitumor activity in advanced colorectal cancer (ACC). Proc Am Soc Clin Oncol 13:A584.

194. Pazdur R, Casper ES, Meropol NJ, Fuchs C, Kennealey GT (1994) Phase II trial of Tomudex

(ZD1694), a thymidylate synthase inhibitor, in advanced pancreatic cancer. Proc Am Soc Clin Oncol 13:A613.

195. Zalcberg J, Cunningham D, Green M, Francois E, van Cutsem E, Schornagel J, Adenis A, Seymour L, Azab M (1995) The final results of a large phase II study of the potent thymidylate synthase (TS) inhibitor Tomudex (ZD1694) in advanced colorectal cancer. Proc Am Soc Clin Oncol 13:A494.

196. Webber SE, Bleckman TM, Attard J, Deal JG, Kathardekar V, Welsh KM, Webber S, Janson CA, Matthews DA, Smith WW, Freer ST, Jordon SR, Bacquet RJ, Howland EF, Booth CLJ, Ward RW, Hermann SM, White J, Morse CA, Hilliard JA, Bartlett CA (1993) Design of thymidylate synthase inhibitors using protein crystal structures: The synthesis and biological evaluation of a novel class of 5-substituted quinazolinones. J Med Chem 36:733–746.

197. Varney MD, Marzoni GP, Palmer CL, Deal JG, Webber S, Welsh KM, Bacquet RJ, Bartlett CA, Morse CA, Booth CLJ, Herrmann SM, Howland EF, Ward RW, White J (1992) Crystal-structure-based design and synthesis of benz[cd]indole-containing inhibitors of thymidylate synthase. J Med Chem 35:663–676.

198. Webber S, Johnston A, Shetty B, Webber SE, Welsh K, Hilliard J, Kosa M, Morse C, Soda K (1993) Preclinical studies on AG-337, a novel lipophilic thymidylate synthase inhibitor. Proc Am Assoc Cancer Res 34:1622.

199. Rafi I, Taylor GA, Calvete JA, Balmanno K, Boddy AV, Bailey NB, Lind MJ, Newell D, Calvert AH, Johnston A, Clendeninn NJ (1995) A phase I clinical study of the novel antifolate AG337 given by a 5 day continuous infusion. Proc Am Assoc Cancer Res 36:1433.

200. Calvete JA, Balmanno K, Rafi I, Newell DR, Taylor GA, Boddy AV, Lind MJ, Bailey NB, Calvert AH, Webber S, Johnson A, Clendeninn NJ (1995) Pre-clinical and clinical studies of the novel thymidylate synthase inhibitor, AG337, given by oral administration. Proc Am Assoc Cancer Res 36:2262.

201. Webber S, Shetty B, Johnston A, Welsh K, Varney M, Deal J, Morse C, Soda K (1992) In vitro properties and antitumor activity of AG-331, a novel lipophilic thymidylate synthase inhibitor. Proc Am Assoc Cancer Res 33:2466.

202. O'Connor BM, Webber S, Jackson RC, Galivan J, Rhee MS (1994) Biological activity of a novel rationally designed lipophilic thymidylate synthase inhibitor. Cancer Chemother Pharmacol 34:225–229.

203. Giantonio B, Qian M, Gallo J, DiMaria D, Legerton K, Johnston AL, Clendeninn NJ, O'Dwyer PJ (1995) Phase I trial of AG-331 as a 5-day continuous infusion. Proc Am Soc Clin Oncol 14:1562.

204. Taylor EC, Harrington PJ, Fletcher SR, Beardsley GP (1989) Synthesis of the antileukemic agents, 5,10-deazaaminopterin and 5,6,7,8 dideazatertrahydroaminopterin. J Med Chem 28:914–921.

205. Beardsley GP, Moroson BA, Taylor EC, Moran RG (1985) A new folate antimetabolite, 5,10-dideaza-5,6,7,8-tetrahydrofolate is a potent inhibitor of de novo purine synthesis. J Biol Chem 264:328–333.

206. Beardsley GP, Taylor EC, Grindey GB, Moran RG (1986) Deaza derivatives of tetrahydrofolic acid. A new class of folate antimetabolites. In BA Cooper, VM Whitehead, eds. Chemistry and Biology of the Pteridines. Berlin: Walter de Gruyter, pp 953–957.

207. Moran RG, Baldwin SW, Taylor EC, Shih J (1989) The 6S- and 6R-diastereomers of 5,10-dideaza-5,6,7,8-tetrahydrofolate are equiactive inhibitors of de novo purine synthesis. J Biol Chem 264:21047–21049.

208. Pizzorno G, Moroson BA, Cashmore AR, Beardsley GP (1991) Effects of 5,10-dideaza-5,6,7,8-tetrahydrofolate on nucleotide metabolism in CCRF-CEM cells. Cancer Res 51:2291–2295.

209. Russello O, Moroson BA, Cross AD, Pizzorno G, Beardsley GP (1992) Kinetics of inhibition of GARTF and AICARTF by DDATHF polyglutamates in the presence of the natural substrates. Proc Am Assoc Cancer Res 33:A2465.

210. Pizzorno G, Sokoloski JA, Cashmore AR, Moroson BA, Cross AD, Beardsley GP (1991) Intracellular metabolism of 5,10-dideazatetrahydrofolic acid in human leukemia cell lines. Mol Pharmacol 39:85–89.

211. Pizzorno G, Moroson BA, Cashmore AR, Russello O, Mayer JR, Galivan J, Bunni MA, Priest DG, Beardsley GP (1995) Multifactorial resistance to 5,10-dideazatetrahydrofolic acid in cell lines derived from human lymphoblastic leukemia CCRF-CEM. Cancer Res 55:566–573.

212. Tse A, Moran RG (1994) Control of the polyglutamation of 5,10-dideazatetrahydro folate by intracellular folate pools: A novel mechanism of resistance to antifolates. Proc Am Assoc Cancer Res 35:304.

213. Pizzorno G, Cashmore AR, Moroson BA, Cross AD, Smith AK, Marling-Cason M, Kamen BA, Beardsley GP (1993) 5,10-Dideazatetrahydrofolic acid (DDATHF) transport in CCRF-CEM and MA104 cell lines. J Biol Chem 268:1017–1023.
214. Muggia F, Martin T, Ray M, Leichman CG, Grunberg S, Gill I, Moran R, Dyke R, Grindey G (1990) Phase-I study of weekly 5,10-dideazatetrahydrofolate (LY 264618, DDATHF-B). Proc Am Soc Clin Oncol 9:A285.
215. Nelson R, Butler F, Dugan W Jr, David-Land C, Stone M, Dyke R (1990) Phase I clinical trial of LY264618 (dideazatetrahydrofolic acid: DDATHF). Proc Am Soc Clin Oncol 9:A293.
216. Young C, Currie V, Baltzer L, Trochanowski B, Eton O, Dyke R, Bowsher R (1990) Phase I and clinical pharmacologic study of LY264618, 5,10-dideazatetrahydrofolate. Proc Am Assoc Cancer Res 31:A1053.
217. Sessa C, Gumbrell L, Hatty S, Kern H, Cavalli F (1990) Phase I study of 5,10-dideazatetrahydrofolic acid (LY264618; DDATHF) given daily for 3 consecutive days. Ann Oncol 1(Suppl):38–42.
218. Ray MS, Muggia FM, Leichman CG, Grunberg SM, Nelson RL, Dyke RW, Moran RG (1993) Phase I study of (6R)-5,10-dideazatetrahydrofolate: A folate antimetabolite inhibitory to de novo purine synthesis. J Natl Cancer Inst 85:1154–1159.
219. Grindey GB, Alati T, Shih C (1991) Reversal of the toxicity, but not the antitumor activity of Lometrexol by folic acid. Proc Am Assoc Cancer Res 32:A324.
220. Wedge SR, Laohavinij S, Taylor G, Newell DR, Charlton CJ, Proctor M, Chapman F, Simmons D, Oakey A, Gumbrell L, Calvert AH (1993) Modulation of lometrexol toxicity by oral folic acid administration: A Phase I study. Proc Am Assoc Cancer Res 34:A1629.

9. HUMAN IMMUNODEFICIENCY VIRUS REPLICATION IN THE PRESENCE OF ANTIRETROVIRAL DRUGS: ANALOGIES TO ANTINEOPLASTIC DRUG RESISTANCE

ROGER K. STRAIR AND DANIEL J. MEDINA

Oncologists commonly care for patients with human immunodeficiency virus (HIV)–associated malignancies. In fact, the management of HIV-infected patients with Kaposi's sarcoma, non-Hodgkin's lymphoma, or squamous cell carcinoma of the cervix is common in many oncology practices. In addition, many hematologists care for patients with hemophilia and HIV infection, or patients with HIV-associated hematologic disorders, such as immune thrombocytopenia, antiphospholipid antibodies, chronic cytopenias, and thrombotic thrombocytopenic purpura.

In addition to this high level of clinical interaction with HIV-infected patients, there are many features of the biology of HIV infection that are familiar to hematologists and oncologists. For example, the development of genetic and phenotypic diversity in HIV contributes to disease progression and the ultimate resistance of the virus to antiretroviral therapy. A similar generation of diversity occurs during tumor development and allows tumors to evolve and survive a variety of selective pressures. Most tumors are believed to be derived from a single mutated malignant cell, and the growth advantage of this cell results in additional cell divisions. Subsequent mutations that arise during these cell divisions facilitate clonal evolution in response to environmental, immunologic, and therapeutic selection. The result is often populations of cells that continue to replicate, induce angiogenesis, avert immune surveillance, become increasingly invasive, metastasize, and become resistant to antitumor therapy.

In malignancies the mutation rate associated with cell division contributes to the heterogeneity of the tumor. In fact, inherited mutations associated with the DNA repair machinery can predispose to malignancy, and there are likely to be other non-inherited alterations of the malignant cell, for example, acquired mutations, that contribute to an increased mutation rate in these cells. Even if the mutation rate is not increased in malignant cells, the relatively high rate of cell division in these cells provides multiple opportunities for the generation and accumulation of mutations. For example, the spontaneous mutation rate is estimated to be 10^{-9}/nucleotide/cell division. Therefore, a gene with an average coding sequence will undergo one base pair change in the coding sequence every 10^6 cell divisions. Under these conditions a small tumor containing 10^8 cells might have at least 100 cells with a mutation in that individual coding sequence [1]. Some of these mutations may be selected for, some may be selected against, and some will be neutral. Over the course of time, positively selected mutations will accumulate and the heterogeneity introduced into the tumor by these mutations will make a major contribution to the phenotypic diversity of the tumor. Continued replication ensures ongoing generation of diversity and evolution. Resistance to many natural defenses, as well as resistance to chemotherapy and radiation therapy, may ultimately develop as a consequence of this diversity.

Diversity is also a major contributory factor to the pathogenesis of HIV infection. Acute infection is accompanied by a burst of viral replication that generates a wide range of HIV genetic variants. In contrast to the mutation rate of genomic cellular DNA, the mutation rate of HIV is much higher, estimated to be 10^{-4} to 10^{-3}/nucleotide/replication cycle [2–4]. This high mutation rate is partially ascribed to the absence of an editing of errors in the reverse transcription of the viral RNA. This strikingly high mutation rate ensures the rapid generation of diversity and the rapid evolution of the virus in the face of selective pressures, such as the host immune system or antiretroviral therapy [5,6]. In addition, the viral DNA integrates into the host cell DNA and replicates along with cellular genes. This conservative replication allows the HIV genome to be preserved without rapid mutation. If the integrated viral DNA can produce infectious virus (i.e., it has not undergone deleterious mutations), it will serve as the template for additional mutations during subsequent cycles of infection of other cells by its progeny virions. If, however, the integrated virus is defective as a consequence of the mutations it has undergone, it will not produce infectious progeny and will often be a genetic dead end. This system ensures the preservation of functional viruses in the face of very high mutation rates [5,6]. Analogous to the clonal evolution of tumors, viruses that accumulate in the population undergo further mutation and become the templates for continued evolution. In addition, some HIV-infected cells may be latently infected, not producing viral products that target the cell for immune-mediated death. This may allow the preservation of diverse viral genomes in the face of a functional immune system. Furthermore, the presence of various host cell tropisms for the diversifying variants of HIV generates several lineages of HIV within a given patient. This allows an even greater diversity of HIV. These physiologic lineages may be analogous to anatomic lineages that develop when a tumor becomes metastatic.

HIV and tumor cells both accumulate adaptive mutations that allow the aversion of natural restrictive processes, such as the immune system or anatomical/physiologic boundaries. The number of tumor cells in many disseminated malignancies may reach 10^{12}, and the numbers of cells with multiple mutations and evolving mutations is likely to be very high and may contribute to resistance to antineoplastic therapy. Similarly, the number of viral genomes in advanced HIV infection is likely to be very high, and with the high rate of viral mutation the virus is extraordinarily adept at responding to selective pressures. The gradual destruction of the immune system makes advanced HIV infection that much more adaptable, allowing higher rates of replication, an increased number of mutant viruses, and a greater capacity to avert antiviral therapy.

The pharmacologic therapy of HIV infection can readily focus on processes such as reverse transcription that are unique to the virus. The ability to target processes unique to HIV or to classes of viruses of which HIV is a member has generated limited optimism in some who design anti-HIV therapies. They argue that HIV has several unique processes that should be able to be targeted, and, even if eradication of the virus is not possible, it may be feasible to inhibit these processes for prolonged periods of time. In contrast, the skeptics cite the extreme diversity of the virus and the possibility that even these unique processes share common features with cellular processes. Such shared features may make it difficult to completely inhibit viral functions without causing significant cellular toxicity. New antiviral approaches with similarities to new antineoplastic therapies are actively being studied: combinations of drugs, genetic therapies, specific therapies targeted at the destruction of specific cells (infected cells or neoplastic cells), and attempts to modulate the immune system are currently undergoing preclinical or clinical evaluation. These similarities between antiviral and antineoplastic therapy have fostered many scientific interactions between investigators focusing on these fields. These interactions ensure that the ramifications of biological and technical advances in antineoplastic therapy will be investigated in HIV therapy and vice versa. This has expanded the force of scientists working in these fields and has resulted in a large patient care and research-based community that is interactive and will hopefully benefit both patients with neoplastic diseases and patients with HIV infection.

One area in which this type of collaboration is evident is in the design of antiviral chemotherapy. In addition to the testing of new drugs and new drug combinations, some pharmacologists and virologists are using the same principles utilized in oncology drug development to develop new treatments for HIV-infected patients. Antiretroviral therapy like antineoplastic therapy must confront a multitude of obstacles. In addition to the ultimate development of genetic drug resistance, pharmacologic sanctuaries in which the drug is not active may be a major therapeutic problem in the treatment of HIV-infected patients and in the treatment of patients with malignancies. In addition, the host cells for HIV infection are varied, and sanctuary growth may, in some cases, be less anatomic than due to differences in the biochemistry of the varied cells that are potential hosts for HIV infection. Furthermore, the size of the sanctuary may change over time, perhaps due to selective pressures imposed by drug treatment or other mechanisms that may contribute to the evolution of cell types in the presence of the drug.

This chapter reviews some of the common mechanisms responsible for the failure of antiviral agents to eradicate HIV infection. While most of this failure is ultimately due to the selection of HIV that contain mutations that encode resistance to the antiviral drug, a comparison of two inhibitors of the viral reverse transcriptase (RT) indicates that the capacity of the virus to replicate in the presence of antiviral agents can derive from diverse mechanisms. Analogies between these mechanisms and the selective processes that result in the resistance of tumors to antineoplastic therapy are emphasized.

FEATURES OF THE RETROVIRAL REPLICATIVE CYCLE CONTRIBUTING TO GENETIC HETEROGENEITY

When a retrovirus infects a cell, it undergoes a cycle of reverse transcription that converts the two copies of genomic viral RNA into a single copy of double-stranded DNA [7–9]. This process of reverse transcription is error prone, perhaps as a consequence of polymerization by a viral enzyme, RT, that lacks a $3'-5'$ exonuclease activity. In the absence of such an exonuclease, misincorporated nucleotides cannot be removed and mutations result. The RT of HIV is estimated to be even more error prone than the RT of other retroviruses. In fact, the genome of HIV contains approximately 10^4 nucleotides, and it has been estimated that 1–10 mutations are introduced during each cycle of reverse transcription [2–4].

The product of reverse transcription is a DNA molecule that is integrated into the host cell genomic DNA. This integrated proviral DNA is replicated along with cellular DNA in cells that are dividing. Few mutations are induced in proviral DNA during this host cell replication. The proviral DNA serves as the template for the production of viral RNA, which has several possible fates. Host cell RNA polymerase II transcribes the proviral DNA in a process that may introduce mutations into the viral RNA. Some of the viral RNA is processed into mRNA, which is translated into viral proteins. Other molecules of viral RNA remain full length and are either translated into other viral proteins or are packaged into virions as genomic RNA. These virions are released and can infect new host cells.

The bulk of HIV heterogeneity appears to derive from error-prone reverse transcription. Additional mutations may result from transcription of the proviral DNA by host cell RNA polymerase, but few mutations are likely to be introduced during DNA replication of the integrated proviral DNA. The process of reverse transcription results in a high mutation rate and extensive genetic heterogeneity. The production of progeny virions assures the continued generation of mutations during subsequent infection and reverse transcription. The result is rapid evolution and the production of a quasispecies with an extensive array of genetic variants. Variants that are defective or are selected against may result in the formation of proviruses, but infectious progeny will not be produced and the variant will become very under-represented in the population of viruses. Viruses that are selected predominate in the population, undergo repeated infectious cycles, and serve as templates for additional mutations (continued evolution) [7–10]. This entire process is highly analogous to tumor evolution and explains the capacity of HIV to respond to a broad range of selective pressures, including antiretroviral therapy, with the outgrowth of genetically altered virus.

DRUG-RESISTANCE MUTATIONS IN HIV

Genetic resistance to virtually every antiviral drug that has been used against HIV has ultimately emerged during therapy [11]. For many of the drugs, resistance can be encoded by several distinct mutations. In addition, crossresistance to other drugs may be induced by some mutations, and mutations encoding resistance to one drug may interfere with the resistance to different drugs induced by other mutations. These interactions establish complex patterns of clonal selection and evolution during the selective pressures of drug therapy. Combination therapy with multiple antiviral agents can result in particularly complicated patterns of viral evolution.

RESISTANCE TO AZT (ZIDOVUDINE)

The HIV RT is the target of many currently used antiretoviral drugs. Reverse transcriptase is an attractive target for antiviral therapy because reverse transcription is an essential step in retroviral replication that is unique to the virus. $3'$-Azido-$3'$-deoxythymidine (AZT) was the first nucleoside analog demonstrated to have activity against HIV [12–14]. The active metabolite of AZT is AZT triphosphate (AZTTP), which inhibits RT in vitro by either competitive inhibition with the normal substrate, thymidine triphosphate (TTP), or by incorporation into the viral DNA, resulting in chain termination. In either case, viral DNA production is blocked, resulting in an aborted infection. Clinical studies with AZT have indicated that AZT has a beneficial effect in a variety of HIV-related clinical states [14–16]. An initial report from the European Concorde study has raised questions about whether early initiation of AZT in the asymptomatic state has any effect on survival [17].

Reports describing the isolation of virus resistant to AZT appeared shortly after AZT entered clinical use. The first report of AZT-resistant virus described isolates from 33 patients who had been treated with AZT for various periods of time [18]. Virus isolated from patients never treated with AZT was uniformly inhibited by very low concentrations of AZT ($IC_{50} < 0.05\,\mu M$). Similarly, virus isolated from patients receiving AZT treatment for less than 6 months generally remained very susceptible to AZT. In contrast, virus isolated from patients treated with AZT for greater than 6 months often exhibited some degree of AZT resistance. The extent of resistance correlated with the duration of AZT therapy, and progressive increases in resistance were noted in some patients.

Additional studies have confirmed and extended the findings of this initial report. An analysis of patients treated at various clinical stages of HIV disease demonstrated that AZT resistance appeared earlier in patients with more advanced disease. After 1 year of AZT therapy, 89% of patients with advanced disease and 31% of patients with early-stage disease had AZT-resistant isolates [19]. Using a different methodology to detect AZT-resistant virus, one study has demonstrated AZT-resistant virus in some untreated patients who became infected prior to the availability of AZT [20]. Since there can be so many different HIV variants in a patient, it is not surprising that AZT-resistant viruses exist in these untreated patients; however, the ability to detect these resistant viruses will depend upon their prevalence in an unselected population of HIV. The prevalence of AZT-resistant viruses in untreated patients is likely to be highest in those who have been infected by virus from HIV-infected patients treated with AZT.

Genetic analyses of AZT-resistant virus isolates have demonstrated that several mutations, alone and in combination, in the RT gene are the cause of AZT resistance [21–27]. The importance of these mutations was proven by experiments that introduced these mutations into cloned laboratory strains of virus. These genetically engineered viruses became resistant to AZT, proving that AZT resistance was caused by these mutations in the RT gene. The mutations result in structural changes in RT that are likely to alter interactions with AZTTP. These extremely important studies established that virus isolated from patients on long-term AZT therapy can be resistant to AZT as a consequence of specific mutations in the RT gene.

With the identification of the mutations responsible for AZT resistance, it became possible to develop sensitive molecular techniques to detect these mutations directly in clinical samples [25–27]. In one study, specimens from 168 patients were subjected to genetic analysis. Specific mutations (corresponding to amino acids 70 and 215) generally occurred earliest after initiation of AZT and were associated with relatively small degrees of AZT resistance [25]. Additional mutations (corresponding to amino acids 67 and 219) subsequently appeared, and in combination with the other mutations resulted in a higher level of AZT resistance. Other analyses have defined additional mutations contributing to AZT resistance [22].

MECHANISMS OF AZT RESISTANCE

The mechanism by which AZT-resistant virus becomes refractory to AZT is unknown. Mutations in RT are sufficient to cause resistance when introduced into laboratory strains of virus, indicating that alterations of the structure of RT induce resistance to AZT. It has not , however, been possible to unequivocally demonstrate that the mutated RT has significantly reduced sensitivity to AZTTP in in-vitro assays [62]. Therefore, it is possible that these in vitro assays do not accurately reflect the functioning of the enzyme in vivo. Alternatively, AZT action is partially mediated by metabolites other than AZTTP, or the antiretroviral effects of AZT are mediated by RT at a step other than reverse transcription.

Two groups of investigators have recently been able to "crystallize" HIV-1 RT [28,29]. The crystallization of RT has allowed x-ray diffraction to be used to develop a detailed three-dimensional model of RT structure. Such a model of RT has provided considerable information about the location of the active polymerization site and the sites at which the viral RNA, viral DNA, and primers for reverse transcription interact with the enzyme. The definition and structural orientation of these sites within RT has allowed a correlation of mutations with the structure of the enzyme. While some inhibitors have been shown to bind to RT near the active site, the widely distributed mutations that result in AZT resistance (mutations corresponding to amino acids 41, 67, 70, 215, and 219) do not appear to directly involve the active site for polymerization and are more likely to alter the way in which HIV-1 RT interacts with viral RNA, viral DNA, or primer RNA. These altered interactions may cause a structural change in the enzyme that reduces the efficacy of AZTTP as an inhibitor of RT [30]. The availability of the three-dimensional structure of HIV-1 RT will provide considerable information about the biology of the enzyme. In addition, the availability of this information will allow inhibitors to be designed on the basis of the molecular features of the active site of the enzyme. This may make it possible to design drugs targeted to the active site in such a way that mutations that interfere with an interaction between the drug and RT interfere with the functioning of the enzyme to a great enough degree to disable the virus.

RESISTANCE TO NON-NUCLEOSIDE REVERSE TRANSCRIPTASE INHIBITORS SUCH AS NEVIRAPINE

The anti–HIV-1 drug nevirapine is a member of a class of antiviral agents known as non-nucleoside reverse transcriptase inhibitors (NNRTIs). These agents are active against HIV-1 but do not have activity against other retroviruses. HIV variants that are resistant to nevirapine and other NNRTIs can be readily selected in cell culture and emerge after a short time in patients undergoing treatment with these drugs [31–35]. As with AZT, multiple mutations in RT can encode resistance to the NNRTIs. However, unlike the mutations that encode AZT resistance, relatively high level resistance can be found in HIV with only a single mutation in RT. This association of high-level resistance with only single mutations explains why many members of this class of antiretroviral agents are limited by the very rapid emergence of drug-resistant variants.

HIV-1 KINETICS DURING ANTIRETROVIRAL THERAPY WITH NEVIRAPINE OR AZT

Recent clinical studies have quantitated the antiviral response that occurs in the setting of antiretroviral therapy. These studies have taken advantage of the ability to accurately determine the amount of viral RNA present in plasma. The initial studies demonstrated that shortly after the initiation of therapy with nevirapine, there is a rapid decline in the amount of viral RNA in plasma [34,35]. The half-life of the viral RNA is approximately 2 days, indicating that neither the half-life of the virus particles nor the half-life of cells producing the bulk of the virus can exceed 2 days. This model of HIV-1 kinetics suggests rapid and continuous viral replication and rapid cellular turnover throughout the course of the infection. A detailed analysis of viral RNA after the initiation of nevirapine indicated that after the initial decline in viral RNA there was a rapid rebound in the amount viral RNA in plasma.

Characterization of this RNA and the virions from which it was derived indicated that the rebound in viral RNA was due to the rapid emergence of drug-resistant variants containing well-characterized mutations that result in nevirapine resistance. After 2 weeks of nevirapine therapy, the bulk of viral RNA already contained mutations encoding resistance to nevirapine.

These studies indicate the rapid selection of a drug-resistant variant that must have pre-existed within the unselected viral population at a relatively high frequency. Estimates based upon another kinetic analysis have indicated the presence of similar drug-resistant variants at a frequency of approximately 1 in 750 HIV-1 virions [35]. The rapid selection of pre-existing nevriapine-resistant HIV-1 variants is in agreement with in vitro studies that indicate the rapid selection of nevirapine-resistant viruses during tissue culture infections in the presence of nevirapine [33]. In vitro studies of the prevalence of unselected resistance to a functionally and biologically related RT inhibitor have also indicated a similar prevalence of unselected drug-resistant variants [36]. Therefore, the failure of nevirapine therapy is likely to be a direct consequence of extensive HIV-1 genetic heterogeneity that results in a high prevalence of nevirapine-resistant variants prior to the initiation of nevirapine therapy.

A similar analysis of HIV-1 plasma RNA levels after the initiation of zidovudine (AZT) has indicated more complex dynamics [37]. In that study there was a similar initial decline and subsequent rebound in viral RNA shortly after initiating AZT therapy. A characterization of the viral RNA associated with the early rebound indicated there were no corresponding mutations that are known to encode resistance to AZT. Therefore, in contrast to HIV kinetics during nevirapine therapy, the early rebound in viral RNA during AZT treatment was not due to the emergence of drug-resistant HIV. These more complex dynamics may be a consequence of a variety of pharmacologic, cellular, and viral features.

The mutations associated with AZT resistance may be present in the initial (unselected) viral population at much lower levels than those that encode nevirapine resistance. Certainly, viral variants with high-level AZT resistance contain multiple mutations and emerge/evolve over several months to years; these variants containing multiple mutations would be expected to either be present at very low levels in the initial population or to develop in a stepwise fashion during selection. While the slow emergence of resistant variants can be explained by a low prevalence of AZT-resistant variants, the need for superimposed mutations, or selection against the emergence of these variants, the early outgrowth of AZT-sensitive virus in the presence of AZT must be explained by virologic, cellular, or pharmacologic features that result in the ability of HIV-1 that is genotypically and phenotypically sensitive to AZT to replicate in the presence of AZT.

DIVERSE MECHANISMS CAN CONTRIBUTE TO THE ABILITY OF HIV-1 TO REPLICATE IN THE PRESENCE OF ANTIVIRAL DRUGS

The ability of HIV-1 to continue to replicate in the presence of an antiviral drug is known as *viral breakthrough*. Viral breakthrough can occur by several different mechanisms. The predominant mechanism resulting in viral breakthrough infection in the presence of nevirapine is the selection and outgrowth of virus-containing mutations that result in nevirapine resistance. The virions that emerge contain well-characterized RT mutations, which result in the production of a RT that is not inhibited by nevirapine.

The ultimate ability of HIV-1 to replicate in the presence of AZT is also a consequence of the emergence of AZT-resistant virus. However, early in the course of AZT treatment, the circulating virus is not resistant to AZT. This early HIV breakthrough in the presence of AZT therefore represents virus that can avert the selective pressure of AZT. The kinetic studies described earlier have not only determined the patterns of HIV breakthrough infection but have indicated a very rapid turnover of HIV virions and cells producing large amounts of virus. This dynamic model of repeated cycles of infection, without major amounts of virus being produced by latently infected cells, implies that circulating virus predominantly represents virus that is actively replicating. Therefore, the emergence of AZT-sensitive virus after the initiation of AZT is very likely to represent virus that is actively replicating.

Since the emergence of resistant virus containing mutations in the RT gene does not explain early HIV replication in the presence of AZT, alternate mechanisms must be responsible for such replication. The potential mechanisms contributing to viral breakthrough in the absence of the development of genetic drug resistance may include pharmacologic [38,39], virologic [40,41], and cellular parameters, including host cell heterogeneity in the uptake and/or metabolism of the drug [44–48,59,60]. This cellular heterogeneity is directly analogous to the tumor cell heterogeneity that often complicates antineoplastic therapy in that it may result in a subset of the cellular population in which the drug is ineffective. For example, a cell deficient in thymidine kinase would have a diminished capacity to phosphorylate AZT to its active triphosphate and would be refractory to the antiretroviral effects of AZT. This would allow virus with an AZT-sensitive genotype to replicate in the presence of AZT.

Alternatively, there could be host cell heterogeneity in the levels of TTP that compete with AZTTP. Furthermore, cellular nucleases capable of removing chain-terminating nucleoside analogs may be present and could conceivably reverse the antiretroviral effects of some drugs [49]. Other factors contributing to viral breakthrough may involve virologic features related to viral load or viral phenotype (in addition to genetic drug resistance). Similarly, a component of viral reverse transcription may occur extracellularly (intravirion reverse transcription), in the absence of exposure to AZTTP, that is intracellular [41]. In addition, there may be complex pharmacologic features related to drug accumulation, disposition, and efficacy [38,39]. To a certain degree, these latter pharmacologic features may overlap considerably with both viral and cellular factors that contribute to viral breakthrough. Notably, drugs like nevirapine do not require cellular activation, and "cellular resistance" to the antiretroviral effects of these drugs is therefore less likely than "cellular resistance" to the antiviral effects of nucleoside analog RT inhibitors, such as AZT, ddC, ddI, and d4T, all of which must be phosphorylated to an active intracellular triphosphate.

"Cellular resistance" to the antiretroviral effects of AZT and ddC has been described and has been ascribed to metabolic/enzymatic alterations in the specific cell types analyzed [42,43]. For example, a relative inefficacy of AZT in some cells has been reported and ascribed to reduced levels of the kinases necessary for nucleoside phosphorylation [44–46,50]. A clinical role of this inefficacy over a period of time has been suggested by some studies that indicate variations in the levels of intracellular phosphorylated AZT over time [52,56]. In other studies the selection of cells in very high concentrations of AZT (and in some studies, BrdU) for prolonged periods of time has resulted in the outgrowth of cells with resistance to the cytotoxic and antiviral effects of AZT, and the selected cells may be deficient in thymidine kinase [51–56]. Furthermore, expression of the multidrug resistance (mdr) gene product has been linked to "cellular resistance" to the antiretroviral effects of nucleoside analog RT inhibitors [63]. Studies such as these that select cells in high concentrations of AZT or subject cells to BrdU emphasize changes that might occur in highly selected cells over a period of time, but the contribution of such cells to early or late viral breakthrough infection is unclear, and the relevance of the generally rigorous selection process (with prolonged exposures to very high concentrations of AZT) to clinical HIV infection and treatment is in question.

With respect to potential biochemical mechanisms allowing drug-sensitive virus to replicate in the presence of a drug, there are several features of the intracellular metabolism of the nucleoside analog reverse transcriptase inhibitors that could contribute to the resistance of some cells to the antiretroviral effects of these drugs. For example, resting cells can initiate reverse transcription, but completion of reverse transcription may require cellular activation [57,58]. As mentioned earlier, cellular activation and the growth state of the cell are also important determinants of nucleoside pools and the levels of enzymes necessary to produce the natural nucleoside triphosphates [44–48,51,59,60]. The sizes of these pools and the ability to phosphorylate natural nucleosides and the nucleoside analogs could have profound effects on the efficacy of the nucleoside analogs in different cells and cell types in a population of cells. In addition, more complex mechanisms contributing to alterations in drug activation and nucleotide pool sizes may occur. For example, one study has indicated that very high concentrations of AZT induce DNA hypermethylation, and epigenetic deficiencies in thymidine kinase can result. These cells could conceivably be refractory to the antiretroviral effects of AZT as a consequence of these epigenetic alterations of thymidine kinase levels [54,55].

IMPORTANCE OF EARLY VIRAL BREAKTHROUGH IN THE PRESENCE OF ANTIVIRAL DRUGS

In contrast to the rapid selection of nevirapine-resistant HIV, early viral breakthrough in the presence of AZT is generally due to infection with drug-sensitive virus. A variety of cellular, pharmacologic, and viral mechanisms may allow AZT-sensitive virus to replicate in the presence of AZT. With continued growth there is amplification of viral variants with genetic resistance because the genetically resistant virus can infect any suitable target cell and is not subject to the antiviral constraints of AZT. Therefore, whatever sanctuary is responsible for early AZT-sensitive HIV infection in the presence of AZT limits viral replication to a subset of cells, viruses, or locales. The emergence of genetic resistance generates HIV without these limitations to replication. This gives a relative growth advantage to genetically resistant virus. Subsequent additional mutations or recombination events result in viruses with multiple mutations that encode high-level AZT resistance. The initial events that allow a population of nonresistant or partially resistant virus to replicate provide a pool of virus in which additional mutations and recombination events can occur. These additional events may contribute to the development of the additional mutations that result in high-level resistance. Reversal of the early viral breakthrough by genetically sensitive virus could conceivably delay, or even prevent, the outgrowth of highly resistant virus with multiple mutations by not allowing nonresistant or only partially resistant virus (with single mutations) to replicate.

IN VITRO SYSTEMS TO DEMONSTRATE AND CHARACTERIZE EARLY BREAKTHROUGH

There are currently few ways to quantitate and characterize early breakthrough virus infection in the presence of antiviral drugs. Furthermore, it is difficult to rapidly isolalte and characterize cells that are infected early during drug treatment. This characterization is essential because it may demonstrate the mechanism of early viral breakthrough (including "cellular resistance" to the antiviral effects of drugs) and provide clues to reversing this early breakthrough.

One system that has recently been developed has involved the use of defective recombinant HIV that encode reporter genes. This approach is useful because it allows the both the quantitative analysis of a single cycle of infection and the isolation of cells that have been infected [36,61]. In addition, these analyses allow estimations of the prevalence of genetic drug resistance in unselected populations of HIV. Experiments that have been performed in the presence of a non-nucleoside reverse transcriptase inhibitor (which is biologically similar to nevirapine) have demonstrated that early HIV breakthrough occurs as a consequence of infection by virus that is resistant to the drug [36]. The prevalence of this breakthrough infection is similar to that calculated from the clinical studies described earlier [35].

When the same system was used to analyze HIV breakthrough infection in the presence of AZT, it was found that early infection was not likely to be occurring as a consequence of drug resistance [61]. An analysis of cells that were infected during the first cycle after initation of AZT indicated that some of the cells were refractory to the antiviral effects of AZT. The cells were labeled as having "cellular resistance" to the antiviral effects of AZT, and the relaltive inefficacy of AZT as an antiviral agent in these cells has been documented with other replication-defective viruses as well as with replication-competent (nondefective) HIV-1. In addition, cellular resistance to the antiviral effects of the other nucleoside analogs has been demonstrated in other cells in the population that was studied. Recent studies have extended these results and have demonstrated that other cell types have a similar prevalence of cells with resistance to the antiviral effects of AZT.

The ability to isolalte the cells that were infected by AZT-sensitive virus in the presence of AZT allowed biochemical analyses of the mechanisms resulting in the inefficacy of AZT to be undertaken. An analysis of a cell line derived from one such infected cell has indicated excessive conversion of ^{3}H-thymidine into TTP and decreased accumulation of AZTTP. These biochemical parameters may explain the relative inefficacy of AZT in these cells and suggest that interventions to decrease levels of TTP may increase AZT efficacy in these cells. The analysis of many such clones may help determine the predominant mechanisms responsible for the ability of AZT-sensitive virus to replicate in the presence of AZT. These in vitro studies indicate that early infection in the presence of nucleoside analogs is often the result of drug-sensitive virus infecting cells in which the antiviral agent is ineffective. When interpreted in the context of clinical studies indicating that early viral replication after initiation of AZT is not due to the emergence of AZT-resistant virus, the in vitro studies may provide a clinically relevant model of early viral breakthrough infection in the presence of AZT. Reversal of the mechanisms allowing this early infection may result in improved antiretroviral therapy as a consequence of more prolonged suppression of viral replication and delayed emergence of genetically AZT-resistant HIV. Studies with the other nucleoside analogs indicate that cellular resistance to the antiviral effects of some of these drugs commonly occurs.

SUMMARY

There are many analogies between antineoplastic therapy and antiviral therapy. For each there may be sanctuary sites in which the drug is ineffective because of decreased accumulation of the active form of the drug or increased competition by naturally occurring inhibitors. These sanctuaries may be restricted to anatomic or biochemical subsets of the population. A knowledge of these sanctuaries is essential to an understanding of the failure of therapy and for the design of more effective treatments. Eradication of these sanctuary sites may be important because they may be responsible for the viral replication or tumor cell division that continues to generate the diversity that drives clonal evolution. Ultimately, diversity as a consequence of the accumulation of mutations results in the selection of resistant viral or tumor cell variants and the failure of drug therapy. Maximizing therapy in an attempt to diminish the rate of generation of this diversity may result in better clinical outcomes, including a delay in the generation of variants with genetic drug resistance.

REFERENCES

1. Lewin B (1987) Genes III. New York: John Wiley.
2. Roberts JD, Bebenek K, Kunkel TA (1988) The accuracy of reverse transcriptase from HIV-1. Science 242:1171.
3. Katz RA, Skalka AM (1990) Generation of diversity in retroviruses. Ann Rev Genet 24:409.
4. Preston BD, Poiesz BJ, Loeb LA (1988) Fidelity of HIV-1 reverse transcriptase. Science 242:1168.
5. Varmus HE (1988) Retroviruses. Science 240:1427.

6. Hu WS, Temin HM (1990) Retroviral recombination and reverse transcription. Science 250:1227.
7. Cullen BR (1991) Human immunodeficiency virus as a prototypic complex retrovirus. J Virol 65:1053–1056.
8. Luciw PA, Leung NJ (1992) Mechanism of retroviral replication. In JA Levy, ed. The Retroviridae, Vol. 1. New York: Plenum Press, pp 159–298.
9. Temin HM (1989) Retrovirus variation and evolution. Genome 31:17.
10. Myers G, Pavlakis GN (1992) Evolutionary potential of complex retroviruses. In JA Levy, ed. The Retroviridae, Vol. 1. New York: Plenum Press, pp 51–104.
11. Strair RK, Mellors JW (1994) Resistance of HIV-1 to antiretroviral drugs. AIDS Updates.
12. Mitsuya H, Weinhold KJ, Furman PA, et al. (1985) 3'-azido-3'-deoxythymidine (BWA509U): An antiviral agent that inhibits the infectivity and cytopathic effect of human T-lymphotropic virus type III/lymphadenopathy associated virus in vitro. Proc Natl Acad Sci USA 82:7096–7100.
13. Mitsuya H, Broder S (1986) Inhibition of the in vitro infectivity and cytopathic effect of human T-lymphotropic virus type III/lymphadenopathy associated virus (HTLV III/LAV) by 2',3'-dideoxynucleosides. Proc Natl Acad Sci USA 83:1911–1915.
14. Richman DD (1992) Antiretroviral therapy: Azidothymidine and other deoxynucleoside analogues. In VT DeVita, S Hellman, SA Rosenberg, eds. AIDS: Etiology, Diagnosis, Treatment and Prevention. Philadelphia: JB Lippincott, pp 373–387.
15. Fischl MA, Richman DD, Grieco MH, et al. (1987) The efficacy of azidothymidine AZT in the treatment of patients with AIDS and the AIDS related complex. A double blind placebo controlled trial. N Engl J Med 317:185–191.
16. Ioannidis JP, Cappelleri JC, Lau J, Skolnik PR, Melville B, Chalmers TC, Sacks HS (1995) Early or deferred zidovudine therapy in HIV-infected patients without an AIDS-defining illness. Ann Intern Med 122:856–866.
17. Aboulker JP, Swart AM (1993) Preliminary analysis of the Concorde trial. Lancet 341:889–890.
18. Larder BA, Darby G, Richman DD (1989) HIV with reduced sensitivity to zidovudine (AZT) isolated during prolonged therapy. Science 243:1731–1734.
19. Richman DD, Grimes JM, Lagakos SW (1990) Effect of stage of disease and drug dose on zidovudine susceptibilities of isolates of human immunodeficiency virus. J Acquir Immune Defic Syndr 3:743–746.
20. Mohri H, Singh MK, Ching WTW, Ho DD (1993) Quantitation of zidovudine resistant human immunodeficiency virus type 1 in the blood of treated and untreated patients. Proc Natl Acad Sci USA 90:25–29.
21. Larder BA, Kemp SD (1989) Multiple mutations in HIV-1 reverse transcriptase confer high-level resistance to zidovudine (AZT). Science 246:1155–1158.
22. Kellam P, Boucher CA, Larder BA (1992) Fifth mutation in human immunodeficiency virus type 1 reverse transcriptase contributes to the development of high-level resistance to zidovudine. Proc Natl Acad Sci USA 89:1934–1938.
23. Dianzani F, Antonelli G, Turriziani O, Dong G, Capobianchi MR, Riva E (1992) In vitro selection of human immunodeficiency virus type 1 resistant to 3'-azido-3'-deoxythymidine. Antiviral Res 18:39–52.
24. Gao Q, Gu Z, Parniak MA, Li X, Wainberg MA (1992) In vitro selection of variants of human immunodeficiency virus type 1 resistant to 3'-azido-3'-deoxythymidine and 2',3'-dideoxyinosine. J Virol 66:12–19.
25. Richman DD, Guatelli JC, Grimes J, Tsiatis A, Gingeras T (1991) Detection of mutations associated with zidovudine resistance in human immunodeficiency virus by use of the polymerase chain reaction. J Infect Dis 164:1075–1081.
26. Boucher CAB, Tersmette M, Lange MA, et al. (1990) Zidovudine sensitivity of human immunodeficiency viruses from high-risk, symptom-free individuals during therapy. Lancet 336:585–590.
27. Boucher CAB, O'Sullivan E, Mulder JW, et al. (1992) Ordered appearance of zidovudine resistance mutations during treatment of 18 human immunodeficiency virus positive subjects. J Infect Dis 165:105–110.
28. Kohlstaedt LAW J, Friedman JM, Rice PA, Steitz TA (1992) Crystal structure at 3.5 A resolution of HIV-1 reverse transcriptase complexed with an inhibitor. Science 256:1783–1790.
29. Jacobo-Molina A, Ding J, Nanni RG, et al. (1993) Structure of HIV-1 reverse transcriptase complexed with double stranded DNA at 3.0 A resolution shows bent DNA. Proc Natl Acad Sci USA 90:6320–6324.
30. Boyer PL, Tantillo C, Jacobo-Molina A, et al. (1993) Structural and biochemical analysis shows nucleoside analog resistance of HIV-1 RT variants involves alterations in template: primer positioning. Third Workshop on Viral Resistance, Gaithersburg, Maryland.

31. Richman DD and the ACTG 164/168 Study Team (1993) Nevirapine resistance during clinical trials. Second International HIV-1 Drug Resistance Workshop. Noordwijk, the Netherlands.
32. Saag MS, Emini EA, Laskin OL, et al. (1993) A short-term clinical evaluation of L-697,661, a non-nucleoside inhibitor of HIV-1 reverse transcriptase. N Engl J Med 329:1065–1072.
33. Richman D, Shih CK, Lowy I, et al. (1991) Human immunodeficiency virus type 1 mutants resistant to nonucleoside inhibitors of reverse transcriptase arise in tissue culture. Proc Natl Acad Sci USA 88:11241–11244.
34. Wei X, Ghosh SK, Taylor ME, Johnson VA, Emini EA, Deutsh P, Lifson JD, Bonhoeffer S, Nowak MA, Hahn BH, Saag MS, Shaw GM (1995) Viral dynamics in HIV-1 infection. Nature 373:117.
35. Havlir D, Eastman S, Richman DD (1995) HIV-1 kinetics: Rates of production and clearance of viral populations in asymptomatic patients treated with nevirapine. Abstract 229. Second National Conference: Human Retroviruses and Related Infections.
36. Strair RK, Medina DJ, Nelson CJ, Graubert T, Mellors JW (1993) Recombinant retrviral systems for the analysis of drug-resistant HIV. Nucleic Acids Res 21:4836–4842.
37. Loveday C, Kaye S, Tenant-Flowers M, Semple M, Ayliffe U, Weller IVD, Tedder RS (1995) HIV-1 RNA serum-load and resistant viral genotypes during early zidovudine therapy. Lancet 345:820–824.
38. Dudley MN (1995) Clinical pharmacokinetics of nuclleoside antiretroviral agents. J Infect Dis 171(Suppl 2):S99–S112.
39. Stretcher BN, Pesce AJ, Frame PT, Stein DS (1994) Pharmacokinetics of zidovudine phosphorylation in peripheral blood mononuclear cells from patients infected with human immunodeficiency virus. Antimicrob Agents Chemother 38:1541–1547.
40. Spira AI, Ho DD (1995) Effect of different donor cells on human immunodeficiency virus replication and selection in vitro. J Virol 69:422.
41. Zhang H, Bagasra O, Niikura M, Poiesz BJ, Pomerantz RJ (1994) Intravirion reverse transcripts in the peripheral blood plasma on human immunodeficiency virus type 1-infected individuals. J Virol 68:7591.
42. Hostetler KY, Richman DD, Carson DA, et al. (1992) Greatly enhanced inhibition of human immunodeficiency virus type 1 replication in CEM and HT4-6C cells by 3'-deoxythymidine diphosphate dimyristoylglycerol, a lipid prodrug of 3'-deoxythymidine. Antimicrob Agents Chemother 36:2025–2029.
43. Balzarini J, Cooney DA, Dalal M (1987) 2',3'-Dideoxycytidine: Regulation of its metabolism and antiretroviral potency by natural pyrimidine nucleosides and by inhibitors of pyrimidine nuclleotide synthesis. Mol Pharmacol 32:798.
44. Furman PH, Fyfe JA, St. Clair MH, et al. (1986) Phosphorylation of 3'-azido-3'-deoxythymidine and selective interaction of the 5'-triphosphate with human immunodeficiency virus reverse transcriptase. Proc Natl Acad Sci USA 83:8333–8337.
45. Gao W-Y, Shirasaka T, Johns DG, Broder S, Mitsuya H (1993) Differential phosphorylation of azidothymidine, dideoxycytidine and dideoxyinosine in resting and activated peripheral blood mononuclear cells. J Clin Invest 91:2326–2333.
46. Johnson MA, Ahluwalia G, Connelly MC (1988) Metabolic pathways for the activation of the antiretroviral agent 2,',3'-dideoxyadenosine in human lymphoid cells. J Biol Chem 263:15354.
47. Richman DD, Kornbluth RS, Carson DA (1987) Failure of dideoxynucleosides to inhibit human immunodeficiency virus replication in cultured human macrophages. J Exp Med 166:1144.
48. Perno CF, Yarchoan R, Cooney DA, et al. (1988) Inhibition of human immunodeficiency virus replication in fresh and cultured human peripheral blood monocytes/macrophages by azidothymidine and related 2',3'-dideoxynucleosides. J Exp Med 168:1111.
49. Skalski V, Chang CN, Dutschman GE, Liu SH, Cheng YC (1993) Identification of a human cytosolic exonuclease: Implication in multidrug resistance. Third Workshop on Viral Resistance, Gaithersburg, Maryland.
50. Mukherji E, Au JLS, Mathes LE (1994) Differential antiviral activities and intracellulalr metabolism of 3'-azido-3'-deoxythymidine and 2',3'-dideoxyinosine in human cells. Antimicrob Agents Chemother 38:1573–1579.
51. Dianzani F, Antonelli G, Torriziani O, Riva E, Simeoni E, Sagnoretti C, Stroselle S, Cianfriglia M (1994) Zidovudine induces the expression of cellular resistance affecting its antiviral activity. AIDS Res Hum Retroviruses 10:1471.
52. Agarwal RP, Mian AM (1991) Thymidine and zidovudine metabolism in chronically zidovudine-exposed cells in vitro. Biochem Pharmacol 42:905–911.
53. Riva E, Turriziani O, Simeoni E, Di Marco P, Bellarosa D, Romagnoli G, Cianfriglia M, Antonelli

G, Dianzani F (1994) Cellular resistance induced by in vitro AZT-treatment of CEM cells. Int Conf AIDS 10:104 (abstract no. PA0297).

54. Wu S, Liu X, Solorzano MM, Kwock R, Avramis VI (1995) Development of Zidovudine resistance in Jurkat T cells is associated with decreased expression of the thymidine kinase gene and hypermethylation of the 5′ end of the human TK gene. J AIDS Human Retroviruses 8:1.

55. Nyce J, Leonard S, Canupp D, Schulz S, Wong S (1993) Epigenetic mechanisms of drug resistance: Drug induced DNA hypermethylation and drug resistance. Proc Natl Acad Sci USA 90:2960–2964.

56. Avramis VI, Kwock R, Solorzano MM, Gomperts E (1993) Evidence of in vitro development of drug resistance to azidothymidine in T-lymphocytic leukemia cell lines and in pediatric patients with HIV-1 infection. J Acqu Immune Defic Syndr 6:1287–1293.

57. Zack JA, Haislip AM, Krogstad P, Chen IS (1992) Incompletely reverse-transcribed human immunodeficiency virus type 1 genomes in quiescent cells can function as intermediates in the retroviral life cycle. J Virol 66:1717–1725.

58. Bukrinsky MI, Stanwick TL, Dempsey MP, Stevenson M (1992) Quiescent T lymphocytes as an inducible virus reservoir in HIV-1 infection. Science 254:423–427.

59. Hao Z, Cooney DA, Hartman NR, Perno CF, Fridland A, DeVico AL, et al. (1988) Factors determining the activity of 2′,3′-dideoxynucleotides in suppressing HIV in vitro. Mol Pharmacol 34:431.

60. Tornevik Y, Jacobsson B, Britton S, Eriksson S (1991) Intracellular metabolism of 3′-azidothymidine in isolalted human peripheral blood mononuclear cells. AIDS Res Hum Retroviruses 7:751–759.

61. Medina DJ, Tung PP, Lerner-Tung MB, Nelson CJ, Mellors JW, Strair RK (1995) Sanctuary growth of HIV in the presence of 3′-azido-3′-deoxythymidine. J Virol 69:1606–1611.

62. Lacey SF, Reardon JE, Furfine ES, et al. (1992) Biochemical studies on the reverse transcriptase and RNase H activities from human immunodeficiency virus strains resistant to 3′-azido-3′-deoxythymidine. J Biol Chem 267:15789–15794.

63. Antonelli G, Turriziano O, Cianfriglia M, Riva E, Dong G, Fattorossi A, Dianzani F (1992) Resistance of HIV-1 to AZT might also involve the cellular expression of multidrug resistance P-glycoprotein. AIDS Res Hum Retroviruses 8:1839–1844.

V. TOPOISOMERASES

10. CELLULAR RESISTANCE TO TOPOISOMERASE POISONS

ERIC H. RUBIN, TSAI-KUN LI, PU DUANN, AND LEROY F. LIU

It is now known that several antimicrobial and antitumor drugs destroy cells by interacting with cellular DNA topoisomerases. These enzymes are ubiquitous in nature and are required for the regulation of DNA structure (topology) in the cell. Specifically, DNA topoisomerases regulate the coiling of the DNA double helix, a parameter critical for processes such as replication and transcription. Topoisomerases alter DNA coiling by transiently cleaving DNA. They have been defined mechanistically as type I if they nick a single strand of the DNA double helix and type II if they cleave both strands. The discovery of antitumor drugs that specifically target topoisomerases has not only led to an improved understanding of tumor cell biology but has also fostered the rapid development of new anticancer drugs. This chapter reviews the anticancer drugs that target topoisomerases and focuses on cellular mechanisms of resistance to these drugs.

TOPOISOMERASE CATALYSIS

A type I topoisomerase, topo I, and two type II topoisomerase isozymes, topo IIα and β, have been found in mammalian cells [1–4]. Topo I is a 100 kDa protein, and topo IIα and β are 170 and 180 kDa, respectively. The two topo II isozymes are coded by genes on separate chromosomes and appear to have different cellular functions. For example, levels of topo IIα increase following growth stimulation and appear to peak during the S/G_2 phases of the cell cycle [4]. In contrast, topo IIβ levels appear to increase during growth cessation [4]. Topo IIα and IIβ are also distinguishable in terms of enzyme processivity and in reactivity with certain drugs

243

[4]. Moreover, topo IIβ but not topo IIα is localized exclusively in the nucleolus [5].

The catalytic cycle for both the type 1 and 2 enzymes involves the sequential steps of DNA binding, DNA cleavage, and DNA religation (Figure 10–1) [6,7]. Both enzymes appear to prefer bent or supercoiled DNA as substrates, and both cleave DNA by the formation of a covalent bond between a tyrosine residue and a phosphoryl group in the DNA backbone. Moreover, this DNA–topo reaction intermediate (often referred to as the *cleavable complex*) may be isolated using either enzyme with protein denaturants. However, topo II enzymes cleave both strands of DNA and function as homodimers, whereas topo I nicks one strand only and acts as a monomer. Topo II isozymes also require binding and hydrolysis of ATP for activity, whereas topo I does not. In addition, the topo II enzymes form a covalent link with the 5'-ends of the cleaved DNA, whereas topo I links with the 3'-end.

Importantly, the ability of topo II isozymes to cleave both strands of DNA allows these enzymes, but not topo I, to solve certain DNA topology problems. Most notable among these is the problem of interlinked DNA rings following replication of circular DNA. Separation of these rings, or *decatenation*, requires cleavage of both DNA strands [8]. Linear DNA organized into chromosomes likely presents a similar topological problem following replication. The unique ability of topo II to resolve this problem is consistent with the finding that yeast lacking topo II are unable to undergo mitosis [9]. In contrast, yeast do not require topo I for cell cycle progression, and cells devoid of this enzyme are nearly normal, suggesting that either topo I is not essential or that topo II may perform the functions of topo I in these cells [10,11]. This apparent capacity for substitution may not hold true for all eukaryotes, since topo I is required in *Drosophila* development [12]. Currently, it is uncertain whether topo I is required for mammalian cell viability.

CYTOTOXICITY OF TOPOISOMERASE POISONS

It is now clear that several naturally occurring and synthetic cytotoxic compounds interact specifically with DNA topoisomerases. Topoisomerase-linked DNA strand breaks can be detected shortly after cellular exposure to these drugs. This effect is believed to result from inhibition of the religation step of the topoisomerase catalytic cycle, leading to accumulation of the cleaved DNA–enzyme intermediate [13–20]. Some of the topo drugs appear to accomplish this effect by binding DNA, which may result in misalignment of the two ends of the cleaved DNA in the topo–DNA complex [21,22]. This misalignment may prevent the enzyme from religating the two strands. However, other drugs, such as camptothecin, do not bind DNA alone, and the method by which these drugs intefere with the topo catalytic cycle is unclear. A possible explanation is that these drugs are in fact capable of binding DNA, but only in the presence of the topo–DNA complex.

In the case of drugs that interact with topo I, yeast strains lacking topo I have been used to demonstrate clearly that topo I is necessary for the cytotoxic effects of these drugs [23]. This experiment cannot be done with topo II, since deletion of this gene in yeast is lethal. However, studies with yeast strains containing temperature-

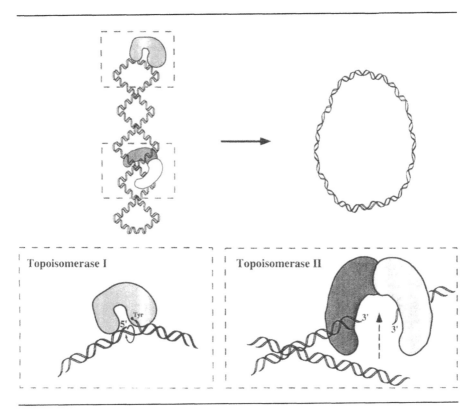

Figure 10–1. Catalytic cycle of topoisomerase I and II. Both enzymes are capable of relaxing a supercoiled DNA substrate (upper part of the figure). The mechanism of each enzyme is shown in greater detail in the lower part of the figure.

sensitive topo II alleles suggest that topo II is required for the lethal effects of drugs that interact with this enzyme [24]. For both topo I and topo II drugs, cytotoxicity is believed to result from drug-induced accumulation of the cleavable complex intermediate. Thus, these drugs are most appropriately referred to as *topoisomerase poisons*, since their effects are enhanced in the presence of greater amounts of enzyme [25]. In constrast, drugs that inhibit topoisomerase activity without stabilizing the cleavable complex have been referred to as *inhibitors*. Since topoisomerase II appears to be required for cell viability, topo II inhibitors are expected to be cytotoxic. In contrast, since it is unclear whether topo I is required for mammalian cell viability, it is uncertain whether inhibition of this enzyme will lead to cell death.

All of the drugs in current clinical use that interact with topoisomerases are poisons. The events following drug-stabilized topo I or topo II DNA cleavage that result in cell death are not completely understood. It appears that stabilization of the cleavable complex intermediate is necessary but not sufficient for cell death induced by topoisomerase poisons [26]. Current models suggest that collisions between cleavable complexes and certain DNA enzymes, such as DNA and/or RNA poly-

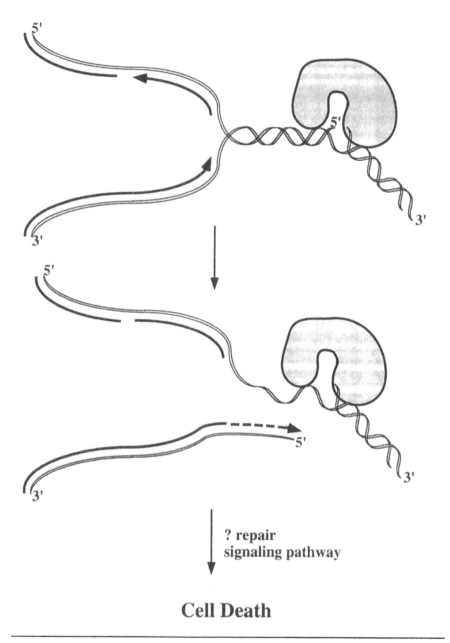

Figure 10–2. Model of collison between drug-stabilized topo I cleavable complexes and DNA replication forks.

merases, lead to irreversible double-strand breaks in DNA that are important to the cytotoxicity of these agents [27–29] (Figure 10–2). Additional parameters, such as the status of cellular DNA repair pathways, p53, and other proteins involved in apoptosis, also appear to be important in determining the toxicity of topoisomerase poisons [30,31].

This model of cytotoxicity mediated by topoisomerase poisons can be used to predict potential mechanisms of cellular resistance to these drugs (Table 10–1). Specific mechanisms that have been shown to occur in resistant cells are discussed in detail in the remainder of this chapter.

RESISTANCE TO DRUGS THAT TARGET TOPOISOMERASE II

Several antineoplastic compounds are now known to interfere with the topo II catalytic cycle by stabilizing the cleavable complex reaction intermediate. This effect does not appear to be lethal to the cell in itself, but may be converted to a lethal event by interactions between the stabilized cleavable complex and the replication or transcriptional machinery. Although the topo II poisons include drugs with different chemical structures, they may be grouped according to whether or not they are capable of inserting between adjacent base pairs of duplex DNA (intercalating). Examples of intercalating drugs include the anthracyclines, the aminoacridines (amsacrine), the anthracenediones (mitoxantrone), the ellipticines, and the actinomycins (Figure 10–3). Examples of non-intercalating topo II poisons include the podophyllotoxin derivatives etoposide and teniposide (Figure 10–3). Topo II poisons may also be classified depending upon whether or not ATP stimulates drug-induced DNA cleavage by the enzyme. Topo II poisoning by the drugs listed earlier is ATP dependent, whereas poisoning by amonafide, batracyclin, and menadione is ATP independent (Figure 10–3). Since ATP is believed to alter the conformation of topo II [32], whether drug-induced cleavage is affected by ATP likely reflects the preference of the drug for interacting with a particular conformation of topo II [33]. Nevertheless, regardless of drug structure, all of these agents appear to affect topo II by blocking the religation step of the catalytic cycle [33,34].

Several cell lines have been selected for resistance to the ATP-dependent topo II poisons [35–56; for review see 57]. Characterization of the resistant cells indicate that one or more of the following phenomena are involved: (1) removal of the drug from the cell, (2) downregulation or cellular redistribution of topo II, or (3) mutation of topo II. The prototypic example of drug removal involves P-glycoprotein, which may be overexpressed in drug-resistant cells [58]. This 170-kDa transmembrane protein appears to bind to and efflux from the cell structurally diverse

Table 10–1. Possible cellular mechanisms of resistance to topoisomerase poisons

1. Decreased intracellular drug levels
2. Decreased cellular topoisomerase content
3. Drug interaction with the topoisomerase–DNA complex is impaired
4. Lethal effects of drug-induced topoisomerase-mediated DNA cleavage are abrogated

A. Intercalators

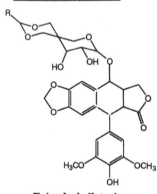

Anthracyclines

Doxorubicin	$R_1 = CH_2OH$ $R_2 = OCH_3$
Daunorubicin	$R_1 = CH_3$ $R_2 = OCH_3$
Idarubicin	$R_1 = CH_3$ $R_2 = H$

Amsacrine

Mitoxantrone

Ellipticine

Actinomycin D

B. Non-intercalators

Epipodophyllotoxins

Etoposide R =CH₃

Teniposide R =

C. Non-ATP-dependent

Amonafide

Batracyclin

Menadione

Figure 10–3. Topoisomerase II poisons.

hydrophobic compounds (see Chapter 1). Since many drugs derived from natural products are substrates for this protein, it is not surprising that most of the topo II poisons, which are derived from naturally occurring sources, are affected by P-glycoprotein. Moreover, other proteins with similar function, such as the multidrug resistance-associated protein (MRP), have been implicated in cellular resistance to topo II poisons (see Chapter 2) [53].

Since topo II is required for cell survival, large decreases in topo II protein content or catalytic activity would not be expected as a mechanism of resistance to topo II poisons. Nevertheless, cell lines resistant to topo II poisons have been shown to express severalfold lower levels of nuclear [41,44,50] or total cellular [54,55] topo II protein relative to wild-type cells. The decrease in topo II protein expression may involve topo IIα, topo IIβ, or both [3,56,59]. The mechanisms by which topo II is reduced in these cells may involve genomic rearrangements leading to loss of allelic expression [60]. In addition, nuclear topo II content may be decreased by mutations affecting nuclear localization sequences that are present in the carboxyl region of the protein [52]. This type of mutation may allow topo II to function normally during mitosis because of the breakdown of the nuclear envelope during this phase of the cell cycle [52].

Downregulation of topo II protein may also be accompanied by a compensatory increase in catalytic activity. For example, despite a 10-fold decrease in enzyme content, the topo II catalytic activity of nuclear extracts from etoposide-resistant cells was found to be similar to that of wild-type cells [44]. This finding may relate to increased phosphorylation of topo II in the resistant cells, since phosphorylation is known to augment enzyme activity [61,62]. Post-translational modifications in topo II have also been postulated to affect interactions with topo II poisons. For example, in vitro studies have shown that phosphorylation of topo II by either casein kinase II or protein kinase C modestly decreases the formation of drug-stabilized cleavable complex [63].

Mutations in topo IIα that confer enzymatic drug resistance have been found in several vertebrate cell lines selected for resistance to a variety of topo II poisons (Figure 10–4). These mutations cluster in two conserved regions of the topo IIα gene: One is located near the consensus ATP-binding region and includes a dinucleotide binding motif [47,64–66]. Studies using yeast indicate that some mutations in this region may confer a dominant form of cellular drug resistance, perhaps as a result of heterodimer formation between wild-type and mutant proteins [67]. The other region that commonly contains mutations in drug-resistant cell lines is near the active site tyrosine residue (amino acid 805) [68,69]. In addition, a third region involved in drug resistance has recently been identified in the carboxyl terminus of the yeast topo II protein [70]. In most cases, enzymes containing mutations in these regions exhibit either crossresistance or collateral sensitivity to other topo II poisons, suggesting that these regions comprise a common domain involved in the interaction with topo II poisons.

This non–P-glycoprotein–mediated crossresistance to other drugs has been described as *atypical multidrug resistance* [71]. Taken together, these studies suggest that

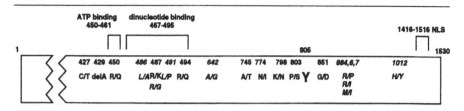

Figure 10–4. Drug-resistant human and yeast topoisomerase II mutations. Mutations are denoted by plain text if they were identified in human cells and by italics if they were identified in yeast. Other known strutural features of the enzyme are also indicated, including the position of the active-site tyrosine.

certain sequences that are discontinuous in the topo II amino acid sequence may be contiguous in the three-dimensional structure of topo II and form a drug binding site [72]. Alternatively, some or all of these mutations may not represent a true drug binding site, but may affect topo II catalytic activity and steady-state enzyme–DNA cleavable complex formation so that in the presence of any drug there is a decrease in the amount of drug–enzyme–DNA ternary complex [73]. Proof of these conjectures awaits a detailed structural analysis of eukaryotic topo II.

The hypothesis that mutations conferring drug resistance to topo II poisons alter topo II catalysis is supported by the finding that many of these mutations occur in highly conserved regions of the protein. Indeed, certain mutations near the active site tyrosine that confer drug resistance have been shown to alter the temperature dependence of the enzyme [68]. Mutations near the region containing the ATP-binding motif have also been shown to affect topo II catalytic activity. For example, a glutamine for arginine mutation at amino acid 450 has been suggested to decrease enzyme affinity for ATP [65]. Moreover, studies with yeast topo II indicate that mutations in this region that confer drug resistance can also affect the plasmid relaxation activity of the enzyme [73]. Regarding the mutation described in the carboxyl region of topo II, purified enzyme containing this mutation has been shown to exhibit impaired noncovalent DNA binding [70].

An additional mutation in topo IIα has been described that appears to involve a unique resistance mechanism. Cleavable complex formation by crude cell extracts in the presence of etoposide was found to be greatly reduced in a human melanoma cell line resistant to this drug [51,74]. However, when nuclear extracts were analyzed, the topo II activity from the resistant cell line was found to exhibit wild-type activity and sensitivity to etoposide. Sequencing of topo IIα cDNAs from the resistant cells indicated that a single mRNA was expressed and contained an alteration resulting in deletion of an alanine at position 429. The mechanism by which this deletion confers cellular but not enzymatic resistance is unknown, although it may involve alterations in topo II nuclear location or in interactions between this enzyme and other proteins.

It should be emphasized that the relative importance of topo IIα and IIβ in the cytotoxicity of topo II poisons is unclear. Since both enzymes may be affected by these drugs [4], both may serve as cellular targets, and thus alterations in both may be required for resistance. Indeed, resistant cell lines containing alterations in both topo IIα and IIβ have been described [56,59]. However, a recent analysis of six leukemic cell lines found a direct correlation between topo IIβ protein content and sensitivity to daunorubicin, suggesting that topo IIβ may be particularly important in mediating the cytotoxic effects of this drug [75]. Notably, mutations conferring drug resistance in topo IIβ have not been reported.

RESISTANCE TO DRUGS THAT TARGET TOPOISOMERASE I

It has only recently been appreciated that topo I is also a target for several naturally occurring and synthetic compounds [20,25]. Similar to topo II, there are structurally diverse compounds that are capable of poisoning topo I in an apparently similar fashion (Figure 10–5). Some of these compounds are known to interact with the DNA minor groove, and thus share a general capacity for DNA binding with the intercalating topo II poisons [76,77]. Indeed, certain DNA-binding compounds, such as intoplicine, saintopin, and actinomycin D, are capable of poisoning both topo I and II [78–80].

Camptothecin is the best known topo I poison, and this drug and its derivatives are the only such compounds in clinical use. Camptothecin was isolated from the Chinese tree *Camptotheca acuminata* and underwent clinical testing prior to its identification as a topo I poison [81–83]. Currently, the derivatives topotecan, CPT-11, 9-aminocamptothecin, and 9-nitrocamptothecin have been synthesized and are being evaluated in clinical trials [84].

Camptothecin specifically interacts with topo I, leading to enzyme-linked DNA single-strand breaks [17,20]. Since this drug is predominantly cytotoxic for cells in S phase, a model of collision of the DNA replication machinery with camptothecin-stabilized DNA breaks has been proposed as a mechanism whereby lethal double-strand breaks are generated (Figure 10–2) [27,29]. More recent studies suggest that similar interactions may occur between these breaks and the transcriptional machinery [Wu and Liu, unpublished observations]. This finding may explain the toxic effects of camptothecin that have been observed outside of the S phase of the cell cycle [85].

At this time, camptothecin is the only topo I poison for which cellular resistance mechanisms have been reported. Resistance to camptothecin has been generated by continuous exposure of cells to drug or by treatment with a mutagenizing agent followed by selection in the presence of the drug. Similar to studies with topo II poisons, resistance appears to result from one or more of the following events: (1) removal of the drug from the cancer cell, (2) decrease in topo I protein, or (3) mutation of topo I.

Unlike resistance to topo II poisons, P-glycoprotein has not been found to be important in the cellular resistance to most camptothecins [86]. Despite the fact that many camptothecin derivatives are hydrophobic, these compounds are apparently not good substrates for P-glycoprotein. However, in studies using cell lines that overexpress P-glycoprotein, a differential response to certain camptothecin deriva-

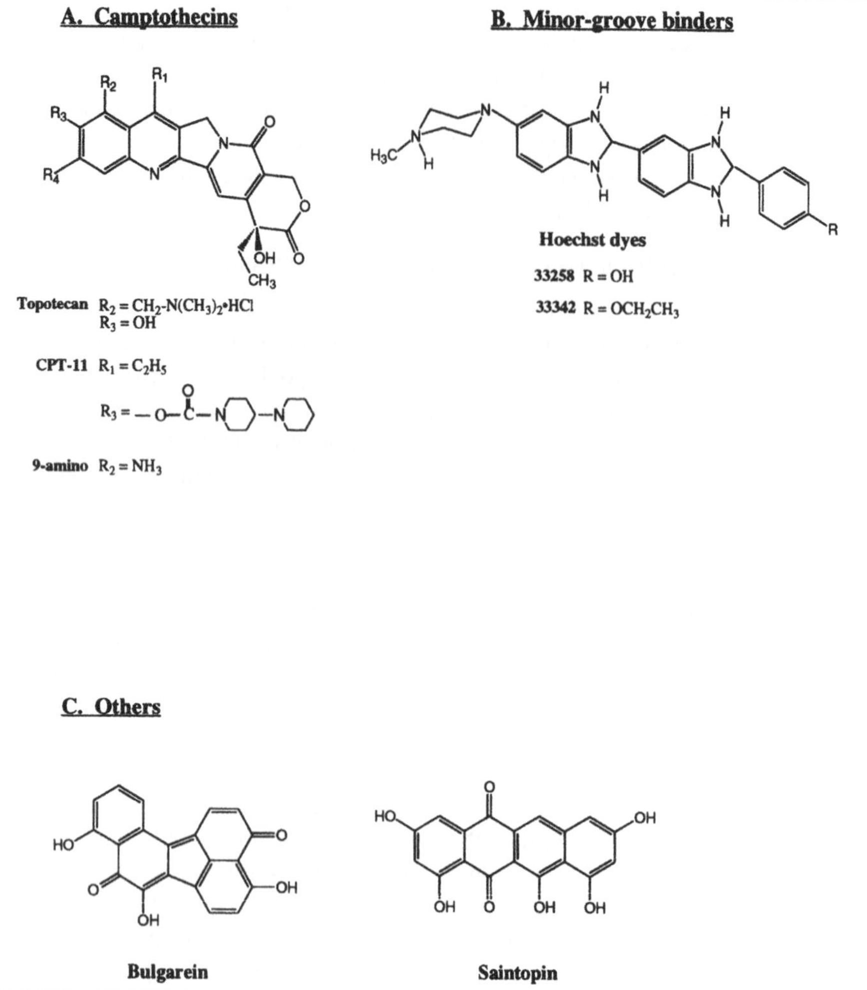

A. Camptothecins

Topotecan $R_2 = CH_2\text{-}N(CH_3)_2 \cdot HCl$
            $R_3 = OH$

CPT-11 $R_1 = C_2H_5$

9-amino $R_2 = NH_3$

B. Minor-groove binders

Hoechst dyes

33258 R = OH

33342 R = OCH_2CH_3

C. Others

Bulgarein

Saintopin

Figure 10–5. Topoisomerase I poisons.

tives has been reported. Charged derivatives such as topotecan were found to be less cytotoxic to these cells than neutral camptothecin derivatives, suggesting that topotecan may be affected by P-glycoprotein [87,88]. Similarly, xenografts resistant to drugs commonly affected by P-glycoprotein exhibit crossresistance to topotecan but not to CPT-11 [89]. However, it should be emphasized that the relative effect of P-glycoprotein on topotecan is small compared with its effect on topo II poisons, and it is unlikely that P-glycoprotein is important in clinical resistance to camptothecins [88].

Several mammalian cell lines resistant to camptothecin exhibit decreased levels of topo I [90–97]. In some cases, this appears to result from alterations in the topo I

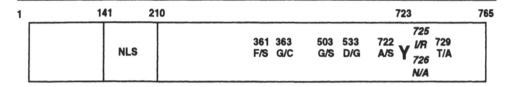

Figure 10–6. Drug-resistant human and yeast topoisomerase I mutations. Mutations are denoted by plain text if they were identified in human cells and by italics if they were identified in yeast. Other known strutural features of the enzyme are also indicated, including the position of the active-site tyrosine.

genome, leading to loss of allelic expression [60,92]. Hypermethylation of topo I genes has also been implicated as a mechanism of transcriptional silencing in camptothecin-resistant cell lines [60,92]. Other mechanisms by which topo I levels or activity may be downregulated involve post-transcriptional events. Recent work suggests that in the presence of camptothecin, cellular protein levels of topo I diminish rapidly [98]. This phenomenon may involve degradation of topo I, perhaps involving the ubiquitin pathway [D'Arpa, unpublished observations]. Since rapid decreases in topo I have been observed in peripheral blood mononuclear cells obtained from patients treated with camptothecins [99], this mechanism may be important in determining the clinical effects of these drugs.

The topo I protein may also be modified by poly(ADP-ribosyl)ation [100] or phosphorylation [101–106]. These effects have been shown to alter the sensitivity of topo I to camptothecin in in vitro assays, and thus may represent additional mechanisms of cellular resistance. However, neither of these post-translational modifications have been directly linked to cellular drug resistance.

Certain cell lines resistant to camptothecin have been found to harbor mutations in topo I that confer resistance to the drug [107–111]. The mutations cluster in three highly conserved regions of the protein (Figure 10–6). One region is near tyrosine 723, which is the residue that is covalently linked to DNA in the cleavable complex intermediate. As expected, mutations in this region have been found to impair the catalytic activity of the enzyme [108,111]. Another site encompasses amino acids 500–530. This region also appears to be important in topo I catalytic activity, since mutations in this region alter the ability of the enzyme to relax supercoiled DNA [109,112].

The G503S mutation exhibits a decrease in plasmid relaxation activity [109], whereas the D533G mutation exhibits increased activity with an apparent enhancement of the religation function of the enzyme [112]. Although the mechanism by which the D533G mutation produces this effect is unclear, this mutation may alter the topo I-DNA interaction so that camptothecin can no longer enter the complex. The third site involved in drug resistance involves the 361–363 region of topo I. Certain mutations in this area appear to confer drug resistance without significantly affecting plasmid relaxation activity [110,113]. This may be accomplished by a subtle change in the manner in which the enzyme interacts with DNA, resulting in loss of the association with camptothecin but preservation of catalytic activity. Indeed, studies with bacterially expressed enzymes indicate that mutations in this region can affect DNA cleavage by the enzyme [114]. Further work is necessary to define the role of the regions near 533 and 361 in the topo I catalytic cycle, and the mechanisms by which mutations in these regions confer resistance to camptothecin.

Notably, there have been no reports of a complete lack of topo I in CPT-resistant vertebrate cells. If topo I were dispensable for cell survival (as it is in yeast), one might expect to observe loss or mutagenic inactivation of the topo I protein in some resistant cell lines. The fact that such cell lines have not been found suggests that topo I is required for survival in higher eukaryotic cells. Indeed, as is discussed later, topo II activity is often increased in CPT-resistant cells with decreased topo I activity, perhaps to compensate for the loss of topo I activity.

CROSSRESISTANCE AND COLLATERAL SENSITIVITY TO TOPOISOMERASE POISONS

Collateral alterations in topo I or II have been found in several cell lines selected for resistance to a variety of DNA-damaging agents. Among the best characterized alterations is a reciprocal change in one enzyme in cell lines selected for resistance to a poison of the other enzyme. For example, cell lines selected for resistance to camptothecin often demonstrate collateral sensitivity to topo II poisons and increases in topo II enzyme activity or content [90,92,94,95,110,115,116]. Similarly, reciprocal changes in topo I activity have been observed in studies of cell lines resistant to topo II poisons [49,60,117]. Although the cellular mechanisms underlying these phenomenona are unknown, these findings suggest that sequential exposure to topo poisons may be used as a strategy for combination therapy. Indeed, this conjecture has been supported by the finding that sequential exposure of colon carcinoma cells to camptothecin and etoposide leads to additive cytotoxicity [118]. Importantly, the timing of drug administration is critical, since coadministration may produce antagonistic effects [119]. This finding may be explained by the fact that the cytotoxicity of both topo I and II poisons appears to require replication and/or transcription. Thus, inhibition of these processes by one drug may interfere with the effects of the other.

Studies of cell lines resistant to drugs not known to poison topoisomerases, such as alkylating agents, have yielded the interesting observation that these cells may contain alterations in topoisomerases. Cells resistant to nitrogen mustard have been shown to exhibit enhanced sensitivity to topo II poisons, associated with an increase in topo II enzyme activity [120]. Similar findings have been reported in a cell line resistant to melphalan, in which collateral sensitivity to topo II poisons was exhibited coincident with an increase in topo II protein levels [121]. This same cell line was found to be crossresistant to topotecan and to have diminished levels of topo I protein. A cisplatinum-resistant cell line has also been found to exhibit crossresistance to a camptothecin derivative [122]. In contrast, other cell lines resistant to cisplatinum exhibit collateral sensitivity to camptothecin [123,124]. In one case, this phenomenon was related to an increase in topo I mRNA and protein [124]. Taken together, these findings suggest that topoisomerases may be involved in the development of cellular resistance or sensitivity to diverse anticancer agents. Since topoisomerases appear to be required for most processes involving DNA, it is possible that the DNA damage produced by many anticancer drugs may depend in part on topoisomerase activity for either conversion to lethality or repair.

In summary, although topo poisons are becoming increasingly important in cancer chemotherapy, it appears that cancer cells possess multiple mechanisms that may allow them to survive exposure to these drugs. Studies of these mechanisms have not only provided insight into the biology of topoisomerases but have also suggested potential strategies to overcome resistance. For the most effective clinical use of topoisomerase poisons, cellular resistance mechanisms must continue to be studied and the results translated to the clinic.

REFERENCES

1. Liu LF, Liu C, Alberts BM (1980) Type II DNA topoisomerases: Enzymes that can unknot a topologically knotted DNA molecule via a reversible double-strand break. Cell 19:697–707.
2. Liu LF, Miller KG (1981) Eukaryotic DNA topoisomerases: Two forms of type I DNA topoisomerases from HeLa cell nuclei. Proc Natl Acad Sci USA 78:3487–3491.
3. Drake FH, Zimmerman JP, McCabe FL, Bartus HF, Per SR, Sullivan DM, Ross WE, Mattern MR, Johnson RK, Crooke ST, Mirabelli CK (1987) Purification of topoisomerase II from amsacrine-resistant P388 leukemia cells. J Biol Chem 262:16739–16747.
4. Drake FH, Hofman GA, Bartus HF, Mattern MR, Crooke ST, Mirabelli CK (1989) Biochemical and pharmacological properties of p170 and p180 forms of topoisomerase II. Biochemistry 28:8154–8160.
5. Negri C, Scovassi AI, Braghetti A, Guano F, Astaldi Ricotti GCB (1993) DNA topoisomerase IIβ: Stability and distribution in different animal cells in comparison to DNA topoisomerase I and IIα. Exp Cell Res 206:128–133.
6. Champoux JJ (1994) Mechanism of catalysis by eukaryotic DNA topoisomerase I. In LF Liu, ed. DNA Topoisomerases: Biochemistry and Molecular Biology. San Diego, CA: Academic Press, pp 71–79.
7. Anderson AH (1994) The DNA binding, cleavage, and religation reactions of eukaryotic topoisomerases I and II. In LF Liu, ed. DNA Topoisomerases: Biochemistry and Molecular Biology. San Diego, CA: Academic Press, pp 83–97.
8. Wang JC (1985) DNA topoisomerases. Annu Rev biochem 54:665–697.
9. DiNardo S, Voelkel K, Sternglanz R (1984) DNA topoisomerase II mutant of *Saccharomyces cerevisiae*: Topoisomerase II is required for segregation of daughter molecules at the termination of DNA replication. Proc Natl Acad Sci USA 81:2616–2620.
10. Uemura T, Yanagida M (1984) Isolation of type I and II DNA topoisomerase mutants from fission yeast: Single and double mutants show different phenotypes in cell growth and chromatin organization. EMBO J 3:1737–1744.
11. Christman MF, Dietrich FS, Fink CR (1988) Mitotic recombination in the rDNA of S. cerevisiae is suppressed by the combined action of DNA topoisomerase I and II. Cell 55:413–425.
12. Lee M, Brown S, Chen A, Hsieh T (1993) DNA topoisomerase I is essential in *Drosophila melanogaster*. Proc Natl Acad Sci USA 90:6656–6660.
13. Ross WE, Glaubiger DL, Kohn KW (1978) Protein-associated DNA breaks in cells treated with Adriamycin or ellipticine. Biochem Biophys Acta 519:23–30.
14. Liu LF, Rowe TC, Yang L, Tewey KM, Chen GL (1984) Cleavage of DNA by mammalian DNA topoisomerase II. J Biol Chem 258:15365–15370.
15. Ross WE, Rowe T, Glisson B, Yalowich J, Liu LF (1984) Role of topoisomerase II in mediating epipodophyllotoxin-mediated DNA cleavage. Cancer Res 44:5857–5800.
16. Tewey KM, Chen GL, Nelson EM, Liu LF (1984) Intercalative antitumor drugs interfere with the breakage-reunion reaction of mammalian DNA topoisomerase II. J Biol Chem 259:9182–9187.

17. Hsiang Y, Hertzberg R, Hecht S, Liu LF (1985) Camptothecin induces protein-linked DNA breaks via mammalian DNA topoisomerase I. J Biol Chem 260:14873–14878.
18. Rowe TC, Chen GL, Hsiang Y, Liu LF (1986) DNA damage by antitumor acridines mediated by mammalian DNA topoisomerase II. Cancer Res 46:2021–2026.
19. Mattern MR, Mong S, Bartus HF, Mirabelli CK, Crooke ST, Johnson RK (1987) Relationship between the intracellular effects of camptothecin and the inhibition of DNA topoisomerase I in cultured L1210 cells. Cancer Res 47:1793–1798.
20. Hsiang Y, Liu L (1988) Identification of mammalian DNA topoisomerase I as an intracellular target of the anticancer drug camptothecin. Cancer Res 48:1722–1726.
21. Liu LF (1990) Anticancer drugs that convert DNA topoisomerases into DNA damaging agents. In NR Cozzarelli, JC Wang, ed. DNA Topology and its Biological Effects. Cold Spring Harbor, NY: Cold Harbor Laboratory Press, pp 371–389.
22. D'Arpa P, Liu LF (1989) Topoisomerase-targeting antitumor drugs. Biochim Biophys Acta 989:163–177.
23. Bjornsti M, Benedetti P, Vigilanti G, Wang J (1989) Expression of human DNA topoisomerase I in yeast cells lacking yeast DNA topoisomerase I: Restoration of sensitivity of the cells to the antitumor drug camptothecin. Cancer Res 49:6318–6323.
24. Nitiss JL, Liu YX, Hsiung Y (1993) A temperature sensitive topoisomerase II allele confers temperature dependent drug resistance to amsacrine and etoposide: A genetic system for determining the targets of topoisomerase II inhibitors. Cancer Res 53:89–93.
25. Liu LF (1989) DNA topoisomerase poisons as antitumor drugs. Annu Rev Biochem 58:351–375.
26. D'Arpa P (1994) Determinants of sensitivity to topoisomerase-targeting antitumor drugs. In LF Liu, ed. DNA Topoisomerases: Topoisomerase-Targeting Drugs. San Diego, CA: Academic Press, pp 127–137.
27. Hsiang Y, Lihou M, Liu L (1989) Arrest of replication forks by drug-stabilized topoisomerase I-DNA cleavable complexes as a mechanism of cell killing by camptothecin. Cancer Res 49:5077–5082.
28. D'Arpa P, Beardmore C, Liu LF (1990) Involvement of nucleic acid synthesis in cell killing mechanisms of topoisomerase poisons. Cancer Res 50:6919–6924.
29. Tsao Y, Russo A, Nyamuswa G, Silber R, Liu LF (1993) Interaction between replication forks and topoisomerase I-DNA cleavable complexes: Studies in a cell-free SV40 DNA replication system. Cancer Res 53:5908–5914.
30. Squires S, Ryan AJ, Strutt HL, Johnson RT (1993) Hypersensitivity of Cockayne's syndrome cells to camptothecin is associated with the generation of abnormally high levels of double strand breaks in nascent DNA. Cancer Res 53:2012–2019.
31. Lowe S, Bodis S, McClatchey A, Remington L, Ruley HE, Fisher DE, Housman DE, Jacks T (1994) p53 status and the efficacy of cancer therapy in vivo. Science 266:807–810.
32. Roca J, Wang JC (1994) DNA transport by a type II DNA topoisomerase: Evidence in favor of a two-gate mechanism. Cell 77:609–616.
33. Chen AY, Liu LF (1994) DNA topoisomerases: Essential enzymes and lethal targets. Annu Rev Pharmacol Toxicol 34:191–218.
34. Osheroff N, Corbett AH, Robinson MJ (1994) Mechanism of action of topoisomerase II-targeted antineoplastic drugs. In LF Liu, ed. DNA Topoisomerases: Topoisomerase-Targeting Drugs. San Diego CA: Academic Press, pp 105–119.
35. Glisson B, Gupta R, Smallwood-Kentro S, Ross W (1986) Characterization of acquired epipodophyllotoxin resistance in a Chinese Hamster ovary cell line: Loss of drug-stimulated DNA cleavage activity. Cancer Res 46:1934–1938.
36. Danks MK, Yalowich JY, Beck WT (1987) Atypical multiple drug resistance in a human leukemic cell line selected for resistance to teniposide (VM-26). Cancer Res 47:1297–1301.
37. Charcosset JY, Saucier JM, Jacquemin-Sablon A (1988) Reduced DNA topoisomerase II cleavage activity and drug-stimulated DNA cleavage in 9-hydroxyellipticine resistant cells. Biochem Pharmacol 37:2145–2149.
38. Zjilstra JG, de Vries EGG, Mulder NH (1987) Multifactorial drug resistance in an Adriamycin-resistant human small cell lung carcinoma line. Cancer Res 47:1780–1784.
39. Per SR, Mattern MR, Mirabelli CK, Drake FH, Johnson RK, Crooke ST (1987) Characterization of a subline of p388 leukemia resistant to amsacrine: Evidence of altered topoisomerase II function. Mol Pharmacol 32:17–25.
40. Zwelling LA, Hinds M, Chan D, Mayes J, Sie KL, Parker E, Silberman L, Radcliff A, Beran M, Blick M (1989) Characterization of an amsacrine-resistant line of human leukemia cells. J Biol Chem 264:16411–16420.

41. Deffie AM, Batra JK, Goldenberg GJ (1989) Direct correlation between DNA topoisomerase II activity and cytotoxicity in adriamycin-sensitive and resistant P388 leukemia cell lines. Cancer Res 49:58–62.
42. Harker WG, Slade DL, Dalton WS, Meltzer PS, Trent JM (1989) Multidrug resistance in mitoxantrone-selected HL-60 leukemia cells in the absence of P-glycoprotein overexpression. Cancer Res 49:4542–4549.
43. Dietel M, Arps H, Lage H, Niendorf A (1990) Membrane vesicle formation due to acquired mitoxantrone resistance in human gastric carcinoma cell line EPG85-257. Cancer Res 50:6100–6106.
44. Takano H, Kohno K, Ono M, Uchida Y, Kuwano M (1991) Increased phosphorylation of DNA topoisomerase II in etoposide-resistant mutants of human cancer KB cells. Cancer Res 51:3951–3957.
45. Rappa G, Lorico A, Sartorelli AC (1992) Development and characterization of a WEHI-3B D⁺ monomyelocytic cell line resistant to novobiocin and cross-resistant to other topoisomerase II-targeted drugs. Cancer Res 52:2782–2790.
46. Cole SPC, Chanda ER, Dicke FP, Gerlach JH, Mirski SEL (1991) Non-P-glycoprotein-mediated multidrug resistance in a small cell lung cancer cell line: Evidence for decreased susceptibility to drug-induced DNA damage and reduced levels of topoisomerase II. Cancer Res 51:3345–3352.
47. Lee M, Wang JC, Beran M (1992) Two independent amsacrine-resistant human myeloid leukemia cell lines share an identical point mutation in the 170 kDa form of human topoisomerase II. J Mol Biol 223:837–843.
48. Patel S, Austin CA, Fisher LM (1990) Development and properties of an etoposide-resistant human leukaemic CCRF-CEM cell line. Anticancer Drug Des 5:149–157.
49. Lefevre D, Riou JF, Ahomadegbe JC, Zhou D, Bernard J, Riou G (1991) Study of molecular markers of resistance to m-AMSA in a human breast cancer cell line. Decrease of topoisomerase II and increase of both topoisomerase I and acidic glutathione S-transferase. Biochem Pharm 41:1967–1979.
50. Friche E, Danks MK, Schmidt CA, Beck WT (1991) Decreased DNA topoisomerase II in daunorubicin-resistant Ehrlich ascites tumor cells. Cancer Res 51:4213–4218.
51. Campain JA, Padmanabhan R, Hwang J, Gottesman MM, Pastan I (1993) Characterization of an unusual mutant of human melanoma cells resistant to anticancer drugs that inhibit topoisomerase II. J Cell Physiol 155:414–425.
52. Mirski SEL, Cole SPC (1995) Cytoplasmic localization of a mutant M, 160,000 topoisomerase IIα is associated with the loss of putative bipartite nuclear localization signals in a drug-resistant human lung cancer cell line. Cancer Res 55:2129–2134.
53. Grant CE, Valdimarsson G, Hipfner DR, Almquist KC, Cole SPC, Deeley RG (1994) Overexpression of multidrug resistance-associated protein (MRP) increases resistance to natural product drugs. Cancer Res 54:357–361.
54. Ferguson PJ, Fisher MH, Stephenson J, Li D, Zhou B, Cheng YC (1988) Combined modalities of resistance in etoposide-resistant human KB cell lines. Cancer Res 48:5956–5964.
55. de Jong S, Kooistra AJ, de Vries EGE, Mulder NH, Zijlstra JG (1993) Topoisomerase II as a target of VM-26 and 4′-(9-acridinylamino)methanesulfon-m-aniside in atypical multidrug resistant human small cell lung carcinoma cells. Cancer Res 53:1064–1071.
56. Chen M, Beck WT (1995) DNA topoisomerase II expression, stability, and phosphorylation in two VM-26-resistant human leukemic CEM sublines. Oncol Res 7:103–111.
57. Beck WT, Danks MK, Wolverton JS, Chen M, Granzen B, Kim R, Parker Suttle D (1994) Resistance of mammalian tumor cells to inhibitors of DNA topoisomerase II. In LF Liu, ed. DNA Topoisomerases: Topoisomerase-Targeting Drugs. San Diego, CA: Academic Press, pp 145–169.
58. Endicott JA, Ling V (1989) The biochemistry of P-glycoprotein-mediated multidrug resistance. Annu Rev Biochem 58:137.
59. Harker WG, Slade DL, Parr RL, Feldhoff PW, Sullivan DM, Holguin MH (1995) Alterations in the topoisomerase IIα gene, messenger RNA, and subcellular protein distribution as well as reduced expression of the DNA topoisomerase IIβ enzyme in a mitoxantrone-resistant HL-60 human leukemia cell line. Cancer Res 55:1707–1716.
60. Tan KB, Mattern MR, Eng W, McCabe FL, Johnson RK (1989) Nonproductive rearrangement of DNA topoisomerase I and II genes: Correlation with resistance to topoisomerase I inhibitors. J Natl Cancer Inst 81:1732–1735.
61. Ackerman P, Glover CVC, Osheroff N (1985) Phosphorylation of DNA topoisomerase II by casein kinase II: Modulation of eukaryotic topoisomerase II activity in vitro. Proc Natl Acad Sci USA 83:3164–3168.

62. Sahyoun N, Wolf M, Besterman J, Hsieh TS, Sander M, LeVine H, Chang KJ, Cuatrecasas P (1986) Protein kinase C phosphorylates topoisomerase II: Topoisomerase activation and its possible role in phorbol ester-induced differentiation of HL-60 cells. Proc Natl Acad Sci USA 83:1603–1607.

63. DeVore RF, Corbett AH, Osheroff N (1992) Phosphorylation of topoisomerase II by casein kinase II and protein kinase C: Effects on enzyme-mediated DNA cleavage/religation and sensitivity to the antineoplastic drugs etoposide and 4'-(9-acridinylamino)methane-sulfon-m-anisidide. Cancer Res 52:2156–2161.

64. Hinds M, Deisseroth K, Mayes J, Altschuler E, Jansen R, Ledley FD, Zwelling LA (1991) Identification of a point mutation in the topoisomerase II gene from a human leukemia cell line containing an amsacrine-resistant form of topoisomerase II. Cancer Res 51:4729–4731.

65. Bugg BY, Danks MK, Beck WT, Suttle DP (1991) Expression of a mutant DNA topoisomerase II in CCRF-CEM human leukemic cells selected for resistance to teniposide. Proc Natl Acad Sci USA 88:7654–7658.

66. Chan VTW, Ng S, Eder JP, Schnipper LE (1993) Molecular cloning and identification of a point mutation in the topoisomerase II cDNA from an etoposide-resistant Chinese hamster ovary cell line. J Biol Chem 268:2160–2165.

67. Nitiss JL, Vilalta PM, Wu H, McMahon J (1994) Mutations in the gyrB domain of eukaryotic topoisomerase II can lead to partially dominant resistance to etoposide and amsacrine. Mol Pharmacol 46:773–777.

68. Jannatipouri M, Liu Y, Nitiss JL (1993) The top2-5 mutant of yeast topoisomerase II encodes an enzyme resistant to etoposide and amsacrine. J Biol Chem 268:18586–18592.

69. Patel S, Fisher LM (1992) Novel selection and genetic characterisation of an etoposide-resistant human leukaemic CCRF-CEM cell line. Br J Cancer 67:456–463.

70. Elsea SH, Hsiung Y, Nitiss JL, Osheroff N (1995) A yeast type II topoisomerase selected for resistance to quinolones. J Biol Chem 270:1913–1920.

71. Beck WT, Cirtain MC, Danks MK, Felsted RL, Safa AR, Wolverton JS, Suttle DP, Trent JM (1987) Pharmacological, molecular, and cytogenetic analysis of "atypical" multidrug-resistant human leukemic cells. Cancer Res 47:5455–5460.

72. Huff AC, Kreuzer KN (1990) Evidence for a common mechanism of action for antitumor and antibacterial agents that inhibit type II DNA topoisomerases. J Biol Chem 265:20496–20505.

73. Wasserman RA, Wang JC (1994) Mechanistic studies of amsacrine-resistant derivatives of DNA topoisomerase II. J Biol Chem 269:20943–20951.

74. Campain JA, Gottesman MM, Pastan I (1994) A novel mutant topoisomerase IIα present in VP-16-resistant human melanoma cell lines has a deletion of alanine 429. Biochemistry 33:11327–11332.

75. Brown GA, McPherson JP, Gu L, Hedley DW, Toso R, Deuchars KL, Freeman MH, Goldenberg GJ (1995) Relationship of DNA polymerase IIa and b expression to cytotoxicity of antineoplastic agents in human acute lymphoblastic leukemia cell lines. Cancer Res 55:78–82.

76 Chen AY, Yu C, Bodley A, Peng LF, Liu LF (1993) A new mammalian DNA topoisomerase I poison Hoechst 33342: Cytotoxicity and drug resistance in human cell cultures. Cancer Res 53:1332–1337.

77. Chen AY, Yu C, Gatto B, Liu LF (1993) DNA minor groove-binding ligands: A different class of mammalian DNA topoisomerase I inhibitors. Proc Natl Acad Sci USA 90:8131–8135.

78. Trask DK, Muller MT (1988) Stabilization of type I topoisomerase-DNA covalent complexes by actinomycin D. Proc Natl Acad Sci USA 85:1417–1421.

79. Poddevin B, Riou J, Lavelle F, Pommier Y (1993) Dual topoisomerase I and II inhibition by intoplicine (RP-60475), a new antitumor agent in early clinical trials. Mol Pharmacol 44:767–774.

80. Leteurtre F, Fujimori A, Tanizawa A, Chabra A, Mazumder A, Kohlhagen G, Nakano H, Pommier Y (1994) Saintopin, a dual inhibitor of DNA topoisomerases I and II, as a probe for drug-enzyme interactions. J Biol Chem 28702–28707.

81. Gottlieb JA, Guarino AM, Call JB, Oliverio VT, Block JB (1970) Preliminary pharmacologic and clinical evaluation of camptothecin sodium (NSC-100880). Cancer Chemother Rep 54:461–470.

82. Gottlieb JA, Luce JK (1972) Treatment of malignant melanoma with camptothecin (NSC-100880). Cancer Chemother Rep 56:103–105.

83. Moertel CG, Schutt AJ, Reitemeier RJ, Hahn RG (1972) Phase II study of camptothecin (NSC-100880) in the treatment of advanced gastrointestinal cancer. Cancer Chemother Rep 56:95–101.

84. Slichenmeyer WJ, Rowinsky EK, Donehower RC, Kaufmann SH (1993) The current status of camptothecin analogues as antitumor agents. J Natl Cancer Inst 85:271–291.

85. Del-Bino GD, Lassota P, Darzynkiewicz Z (1991) The S-phase cytotoxicity of camptothecin. Exp Cell Res 193:27–35.
86. Tsuruo T, Matsuzaki T, Matsushita M, Saito H, Yokokura T (1988) Antitumor activity of CPT-11, a new derivative of camptothecin, against pleiotropic drug resistant tumors in vitro and in vivo. Cancer Chemother Pharmacol 21:71–74.
87. Chen AY, Yu C, Potmesil M, Wall ME, Wani MC, Liu LF (1991) Camptothecin overcomes MDR1-mediated resistance in human KB carcinoma cells. Cancer Res 51:6039–6044.
88. Hendricks CB, Rowinsky EK, Grochow LB, Donehower RC, Kaufmann SH (1992) Effect of P-glycoprotein expression on the accumulation and cytotoxicity of topotecan (SK&F 104864), a new camptothecin analogue. Cancer Res 52:2268–2278.
89. Houghton PJ, Cheshire PJ, Hallman JC, Bissery MC, Mathieu-Boue A, Houghton JA (1993) Therapeutic efficacy of the topoisomerase I inhibitor 7-ethyl-10-(4-[1-piperidino]-1-piperidino)-carbonyloxy-camptothecin against human tumor xenografts: Lack of cross-resistance in vivo in tumors with acquired resistance to the topoisomerase I inhibitor 9-dimethylaminomethyl-10-hydroxycamptothecin. Cancer Res 53:2823–2829.
90. Gupta RS, Gupta R, Eng B, Lock RB, Ross WE, Hertzberg RP, Caranfa MJ, Johnson RK (1988) Camptothecin-resistant mutants of Chinese hamster ovary cells containing a resistant form of topoisomerase I. Cancer Res 48:6404–6410.
91. Sugimoto Y, Tsukahara S, Oh-hara T, Isoe T, Tsuruo T (1990) Decreased expression of DNA topoisomerase I in camptothecin-resistant tumor cell lines as determined by a monoclonal antibody. Cancer Res 50:6925–6930.
92. Eng WK, McCabe FL, Tan KB, Mattern MR, Hofmann GA, Woessner RD, Hertzberg RP, Johnson RK (1990) Development of a stable camptothecin-resistant subline of P388 leukemia with reduced topoisomerase I content. Mol Pharmacol 38:471–480.
93. Kanzawa F, Sugimoto Y, Minato K, Kasahara K, Bungo M, Nakagawa K, Fujiwara Y, Liu LF, Saijo N (1990) Establishment of a camptothecin analogue (CPT-11)-resistant cell line of human non-small lung cancer: Characterization and mechanism of resistance. Cancer Res 50:5919–5924.
94. Woessner RD, Eng W, Hofmann GA, Rieman DJ, McCabe FL, Hertzberg RP, Mattern MR, Tan KB, Johnson RK (1992) Camptothecin hyper-resistant P388 cells: Drug-dependent reduction in topoisomerase I content. Oncol Res 4:481–488.
95. Chang J, Dethlefsen LA, Barley LR, Zhou B, Cheng Y (1992) Characterization of camptothecin-resistant Chinese hamster lung cells. Biochem Pharmacol 43:2443–2452.
96. Madelaine I, Prost S, Naudin A, Riou G, Lavelle F, Riou J (1993) Sequential modifications of topoisomerase I activity in a camptothecin-resistant cell line established by progressive adaptation. Biochem Pharmacol 45:339–348.
97. Kapoor R, Slade DL, Fujimori A, Pommier Y, Harker WG (1995) Altered topoisomerase I expression in two subclones of human CEM leukemia selected for resistance to camptothecin. Oncol Res 7:83–95.
98. Beidler DR, Cheng Y (1995) Camptothecin induction of a time and concentration-dependent decrease of topoisomerase I and its implication in camptothecin activity. Mol Pharmacol 47:907–914.
99. Rubin E, Wood V, Bharti A, Trites D, Lynch C, Hurwitz S, Bartel S, Levy S, Rosowsky A, Toppmeyer D, Kufe D (1995) A phase I and pharmacokinetic study of a new camptothecin derivative, 9-aminocamptothecin. Clin Cancer Res 1:269–276.
100. Ferro AM, Olivera BM (1984) Poly (ADP-ribosylation) of DNA topoisomerase I from calf thymus. J Biol Chem 259:547–554.
101. Durban E, Mills JS, Roll D, Busch H (1983) Phosphorylation of purified Novikoff hepatoma topoisomerase I. Biochem Biophys Res Commun 111:897–905.
102. Tse-Dinh Y, Wong T, Goldberg AR (1984) Virus- and cell-encoded tyrosine protein kinases inactivate DNA topoisomerases in vitro. Nature 312:785–786.
103. Durban E, Goodenough M, Mills J, Busch H (1985) Topoisomerase I phosphorylation in vitro and in rapidly growing Novikoff hepatoma cells. EMBO J 4:2921–2926.
104. Pommier Y, Kerrigan D, Hartman KD, Glazer RI (1990) Phosphorylation of mammalian DNA topoisomerase I and activiation by protein kinase C. J Biol Chem 265:9418–9422.
105. Samuels DS, Shimizu N (1992) DNA topoisomerase I phosphorylation in murine fibroblasts treated with 12-o-tetradecanoylphorbol-13-acetate and in vitro by protein kinase C. J Biol Chem 267:11156–11162.
106. Cardellini E, Durban E (1993) Phosphorylation of human topoisomerase I by protein kinase C in

vitro and in phorbol 12-myristate 13-acetate-activated HL-60 promyelocytic leukaemia cells. Biochem J 291:303–307.

107. Tamura H, Kohchi C, Yamada R, Ikeda T, Koiwai O, Patterson E, Keene J, Okada K, Nishikawa K, Andoh T (1990) Molecular cloning of a cDNA of a camptothecin-resistant human DNA topoisomerase I and identification of mutation sites. Nucleic Acids Res 19:69–75.

108. Kubota N, Kanzawa F, Nishio K, Takeda Y, Ohmori T, Fujiwara Y, Terashima Y, Saijo N (1992) Detection of topoisomerase I gene point mutation in CPT-11 resistant lung cancer cell line. Biochem Biophys Res Commun 188:571–577.

109. Tanizawa A, Bertrand R, Kohlhagen G, Tabuchi A, Jenkins J, Pommier Y (1993) Cloning of Chinese hamster DNA topoisomerase I cDNA and identification of a single point mutation responsible for camptothecin resistance. J Biol Chem 268:25463–25468.

110. Rubin E, Pantazis P, Bharti A, Toppmeyer D, Giovanella B, Kufe D (1994) Identification of a mutant human topoisomerase I with intact catalytic activity and resistance to 9-nitro-camptothecin. J Biol Chem 269:2433–2439.

111. Fujimori A, Harker WG, Kohlhagen G, Hoki Y, Pommier Y (1995) Mutation of the catalytic site of topoisomerase I in CEM/C2, a human leukemia cell line resistant to camptothecin. Cancer Res 55:1339–1346.

112. Gromova II, Kjeldsen E, Svestrup JQ, Alsner J, Christiansen K, Westergaard O (1993) Characterization of an altered DNA catalysis of a camptothecin-resistant eukaryotic topoisomerase I. Nucleic Acids Res 21:593–600.

113. Benedetti P, Fiorani P, Capuani L, Wang JC (1993) Camptothecin resistance from a single mutation changing glycine 363 of human DNA topoisomerase I to cysteine. Cancer Res 53:4343–4348.

114. Rubin E, Hsiang Y, Bharti A, Kufe D (1995) Involvement of amino acids near position 361 in the human topoisomerase I catalytic cycle and in resistance to camptothecin. Proc Assoc Cancer Res 36:abst2692.

115. Sugimoto Y, Tsukahara S, Oh-hara T, Liu LF, Tsuruo T (1990) Elevated expression of DNA topoisomerase II in camptothecin-resistant human tumor cell lines. Cancer Res 50:7962–7965.

116. Tanizawa A, Pommier Y (1992) Topoisomerase I alteration in a camptothecin-resistant cell line derived from Chinese hamster DC3F cells in culture. Cancer Res 52:1848–1854.

117. Riou J, Grondard L, Petitgenet O, Abitbol M, Lavelle F (1993) Altered topoisomerase I activity and recombination activating gene expression in a human leukemia cell line resistant to doxorubicin. Biochem Pharmacol 46:851–861.

118. Bertrand R, O'Connor PM, Kerrigan D, Pommier Y (1992) Sequential administration of camptothecin and etoposide circumvents the antagonistic cytotoxicity of simultaneous drug administration in slowly growing human colon carcinoma HT-29 cells. Eur J Cancer 28A:743–748.

119. Kaufmann SH (1991) Antagonism between camptothecin and topoisomerae II-directed chemotherapeutic agents in a human leukemia cell line. Cancer Res 51:1129–1136.

120. Tan KB, Mattern MR, Boyce RA, Schein PS (1987) Elevated DNA topoisomerase II activity in nitrogen mustard resistant human cells. Proc Natl Acad Sci USA 84:7668–7671.

121. Friedman HS, Dolan ME, Kaufmann SH, Colvin OM, Griffith OW, Moschel RC, Schold SC, Bigner DD, Ali-Osman F (1994) Elevated DNA polymerase a, DNA polymerase b, and DNA topoisomerase II in a melphalan-resistant rhabdomyosarcoma xenograft that is cross-resistant to nitrosoureas and topotecan. Cancer Res 54:3487–3493.

122. Niimi S, Nakagawa K, Sugimoto Y, Nishio K, Fujiwara Y, Yokoyama S, Terashima Y, Saijo N (1992) Mechanism of cross-resistance to a camptothecin analogue (CPT-11) in a human ovarian cancer cell line selected by cisplatin. Cancer Res 52:328–333.

123. Boscia R, Korbut T, Holden S, Ara G, Teicher B (1993) Interaction of topoisomerase I inhibitors with radiation in cis-diamminedichloroplatinum (II)-sensitive and -resistant cells in vitro and in the FSAIIC fibrosarcoma in vivo. Int J Cancer 53:118–123.

124. Kotoh S, Naito S, Yokomizo A, Kumazawa J, Asakuno K, Kohno K, Kuwano M (1994) Increased expression of DNA topoisomerase I gene and collateral sensitivity to camptothecin in human cisplatin-resistant bladder cancer cells. Cancer Res 54:3248–3252.

VI. RESISTANCE TO ENDOCRINE THERAPIES

11. ACQUISITION OF AN ANTIESTROGEN-RESISTANT PHENOTYPE IN BREAST CANCER: ROLE OF CELLULAR AND MOLECULAR MECHANISMS

ROBERT CLARKE, TODD SKAAR, FABIO LEONESSA, BRENDA BRANKIN, MATTIE JAMES, NILS BRÜNNER, AND MARC E. LIPPMAN

It is estimated that almost 11% of all women living to age 80 will develop breast cancer [1]. The annual worldwide incidence of breast cancer is estimated to be one million by the year 2000 [1]. The factors responsible for the genesis of breast cancer remain unclear, but estrogens have been strongly implicated [2]. Estrogens may function as carcinogens and/or cocarcinogens [2,3], but it is their role as promoters of the growth of estrogen-dependent and estrogen-responsive tumors through activation of their nuclear receptors [2] that has provided a rationale for the design of therapeutic strategies, that is, antiestrogens.

Ablative endocrine therapies for breast cancer, for example, ovariectomy, have been in widespread use since Beatson first reported remissions in premenopausal breast cancer in 1896 [4]. However, these approaches have largely been replaced by additive therapies, for example, antiestrogens (putative competitive inhibitors of estrogens), aromatase inhibitors (inhibitors of estrogen biosynthesis), and luteinizing hormore–releasing hormore (LHRH) agonists/antagonists (inhibitors of gonadotropin secretion and lowering serum estrogen levels). The antiestrogens are among the most widely administered of these compounds, particularly the triphenylethylene Tamoxifen (TAM).

The original triphenylethylene and related compounds were originally formulated as fertility drugs. MER-25 (ethamoxytriphetol) was one of the earliest of the nonsteroidal antiestrogen to receive attention. It was produced in 1954 and subsequently was shown to possess activity in patients with breast cancer [5], but toxicity prevented its further development. The utility of a related triphenylethylene (clomiphene) [6] also was demonstrated, establishing a potential role for anti-estrogenic compunds in breast cancer. However, it was not until the introduction of TAM (ICI 46474) that the nature of endocrine manipulation as a treatment for breast cancer significantly changed.

It has been 25 years since the first report of the clinical efficacy of the triphenylethylene antiestrogen TAM by Cole et al. in 1971 [7]. In the 17 years between 1971 and 1988, it has been estimated that the total exposure to TAM was greater than 1.5 million patient years [8]. Currently, this exposure is likely to approximate 8 million. Despite the considerable experience with TAM, its precise mechanism(s) of action, and the mechanisms that confer resistance remain largely unknown.

Major advantages of endocrine therapies, and antiestrogenic treatments in particular, include their low toxicity relative to cytotoxic chemotherapy, the ability to identify potential responders based on the expression of steroid hormone receptors, and the additional beneficial effects on osteoporosis, cardiovascular tissues, and several other symptoms associated with menopause. Response rates among patients with receptor-positive tumors is high [9,10], and there is clear evidence of increases in disease-free and overall survival following antiestrogen therapy, for example, in patients with early-stage disease [11,12]. An ability to prevent or overcome antiestrogen resistance could have significant implications for the management of patients with breast cancer.

MULTIPLE RESISTANCE PHENOTYPE IN BREAST CANCER

Despite being an initially responsive disease [13], most drug-responsive breast tumors, either spontaneously or following the selective pressure of systemic therapies, acquire a phenotype of multiple metastatic lesions that are resistant to all endocrine and cytotoxic therapies [14–17]. It is the development of a multiple resistance phenotype in patients with metastatic disease that is primarily responsible for the failure of current breast cancer therapies.

The mechanisms that confer a multiple resistance phenotype are unclear but are likely to involve multiple molecular mechanisms. For cytotoxic drugs, the gp170 product of the MDR1 (multidrug resistance) gene [18], the multidrug resistance associated protein (MRP) [19], and the altered expression of detoxification (e.g., superoxide dismultases, glutathione transferases) [20,21], stress (e.g., heat shock proteins) [22], and other genes (e.g., topoisomerases) [23] likely contribute. The mechanisms that confer resistance to endocrine therapies are less well understood and may be equally diverse. However, it seems likely that a multiple hormone resistance phenotype (MHR) exists, analogous in some ways to the multidrug resistance phenotype.

The precise contribution of each potential resistance mechanism is unclear, and it is likely that more than one resistance mechanism, for example, loss of steroid hormone receptor expression conferring a MHR component, or overexpression of gp170 conferring a multiple cytotoxic drug resistance component, can operate either within the same tumor cell subpopulation and/or within different subpopulations of the same tumor. Thus, treating a multiple resistance phenotype comprised of both endocrine resistance and cytotoxic drug resistance components may ultimately require the development of novel therapies targetting several resistance mechanisms. A better understanding of how cells become resistant and how this resistance can be prevented, delayed, or overcome are preprequisites for the development of such strategies.

ANTIESTROGENS: MECHANISMS OF ACTION, PARTIAL AGONISTS, PURE ANTAGONISTS, AND SPECIES AND TISSUE SPECIFICITY

The most important function of antiestrogens is likely to be their competitive antagonism of estrogen binding to ER. This has been widely reported and reviewed [24,25]. However, other mechanisms that operate essentially independently of ER-mediated events may also contribute (Table 11–1). These include the ability of TAM to inhibit the activity of the intracellular signal transduction molecules protein kinase C [26] and calmodulin [27], changes in membrane structure/function [28], de novo production of estrogens [29], and endocrine perturbations [30]. The extent to which each or all of these contribute to the diverse effects of antiestrogens in clinical situations largely remains to be established. We discuss each of these in more detail in terms of their potential contribution to resistance in later sections.

The biological activities of antiestrogens, particularly the nonsteroidal antiestrogens, are marked by significant differences in both species-specific and tissue-specific responses. For example, TAM is clearly a partial agonist, producing both estrogenic and antiestrogenic effects. MCF-7 breast cancer cells elicit a mitogenic

Table 11–1. Suggested mechanisms of resistance to antiestrogens

Systemic/local effects	Increased serum estrogens	Alterations in the gonadal/pituitary axis Increased de novo synthesis in peripheral tissues or the tumor
	Altered immune competence	Loss of TAM induction of NK activity
	Production of estrogenic metabolites	Altered hepatic (or tumor cell metabolism)
Biochemical pharmacology	Altered transport	Reduced intratumor levels
	Reduced bioavailability	Elevation of antiestrogen binding site levels
	Mutations in ER	Constitutively active, non–ligand binding mutants
	Reduced expression of inhibited/inhibitory targets	Loss of a requirement for ER, or selection for ER-negative cells
	Increased expression of inhibited/inhibitory targets	Protein kinase C; calmodulin
Growth factors	Reduced secretion or sensitivity to inhibitory factors	TGFβ/TGFβ-receptor autocrine loop
	Increased secretion or sensitivity to mitogenic factors	TGFα/EGF-receptor autocrine loop

ER = estrogen receptor; TGF = transforming growth factor; TAM = tamoxifen; NK = natural killer.

response when treated with low doses of TAM in the absence of physiological concentrations of estrogen [31]. At higher concentrations, or in the presence of estrogens, these cells are growth inhibited [31]. This in vitro dose–response profile may mimic that seen in those patients who initially exhibit tumor flare [32,33], which is frequently followed by a beneficial clinical response [32]. Steady-state levels of TAM in patient sera are not reached for up to 4 weeks [34,35], and the initially low levels may be mitogenic. Once the elevated levels at steady state are reached, the antagonist properties of TAM could predominate, accounting for the subsequent remissions.

TAM produces an estrogenic stimulation of both rat [36] and human vaginal epithelium [37]. The ability to induce significant agonist effects in some tissues, when administered at doses that inhibit breast tumors, may contribute to the most serious side effect attributed to TAM, induction of endometrial adenocarcinomas. Several studies on the long-term administration of TAM have reported an increased incidence of endometrial cancer [38]. These observations have lead to concerns regarding the use of TAM as a chemopreventive agent for women at high risk of breast cancer.

There is marked species specificity for responses to TAM [39–41]. In mice, TAM is an agonist in essentially all tissues that are capable of responding, for example, TAM produces a threefold increase in uterine weight [42]. In rats, the effects of TAM are tissue specific, with TAM failing to stimulate uterine epithelial proliferation and to inhibit proliferation induced by E2 [36]. Estrogenic effects are observed in vaginal tissues [36], while the growth of mammary tumors is inhibited.

The laboratories that initially developed TAM have recently produced a new series of steroidal antiestrogens. These compounds, which are C7-acyl–substituted analogues of 17β-estradiol, appear to be substantially different from the triphenylethylenes, and potentially represent a major development for the management of endocrine-responsive breast cancer. Two analogues have received considerable attention: ICI 182,780, which already has begun clinical trials in Europe (ICI 182,780), and its predecessor, ICI 164,384. These compounds have a higher affinity for estrogen receptors (ER) than TAM and are devoid of significant agonist activities in most of the models studied to date [43,44]. However, it is unlikely that long-term use of these compunds will produce the beneficial effects on osteoporosis and coronary heart disease associated with the partial agonist properties of TAM and the other triphenylethylenes.

With such diverse possible mechanisms of antiestrogenic action, particularly for TAM and the other triphenylethylene antiestrogens, it is likely that a single mechanism of action will inadequately account for all biological responses. Even in the growth regulation of breast cancer, it seems most likely that several mechanisms will operate, each with its own dose–response relationship/K_i. Thus, the overall inhibition of proliferation will reflect the effects of multiple overlapping mechanisms.

HORMONE INDEPENDENCE AND ANTIESTROGEN RESISTANCE

The growth of several human breast cancer cell lines in vivo and in vitro is dependent upon estrogenic stimulation. We have previously suggested that these cells represent an early phenotype (hormone dependent) in the malignant progression of human breast cancer, and have hypothesized that hormone-dependent cells can progress to a phenotype in which hormones are no longer a requisite for growth (hormone independent) [14,15]. To address this hypothesis and to assess the potential relationship between hormone independence and antiestrogen responsiveness, we selected hormone-dependent cells for growth in vivo in the mammary fat pads of ovariectomized athymic nude mice [45]. These mice have serum steroid levels similar to those found in postmenopausal women [46,47]. Following one in vivo selection, we obtained the MCF7/MIII population [45], and a further selection of these cells produced the MCF7/LCC1 population [48]. These cells do not require estrogens for proliferation either in vivo or in vitro. However, growth in vivo but not in vitro can be further stimulated by estrogen supplementation [45,48].

We studied the hormone-independent populations for their sensitivity to drugs representative of several of the major classes of antiestrogens, for example, the steroidal antiestrogens ICI 164,384 and ICI 182,780 [31,49], the triphenylethylene 4-hydroxytamoxifen [31,48,50], the benzothiophene LY 117,018, and another non-steroidal compound, nafoxidine [31]. All drugs produce a similar dose-dependent inhibition of the anchorage-independent growth of parental (MCF-7) and hormone-independent cells (MCF7/MIII; MCF7/LCC1) that is either fully or partially reversed by estrogen. Since fully estrogen-dependent cells would rarely arise and survive in a postmenopausal woman, the intermediate hormone-independent and hormone-responsive phenotype exhibited by the MCF7/MIII and MCF7/LCC1 cells may be among the predominant endocrine-responsive phenotypes in breast cancer patients. These data clearly suggest that an acquired independence from estrogens for proliferation can arise independently of an acquired antiestrogen resistance.

PHARMACOLOGY OF ANTIESTROGENS AND RESISTANCE

Triphenylethylenes including TAM are extensively metabolized in the liver, and several of these differ markedly from the parental drug in their affinity for ER and agonist/antagonist properties. The major metabolite is N-desmethylTAM, the plasma levels of which frequently exceed those of TAM [34]. This metabolite is comparable with TAM with respect to its biological activity. The primary amine results from further demethylation, with subsequent deamination yielding the primary alcohol [51]. Hydroxylation produces 4-hydroxy TAM, another major metabolite, and the less important 3,4-dihydroxyTAM. The 4-hydroxy metabolite has a higher potency and affinity for ER and has been widely studied [52,53]. TAM and N-desmethylTAM constitute the major species in both plasma and tissues in humans [34]. The metabolic profile is different in other species. For example, TAM is hydroxylated more readily in the mouse [54]. Interspecies differences in triphenylethylene metabolism should be adequately considered in the design of animal studies.

An increased metabolism of TAM to agonistic metabolites has been implicated as a potential resistance mechanism [55,56]. Estrogenic metabolites could compete with the major antiestrogenic metabolites and produce an apparent "TAM-stimulated" phenotype. This phenotype has been observed in several human tumor xenograft models of breast cancer [57,58] and in cells transfected with the ER gene [59] or a fibroblast growth factor (kFGF) [60]. However, studies with non-isomerizable TAM analogues that cannot be metabolized to the major estrogenic metabolites still produce a TAM stimulation [61]. These data suggest that estrogenic TAM metabolites are unlikely to be responsible for this phenotype.

While TAM metabolism does not appear to be a major resistance mechanism, withdrawal responses to TAM have been documented, providing indirect clinical evidence for a "TAM-stimulated" phenotype. The frequency with which these occur is unclear. Most reports are single case studies or small studies [62–64]. This phenomenon is quite different from tumor flare, in which continuation of TAM treatment can induce clinical responses [32]. The frequency and relevance of TAM withdrawal responses awaits the outcome of clinical studies designed to better characterize this response pattern.

One common drug resistance mechanism is an altered ability of cells to accumulate drug, generally produced by perturbations in the function/expression of a membrane transporter. This can produce an altered rate or capacity for influx, for example, reduced activity of the folate transporter reduces methotrexate accumulation [65]; the gp170 product of the MDR1 gene effluxes *Vinca* alkaloids, anthracyclines, and several other classes of drugs [66]. The precise mechanism through which steroidal and triphenylethylene compounds enter cells is unknown, although it seems most likely that simple diffusion through the plasma membrane predominates.

Despite the apparent lack of a membrane transporter there is some evidence to suggest that resistant breast tumors exhibit reduced cellular accumulation. Lower intratumor TAM concentrations in patients with acquired resistance have been reported [56,67], despite their being no difference in serum levels [67]. We and others have demonstrated that TAM can reverse the effects of the gp170 multidrug resistance transporter [68,69], suggesting that TAM may be a substrate. There also is limited clinical evidence suggesting an association between gp170 expression and clinical resistance to TAM [70]. However, TAM is not effluxed by gp170 (Figure 11–1), and overexpression of gp170 does not confer resistance to TAM [71]. Thus, the precise mechanism for any altered TAM accumulation in breast tumors remains unknown.

ENDOCRINOLOGY OF ANTIESTROGENS AND RESISTANCE

The ovarian–pituitary axis is an important endocrinologic target for antiestrogens. In premenopausal women, the release of estrogen and progesterone is under the regulation of the gonadotropins luteinizing hormone (LH) and follicle stimulating hormone (FSH). The secretion of gonadotropins from the anterior pituitary is regulated both by steroids (negative feedback) and by the gonadotropin releasing hormone secreted from the hypothalamus. The release of gonadotropin releasing hormone also is inhibited by steroids. Antiestrogens can potentially interfere with the estrogenic regulation of both gonadotropin releasing hormone and the gonadot-

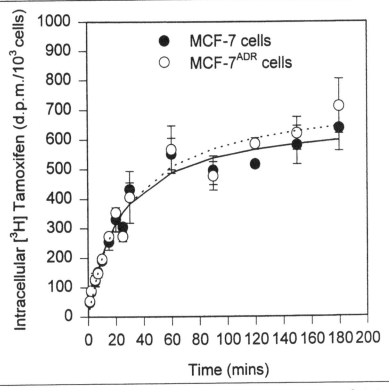

Figure 11–1. Accumulation of [³H]TAM in the gp170-expressing MCF-7ADR cells (O, broken line) and their parental MCF-7 cells (●, solid line) [71]. The curves were obtained by fitting y = Bmax (T/T + K$_{in}$) to the data points, such that Bmax = maximum intracellular ligand concentration, T = time, and K$_{in}$ = time required to achieve 50% total intracellular drug accumulation [68].

ropins. This may explain the relatively poor response rate to TAM, particularly in premenopausal women. TAM produces an increase in serum estrogen levels in the presence of normal to slightly elevated gonadotropin levels [30]. Increased sex steroid levels can also occur in postmenopausal women [72], in whom there is an apparent triphenylethylene-induced increase in dehydroepiandrosterone, estradiol, and estrone. These are probably derived from an elevated production of adrenal androgens that are subseqeuntly metabolized to estrogens. The presence of elevated circulating levels of estrogens could compete with antiestrogens for binding to ER. This would produce an "apparent resistance," since the cells could retain mechanistic sensitivity to antiestrogens but would fail to regress. Aromatase inhibitors and LHRH antagonists would prevent/reverse this form of resistance by inhibiting estrogen biosynthesis and release.

It has been suggested that another form of antiestrogen resistance could arise from the local production of an excess of estrogenic metabolites [29]. There are at least two enzymes that are critical in this process. The P450 aromatase enzyme can aromatize the A-ring of specific androgens to produce estrogens. In postmenopausal women this activity is greatest in peripheral adipose tissues, with some breast tumor cells also expressing significant aromatase activity [73]. The primary estrogen produced in postmenopausal women is estrone, with the biologically inactive sulfate metabolite, as generated by the sulfotransferase enzyme, being the predominant estrogen in serum. The biologically active estrogens are produced by the release of the sulfate group, a reaction driven by the sulfatase enzyme. Many breast tumors express significant sulfatase activity [74]. Alone or together, the aromatase and sulfatase enzymes could produce sufficient intratumor levels of estrogens to effectively compete with available antiestrogenic compounds. This would produce an "apparent resistance" similar to that resulting from elevated serum estrogen levels. Such tumors may be sensitive to aromatase and/or sulfatase inhibitors alone or in combination with antiestrogens.

It is difficult to assess the frequency with which this form of resistance may arise. There is evidence that the addition of aminoglutethimide (aromatase inhibitor) and danazol (sulfatase inhibitor) to TAM can increase the response rate relative to TAM alone [75]. However, the duration of response is less than that produced by TAM alone, implying that resistance is more rapidly acquired with a combination regimen [75]. The mechanism for an accelerated acquisition of resistance in these combination regimens remains to be determined.

ESTROGEN AND PROGESTERONE RECEPTORS IN ANTIESTROGEN RESPONSE AND RESISTANCE

In contrast to the cytotoxic therapies available for breast cancer, it is possible to identify those patients with a high probability of obtaining a response to antiestrogen treatment. Approximately 30% of all breast tumors will respond to antiestrogens. However, if both the ER and prostaglandin receptor (PGR) proteins are expressed in tumors not exposed to other endocrine therapies, the response rate rises to >60% in postmenopausal women [9,10,76]. A response to a prior endocrine manipulation [77,78] also indicates a likely further response to an antiestrogen. Age and menopausal status are important indicators of response, since women over 50 years demonstrate responses more frequently than younger women [8]. Antiestrogens have been relatively disappointing in premenopausal women, in whom other endocrine manipulations, for example, LHRH analogues, generate more frequent and/or better responses.

The marked intratumor heterogeneity of steroid hormone receptor expression [79,80] suggests that most tumors already contain resistant cells, an observation predicted by the Goldie–Coldman hypothesis [81]. Thus, one mechanism of resistance could be a selection by antiestrogens for the ER-negative subpopulations [25]. There is some evidence in support of this hypothesis [82,83]. However, many patients who respond and subseqeuntly fail on TAM do so while still expressing both ER and PGR [83]. This phenotype is minicked in the TAM-resistant MCF7/LCC2 model, which was generated by selection against 4-hydroxytamoxifen and retains ER and PGR expression [50]. Approximately one third of ER/PGR-positive patients are already resistant and fail to respond to TAM. These observations suggest that a significant proportion of tumors retain ER/PGR expression but the functionality of these receptor systems is, in some way, impaired. A more reliable marker for a functional ER system than PGR expression may better identify those ER/PGR-positive tumors that are resistant and facilitate an early detection of resistance. Currently, no such marker(s) exist.

Since the ER is the primary target for antiestrogens, alterations in its expression, ligand binding characteristics, and/or function could influence responsivity to antiestrogens. There have been several reports of mutations in the ER gene in breast cancer. However, it has been more difficult to determine the likely functional significance, at least from a clinical perspective, than it has been to identify such mutant receptors. Almost without exception, when mutant receptors are found they are coexpressed with significant levels of wild-type receptor [84]. Thus, dominant negative mutants are more likely to have biological function. Such mutants could function either by binding wild-type receptor and squelching/preventing transcriptional activation, even when bound to DNA, or be transcriptionally inactive and compete with wild-type receptor for DNA binding.

There are some clear examples of ER mutants that exhibit these properties: a truncated ER that comprises exons 1 and 2, and an unrelated sequence homologous to the transposable element LINE 1 [84–86]. Higher levels of this variant relative to the wild-type ER are found in tumors predicated to exhibit a relatively poor prognosis [86]. Wang and Miksicek [87] have identified an exon 3 deletion mutant in T47D cells. The ERδE3 mutant functions as a dominant negative, inhibiting wild-type receptor function. Similarly, Fuqua et al. [88] have described a truncated ER that lacks exon 7, is transcriptionally inactive, and can prevent wild-type ER from binding to an estrogen response element (ERE). This mutant is abundant in some ER+/PGR− breast tumors, and could at least partly account for the lack of PGR expression in the presence of ER. In contrast, an exon 5 deletion mutant has been described that is transcriptionally active in the absence of ligand [89]. Koehorst et al. [90] have identified an alternatively spliced exon 4 deletion mutant in MCF-7 cells and meningiomas, but this variant appears silent, since it neither binds E2 nor to an ERE. A $Val_{400} \rightarrow Gly_{400}$ point mutation can switch the ER function from antagonist to agonist when occupied with 4-hydroxytamoxifen [91]. This phenotype could explain the acquired TAM-stimulated phenotype observed in some human xenograft models [57,58], and also could account for clinical TAM withdrawal responses.

The presence of ER mutant proteins in human breast tumors and their function in in-vitro transcription analyses is insufficient to clearly determine their function in vivo. However, the presence of dominant receptors does establish the principle that such molecules could have significant clinical relevance. The ability of such variants to essentially sequester wild-type receptors could induce resistance to antiestrogens by depriving them of their functionally active molecular targets. The ability of mutant ER to switch perception of antiestrogens from antagonist to agonist, while not producing resistance per se, would produce a clinical response pattern requiring cessation of treatment.

ROLE OF NON-ESTROGEN RECEPTOR-MEDIATED EVENTS IN RESISTANCE

Triphenylethylene compounds have been shown to interact with several proteins other than ER. These include the potential signal transduction molecules calmodulin and protein kinase C (PKC), and a binding site that appears to provide some specificity for triphenylethylenes. The precise role of these molecules remains largely unproven, although some or all could contribute to antiestrogen responsiveness and resistance.

The calcium binding protein calmodulin has been implicated in some signal transduction pathways that can influence the intracellular activities of calcium. Calmodulin is involved in cyclic nucleotide metabolism, and a recent report has described the ability of cAMP to potentially stimulate ER-mediated transcription in vitro [92]. Intracellular calmodulin levels are higher in ER-positive tumors [93], and these also are more sensitive than ER-negative tumors to the inhibitory effects of antiestrogens. However, the apparent in vivo tissue concentrations of TAM do not appear to approach the IC_{50} for the inhibition of Ca^{2+} uptake and enzyme function ($\sim 9\,\mu M$) [94]. Until there is clear evidence that tissue levels of TAM are significantly elevated above serum levels and can approach those required to inhibit calmoduin, the role of calmodulin as a signal transduction molecule for TAM will remain unclear. Currently, a contributory role for altered calmodulin levels/activity in antiestrogen resistance cannot excluded.

Protein kinase C has been implicated as a signal transduction molecule in the regulation of cellular proliferation in several systems. Inactivation of PKC could contribute to the growth inhibition induced by antiestrogens. TAM, and probably several other related triphenylethylenes, bind to PKC and inhibit its activity [95,96]. However, the IC_{50} is $25\,\mu M$ [95], a concentration up to 10-fold greater than the clinically achievable plasma levels of TAM [34,97]. Furthermore, the more potent metabolite 4-hydroxytamoxifen does not appear to bind directly to PKC [96]. Thus, the precise role of PKC as a signal transduction molecule for TAM remains unclear. It is conceivable, however, that alterations in the level or function of PKC, and/or its affinity for TAM, may contribute to antiestrogen resistance in a manner yet to be clearly elucidated. For example, some PKC activities may be dependent on its plasma membrane environment, and these may be influenced by the structural membrane modifications induced by TAM that are observed at $1\,\mu M$ TAM [28,98].

A novel intracellular binding site for the triphenylethylenes has been described. Antiestrogen binding sites (AEBS) appear to be microsomal, high-affinity, saturable binding proteins, for which TAM has a significantly higher affinity than estrogen [99]. These proteins are probably not directly involved in mediating a signal induced by TAM, since the biological potency of antiestrogens does not correlate with their affinity for AEBS [99]. However, their ability to seqester free drug could reduce intracellular bioavailability and thereby induce resistance.

The interactions between steroids and cellular membranes has been known for many years. Thirty-five years ago Wilmer [100] proposed that steroids would partition into membranes with their more hydrophilic moieties associated with the aqueous phase and/or any local polar groups. Using polarization of fluorescence analyses, we have demonstrated the ability of both E2 and TAM to decrease the fluidity in MCF-7 (ER-positive) and MDA-MB-436 (ER-negative) human breast cancer cells. These decreases in membrane fluidity correlate with the ability of high-dose E2 and TAM to inhibit the rates of DNA synthesis and cellular proliferation [28]. Many membrane proteins have a chemical requirement for their lipid environment to function [101], and a decreased mobility within the membrane could alter their function. Resistance could be conferred by a loss of sensitivity to changes in membrane structure, or by modifications in membrane organization. Cells also could switch to signal transduction pathways triggered by events not requiring membrane proteins, or at least not requiring the function of membrane proteins influenced by TAM. For example, we have shown that the estrogenic regulation of phosphoinositol turnover [102], which occurs primarily in the plasma membrane, is lost when cells become independent of estrogen for growth [48].

CROSSRESISTANCE AMONG ANTIESTROGENS

Until recently, there were few compelling reasons to be concerned with the potential for crossresistance among antiestrogens. Most drugs available for clinical use were triphenylethylene analogues representing relatively minor modifications to the structure of TAM, for example, Toremifene (chloro-Tamoxifen) and Droloxifen (3-hydroxytamoxifen). There has been little compelling evidence that these drugs have any consistently significant differences in either their potencies or response patterns in experimental models and breast cancer patients, or that they have substantial differences in their mechanisms of action. However, the new generation of steroidal antiestrogens does appear to exhibit significant differences from the triphenylethylenes in its potencies and molecular mechanisms.

Since the steroidal antiestrogens have not been widely used in the clinic, there are little data regarding their possible crossresistance with the triphenylethylenes. We have begun to address this issue in our experimental in vitro and in vivo models. The MCF7/LCC2 cells were selected for resistance to 4-hydroxytamoxifen. When screened for their responsiveness to ICI 182,780 [50] and ICI 164,384 [49], we found that they are not crossresistant and exhibit a dose–response relationship similar to their parental cells (MCF7/LCC1). This suggested that patients who responded and then failed TAM could respond to a steroidal antiestrogen [15]. There is some preliminary evidence to support this prediction. Patients who initially responded to TAM and subsequently failed have been included in the phase I trial of ICI 182,780. Significantly, several of these patients are now exhibiting responses to the steroidal compound [103].

We have recently isolated cells resistant to ICI 182,780, designated MCF7/LCC9 [104]. These cells appear crossresistant to TAM, even though they only have been exposed to ICI 182,780. This suggests that primary treatment with the more potent steroidal compounds may preclude subsequent response to a triphenylethylene. While there are no clinical data as yet to support this, there are other reasons to consider scheduling. It seems likely that the Goldie–Coldman hypothesis [81] could apply to endocrine therapies as it does to cytotoxic therapies. Day's modification of this hypothesis suggests that the sequential, rather than alternating, administration of drugs may be more effective. Furthermore, he predicted that the greatest benefit would be derived by administering the lesser potent of two drugs first, followed by the more potent drug [105,106]. Thus, following this rationale, patients may be better served by initial treatment with TAM, from which they also will obtain the benefits on cardiovascular performance and bone resorption, with crossover to ICI 182,780 upon relapse/progression.

MOLECULARMECHANISMS OF ANTIESTROGEN ACTION AND RESISTANCE: GENE NETWORKS

Our studies with hormone-independent and antiestrogen-resistant variants of the MCF-7 cell line clearly suggest that an acquired independence from estrogens for proliferation can arise independently of an acquired antiestrogen resistance. However, it is unclear mechanistically why these two potentially interdependent phenotypes should arise independently, particularly since it is widely accepted that a major action of the antiestrogens is as competitive antagonists for estrogens. These compounds clearly compete with estrogens for binding to ER, and thereby interfere with the estrogen-induced regulation of specific genes, for example, TAM inhibits the estrogen-induced expression of transforming growth factor alpha (TGFα) [107] and reverses the estrogen-induced transcriptional inhibition of TGFβ [108].

It is now apparent that TAM and other antiestrogens can regulate gene transcription in the apparent absence of estrogens. Indeed, these compounds can inhibit the proliferation of breast cancer cells growing in vitro in the apparent absence of estrogens in a manner that is reversed by estrogens, and with a dose–response relationship that reflects their affinity for ER. As indicated earlier, TAM also can function as a partial agonist. Together, these observations strongly suggest both that an antiestrogen–ER complex can be transcriptionally active and that the genes that are regulated, particularly the network of genes associated with cell proliferation, may be those that also are regulated by estrogens [109].

We hypothesized that the acquisition of a hormone-independent phenotype is conferred by the altered regulation of specific genes, for example, apparent constitutive induction/upregulation or constitutive repression/downregulation of genes that are normally induced/repressed estrogen regulated [110]. Antiestrogen resistance would not be acquired per se if the altered regulation of these genes enabled them to retain an ability to be regulated by antiestrogens and/or signals originating through other transduction pathways [109]. Thus, cells that have escaped from a dependence upon estrogen by altering the regulation of specific estrogen-regulated genes may still retain sensitivity to antiestrogens.

We have obtained some evidence in support of these hypotheses. The expression of several estrogen-regulated genes is clearly altered in the hormone-independent and hormone-responsive MCF7/MIII and MCF7/LCC1 cells. For example, pS2 mRNA is expressed in MCF7/LCC1 cells growing in the absence of estrogen at levels equivalent to that induced by estrogen in the hormone-dependent MCF-7 cells [48]. The baseline level of progesterone receptor protein but not mRNA expression also is significantly increased in the hormone-independent cells [48], while the regulation of ER and epidermal growth factor (EGF)-receptor expression appears essentially equivalent in the hormone-dependent and hormone-independent cells [45]. Preliminary data suggest that the expression of some of the genes that are upregulated in the absence of estrogen can still be inhibited by antiestrogens in the hormone-independent MCF7/LCC1 cells. These patterns of gene regulation clearly support our hypotheses, and provide at least one potential mechanistic explanation of how, at the molecular level, hormone independence and antiestrogen resistance can be independent but interrelated phenotypes.

These hypotheses would suggest that resistance to one antiestrogen may produce cross-resistance to others. Thus, the non-crossresistance phenotype of the TAM-resistant MCF7/LCC2 cells, that is, their sensitivity to steroidal antiestrogens, requires further consideration. There is good evidence indicating that the results of antiestrogen–ER interactions are different for triphenylethylene and steroidal antiestrogens. TAM can induce ER dimerization and DNA binding, and perhaps enable regulation of those functions mediated through the activity of only one of the two putative transcriptional activation functions of ER (estrogens activate both transcriptional activation functions). In contrast, the steroidal antiestrogens may inhibit ER dimerization [111] and alter receptor turnover [112]. These differences could result in some genes being regulated by triphenylethylene but not steroidal antiestrogens and/or vice versa. The steroidal antiestrogens also are significantly more potent than the triphenylethylenes and apparently function as agonists rather than partial agonists. Thus, some genes may be regulated by both classes of compound but not in the same direction. Other genes may be regulated in the same direction, but the potency of the triphenylethylenes may not be sufficient to produce a biologically meaningful degree of regulation.

It is evident that both steroidal and triphenylethylene antiestrogens inhibit cell proliferation, and these events are likely to primarily originate from signals transduced through the transcriptional activity of the ER system. There appears to be considerable redundancy in the regulatory mechanisms that control cell proliferation [113]. While there ultimately could prove to be a relatively small number of core functional genes/proteins driving proliferation, there are likely to be many signaling pathways that feed into this core but produce the same end result. The ER system could influence proliferation by regulating several signaling pathways; these could include signals that suppress or stimulate proliferation. While cells could initially rely on one ER pathway, they may be able to readily adapt to the utilization of another. Triphenylethylenes like TAM could regulate one or more, but not all, pathways, while steroidal compounds effectively shut down all estrogenic pathways. This would enable cells to acquire resistance to TAM while retaining sensitivity to ICI 182,780, but would ensure that cells that become resistant to ICI 182,780 are crossresistant to other antiestrogens.

What remains to be determined are the critical players in these regulatory networks. Not all events may occur at the transcriptional level. PGR protein, but not steady-state mRNA levels, are changed in the MCF7/LCC1 cells [48], clearly implicating post-transcriptional events. One of the challenges in the coming years will be to identify those genes/proteins that are regulated by estrogens and antiestrogens, and whose action ultimately is to regulate the complex machinery of cell cycle progression.

MOLECULAR MECHANISMS OF ANTIESTROGEN ACTION AND RESISTANCE: REGULATION OF GENE NETWORKS

We have hypothesized that several potentially interrelated gene regulatory networks may be involved in both the non-crossresistance phenotype of the MCF7/LCC2 and the crossresistant phenotype of the MCF7/LCC9 cells. This implies an ability of different antiestrogens to differentially regulate the same genes. Since these cells can be growth inhibited by antiestrogens in the absence of E2 in a manner that can be reversed by addition of excess E2, it seems likely that interactions with an ER system that has transcriptional activity in the absence of ligand are involved. There are several observations that provide direct and indirect support for our hypothesis. For example, Tzukerman et al. [114] have described both transcriptional activator and repressor activities of the wild-type human ER, in the absence of ligand, in cells transiently transfected with an ERE-CAT reporter construct. While the nonsteroidal antiestrogens clearly activate ER in the absence of ligand, this has not been widely reported for the steroidal antiestrogens. However, there is one report of activation of an ERE in cells expressing an ER mutant [115]. It seems most likely that the steroidal antiestrogens, through their ability to alter ER turnover and dimerization [111,112], could still regulate the constitutive activity of ER that occurs in the absence of ligand. These observations provide a potential explanation for growth inhibition, in the absence of E2, by both triphenylethylene and steroidal antiestrogens.

The nature of a specific gene's response to an activate ER-driven transcription complex at its promoter appears complex. For example, gene transcription regulated by some EREs is clearly agonistic, while other genes are transcriptionally repressed [116,117]. The direction of regulation, that is, repression or expression, is dependent upon the ERE sequence, which ligand is occupying the receptor, and which receptor form is present [116,117]. The function of these EREs also may be influenced by what other proteins are involved in the formation/activation of an ER-driven transcription complex. As indicated later, perturbations in the role/function of accessory proteins could differentially alter the expression of specific genes.

One mechanism for gene networks to be differentially regulated by different antiestrogens, without evoking a receptor mutational hypothesis (described elsewhere in this chapter), would be for the different drugs to induce different conformational states in the receptor protein. Many proteins, including receptors, transcription factors, and enzymes, have specific conformational requirements for their function. Conformation may be regulated by several factors, for example, interaction with a ligand(s), substrate, or cofactor, or by post-translational modifications, including phosphorylation, dephosphorylation, glycosylation, or proteolytic cleavage.

Several post-transcriptional modifications are known to occur with ER. For example, there is clear evidence of a ligand-dependent phosphorylation of ER [92], although the precise function of this is not known. Estrogen receptor and other steroid hormone receptors interact with accessory proteins [118–120], often in a manner that is ligand specific [119,120]. While the precise function of these receptor–protein interactions is unknown, it is tempting to speculate that they contribute to the differential/ligand-specific regulation of transcription. More recently, McDonnell et al. have demonstrated that the conformation of the ER is different when occupied with an estrogen, triphenylethylene antiestrogen, or steroidal antiestrogen. It is suggested that these conformational differences contribute to the differential regulation of transcription [121]. Clearly, we cannot exclude the possibility that some or all these ER modifications may occur, in addition to the possible contribution of mutant receptors. These diverse interactions, and the expression of the proteins that mediate these interactions, may differ with time, for example, development versus adult tissues; with tissue, for example, uterus versus mammary gland; and/or with the changing events driving malignant progression from hormone responsiveness to resistance. However, they provide a mechanistic explanation for the possible differential regulation of the same genes by structurally diverse ER ligands, and at least indirectly support our gene network hypothesis.

CONCLUDING COMMENTS AND FUTURE PROSPECTS

The acquisition of antiestrogen resistance is clearly an important clinical and biological issue. It seems likely that resistance will prove to be a multifaceted phenomenon, with several mechanisms potentially specific for the triphenylethylenes. The ability to identify markers for resistance, particularly markers that can predict the onset of acquired resistance in responders, could greatly improve the clinical management of the disease and provide potential targets for therapeutic intervention. The identification of such markers will require an improvement in our understanding of where the diversity, for example, the non-crossresistance phenotype (MCF7/LCC2), and commonality, for example, the crossresistance phenotype (MCF7/LCC9), of resistance mechanisms occur. Until we reach this understanding, the potential for non-crossresistance between triphenylethylene and steroidal antiestrogens may provide the clinician with improved therapeutic strategies.

ACKNOWLEDGMENTS

This work was supported in part by grants R01-CA58022, P30-CA51008, and P50-CA58185 to R. Clarke from the Public Health Service.

REFERENCES

1. Miller AB, Bulbrook RD (1986) UICC multidisciplinary project on breast cancer: The epidemiology, aetiology and prevention of breast cancer. Int J Cancer 37:173–177.
2. Clarke R, Dickson RB, Lippman ME (1992) Hormonal aspects of breast cancer: Growth factors, drugs and stromal interactions. Crit Rev Oncol Hematol 12:1–23.
3. Li JJ, Mueller GC, Sekely LI (1991) Workshop report from the Division of Cancer Etiology, National Cancer Institute, National Institutes of Health. Current Perspectives and Future Trends in Hormonal Carcinogenesis. Cancer Res 51:3626–3629.
4. Beatson GT (1896) On the treatment of inoperable cases of carcinoma of the mamma: Suggestions from a new method of treatment, with ilustrative cases. Lancet 2:104–107.
5. Kistner RW, Smith OW (1960) Observations on the use of a non-steroidal estrogen antagonist: Mer-25. Surg Forum 10:725–729.
6. Herbst AL, Griffiths CT, Kistner RW (1964) Clomiphene citrate (NSC-35770) in disseminated mammary carcinoma. Cancer Chemother Rep 443:39–41.
7. Cole MP, Jones CTA, Todd IDH (1971) A new antioestrogenic agent in late breast cancer. An early clinical appraisal of ICI 46474. Br J Cancer 25:270–275.
8. Litherland S, Jackson IM (1988) Antioestrogens in the management of hormone-dependent cancer. Cancer Treat Rev 15:183–194.
9. Magdelenat H, Pouillart P (1988) Steroid hormone receptors in breast cancer. In PJ Sheridan, K Blum, MC Trachtenberg, eds. Steroid Receptors and Disease: Cancer Autoimmune, Bone and Circulatory Disorders. New York: Marcel Dekker, pp 435–465.
10. McGuire WL, Clark GM (1983) The prognostic role of progesterone receptor in human breast cancer. Semin Oncol 10:2–6.
11. NATO (1985) Controlled trial of tamoxifen as a single adjuvant agent in the management of early breast cancer. Lancet 2:836–839.
12. Committee (1987) BCT Adjuvant tamoxifen in the management of operable breast cancer: The Scottish trial. Lancet 1:171–175.
13. Henderson IC, Shapiro CL (1991) Adjuvant chemotherapy: An overview. In T Powles, IE Smith, eds. Medical Management of Breast Cancer. London: Dunitz, pp 197–215.
14. Clarke R, Dickson RB, Brünner N (1990) The process of malignant progression in human breast cancer. Ann Oncol 1:401–407.
15. Clarke R, Thompson EW, Leonessa F, Lippman J, McGarvey M, Brünner N (1993) Hormone resistance, invasiveness and metastatic potential in human breast cancer. Breast Cancer Res Treat 24:227–239.
16. Clarke R, Leonessa F (1994) Cytotoxic drugs and hormones in breast cancer: Interactions at the cellular level. In RB Dickson, ME Lippman, eds. Drug and Hormonal Resistance in Breast Cancer: Cellular and Molecular Mechanisms. Chichester, UK: Ellis Horwood, pp 407–432.
17. Leonessa F, Boulay V, Wright A, Thompson EW, Brünner N, Clarke R (1991) The biology of breast tumor progression: Acquisition of hormone-independence and resistance to cytotoxic drugs. Acta Oncol 31:115–123.
18. Barsky SH, Togo S, Garbisa S, Liotta LA (1994) Type IV collagenase immunoreactivity in invasive breast carcinoma. Lancet 1:296–297.
19. Schneider E, Horton JK, Yang CH, Nakagawa M, Cowan KH (1994) Multidrug resistance-associated protein gene overexpression and reduced drug sensitivity of topoisomerase II in a human breast carcinoma MCF7 cell line selected for etoposide resistance. Cancer Res 54:152–158.
20. Zyad A, Bernard J, Clarke R, Tursz T, Brockhaus M, Chouaib S (1994) Human breast cancer cross-resistance to TNF and Adriamycin: Relationship to MDR1, MnSOD and TNF gene expression. Cancer Res 54:825–831.
21. Morrow CS, Chiu J, Cowan KH (1992) Posttranscriptional control of glutathione S-transferase pi gene expression in human breast cancer cells. J Biol Chem 267:10544–10550.
22. Fuqua SAW, Oesterreich S, Hilsenbeck SG, Von Hoff DD, Eckardt J, Osborne CK (1994) Heat shock proteins and drug resistance. Breast Cancer Res Treat 32:67–71.
23. Tuccari G, Rizzo A, Giuffre G, Barresi G (1993) Immunocytochemical detection of DNA topoisomerase type II in primary breast carcinomas: Correlation with clinico-pathological features. Virchows Arch A Pathol Anat Histopathol 423:51–55.
24. Hahnel R, Twaddle E, Ratajczak T (1973) The influence of synthetic anti-estrogens on the binding of tritiated estradiol-17β by cytosols of human uterus and human breast carcinoma. J Steroid Biochem 4:687–695.

25. Clarke R, Lippman ME (1992) Antiestrogens resistance: Mechanisms and reversal. In BA Teicher, ed. Drug Resistance in Oncology. New York: Marcel Dekker, pp 501–536.

26. Nardulli AM, Green GL, O'Malley BW, Katzenellenbogen BS (1988) Regulation of progesterone receptor messenger ribonucleic acid and protein levels in MCF-7 cells by estradiol: Analysis of estrogen's effect on progesterone receptor synthesis and degradation. Endocrinology 122:935–944.

27. Lam H-YP (1984) Tamoxifen is a calmodulin antagonist in the activation of cAMP phosphodi-esterase. Biochem Biophys Res Comm 118:27–32.

28. Clarke R, van den Berg HW, Murphy RF (1990) Tamoxifen and 17β-estradiol reduce the membrane fluidity of human breast cancer cells. J Natl Cancer Inst 82:1702–1705.

29. Pasqualini JR, Nguyen B-L (1991) Estrone sulfatase activity and effect of antiestrogens on transfor-mation of estrone sulfate in hormone-dependent vs. independent human breast cancer cell lines. Breast Cancer Res Treat 18:93–98.

30. Ravdin PM, Fritz NF, Tormey DC, Jordan VC (1988) Endocrine status of premenopausal node-positive breast cancer patients following adjuvant chemotherapy and long-term tamoxifen. Cancer Res 48:1026–1029.

31. Clarke R, Brünner N, Thompson EW, Glanz P, Katz D, Dickson RB, Lippman ME (1989) The inter-relationships between ovarian-independent growth, antiestrogen resistance and invasiveness in the malignant progression of human breast cancer. J Endocrinol 122:331–340.

32. Plotkin D, Lechner JJ, Jung WE, Rosen PJ (1978) Tamoxifen flare in advanced breast cancer. JAMA 240:2644–2646.

33. Clarysse A (1985) Hormone-induced tumor flare. Eur J Cancer Clin Oncol 21:545–547.

34. Etienne MC, Milano G, Fischcel JL, Frenay M, Francois E, Formento JL, Gioanni J, Namer M (1989) Tamoxifen metabolism: Pharmacokinetic and in vitro study. Br J Cancer 60:30–35.

35. Buckely MM-T, Goa KL (1989) Tamoxifen: A reappraisal of its pharmacodynamic and pharmaco-kinetic properties, and therapeutic use. Drugs 37:451–490.

36. Katzenellenbogen BS, Ferguson ER (1975) Antiestrogen action in the uterus: Biological ineffective-ness of nuclear bound estradiol after antiestrogen. Endocrinology 97:1–12.

37. Ferrazzi E, Cartei G, Matarazzo R (1977) Oestrogen-like effect of tamoxifen on vaginal epithelium. Lancet 1:1351–1352.

38. Gusberg SB (1990) Tamoxifen for breast cancer: Associated endometrial cancer. Cancer 65:1463–1464.

39. Pasqualini JR, Sumida C, Giambiagi N (1988) Pharmacodynamic and biological effects of anti-estrogens in different models. J Steroid Biochem 31:613–643.

40. Robertson DW, Katzenellenbogen JA, Long DJ, Rorke EA, Katzenellenbogen BS (1982) Tamoxifen antiestrogens. A comparison of the activity, pharmacokinetics, and metabolic activation of the cis and trans isomers of tamoxifen. J Steroid Biochem 16:1–13.

41. Robinson SP, Langan-Fahey SM, Johnson DA, Jordan VC (1991) Metabolites, pharmacodynamics and pharmacokinetics of tamoxifen in rats and mice compared to breast cancer patients. Drug Metab Dispos Biol Fate Chem 19:36–43.

42. Terenius L (1970) Two modes of interactions between oestrogen and anti-oestrogen. Acta Endocrinol 64:47–58.

43. Thompson EW, Katz D, Shima TB, Wakeling AE, Lippman ME, Dickson RB (1989) ICI 164,384: A pure antagonist of estrogen-stimulated MCF-7 cell proliferation and invasiveness. Cancer Res 49:6929–6934.

44. Wakeling AE, Dukes M, Bowler J (1991) A potent specific pure antiestrogen with clinical potential. Cancer Res 51:3867–3873.

45. Clarke R, Brünner N, Katzenellenbogen BS, Thompson EW, Norman MJ, Koppi C, Paik S, Lippman ME, Dickson RB (1989) Progression from hormone dependent to hormone independent growth in MCF-7 human breast cancer cells. Proc Natl Acad Sci USA 86:3649–3653.

46. Seibert K, Shafie SM, Triche TJ, Whang-Peng JJ, O'Brien SJ, Toney JH, Huff KK, Lippman ME (1983) Clonal variation of MCF-7 breast cancer cells in vitro and in athymic nude mice. Cancer Res 43:2223–2239.

47. Brünner N, Svenstrup B, Spang-Thompsen M, Bennet P, Nielsen A, Nielsen JJ (1986) Serum steroid levels in intact and endocrine ablated Balb\c nude mice and their intact litter mates. J Steroid Biochem 25:429–432.

48. Brünner N, Boulay V, Fojo A, Freter C, Lippman ME, Clarke R (1993) Acquisition of hormone-independent growth in MCF-7 cells is accompanied by increased expression of estrogen-regulated genes but without detectable DNA amplifications. Cancer Res 53:283–290.

49. Coopman P, Garcia M, Brünner N, Derocq D, Clarke R, Rochefort H (1994) Antiproliferative

and antiestrogenic effects of ICI 164,384 in 4-OH-Tamoxifen-resistant human breast cancer cells. Int J Cancer 56:295–300.

50. Brünner N, Frandsen TL, Holst-Hansen C, Bei M, Thompson EW, Wakeling AE, Lippman ME, Clarke R (1993) MCF7/LCC2: A 4-hydroxytamoxifen resistant human breast cancer variant which retains sensitivity to the steroidal antiestrogen ICI 182,780. Cancer Res 53:3229–3232.

51. Kemp JV, Adam HK, Wakeling AE, Slater R (1983) Identification and biological activity of tamoxifen metabolites in human serum. Biochem Pharmacol 32:2045–2052.

52. Jordan VC, Bain RR, Brown RR, Gordon B, Santos MA (1983) Determination and pharmacology of a new hydroxylated metabolite of tamoxifen observed in patient sera during therapy for advanced breast cancer. Cancer Res 43:1446–1450.

53. Katzenellenbogen BS, Norman MJ, Eckert RL, Pelyz SW, Mangel WF (1984) Bioactivities, estrogen receptor interactions, and plasminogen activator-inducing activities of tamoxifen and hydroxytamoxifen isomers in MCF-7 human breast cancer cells. Cancer Res 44:112–119.

54. Jordan VC, Robinson SP (1987) Species-specific pharmacology of antiestrogens: Role of metabolism. Fed Proc 46:1870–1874.

55. Wiebe VJ, Osborne CK, McGuire WL, DeGregorio MW (1992) Identification of estrogenic tamoxifen metabolite(s) in tamoxifen-resistant human breast tumors. J Clin Oncol 10:990–994.

56. Osborne CK, Coronado E, Allred DC, Wiebe V, DeGregorio M (1991) Acquired tamoxifen resistance: Correlation with reduced breast tumor levels of tamoxifen and isomerization of trans-4-hydroxytamoxifen. J Natl Cancer Inst 83:1477–1482.

57. Gottardis MM, Wagner RJ, Borden EC, Jordan CV (1989) Differential ability of antiestrogens to stimulate breast cancer cell (MCF-7) growth in vivo and in vitro. Cancer Res 49:4765–4769.

58. Osborne CK, Coronado EB, Robinson JP (1987) Human breast cancer in athymic nude mice: Cytostatic effects of long-term antiestrogen therapy. Eur J Cancer Clin Oncol 23:1189–1196.

59. Jiang S-Y, Jordan VC (1992) Growth regulation of estrogen receptor negative breast cancer cells transfected with estrogen receptor cDNAs. J Natl Cancer Inst 84:580–591.

60. McLeskey SW, Kurebayashi J, Honig SF, Zwiebel JA, Lippman ME, Dickson RB, Kern FG (1993) Fibroblast growth factor 4 transfection of MCF-7 cells produces cell lines that are tumorigenic and metastatic in ovariectomized or tamoifen-treated athymic nude mice. Cancer Res 53:2168–2177.

61. Wolf DM, Langan-Fahey SM, Parker CP, McCague R, Jordan VC (1993) Investigation of the mechanism of tamoxifen stimulated breast tumor growth; non-isomerizable analogues of tamoxifen and its metabolites. J Natl Cancer Inst 85:806–812.

62. Belani CP, Pearl P, Whitley NO, Aisner J (1989) Tomoxifen withdrawal response: report of a case. Arch Intern Med 149:449–450.

63. McIntosh IH, Thynne GS (1977) Tumor stimulation by anti-oestrogens. Br J Surg 64:900–901.

64. Stein W, Hortobagyi GN, Blumenschein GR (1983) Response of metastatic breast cancer to famoxifen withdrawal: Report of a case. J Surg Oncol 22:45–46.

65. Allegra CJ (1990) Antifolates. In BA Chabner, JM Collins, eds. Cancer Chemotherapy: Principles and Practice. Philadelphia: JB Lippincott, pp 110–153.

66. Pastan I, Gottesman MM, Ueda K, Lovelace E, Rutherford AV, Willingham MC (1988) A retrovirus carrying an MDR1 cDNA confers multidrug resistance and polarized expression of P-glycoprotein in MDCK cells. Proc Natl Acad Sci USA 85:4486–4490.

67. Johnston SRD, Haynes BP, Smith IE, Jarman M, Sacks NPM, Ebbs SR, Dowsett M (1993) Acquired tamoxifen resistance in human breast cancer and reduced intra-tumoral drug concentration. Lancet 342:1521–1522.

68. Leonessa F, Jacobson M, Boyle B, Lippman J, McGarvey M, Clarke R (1994) The effect of tamoxifen on the multidrug resistant phenotype in human breast cancer cells: Isobologram, drug accumulation and gp-170 binding studies. Cancer Res 54:441–447.

69. Ramu A, Glaubiger D, Fuks Z (1984) Reversal of acquired resistance to doxorubicin in P388 murine leukemia cells by tamoxifen and other triparanol analogues. Cancer Res 44:4392–4395.

70. Keen JC, Miller EP, Bellamy C, Dixon JM, Miller WR (1994) P-glycoprotein and resistance to tamoxifen. Lancet 343:1047–1048.

71. Clarke R, Currier S, Kaplan O, Lovelace E, Boulay V, Gottesman MM, Dickson RB (1992) Effect of P-glycoprotein expression on sensitivity to hormones in MCF-7 human breast cancer cells. J Natl Cancer Inst 84:1506–1512.

72. Szamel I, Hindy I, Vincze B, Eckhardt S, Kangas L, Hajba A (1994) Influence of toremifene on the endocrine regulation of breast cancer patients. Eur J Cancer 30A:154–158.

73. Brodie AMH, Santen RJ (1985) Aromatase in breast cancer and the role of aminogluthemide and other aromatase inhibitors. CRC Crit Rev Oncol Hematol 5:361–396.

74. Reed MJ, Owen AM, Lai LC, Coldham NG, Ghilchik MW, Shaikh NA, James VHT (1989) In situ oestrone synthesis in normal breast and breast tumour tissues: Effect of treatment with 4-hydroxyandrostenedione. Int J Cancer 44:233–237.

75. Hardy JR, Judson IR, Sinnett HD, Ashley SE, Coombes RC, Ellin CL (1990) Combination of tamoxifen, aminoglutethimide, danazol and medroxyprogesterone acetate in advanced breast cancer. Eur J Cancer 26:824–827.

76. Ravdin PM, Green S, Dorr TM, McGuire WL, Fabian C, Pugh RP, Carter RD, Rivkin SE, Borst JR, Belt RJ (1992) Prognostic significance of progesterone receptor levels in estrogen receptor-positive patients with metastatic breast cancer treated with tamoxifen: Results of a prospective Southwest Oncology Group study. J Clin Oncol 10:1284–1291.

77. Patterson JS, Edwards DG, Battersby LA (1981) A review of the international clinical experience with tamoxifen. Jpn J Cancer Clin (Suppl):157–183.

78. Vuletic L, Bugarski M, Boberic J, Milosauljevic A, Naumovic P (1981) Treatment of advanced breast cancer with tamoxifen: A pilot study. Rev Endoc Related Cancer 9:533–545.

79. Van Netten JP, Algard FT, Coy P (1985) Heterogeneous estrogen receptor levels detected via multiple microsamples from individual breast tumors. Cancer 56:2019–2024.

80. Van Netten JP, Armstrong JB, Carlyle SS, Goodchild NL, Thormton IG, Brigden ML, Coy P, Fletcher C (1988) Estrogen receptor distribution in the peripheral, intermediate and central regions of breast cancers. Eur J Cancer Clin Oncol 24:1885–1889.

81. Goldie JH, Coldman AJ (1979) A mathematical model for relating the drug sensitivity of tumors to the spontaneous mutation rate. Cancer Treat Rep 63:1727–1733.

82. Encarnacion CA, Ciocca DR, McGuire WL, Clark GM, Fuqua SA, Osborne CK (1993) Measurement of steroid hormone receptors in breast cancer patients on tamoxifen. Breast Cancer Res Treat 26:237–246.

83. Johnston SRD, Saccanti-Jotti G, Smith IE, Newby J, Dowsett M (1995) Change in oestrogen receptor expression and function in tamoxifen-resistant breast cancer. Endocr Related Cancer 2:105–110.

84. Murphy LC, Dotzlaw H (1989) Variant estrogen receptor mRNA species in human breast cancer biopsy samples. Mol Endocrinol 3:687–693.

85. Dotzlaw H, Alkhalaf M, Murphy LC (1992) Characterization of estrogen receptor variant mRNAs from human breast cancers. Mol Endocrinol 6:773–785.

86. Murphy LC, Hilsenbeck SG, Dotzlaw H, Fuqua SAW (1995) Relationship of clone 4 estrogen receptor variant messenger RNA expression to some known prognostic variables in human breast cancer. Clin Cancer Res 1:155–159.

87. Wang Y, Miksicek RJ (1991) Identification of a dominant negative form of the human estrogen receptor. Mol Endocrinol 5:1707–1715.

88. Fuqua SAW, Fitzgerald SG, Allred DC, Elledge RM, Nawaz Z, McDonnel D, O'Malley BW, Greene GL, McGuire WL (1992) Inhibition of estrogen receptor action by a naturally occurring variant in human breast tumors. Cancer Res 52:483–486.

89. Fuqua SAW, Fitzgerald SD, Chamness GC, Tandon AK, McDonnel DP, Nawaz Z, O'Malley BW, McGuire WL (1991) Variant human breast tumor estrogen receptor with constitutive transcriptional activity. Cancer Res 51:105–109.

90. Koehorst SGA, Cox JJ, Donker GH, da Silva SL, Burbach JPH, Thijssen JHH, Blankenstein MA (1994) Functional analysis of an alternatively spliced estrogen receptor lacking exon 4 isolated from MCF-7 breast cancer cells and meningiomas. Mol Cell Endocrinol 101:237–245.

91. Jiang S-Y, Langan-Fahey SM, Stella AL, McCague R, Jordan VC (1992) Point mutation of estrogen receptor (ER) in the ligand-binding domain changes the pharmacology of antiestrogens in ER-negative human breast cancer cells stably expressing complementary DNAs for ER. Mol Endocrinol 6:2167–2174.

92. Aronica SM, Katzenellenbogen BS (1993) Stimulation of estrogen receptor-mediated transcription and alteration in the phosphorylation state of the rat uterine estrogen receptor by estrogen, cyclic adenosine monophosphate, and insulin-like growth factor-I. Mol Endocrinol 7:743–752.

93. Krishnaraju K, Murugesan K, Vij U, Kapur BML, Farooq A (1991) Calmodulin levels in oestrogen receptor positive and negative human breast tumours. Br J Cancer 346–347.

94. Greenberg DA, Carpenter CL, Messing RO (1987) Calcium channel antagonist properties of the antineoplastic antiestrogen tamoxifen in the PC12 neurosecretory cell line. Cancer Res 47:70–74.

95. O'Brian CA, Liskamp RM, Solomon DH, Weinstein IB (1986) Triphenylethylenes: A new class of protein kinase C inhibitors. J Natl Cancer Inst 76:1243–1246.

96. O'Brian CA, Housey GM, Weinstein IB (1988) Specific and direct binding of protein kinase C to an immobilized tamoxifen analogue. Cancer Res 48:3626–3629.
97. Fabian C, Sternson L, Barnet M (1980) Clinical pharmacology of tamoxifen in patients with breast cancer: Comparison of traditional and loading dose schedules. Cancer Treat Rep 64:765–773.
98. Custodio JBA, Almeida LM, Madeira VMC (1993) The anticancer drug tamoxifen induces changes in the physical properties of model and native membranes. Biochim Biophys Acta 123–129.
99. Katzenellenbogen BS, Miller AM, Mullick A, Sheen YY (1985) Antiestrogen action in breast cancer cells: Modulation of proliferation and protein synthesis, and interaction with estrogen receptors and additional antiestrogen binding sites. Breast Cancer Res Treat 5:231–243.
100. Wilmer EN (1961) Steroids and cell surfaces. Biol Rev 36:368–398.
101. Lenaz G, Curatola G, Mazzanti L, Parenti-Castelli G (1978) Biophysical studies on agents affecting the state of membrane lipids: Biochemical and pharmacological implications. Mol Cell Biochem 22:3–32.
102. Freter CE, Lippman ME, Cheville A, Zinn S, Gelmann EP (1988) Alterations in phosphoinositide metabolism associated with 17β-estradiol and growth factor treatment of MCF-7 breast cancer cells. Mol Endocrinol 2:159–166.
103. Nicholson RI, Gee JMW, Anderson E, Dowsett M, DeFriend D, Howell A, Robertson JFR, Blamey RW, Baum M, Saunders C, Walton P, Wakeling AE (1993) Phase I study of a new pure antiestrogen ICI 182,780 in women with primary breast cancer: Immunohistochemical analysis. Breast Cancer Res Treat 27:135.
104. Brünner N, Boysen B, Kiilgaard TL, Frandsen TL, Jirus S, Clarke R (1993) Resistance to 40H-Tamoxifen does not confer resistance to the steroidal antiestrogen ICI 182,780, while acquired resistance to ICI 182,780 results in cross resistance to 40H-TAM. Breast Cancer Res Treat 27:135.
105. Day RS (1986) Treatment sequencing, assymetry and uncertainty: Protocol strategies for combination chemotherapy. Cancer Res 46:3876–3885.
106. Norton L, Day R (1991) Potential innovations in scheduling cancer chemotherapy. In VT DeVita, S Hellman, SA Rosenberg, eds. Important Advances in Oncology. Philadelphia: JB Lippincott, pp 57–73.
107. Bates SE, Davidson NE, Valverius EM, Dickson RB, Freter CE, Tam JP, Kudlow JE, Lippman ME, Salomon S (1988) Expression of transforming growth factor-α and its mRNA in human breast cancer: Its regulation by estrogen and its possible functional significance. Mol Endocrinol 2:543–545.
108. Knabbe C, Lippman ME, Wakefield LM, Flanders KC, Derynck R, Dickson RB (1987) Evidence that transforming growth factor-beta is a hormonally regulated negative growth factor in human breast cancer cells. Cell 48:417–428.
109. Clarke R, Brünner N (1995) Cross resistance and molecular mechanisms in antiestrogen resistance. Endocr Related Cancer 2:59–72.
110. Clarke R, Skaar T, Baumann K, Leonessa K, James MP, Lippman J, Thompson EW, Freter C, Brünner N (1994) Hormonal carcinogenesis in breast cancer: Cellular and molecular studies of malignant progression. Breast Cancer Res Treat 31:237–248.
111. Fawell SE, White R, Hoare S, Sydenham M, Page M, Parker MG (1990) Inhibition of estrogen receptor-DNA binding by the "pure" antiestrogen ICI 164,384 appears to be mdiated by impaired receptor dimerization. Proc Natl Acad Sci USA 87:6883–6887.
112. Dauvois S, Danielian PS, White R, Parker MG (1992) Antiestrogen ICI 164,384 reduces cellular estrogen receptor content by increasing its turnover. Proc Natl Acad Sci USA 89:4037–4041.
113. Murray A, Hunt T (1993) The Cell Cycle. New York: WH Freeman.
114. Tzukerman M, Zhang X-K, Herman T, Wills KN, Graupner G, Pfahl M (1990) The human estrogen receptor has transcriptional activator and repressor functions in the absence of a ligand. New Biologist 2:613–620.
115. Xing H, Haase S, Shapiro DJ (1994) Antiestrogens activate an estrogen receptor mutant exhibiting enhanced binding to the estrogen response element. Biochem Biophys Res Commun 202:888–895.
116. Curtis SW, Korach KS (1991) Uterine estrogen receptor-DNA complexes: Effects of different ERE sequences, ligands, and receptor forms. Mol Endocrinol 5:959–966.
117. Dana SL, Hoener PA, Wheeler DA, Lawrence CB, McDonnell DP (1994) Novel estrogen response elements identified by genetic selection in yeast are differentially responsive to estrogens and antiestrogens in mammalian cells. Mol Endocrinol 8:1193–1207.
118. Yoshinaga SK, Peterson CL, Herskowitz I, Yamamoto KR (1992) Roles of SWI1, SWI2 and SWI3 proteins for transcriptional enhancement by steroid receptors. Science 258:1596–1604.

119. Landel CC, Kushner PJ, Greene GL (1994) The interaction of human estrogen receptor with DNA is modulated by receptor-associated proteins. Mol Endocrinol 8:1407–1419.
120. Halachmi S, Marden E, Martin G, MacKay H, Abbondanza C, Brown M (1994) Estrogen receptor-associated proteins: Possible mediators of hormone-induced transcription. Science 264:1455–1458.
121. McDonnell DP, Clemm DL, Hermann T, Goldman ME, Pike JW (1995) Analysis of estrogen receptor function in vitro reveals three distinct classes of antiestrogens. Mol Endocrinol 9:659–669.

12. ANDROGEN RECEPTOR MUTATIONS IN PROSTATE CANCER

EDWARD P. GELMANN

The incidence of prostate cancer in the United States has risen steadily during the past 10 years. This is due to a combination of factors, including increased use of prostate-specific antigen (PSA) for screening, aging of the population, declining mortality from other causes such as cardiac disease, and environmental and dietary factors that have contributed to prostate carcinogenesis. In 1995 it was estimated that 244,000 new cases of prostate cancer would be diagnosed in the United States and prostate cancer would account for approximately 40,400 deaths in that year [1]. The magnitude of the prostate cancer problem has focused attention on the need for better therapies and effective prevention.

Characterization of the androgen receptor in prostate cancer patients is important because the prostate gland depends on androgens for its development and for the maintenance of its integrity. Individuals with androgen insensitivity syndromes or with 5α-reductase deficiency have minimal or absent development of the prostate gland [2]. In animal models as well, one can demonstrate that androgens are critical for the integrity of the prostate gland. For example, in the rat, castration results in rapid prostatic involution that results from epithelial cell apoptosis within 7 days of androgen ablation [3].

Androgens are the natural tumor promoter of prostate cancer. Studies of eunuchoid individuals have suggested that prostate cancer does not develop in the absence of androgens [4]. Moreover, animal models of prostate carcinogenesis require the presence of functioning testes for the development of prostatic cancer [5,6]. In Lobund-Wistar rats, oral carcinogen administration results in prostate cancer development 8–24 months after carcinogen administration. Castration at the time of carcinogen administration abrogates the experimentally induced prostatic carcinogenesis. Epidemiologic studies have attempted to show that androgens play a critical role in prostate cancer incidence in men. It has been proposed that circulating androgen levels are somewhat higher in African Americans that in Caucasian Americans, which has led to speculations that the elevated androgen levels may contribute to the increased incidence of prostate cancer among African Americans. However, the association between prostate cancer incidence and serum androgen levels is controversial and has not been demonstrated conclusively [7–11].

ANDROGEN EFFECTS ON PROSTATE CANCER

Prostate cancer cells, reminiscent of the androgen responsiveness of prostate epithelium, retain the ability to respond to androgens. It has been known for more than half a century that prostate cancer in most cases retains androgen responsiveness and will undergo regression in response to androgen deprivation [12,13]. Over 80% of men with disseminated prostate cancer will show some clinical response to androgen ablation. However, there is no way to predict which patients will not respond or how long the responding patients will benefit from androgen control of their prostate cancer. Although the median duration of response to hormonal ablation is less than 2 years, response durations range from a few months to many years. The lack of correlation between androgen receptor levels and clinical hormone responsiveness is very different from the situation in breast cancer, another hormone-responsive malignancy. In breast cancer, levels of estrogen receptor predict the likelihood of a clinical response to hormones, and the presence of detectable progesterone receptor, an estrogen-inducible gene, increases the likelihood of a clinical hormonal response [14]. On the other hand, androgen responsiveness in prostate cancer does not correlate with either the presence or the levels of androgen receptor in cancer tissues [15–20]. Furthermore, androgen receptor can still be detected at a time when the patient no longer enjoys clinical remission induced by androgen deprivation.

Clinical use of androgen ablation was formerly reserved for patients with inoperable and most often stage D disease. Androgen suppression by diethylstilbestrol (DES) had been shown to prolong survival of patients with metastatic prostate cancer if used at some time in the course of the disease [21]. Use of DES was superceded by gonadotrophin releasing hormone (GnRH) agonists, which are more expensive than DES but have fewer side effects [22]. Since GnRH agonists do not affect stimulation of prostate cancer by adrenal androgens, GnRH therapy is often supplemented with the antiandrogen flutamide to achieve total androgen blockade [23]. Total androgen blockade is either equivalent to or superior than GnRH agonists alone in sustaining disease-free and overall survival of patients with metastatic prostate cancer [24–27].

Androgen ablation has also been adapted for use in patients with localized prostate cancer. Urologists have attempted to induce regression of localized prostate cancer in order to improve operability and to increase local control rates in patients whose organ involvement may exceed the threshold for operability. A randomized trial of neoadjuvant hormone ablation prior to radical prostatectomy versus prostatectomy alone demonstrated that androgen ablation can downsize local disease. However, no information as yet is available on whether there are any long-term survival benefits of neoadjuvant hormonal therapy prior to radical surgery [23]. Androgen ablation has also been combined with radiation therapy for localized prostate cancer. The Radiation Therapy Oncology Group conducted a study that demonstrated pro-longed disease-free survival for those patients who underwent 3 months of androgen ablation prior to the initiation of definitive radiation therapy [29].

There may be a strong theoretical framework in which to study therapeutic regimens that combine cytotoxic modalities with androgen ablation. Radiation and some chemotherapeutic agents cause cell death by inducing DNA fragmentation that signals activation of apoptotic pathways via *p53* or other genes [30–32]. Androgen withdrawal also induces apoptosis in prostatic cells and in prostate cancer [3]. In fact, the presence of androgens may protect prostatic cancer cells from apoptosis by induction of *bcl*-2 gene expression [33]. Theoretically, androgen abla-tion may enhance apoptosis when used in conjunction with modalities that cause DNA strand breakage. The generation of clinical studies that incorporate androgen ablation with other modalities for treatment of local prostate cancer is just begin-ning. The biggest obstacle to wide acceptance of such trials may be side effects of androgen ablation, most importantly importence. One strategy to address this is intermittent use of androgen ablation that would allow hormone "holidays." Whether this will result in more rapid development of androgen resistance in prostate cancer remains to be seen.

There are many reasons to study the structure and expression of the androgen receptor in prostate cancer. The androgen receptor gene has been mapped to the X chromosome and therefore males have only one copy [34]. Any mutations in the androgen receptor would therefore be immediately manifest if that mutation caused a change in androgen receptor function. Since androgen is the tumor promoter of prostate cancer, one could ask whether prostate cancer patients harbor mutant androgen receptors. Patients with metastatic prostate cancer vary in the degree and duration of their clinical response to androgen ablation. Therefore, one could ask whether structural differences in androgen receptor could explain the differences in clinical responses. Lastly, in vitro studies with the human LNCaP prostate cancer cell line have shown that a single point mutation in the androgen receptor can alter the response to the antiandrogen flutamide, such that the antiandrogen is seen as a receptor agonist [35,36]. In fact, the clinical correlate of this in vitro phenomenon was described recently when it was shown that up to 40% of patients on long-term flutamide therapy will demonstrate prostate cancer regression when treated with flutamide withdrawal [37]. The flutamide withdrawal response in some cases is likely to be the clinical manifestation of spontaneously arising androgen receptor mutations in metastatic prostate cancer sites. Understanding the detailed mutational changes that result from prolonged antiandrogen therapy can contribute to improved under-standing of androgen receptor function and improved design of new antiandrogens for clinical use.

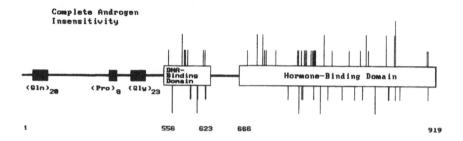

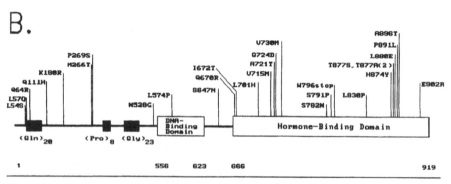

Figure 12–1. Basic structure of the androgen receptor gene. The androgen receptor gene locus on chromosome Xq11-12 contains eight exons. Sizes of the exons in nucleotides are shown in the middle diagram. Exons code for different regions of the protein shown in the lower portion of the figure. The numerical scale at the bottom are amino acid numbers that correspond to the boundaries of the functional regions of the protein. The three regions of amino acid repeats are shown schematically on the amino-terminal region of the protein.

STRUCTURE OF THE ANDROGEN RECEPTOR

The androgen receptor is a member of the family of steroid hormone receptors. That family includes receptors for estrogen, glucocorticoids, retinoids, thyroid hormone, mineralocorticoids, and progesterone [38–40]. These molecules have a common structure and their genes have parallel exonic organization, suggesting that they arose from common ancestry [38]. Androgen receptor structure is illustrated in Figure 12–1. The androgen receptor gene has been mapped to human chromosome

Xq11–12 [34]. The gene is comprised of eight exons. The first and last exons contain sequences that are transcribed into noncoding regions of the mRNA [41]. The mRNA is 10.6 kb in length, of which only 2.8 kb code for the protein. Approximately 1 kb is the 5′ untranslated region and 7 kb are the 3′ untranslated region of the mRNA [42,43]. The first exon codes for the amino-terminal domain of the protein that is responsible for interaction with other transcription factors to carry out the receptor's transactivation functions. The N-terminal domain also contains three regions of amino acid repeats. Polyglutamine and polyglycine repeats of approximately 20 amino acids each vary in length from one individual to another. A polyproline repeat is eight amino acids long. Exons 2 and 3 code for the DNA-binding domain, a region common to all steroid receptors with the highest degree of sequence similarity between the receptors. The DNA-binding region includes eight cysteine residues that constitute two zinc finger domains that interact with the major groove of DNA in the androgen-response element. The androgen-response element is a DNA sequence that is specifically bound by the DNA-binding domain of the androgen receptor. The second zinc finger is also necessary for receptor dimerization that occurs during DNA binding [44,45]. Exons 4–8 code for the steroid hormone-binding domain. The androgen-binding domain is specific for androgen and is highly conserved throughout evolution. For example, the amino acid sequences of the murine and human androgen-binding domains are identical.

More mutations have been described for the androgen receptor than for any other steroid hormone receptor. This is probably because the androgen receptor is not essential for growth or development. Inherited complete and partial androgen insensitivity syndromes have been associated with numerous point mutations in the androgen receptor, the majority of which are located in the hormone-binding domain. Individuals with androgen insensitivity syndromes vary in disease manifestation from phenotypic females associated with complete inactivation of androgen receptor activity to undervirilized males who have partial androgen receptor inactivation.

ANDROGEN RECEPTOR IN PROSTATE CANCER

Androgen receptor mutations could play a role in the origin and pathogenesis of prostate cancer. A known oncogene, v-erbA, identified in the avian erythroblastosis virus, was shown to be the avian homolog of the thyroid hormone receptor and is a member of the steroid hormone receptor family. Therefore, the possibility was raised that other steroid hormone receptors, like the androgen receptor, could be the target for dominant mutations in prostate cancer [40]. Androgen receptor mutations could also result in altered receptor affinity, thereby facilitating prostate cancer promotion by endogenous androgens. Also, androgen receptor mutations may be responsible for the transition of metastatic prostate cancer to hormone independence that results in relapse of metastatic cancer treated with androgen ablation.

Initially studies of the androgen receptor in prostate cancer focused on ligand-binding assays and on measurement of the androgen receptor protein by immunohistochemistry [46–49]. However, it became apparent that deletions of the N-terminus of the androgen receptor could result in a protein devoid of transcriptional activation but capable of high-affinity binding of androgen [50,51]. It was also shown that deletions of the C-terminal steroid-binding domain generated a constitutively active protein without the ability to bind hormone [52]. Therefore, more comprehensive molecular analysis of the androgen receptor was needed and investigators focused on the androgen receptor gene and its mRNA.

Technical considerations in the analysis of androgen receptor in prostate cancer

The discovery and adaptation of the polymerase chain reaction (PCR) has provided a powerful tool for the study of individual genes in human cancer specimens [53]. PCR-based techniques have been used to analyze both androgen receptor DNA and mRNA in prostate tissues. Because PCR is a highly sensitive technique that amplifies specific nucleotide sequences more than a millionfold over all background sequences, it is extremely powerful. However, PCR is also prone to errors introduced by repeated cycles of nucleic acid replication. The enzyme commonly used in PCR reactions, Taq DNA polymerase, has an error rate of approximately 10^{-3} to 10^{-4} nucleotides [54,55]. Therefore, random errors may give false-positive results that suggest the presence of a mutation in the androgen receptor in a fraction of cells.

Analysis of RNA is subject to an even greater error rate. It is attractive to analyze RNA since androgen receptor RNA contains 2.8 kb of coding nucleotides that can be analyzed in one or two PCR reactions, whereas PCR analysis of DNA requires separate PCR reactions of many or most exons. However, mRNA must first be copied into cDNA using reverse transcriptase (RT). Reverse transcriptase copies a DNA strand from an RNA template and during this polymerization has an error rate of 10^{-2} to 10^{-3} nucleotides [56,57]. Although RT introduces random errors in cDNA that can be discerned by careful analysis of multiple PCR reactions, one must always be alert to the possible artifacts introduced into sequence analyses after PCR amplification of a nucleic acid target. Lastly, PCR reactions are so sensitive that minute amounts of contaminating DNA can result in a false-positive result in a sample. For example, if a laboratory used a DNA sample with a known androgen receptor mutation as a positive control and then began to find similar mutations in tumor specimens, there would have to be a high degree of suspicion that coincident mutations in fact resulted from contamination from the control specimen somewhere in the PCR reaction. Therefore, reports of identical mutations found in multiple tissue samples must be scrutinized carefully for the inclusion of appropriate controls and should be confirmed by independent laboratories.

Androgen receptor mutations in primary prostate cancer specimens

The incentive to screen prostate cancer specimens for androgen receptor mutations came from the discovery that the LNCaP human prostate cancer cell line contained a Thr→Ala mutation at codon 877 in the hormone-binding domain of the androgen receptor [36]. Moreover, this mutation altered the response of these cells to the antiandrogen flutamide, which is an androgen receptor agonistic in LNCaP cells [35,36]. It is impossible to determine whether this mutation occurred in culture or during treatment of the LNCaP patient with estrogen, resulting in the development of hormone independence. More recently, a hormone-dependent tumor line, CWR22, derived from a prostate cancer xenograft and propagated in immunodeficient mice, has been found to contain an androgen receptor mutation at codon 874, His→Tyr [58,59]. When the 874 mutant receptor was tested in reporter gene assays, it was found to have an enhanced response of transcriptional activation induced by dihydrotestosterone, an augmented response to dehydroepiandrosterone (DHEA), and agonistic responses to estradiol and hydroxyflutamide [French and Moeller, personal communication]. It also cannot be determined with certainty if this mutation was present in the original material obtained from the patient; however, it was detected in the original CWR22 xenograft tumor.

The first mutational analysis of androgen receptor in primary prostate cancer specimens was published in 1992 [60]. This study focused on exons 5–8, which were first analyzed by denaturing gradient gel electrophoresis (DGGE), which was used to identify abnormal exons for nucleotide sequence analysis. It is possible that the frequency of mutations was understimated by this study because PCR-amplified exons that did not demonstrate aberrant gel migration were not sequenced. Moreover, the DGGE technique was shown to be sensitive to the level of 10%. Any mutations present in fewer than 10% of the cells analyzed would not have been detected. This study reported no androgen receptor mutations in three established prostate cancer cell lines—DU-145, PC-3, and Tsu-Pr1—and in two hormone-independent samples taken from transurethral resections. One of 26 stage B prostate cancers was found to have a Val→Met at 730, a region important for binding to ligand and to heat shock protein 90 [51,52].

Suzuki et al. reported their analysis of androgen receptors in primary and hormone-independent prostate cancer [61]. They used PCR to amplify exons 2–8 of the androgen receptor and to identify putative mutant exons by single-strand conformational polymorphism analysis (SSCP). As with DGGE, exon fragments that did not have aberrant migration in the gel analysis were scored as not having mutations. They found no mutations in seven cases of stage B prostate cancer. In 1 of 8 patients with hormone-independent prostate cancer, they found two separate mutations. The patient's cancerous prostate had a codon 701, Leu→His, mutation. Three separate metastatic sites contained a single mutation that differed from the primary lesion. The metastases all had a codon 877, Thr→Ala, mutation, identical to the mutation in LNCaP. It is noteworthy that LNCaP cell DNA was analyzed simultaneously with the prostatic tissues. It is possible that contamination explained the presence of two separate mutations in the same patient. It is also possible that recurrent tumor in both the prostate and at metastatic sites developed androgen receptor mutations independently during later stages of the disease. However, if three separate metastatic sites all developed the identical codon 877 mutation, as was described by Suzuki et al., one is prompted to conclude that the 877 mutation confers a growth advantage to hormone-independent prostate cancer.

Analysis of another seven specimens from patients with metastatic prostate cancer, four of whom had hormone-independent disease, was added to the literature by Culig et al. [62]. They performed direct sequencing of cDNA transcribed from mRNA extracted from tissues. In one patient with hormone-independent disease, they found a somatic point mutation that caused a Val→Met at position 715. To confirm that this mutation was not the result of a reverse transcription artifact, they investigators repeated the synthesis a second time with *Pyrococcus furiosus* (Pfu) polymerase, which has a proofreading activity. The mutant receptor had similar binding activity to wild-type receptor for a wide range of steroids and nonsteroidal antiandrogens. However, the mutant androgen receptor was found to be functionally different from the wild type in reporter gene assays in which transcriptional activation by progesterone and by androstenedione were enhanced by the codon 715 mutation. This finding was consistent with the premise that androgen receptor mutations conferred some growth advantage to hormone-independent prostate cancer cells. de Winter et al. searched for mutations in exons 2–8 by SSCP analysis of 27 prostate cancer specimens, of which 18 were from patients with hormone-independent metastatic disease [63]. They found no evidence of androgen receptor mutations in these samples. Sharief et al. found a silent mutation at codon 800 (C→T), in one of 22 specimens of hormone-independent prostate cancer and a 877 (Thr→Ala) mutation in a second case [59 and French, personal communication].

The studies described thus far have found a low incidence of somatic androgen receptor mutations in prostate cancer. Because prostate cancer tissue is very heterogeneous and may be made up of predominantly nonmalignant stromal elements, mutations that are present in a subpopulation of tumor cells that represented less than 5% of a specimen cellularity may not have been detected. Taplin and coworkers analyzed bone marrow biopsies of prostate cancer patients for the expression of androgen receptor mRNA by RT-PCR [64]. Patients with metastatic prostate cancer had detectable androgen receptor message in bone marrow taken from sites of known metastases. Although androgen receptor mRNA could be detected in blood samples from normal individuals, it could not be detected in patients who were orchiectomized, had low PSA, and had no bone marrow involvement with prostate cancer [65 and Bubley, personal communication]. They concluded that the androgen receptor mRNA detected by RT-PCR of bone marrow came from metastatic prostate cancer. To address the question of sequencing artifacts introduced by PCR, Taplin and coworkers cloned several independent cDNA fragments and sequenced many receptor clones from each patient. They found a wide scattering of mutations that differed between the clones, but in 5 of 10 patients they found mutations that were present in every clone sequenced. This tedious, but rigorous, approach demonstrated that androgen receptor mutations could be detected in the metastases above a background of sequence errors that were randomly introduced into cDNA transcripts by RT-PCR.

Taplin also found that some metastatic sites contained androgen receptor mutations, whereas the primary tumor samples from the same patient did not. Four mutations found by Taplin included 877 Thr→Ser, 874 His→Tyr, 902 Gln→Arg, and 721 Ala→Thr. A fifth patient had four mutations in the androgen receptor. The 877 and the 874 mutations were compared with wild-type receptor for transcriptional activation in a reporter gene assay. Both estradiol and progesterone activated the mutant receptors but failed to activate the wild-type receptor. This result was consistent with selection for mutations that confer a growth advantage by interactions with other steroid hormones. Another study of androgen receptor in bone metastases from hormone-refractory patients found a somewhat lower frequency of mutations than Taplin et al. Kleinerman et al. described an analysis of five specimens by SSCP analysis of PCR-amplified exons 2–8. They found an exon 8 mutation in one patient [66].

Other investigators have found a more prevalent occurrence of androgen receptor mutations in hormone-independent prostate cancer. Gaddipati et al. performed direct DNA sequencing of PCR-amplified exons 4–8 from 24 specimens [67]. In six samples they found the identical ACT→GCT, Thr→Ala, mutation at codon 877, which is the same mutation that was described in LNCaP cells. Although the investigators performed many experiments to rule out the possibility that their data reflected an artifact of DNA contamination, their data differ from what others have reported it later appeared that the finding resulted from the contamination of the PCR reaction. (Srivastava, personel communication)

Tilley and his coworkers have also found a somewhat higher incidence of androgen receptor gene mutations than have other investigators [68,69]. They analyzed 25 primary prostate cancer specimens, of which 9 specimens were from locally advanced disease and 16 specimens were from patients with metastatic disease (stage D_2). However, none of the patients had begun hormonal therapy. Tilley selected tissue samples carefully by first performing immunostaining with antibodies specific for the amino- or carboxy-termini of the androgen receptor. Areas that had disproportionate staining with the two antibodies were identified and were attributed to possible structural changes in the androgen receptor [70]. Androgen receptor coding sequences were analyzed by SSCP, and individual clones of abnormal SSCP fragments were sequenced in two directions. Single base changes resulting in amino acid changes were seen in 11 (44%) of the samples. Five tumors contained point mutations in more than one exon. The mutations he found are all those including and to the left of the 670, Ile→Thr in the lower panel of Figure 12–2 (see later) plus a 889, Phe→Leu, 828 Leu→Pro, 789 Ser→Pro, and 794 Trp→Stop. This last mutation is the only one in Tilley's series that results in a premature termination codon and has been reported previously in a patient with complete androgen insensitivity [71].

Androgen receptor mutations have been compared in tissues from Japanese and American men. American men have an eightfold higher incidence of prostate cancer than do Japanese men living in Japan. Takahashi et al. studied differences between the two populations in both clinical and latent prostate cancer [72]. They analyzed

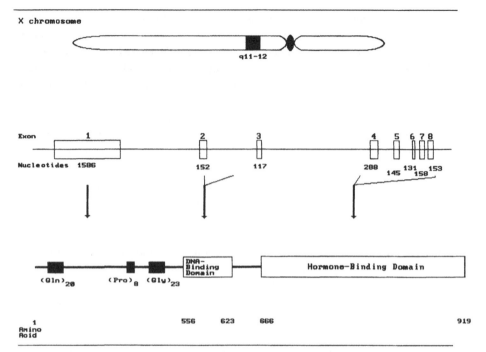

Figure 12-2. *A*: Schematic drawing of the androgen receptor protein on which are indicated all of the published point mutations associated with androgen insensitivity syndromes. On the upper part of panel A are the locations of mutations causing the complete androgen insensitivity syndrome. The lower portion shows the mutations that have been associated with the partial androgen insensitivity syndrome. The different heights of the indicator lines are proportional to the number of mutations (one, two, or three) reported at each amino acid locus. *B*: Location and amino acid substitutions of all of the androgen receptor mutations reported in prostate cancer samples and cited in the text and in Table 1. One-letter amino acid abbreviations indicate the wild-type amino acid on the left of the amino acid number and the mutant amino acid on the right of the amino acid number. Each locus has had only one mutation associated with it, except locus 877, which has had two separate mutations identified in prostate cancer tissues. All amino acid numbers conform to a 919-amino acid protein [42].

exons 2–8 by SSCP and then sequenced DNA from pooled clones of isolated PCR–amplified fragments that gave aberrant results by SSCP analysis. No mutations were found in 64 total cancer samples from both populations. In latent prostate cancer samples, 0 of 43 samples from Americans had mutations and 18 of 79 samples from Japanese men had mutations. The majority of the mutations introduced stop codons and frame shifts in exons 2 and 5, suggesting that they may have resulted in inactivation or attenuation of androgen receptor function. Eight of 18 samples had nonsense mutations or single nucleotide deletions resulting in frame shifts. Of the 10 missense mutations, the majority were in the regions mutated in androgen insensitivity syndromes. These data suggested that latent prostate cancers in Japanese do not progress to clinical cancer in part because androgen-mediated tumor promotion is blocked by inactivation of the androgen receptor. Moreover, of 38 primary prostate cancers from Japanese men, none had detectable androgen receptor mutations. This confirmed that the clinical cancers were susceptible to tumor promotion by androgens.

The data on the incidence of androgen receptor mutations in prostate cancer are summarized in Table 12–1. Except for the reports from Tilley and coworkers, only one other androgen receptor mutation was found in hormone-responsive prostate cancer by other investigators. Because of the heterogeneity of prostate cancer tissues, it is possible that more sensitive techniques or more extensive studies with samples from microdissection may yield a higher percentage of androgen receptor mutations in hormone-dependent disease.

The data on location of androgen receptor point mutations in prostate cancer are summarized in Figure 12–2. The upper panel of Figure 12–2 shows a map of the known point mutations in complete and partial androgen insensitivity syndromes [adapted from 73 and 74]. Mutations are clustered in three regions of the hormone-binding domain. The loci of mutations in prostate cancers are shown in the lower part of the figure. The prostate cancer mutations appear to cluster at the 5′ and 3′ ends of the hormone-binding domain. The limited information available on androgen receptor mutations in prostate cancer suggests that they alter the response of the receptor by sensitizing it to other steroids and nonsteroidal antiandrogens. The androgen insensitivity syndrome mutations are widely distributed throughout the hormone-binding domain and attenuate or abrogate receptor activity. Although some of the mutations in the cancers are at identical sites as the androgen-insensitivity lesions, the clustering of the prostate cancer mutations suggests that there are certain regions of the hormone-binding domain that are targets for mutations that alter receptor response to heterologous molecules.

Results from several laboratories showed that at the current levels of detection,

Table 12–1. Frequency of androgen receptor point mutations in prostate cancer

Reference	Primary prostate cancer	Hormone-independent prostate cancer
Newmark et al. [60]	1/26	0/2
Suzuki et al. [61]	0/7	1/8
Culig et al. [62]	0/3	1/4
de Winter et al. [63]	0/9	0/18
Taplin et al. [64]		5/10
Tilley et al. [68,69 and personal communication]	11/25	
Kleinerman et al. [66]		1/5
Sharief et al. [59]		1/22
Trapman et al. [43]		0/30
Takahashi et al. [72]	0/64	
Total	12/134	9/123

The fractions represent patient specimens that contained one or more mutations in the androgen receptor/total number of patient specimens tested.

10–20% of hormone-refractory cancers have androgen receptor mutations. Two reports suggested that a higher fraction of cancers have androgen receptor mutations. Since androgen receptor mutations may be responsible for aberrant clinical responses to antiandrogens and to other steroid hormones, a 40% rate of androgen receptor mutations would reflect a 40% frequency of response to flutamide withdrawal, as reported by Scher and Kelly [37]. Patients may also have androgen receptor amplification, as suggested by Visakorpi et al., who found amplification in 7 of 23 specimens [75]. Although one could argue that overexpression of the androgen receptor could result in both androgen independence and an aberrant response to steroids, it does not explain the phenomenon of the flutamide-withdrawal response. Moreover, immunohistochemical staining of prostate tissues for androgen receptor have shown general heterogeneity and have been difficult to correlate with tumor stage or progression [16–20]. Since it does not appear that androgen receptor amplification is manifest as a high level of receptor expression, amplification may facilitate the occurrence of androgen receptor mutations. On the other hand, amplification may result in sufficient activation of the androgen receptor to facilitate a response to residual androgens in orchiectomized patients.

Structural considerations regarding exon 1

The androgen receptor contains two nucleotide repeat regions of variable length in exon 1. The more 5′ of these regions contains 11–31 CAG repeats that code for a glutamine repeat. The second is a region of 16–27 GGC codons that code for a glycine repeat. The CAG repeat in the androgen receptor has pathogenic significance, since it is expanded to 40–52 units in patients with X-linked bulbar muscular atrophy [76]. The glutamine and glycine codon repeats have been studied in prostate cancer. Schoenberg et al. found a contraction of the glutamine repeat from 24 to 18 in prostate cancer tissue in 1 of 40 samples [77]. The remainder of the androgen receptor sequence in the tumor tissue was identical to wild-type DNA. This patient was described clinically as having had an agonistic response to flutamide, but the tissue sequencing was done on material from the primary resection and the flutamide agonism was observed more than 4 years after the patient had recurred and had been treated with androgen ablation.

Irvine et al. suggested that there was some disequilibrium in the combination of CAG and GGC repeats in prostate cancer patients [78]. Of the prostate cancer cases analyzed, relatively few of those with longer CAG alleles also had long GGC alleles. However, the number of cases analyzed was small. Moreover, no functional differences of the androgen receptor have been demonstrated to derive from what may be small changes in glutamine and glycine repeat numbers. Scher et al. found no relationship between the CAG repeat length and prostate cancer stage [79].

The lengths of CAG and GGC repeats have been analyzed in larger populations of different racial groups. There appear to be one to two codon differences in the modal repeat lengths found in different races [Danielson, personal communication]. The physiologic significance of these differences is unknown.

CONCLUSIONS

Androgen receptor mutations are currently found in 10% of prostate cancer specimens, more commonly in samples from metastases. It is possible that techniques that enrich for cancer cells in a heterogeneous cell population, such as microdissection, or that amplify cancer-specific nucleic acids, such as androgen receptor mRNA in bone marrow [64], will allow the detection of a higher percentage of mutations in hormone-independent cancer. This author would predict that hormone-independent prostate cancers eventually will be found to have a nearly 50% incidence of androgen receptor mutations. This is based on the results of some investigators cited in this review and also on the clinical observations that approximately 40% of patients on flutamide will have at least a fall in serum PSA levels after flutamide therapy is stopped [37]. A small number of patients will have very dramatic remissions from flutamide withdrawal [37]. It will be important to see if those patients have androgen receptor mutations at specific codons that confer the greatest agonistic response to flutamide.

Response to flutamide, or soon to bicalutamide [80], which has been recently released for sale in the U.S., is not the only important clinical factor for the application androgen receptor structural data. Clinical anecdotes abound on responses of prostate cancer to second-line hormonal therapies, such as corticosteroids, and to adrenal antagonists, such as aminoglutethimide. Some of the mutant androgen receptors already described have been shown to have a more profound activation by adrenal androgens than by hydroxyflutamide. Sartor and colleagues have observed that patients treated with flutamide withdrawal plus aminoglutethimide may have substantial clinical remissions of recurrent prostate cancer [81]. The polyphosphonated naphthylurea suramin has been shown to have occasional activity in hormone-refractory prostate cancer. Suramin's mechanism of action has been postulated to be via binding of peptide ligands of growth factor receptors, thereby inhibiting cell growth [82]. However, since suramin has known adrenal toxicity and is always administered with hydrocortisone supplementation, it is possible that inhibition of adrenal androgen secretion is responsible for the clinical activity of suramin in prostate cancers that have mutant androgen receptors with increased sensitivity to adrenal androgens.

It is more difficult to find a clinical context for androgen receptor amplification in prostate cancer described by Visakorpi et al. [75]. No one has yet shown that androgen receptor expression increases in advanced prostate cancer, nor is there evidence of enhanced androgen binding activity in advanced cancer tissues. It is unclear how an increase in androgen receptor levels would be reflected as androgen independence in advance prostate cancer. One would have to speculate that high intracellular levels of androgen receptor were able to mimic the effects of hormone-bound receptors. It is possible that androgen receptor gene amplification does not result in elevated expression of androgen receptors. In this case we would have yet to understand the effect of androgen receptor gene amplification on the phenotype of prostate cancer.

The results of Takahashi provide great insight into the differences between prostate carcinogenesis in Japan and the United States [72]. These investigators are to be credited with careful analysis of pathologically distinct latent and clinical prostate cancer. There is an 8- to 10-fold difference in the incidence of prostate cancer between Japanese men living in Japan and American men in the United States. Since Japanese who migrated to Hawaii were diagnosed with prostate cancer at a rate that approached that of Caucasians in the United States, it has been assumed that dietary and environmental factors played the major role in prostate carcinogenesis in the United States [83,84]. Now it appears that a significant fraction of latent prostate cancers in Japan have somatic androgen receptor mutations that attenuate androgen activation of receptor. The mechanism for the induction of androgen receptor mutations in latent prostate cancer of Japanese remains to be understood. However, if the result is confirmed, it can be concluded that differences in prostate cancer incidence between Japan and the United States are explained in part by androgen insensitivity of latent prostate cancer in Japan.

Data accumulated during the past 3 years have disclosed important observations about the androgen receptor in prostate cancer. More specific analysis of cancer cells and more extensive series will have to be reported before we know how prevalent androgen receptor mutations are in different phases of prostate cancer. Since mutations appear to cluster at functionally important codons of the androgen receptor, a more detailed understanding of the changes that result from these mutations may bring insight to the design of new androgen agonists and antagonists. Lastly, the implication that prostate-specific androgen insensitivity resulting from somatic mutations in latent prostate cancer is protective against the development of clinical prostate cancer gives further impetus to research in prostate cancer prevention based on androgen antagonists.

ACKNOWLEDGMENTS

I am grateful to colleagues who generously shared unpublished data with me, including Wayne Tilley, Mary-Ellen Taplin, Glenn Bubley, Steve Balk, Frank French, and Mark Danielson. Frank French, Wayne Tilley, Glenn Bubley, and Mary-Ellen Taplin provided helpful comments after critical review of the manuscript. This work was supported, in part, by grant CA57178 from the NCI and by a grant from the CaPCURE Foundation.

REFERENCES

1. Wingo PR, Tong T, Bolden S (1995) Cancer statistics, 1995. CA Cancer J Clin 45:8–30.
2. Griffin JE (1992) Androgen resistance—the clinical and molecular spectrum. N Engl J Med 326:611–618.
3. Kyprianou N, Isaacs JT (1988) Activation of programmed cell death in the rat ventral prostate after castration. Endocrinology 122:552–562.
4. Deaver JB (1922) Enlargement of the prostate: Its history, anatomy, etiology, pathology, clinical causes, symtpoms diagnosis, prognosis, treatment, technique of operations and after-treatment.
5. Pollard M, Luckert PH (1986) Production of autochthonous prostate cancer in Lobund-Wistar rats: By treatments with N-nitroso-N-methylurea and testosterone. J Natl Cancer Inst 77:583–587.

6. Pollard M, Luckert PH (1987) Autochthonous prostate cancer in Lobund-Wistar rats: A model system. Prostate 11:219–227.
7. Ghanadian R, Puah CM, O'Donoghue EPN (1979) Serum testosterone and dihydrotestosterone in carcinoma of the prostate. Br J Cancer 39:696–699.
8. Ahluwalia B, Jackson MA, Jones GW, et al. (1981) Blood hormone profiles in prostate cancer patients in high risk and low risk populations. Cancer 48:2267–2273.
9. Drafta D, Proca E, Zamfir V, et al. (1982) Plasma steroids in benign prostatic hypertrophy and carcinoma of the prostate. J Steroid Biochem 17:689–693.
10. Zumoff B, Levin J, Strain GW, et al. (1985) Abnormal levels of plasma hormones in men with prostate cancer: Evidence toward a "two-disease" theory. Prostate 3:579–588.
11. Nomura A, Heilbrun LK, Stemmermann GN, Judd HL (1988) Prediagnostic serum hormones and the risk of prostate cancer. Cancer Res 48:3515–3517.
12. Huggins C, Hodges CV (1941) Studies on prostatic cancer; effect of castration, of estrogen and of androgen injection on serum phosphatases in metastatic carcinoma of the prostate. Cancer Res 1:293–297.
13. Huggins C, Stevens RE, Hodges CL (1941) Studies on prostatic cancer II. The effect of castration on clinical patients with carcinoma of the prostate. Arch Surg 43:209.
14. Fisher B, Redmond C, Brown A and NSABP investigators (1983) Influences of tumor estrogen and progesterone receptor levels on the responses to tamoxifen and chemotherapy in primary breast cancer. J Clin Oncol 1:227–241.
15. Sadi MV, Walsh PC, Barrack ER (1991) Immunohistochemical study of androgen receptors in metastatic prostate cancer. Cancer 67:3057–3064.
16. Trachtenberg J, Walsh PC (1982) Correlation of prostatic nuclear androgen receptor content with duration of response and survival following hormonal therapy in advanced prostatic cancer. J Urol 127:466.
17. Gonor SE, Lakey WH, McBlain WA (1984) Relationship between concentrations of extractable and matrix-bound nuclear androgen receptor and clinical response to endocrine therapy for prostatic adenocarcinoma. J Urol 131:1196.
18. Benson RC, Gorman PA, O'Brien PC, Holicky EL, Veneziale CM (1987) Relationship between androgen receptor binding activity in human prostate cancer and clinical response to endocrine therapy. Cancer 59:1599.
19. Rennie PS, Bruchovsky N, Goldenberg SL (1988) Relationship of androgen receptors to the growth and regression of the prostate. Am J Clin Oncol 11(Suppl 2):S13.
20. Castellanos JM, Galan A, Calvo MA, Schwartz S (1982) Predicting response of prostatic cancer to endocrine therapy. Lancet 1:448.
21. Prout GR (1976) Endocrine changes after diethylstilbestrol therapy: Effect on prostatic neoplasm and pituitary gonadal axis. Urology 7:148.
22. The Leuprolide Study Group (1984) Leuprolide versus diethylstilbestrol for metastatic prostate cancer. N Engl J Med 311:1281–1286.
23. Labrie F, Dupong A, Belanger A, et al. (1983) New approach in the treatment of prostate cancer: Complete instead of partial withdrawal of androgens. Prostate 4:579–594.
24. Crawford ED, Eisenberger M, McCleod DG, Spaulding JT, Benson R, Dorr FA, Blumenstein BA, Goodman PJ (1989) A controlled trial of leuprolide with and without flutamide in prostatic carcinoma. N Engl J Med 321:419–424.
25. Iversen P, Christensen MG, Friis E, Hornbil P, Hvidt V, Iversen HG, Klaskov P, et al. (1990) A phase III trial of zoladex and flutamide versus orchiectomy in the treatment of patients with advanced carcinoma of the prostate. Cancer 66(Suppl):1058–1066.
26. Newling D, Pavone Macaluse M, Smith P, de Voogt HJ, Robinson MR, Schroder FH, Denis L, Sylveser R (1992) Update of EORTC clinical trials in prostate cancer. The EORTC Genito-Urinary Group. Semin Urol 10:65–71.
27. van Tinteren H, Dalesio O (1993) Systemic overview (metaanalysis) of all randomized trials of treatment of prostate cancer. Cancer 72:3847–3850.
28. Soloway MS, Sharifi R, Wood D, Wajsman Z, McLeod D, Puras A (1995) Randomized comparison of radical prostatectomy alone or preceded by androgen deprivation for cT2b prostate cancer. Proc Am Soc Clin Oncol 14:abstract 644.
29. Pilepich MV, Caplan R, Byhardt RW, Lawton CA, Gallagher MJ, Mesic JB, Hanks GE, Coughlin CT, Porter A (1995) Phase III trial of androgen suppression using goserelin in unfavorable prognosis carcinoma of the prostate treated with definitive radiotherapy (report of RTOG protocol 85-31). Proc Am Soc Clin Oncol 14:abstract 631.

30. Hockenbery D, Nunez G, Milliman C, Schreiber RD, Korsmeyer SJ (1990) Bcl-2 is an inner mitochondrial membrane protein that blocks programmed cell death. Nature 348:334–336.

31. Miyashita T, Reed JC (1993) Bcl-2 oncoprotein blocks chemotherapy-induced apoptosis in a human leukemia cell line. Blood 81:151–157.

32. Kamesaki S, Kamesaki H, Jorgensen TJ, Tanizawa A, Pommier Y, Cossman J (199•) Bcl-2 protein inhibits etoposide-induced apoptosis through its effects on events subsequent to topoisomerase II-induced DNA strand breaks and their repair. SI-MEDL/93373309. Cancer Res 53:••–••.

33. Berchem G, Bosseler M, Sugars LY, Voeller HJ, Zeitlin S, Gelmann EP (1995) Androgens induce resistance to bcl-2-mediated apoptosis in LNCaP prostate cancer cells. Cancer Res 55:735–738.

34. Brown CJ, Goss SJ, Lubahn DB, Joseph DR, Wilson EM, French FS, Willard HF (1989) Androgen receptor locus on the human X chromosome: Regional localization to Xq11-12 and description of a DNA polymorphism. Am J Hum Genet 44:264–269.

35. Wilding G, Chen M, Gelmann EP (1989) Aberrant response in vitro of hormone-responsive prostate cancer cells to antiandrogens. Prostate 14:103–115.

36. Veldscholte J, Ris-Stalper C, Kuiper GGJM (1990) A mutation in the ligand binding domain of the androgen receptor of human LNCaP cells affects steroid binding characteristics and response to anti-androgens. Biochem Biophys Res Commun 173:534–540.

37. Scher HI, Kelly WK (1993) Flutamide withdrawal syndrome: Its impact on clinical trials in hormone-refractory prostate cancer. J Clin Oncol 11:1566–1572.

38. Evans RM (1988) The steroid and thyroid hormone receptor superfamily. Science 240:889–895.

39. O'Malley B (1990) The steroid receptor superfamily: More excitement predicted for the future. Mol Endocrinol 4:363–369.

40. Wahli W, Martinez E (1991) Superfamily of steroid nuclear receptors: Positive and negative regulators of gene expression. FASEB J 5:2243–2249.

41. Kuiper GGJM, Faber TW, van Rooij HC, van der Korput JA, Ris-Stalpers C, Klaassen P, Trapman J, Brinkmann AO (1989) Structural organization of the human androgen receptor gene. J Mol Endoc 2:R1–R4.

42. Lubahn DB, Joseph DR, Sarrinol M, Tan J, Higgs H, Larson RE, French FS, Wilson EM (1988) The human androgen receptor: Complementary deoxyribonucleic acid cloning, sequence analysis and gene expression in prostate. Mol Endocrinol 2:1265–1275.

43. Trapman J, Klaasen P, Kuiper GJ (1988) Cloning, structure and expression of a cDNA encoding the human androgen receptor. Biochem Biophys Res Commun 153:241–248.

44. Luisi BF, Xu WX, Otwinowski Z (1991) Crystallographic analysis of the interaction of the glucocorticoid receptor with DNA. Nature 352:497–505.

45. Hard T, Kellenbach E, Boelens R (1990) Solution structure of the glucocorticoid receptor DNA-binding domain. Science 249:157–160.

46. Ekman P, Snochowski M, Zetterberg A, Hogberg B, Gustafsson JA (1979) Steroid receptor content in human prostatic carcinoma and response to endocrine therapy. Cancer 44:1173.

47. Fentie DD, Lakey WH, McBlain WA (1986) Applicability of nuclear androgen receptor quantification to human prostatic adenocarcinoma. J Urol 135:167.

48. Takeda H, Chodak G, Mutchnik S, Nakamoto T, Chang C (1990) Immunohistochemical localization of androgen receptors with mono- and polyclonal antibodies to androgen receptor. J Endocrinol 126:17.

49. Chodak GW, Kranc DM, Puy LA, Takeda H, Johnson K, Chang C (1992) Nuclear localization of androgen receptor in heterogeneous samples of normal, hyperplastic, and neoplastic human prostate. J Urol 147:798–803.

50. Jenster G, van der Korput HAGM, van Vroonhoven C (1991) Domains of the human androgen receptor involved in steroid binding, transcriptional activation and subcellular localization. Mol Endocrinol 5:1396–1404.

51. Simental JA, Sar M, Lane MV (1991) Transcriptional activation and nuclear targeting signals of the human androgen receptor. J Biol Chem 266:510–518.

52. Danielian PS, White R, Lees JA, Parker MG (1992) Identification of a conserved region required for hormone dependent transcriptional activation by steroid hormone receptors. EMBO J 11:1025–1933.

53. Mullis KB, Faloona FA (1987) Specific synthesis of DNA in vitro via a polymerase chain reaction. Methods Enzymol 155:335–351.

54. Brail L, Fan E, Levin DB, Logan DM (1993) Improved polymerase fidelity in PCR-SSCPA. Mutat Res 303:171–175.

55. Goodman MR, Creighton S, Bloom LB, Petruska J (1993) Biochemical basis of DNA replication fidelity. Crit Rev Biochem Mol Biol 28:83–126.
56. Sooknanan R, Howes M, Read L, Malek LT (1994) Fidelity of nucleic acid amplification with avian myeloblastosis virus reverse transcriptase and T7 RNA polymerase. Biotechniques 17:1077–1080, 1083–1085.
57. Bakhanashvili M, Hizi A (1992) Fidelity of the RNA-dependent DNA synthesis exhibited by the reverse transcriptases of human immunodeficiency virus types 1 and 2 and of murine leukemia virus; mispair extension frequencies. Biochemistry 31:9393–9398.
58. Wainstein MA, He F, Robinson D, Kung HJ, Schwartz S, Giaconia JM, Edgehouse NL, Pretlow TP, Bodner DR, Kursh ED (1994) CWR22: Androgen-dependent xenograft model derived from a primary human prostatic carcinoma. Cancer Res 54:6049–6052.
59. Sharief Y, Wilson EM, Hall SM, Hamil KG, Tan J-A, French FS, Mohler JL (1995) Adrogen receptor gene mutations associated with prostatic carcinoma. Proc Amer Assoc Cancer Res 36:A160S.
60. Newmark JR, Hardy DO, Tonb DC (1992) Androgen receptor gene mutations in human prostate cancer. Proc Natl Acad Sci USA 89:6319–6323.
61. Suzuki H, Sato N, Watabe Y, Masai M, Seino S, Shimazaki J (1993) Androgen receptor gene mutations in human prostate cancer. J Steroid Biochem Mol Biol 46:759–765.
62. Culig Z, Hobisch A, Cronauer MV, Cato ACB, Hittmair A, Radmayr C, Eberle J, Bartsch G, Klocker H (1993) Mutant androgen receptor detected in an advanced-stage prostatic carcinoma is activated by adrenal androgens and progesterone. Mol Endocrinol 0888-8809:1541–1550.
63. de Winter JAR, Janssen PJA, Sleddens HMEB, Verleun-Mooijman MCT, Trapman J, Brinkmann AO, Santerse AB, Schroder FH, van der Kwast TH (1994) Androgen receptor status in localized and locally progressive hormone refractory human prostate cancer. Am J Pathol 144:735–746.
64. Taplin ME, Bubley GJ, Shuster TD, Frantz ME, Spooner AE, Ogata GK, Keer HN, Balk SP (199•) Mutation of the androgen-receptor gene in metastatic androgen-independent prostate cancer. N Engl J Med 332:1393–1398.
65. Quarmby VE, Yarbrough WG, Lubahn DB, French FS, Wilson EM (1990) Autologous down-regulation of androgen receptor messenger ribonucleic acid. Mol Endocrinol 4:22–28.
66. Kleinerman DI, Troncoso P, Pisters LL, Sleddens HMEB, Navone NM, Ordonez NG, van der Kwast TH, Schroeder FH, Brinkmann AO, Logothetis CJ, Hsieh J-T, von Eschenbach AC, Trapman J (1994) Evaluation of androgen receptor expression and structure in bone metastases of prostate carcinoma. Basic Clin Aspects Prostate Cancer A-22.
67. Gaddipati JP, McLeod DG, Heidenberg HB, Sesterhenn IA, Finger J, Moul JW, Srivastava S (1994) Frequent detection of codon 877 mutation in the androgen receptor gene in advanced prostate cancers. Cancer Res 54:2861–2864.
68. Tilley WD, Buchanan G, Hickey TE, Horsfall DJ (1995) Detection of androgen receptor mutations in human prostate cancers by immunohistochemistry and SSCP. Proc Am Assoc Cancer Res 36:abstract 1586.
69. Tilley WD, Buchanan G, Hickey TE, Bentel JM (1996) Mutations in the androgen receptor gene are associated with progression of human prostate cancer to androgen independence. Clin Cancer Res 2:277–285.
70. Tilley WD, Lim-Tio SS, Horsfall DJ, Aspinall JO, Marshall VR, Skinner JM (1994) Detection of discrete androgen receptor epitopes in prostate cancer by immunostaining: Measurement by color video image analysis. Cancer Res 54:4096–4102.
71. Marcelli M, Tilley WD, Wilson CM (1990) A single nucleotide substitution introduces a premature termination codon into the androgen receptor gene of a patient with receptor-negative androgen resistance. J Clin Invest 85:1522–1528.
72. Takahashi H, Furusato M, Allsbrook WC, Nishii H, Wakui S, Barrett JC, Boyd J (1995) Prevalence of androgen receptor gene mutations in latent prostatic carcinomas from Japanese men. Cancer Res 55:1621–1624.
73. Sultan C, Lumbroso S, Poujol N, Belon C, Boudon C, Lobaccaro JM (1993) Mutations of androgen receptor gene in androgen insensitivity syndromes. J Steroid Biochem Mol Biol 46:519–530.
74. Hiipakka RA, Liao S (1995) Androgen receptors and action. In L DeGroot, ed. Endocrinology. Philadelphia: WB Saunders, pp 2336–2350.
75. Visakorpi T, Hyytinen E, Koivisto P, Tanner M, Keinanen R, Palmberg C, Palotie A, Tammela T, Isola J, Kallioniemi OP (1995) In vivo amplification of the androgen receptor gene and progression of human prostate cancer. Nature Genet 9:401–406.

76. La Spada AR, Wilson EM, Lubahn DB (1991) Androgen receptor gene mutations in X-linked spinal and bulbar muscular atrophy. Nature 352:77–79.
77. Schoenberg MP, Hakimi JM, Wang S, Bova GS, Epstein JI, Fischbeck KH, Isaacs WB, Walsh PC, Barrack ER (1994) Microsatellite mutation (CAG24-18) in the androgen receptor gene in human prostate cancer. Biochem Biophys Res Commun 198:74–80.
78. Irvine RA, Yu MC, Ross RK, Coetzee GA (1995) The CAG and GGC microsatellites of the androgen receptor gene are in linkage disequilibrium in men with prostate cancer. Cancer Res 55:1937–1940.
79. Scher H, Hardy DO, Bogenreider T, Amsterdam A, Frank S, Zhang Z-F, Catterall J, Nanus D (1995) Androgen receptor CAG repeat length polymorphisms in patients with prostatic cancer: Association with sensitivity to androgen ablation. Proc Am Soc Clin Oncol 14:abstract 602.
80. Vogelzang NJ, Schellhammer PF, Block NL, Jones MS, Kennealey GT (1995) A randomized double-blind trial in 813 previously untreated metastatic prostate cancer patients comparing a new antiandrogen Casodex (bicalutamide) with Eulexin (flutamide) in combination with luteinizing hormone releasing hormone analogue therapy. Proc Am Soc Clin Oncol 14:abstract 642.
81. Sartor O, Cooper M, Weinberger M, Headlee D, Thibault A, Tompkins A, Steinberg S, Figg WD, Linehan WM, Myers CE (1994) Surprising activity of flutamide withdrawal when combined with aminoglutethimide, in treatment of "hormone-refractory" prostate cancer. J Natl Cancer Inst 86:222–227.
82. Myers C, Cooper M, Stein C, LaRocca R, Walther MM, Weiss G, Choykee P, Dawson N, Steinberg S, Uhrich MM, Cassidy J, Kohler DR, Trepel J, Linehan WM (1992) Suramin: A novel growth factor antagonist with activity in hormone-refractory metastatic prostate cancer. J Clin Oncol 10:881–889.
83. Akazaki K, Stemmerman GN (1973) Comparative study of latent carcinoma of the prostates among Japanese in Japan and Hawaii. J Natl Cancer Inst 50:1137–1144.
84. Hanenszel W, Kurihari M (1968) Studies of Japanese migrants: Mortality from cancer and other diseases among Japanese in the United States. J Natl Cancer Inst 40:43–68.

VII. RESISTANCE TO RETINOIDS

13. RETINOIDS IN CLINICAL CANCER THERAPY

JOSEPHIA R.F. MUINDI

CHEMICAL STRUCTURES OF NATURAL AND SYNTHETIC RETINOIDS

Naturally occurring retinoids

Retinoids constitute a class of naturally occurring and synthetic compounds that are structurally related to vitamin A. The chemical structure of retinoids consists of a cyclic end group (trimethylcyclohexenyl ring) and a dimethyl substituted tetraene chain, ending in a polar hydroxyl, aldehyde, or carboxyl group. Naturally occurring retinoids include vitamin A (all-*trans* retinol) and its oxidative metabolites: retinaldehyde, all-*trans*-retinoic acid (tRA), and 13-*cis*-retinoic acid (13-cRA). Four additional naturally occurring retinoids have been newly discovered in the past 5 years: 9-*cis*-retinoic acid (9-cRA) [1,2], 3,4-didehydroretinoic acid [3], 14-hydroxy retro-retinol [4], and more recently, 9-*cis*, 13-*cis*-retinoic acid [5,6]. The potential for the existence of 11-*cis* and 15-*cis*-retinoic acid is very high [7]. Retinoic acid isomers are generated by changes in the position and chemical nature of the double bonds in the tetraene chain (Figure 1). The clinical use of retinoids in oncology has been dominated by tRA, 13-cRA, and more recently 9-cRA, which are the focus of this discussion. Esters of all-*trans* retinol (vitamin A), particularly retinol palmitate, have also been used as cancer chemopreventive or chemotherapeutic agents [8–10] but will not be discussed in this presentation.

Synthetic retinoids

Chemical substitutions and modifications of either the cyclic group and/or the hydrocarbon chain, including the terminal polar groups, have generated a large

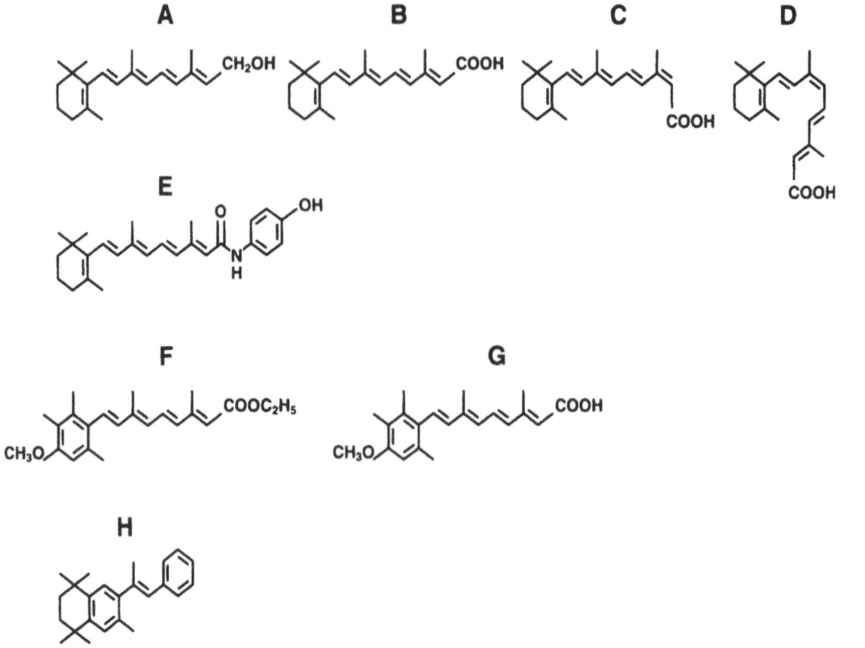

Figure 13–1. Chemical structures of naturally occurring retinoids: All-*trans* retinol (*A*), all-*trans* retinoic acid (*B*), 13-*cis* retinoic acid (*C*), 9-*cis* retinoic acid (*D*), and synthetic retinoids: 4-(N-hydroxyphenyl) retinamide (*E*); aromatic retinoids: etretinate (*F*) and acitretin (*G*); and the arotinoid, temarotene (*H*).

number of synthetic retinoids, which have been clinically evaluated not only as cancer chemotherapeutic and chemopreventive agents but also as therapeutic agents for a variety of human diseases, especially dermatologic disorders [11,12]. Synthetic retinoids have been classified into second (aromatic retinoids) and third generation (arotinoids) based on the part of the chemical structure that is modified. In second generation retinoids, the trimethylcyclohexanyl cyclic ring is replaced by an aromatic ring, while the third generation retinoids contain polyaromatic rings not only in the cyclic head but also in the hydrocarbon chain/polar group. In this classification naturally occurring retinoids belong to the first generation [13]. The only synthetic retinoid in use for the treatment or prevention of cancer in humans is N-(4-hydroxyphenyl)retinamide (4-HPR) (see Figure 13–1) [14]. None of the currently available aromatic retinoids or arotinoids have an established clinical use in the treatment of human malignancies.

SOURCES AND FORMATION OF RETINOIC ACID ISOMERS

Dietary sources

The main source of the dietary retinoids is retinyl esters from animal tissues and carotenoids from vegetables [15]. The beta-carotenoids are oxidatively cleaved at

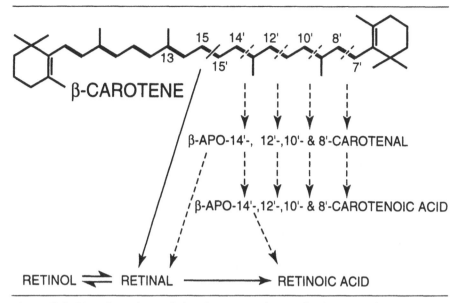

Figure 13–2. Biosynthesis of retinoids from beta-carotene by central and eccentric cleavage mechanism.

either the 15, 15' double bound (central cleavage) or at the terminal double bond of the polyene chain of the beta-carotene (eccentric cleavage) to form retinoids (Figure 13–2). The enzyme, beta-carotene 15, 15' dioxygenase, found in intestinal mucosa and liver, cleaves beta-carotenoids to generate retinaldehydes, which are either reduced to retinol or are further oxidized to retinoic acid [16]. Eccentric cleavage of beta-carotenes generates intermediary apocarotenals, which undergo repeated cycles of oxidative metabolism, similar to fatty acid beta-oxidation, to form retinoic acid [17,18].

Intestinal absorption of retinol is facilitated by special enterocyte cellular retinol binding protein II [CRPB (II)], and the retinol is subsequently esterified in the gastrointestinal mucosal cells [19]. The esterification of retinol is catalyzed by two enzymes: lecithicin retinol acyltransferase (LRAT) and coenzyme A: retinol acyl transferase (ARAT). The retinol–CRBP(II) complex is the preferred substrate for LRAT, while the free retinol in membranes is esterified by ARAT [20,21]. Retinyl esters are transported via the lymphatics and eventually in the blood circulation in the form of chylomicrons. Chylomicron remnants finally deliver retinol esters to the liver parenchymal cells for storage and to other tissues for a variety of physiologic functions. Cellular uptake of chylomicron remnants is mediated via low density lipoprotein receptors. Stored retinol is mobilized by hydrolysis of hepatic esters; the released retinol is carried in circulation bound to specific plasma retinol binding proteins (RBP) to the target cells [22]. Retinoic acid isomers are then synthesized from retinol bound to CRBP(I) in the target cells. CRBPs belong to a superfamily of intracellular protein carriers of hydrophobic ligands that includes cellular retinoic acid binding proteins (CRABPs) and fatty acid binding proteins (FABP).

Carotenoids, particularly the beta-carotenes, exist in *trans*- and several forms of *cis*-isomers depending on the source [23]. The all-*trans* and 13-*cis* isomers account for over 93% and less than 7% of the circulating beta carotenes in humans, respectively, whereas the 9-*cis* isomer is present only in trace amounts [24]. The tissue concentrations of the 9-*cis* isomer are, however, much higher and may reach up to 25% of the total liver beta-carotenes [25]. The natural occurrence of beta-carotene isomers corresponding to the three retinoic acids isomers suggests precursor–product relationship, with the isomerization reaction occurring at either the carotenoid, retinaldehyde, or retinoic acid level. In vitro studies have shown that temperature and light catalyze the interconversion of both beta-carotene and retinoic acid isomers. However, the role of this light- and thermal-dependent isomerization reaction in the whole animal under physiologic conditions remains uncertain. The identification and characterization of retinal isomerase, an enzyme that catalyzes the conversion 11-*cis* to all-*trans* retinal in eye tissues [26,27], suggest that similar enzymatic isomerization reactions may exist in other tissues. Evidence has been reported suggesting that physiologic isomerization of the naturally occurring retinoids takes place at the retinaldehyde level [28,29].

Enzymatic synthesis

Dietary retinoic acid is absorbed from the intestines and transported in the circulation bound to albumin; its cellular uptake is mediated by CRABPs. The contribution and significance of the dietary retinoic acid to cellular retinoic acid pools and function is unknown. It has been suggested that under physiologic conditions, cellular retinoic acid requirements are met by local synthesis from retinol, and probably from beta-carotenes [30–32]. Available experimental data suggest that the retinol–CRPB complex is the preferred substrate for retinoic acid synthesis [33]. Enzymes involved in retinoic acid synthesis from retinol include the cytosolic alcohol dehydrogenases, other unidentified dehydrogenases, and microsomal mixed function oxidase [30,34]. Unlike retinoic acid synthesis mediated by cytosolic NADH-dependent alcohol dehydrogenase, in which no free retinaldehyde is formed, the NADPH-mediated microsomal enzymes generate retinaldehyde, which is further oxidized by cytosolic aldehyde dehydrogenase to retinoic acid [35,36]. However, experimental data indicate that a mixture of cytosolic and microsomal preparations in the presence of NADH and NADPH is six times more efficient at retinoic acid synthesis than the two enzyme systems used separately, suggesting that the two enzymes act synergistically to synthesize retinoic acid. It is not known whether the two enzymatic pathways generate the same or different isomers of retinoic acid.

Oxidative catabolism

Multiple observers have documented that in the presence of NADPH, tRA undergoes progressive oxidative catabolism in microsomes, primarily by cytochrome P-

450–mediated mechanisms, resulting in the sequential formation of 4-hydroxy and 4-oxo retinoic acid and unidentified more polar metabolites. Comparable results have been obtained in microsomes derived from multiple species and tissues, with the highest activity being recorded in the liver and intestines [37–41]. The role of cytochrome P450 in the oxidative catabolism of tRA is supported by increased rates in microsomes derived from experimental animals pretreated with a variety of inducers of different isoforms of cytochrome P450, including ethanol (CYP2E1), dioxin, (CYP1A1 and 1A2), vitamin A (CYP3A2), and phenobarbital (CYP2B4) [42–44]. Furthermore, the oxidative catabolism of tRA in cultured cells and in vivo is inhibited by treatment with ketoconazole and its water-soluble analog, liarozole [45–49]. Ketoconazole and liarazole are known broad inhibitors of cytochrome P-450–mediated reactions, but they also inhibit the 5- and 15-lipoxygenase pathways [50–53]. The importance of the inhibition of lipoxygenase enzymes in cell culture is underscored by the inability of pure cytochrome P450 inhibitors such as triacetyloleandomycin (TAO) and metyrapone to inhibit tRA oxidation [Muindi, unpublished results].

The apparent Km values of cytochrome P-450 enzyme–mediated oxidative metabolism of free tRA, in the presence of traditional cosubstrates of NADPH/(NADH), and molecular oxygen, range from 1 to 24 µM [40,46,54,55]. Since the normal tissue concentrations of tRA range from 40 to 580 pmol/g [30], these Km values may be too high for this enzyme to play significant role in the oxidative catabolism of tRA under physiologic conditions. This has led to the suggestion that the free tRA is not a true substrate, and that other cosubstrates beside reduced pyridines and enzymes other than cytochrome P450 may be involved in the oxidation. Cytochrome P-450 enzymes can also carry out hydroxylation and other oxidative reactions utilizing peroxides, including lipid hydroperoxides (LOOH), through the peroxide shunt. Unlike the NADPH/NADH–mediated reactions. LOOH-mediated oxidations require neither molecular oxygen nor an additional source of electrons [56].

We have recently shown the co-oxidation of tRA by human microsomes genetically enriched with different cytochrome P-450 isoforms in the presence of a variety of LOOH [54]. This rate of tRA co-oxidation is very much faster than that observed with NADPH and is dependent upon the chemical nature of the LOOH used. Lipid hydroperoxides derived from the action of lipoxygenases on arachidonic acid and linolenic acids were particularly efficient in supporting tRA oxidation. Co-oxidation of tRA was observed at submicromolar LOOH concentrations that are potentially achievable in cells. In the presence of LOOH, co-oxidation of tRA has been observed with microsomes genetically enriched with CYP1A1, 1A2, 2B6, 2E1, 2D6, and 3A4 isoforms, indicating the lack of isoform specificity and selectivity of the oxidation, similar to that reported with NADPH as a cosubstrate [57].

Prostaglandin H synthase (PGHS) is another enzyme system that has been shown to co-oxidize tRA and cRA in the presence of LOOH [54,58]. Although, other cellular lipoxygenases might also co-oxidize retinoids, definitive experimental evidence is lacking. The products of tRA co-oxidation by PGHS and cytochrome P-

450 in the presence LOOH are similar to those seen with NADPH; they include polar, 4-oxo- and 4-hydroxy metabolites with trace amounts of 5,6-epoxy retinoic acid [53,57].

There is now strong experimental evidence indicating that tRA bound to CRABP (tRA-CRABP), and not free tRA, is the preferred substrate for cytochrome P450–mediated oxidative catabolism. This conclusion is based on the high affinity of both CRABP(I) and CRABP(II) for the three naturally occurring retinoic acid isomers. Equilibrium dissociation constants for tRA, 9-cRA, and 13-cRA are approximately 10–20 nM, 50–70 nM, and 160–240 nM, respectively [59]. Furthermore, the apparent Km of 1.8 nM for the tRA-CRABP(I) oxidation by testes microsomes is significantly lower than 49 nM for the unbound tRA [60]. To date, no significant difference in the oxidation rates of tRA bound to CRABP(I) and CRABP(II) has been observed. The two CRABPs, however, differ in their tissue distribution: CRABP(I) is predominantly expressed in developing fetal tissues, while CRABP(II) is expressed in adult skin and its expression is modulated by tRA and 9-cRA [61,62]. The two CRABPs also differ in a number of physicochemical properties, including isoelectric point and spectral characteristics [59,60].

The oxidative metabolism of 13-cRA and 9-cRA by isolated microsomal preparations is equally susceptible to cytochrome P450 oxidation. Using NT2/D1 cells that constitutively hypercatabolize tRA, we have observed that tRA is not only oxidized six times faster than 13-cRA but is also sequestered intracellularly, while the bulk of 13-cRA remains outside the cells [Muindi, unpublished observations]. We have attributed these observations to differences in the binding affinity of these isomers to CRABPs. These data are in agreement with the documented physiologic functions of CRABPs, which include modulation of metabolism, facilitation of cellular uptake, sequestration, and intracellular trafficking of various retinoic acid isomers. Overexpression of the CRABP(I) has in the past been shown to sequester and to increase tRA metabolism, resulting in reduced expression of differentiation-specific genes in F9 teratocarcinoma cells [63].

MOLECULAR BIOLOGY OF RETINOIDS

Retinoid signal transduction pathways

The molecular mechanism underlying the multiple biologic effects of both naturally occurring and synthetic retinoids is currently thought to be exerted at the gene transcription level via the retinoid signal transduction pathway [64,65]. There is now indisputable evidence indicating that tRA and 9-cRA are involved in retinoid signal transduction [3,66], although 3,4 didehydroretinoic acid may also be involved [67]. 13-cRA is not rapidly metabolized, poorly translocated to the nucleus and is biologically less active than tRA in signal transduction pathways. These biologic properties of 13-cRA suggest that this isomer functions as a retinoid depot form, from which the biologically active tRA and 9-cRA are generated by isomerization. The generation of tRA and 9-cRA by isomerization from 13-cRA is much faster and may be energetically more economical than their de novo synthesis from retinol or carotenoids.

The retinoid signaling pathway requires protein nuclear receptors that not only translocate tRA and 9-cRA into the nucleus but also facilitate their docking to specific DNA sequences. Two families of retinoid nuclear receptors, retinoic acid receptor (RAR) and retinoid X receptor (RXR), have been identified [2,64,65]. RXR and RAR families belong to a superfamily of nuclear receptors that include thyroid hormone (TR), steroid, vitamin D3 (VDR), and peroxisomal proliferation activating receptors (PPAR) and function as ligand-dependent transcription factors [64,65]. Structural characteristics of the receptor superfamily are shown in Figure 3. The RAR family of the retinoid nuclear receptors has three different subtypes, designated alpha (α), beta (β), and gamma (γ) (Figure 13–4). The RARα has two isoforms, while RARβ has four. All subtypes of RAR bind both tRA and 9-cRA, with a dissociation constant ranging from 1 to 5 nM [68]. Like the RAR family, the RXR family has three subtypes (Figure 13–4) and binds 9-cRA with a dissociation constant of 12 nM [3,66].

Like other members of the superfamily, both RAR and RXR consist of DNA-binding, ligand-binding, receptor-dimerization, and transcription-activation domains. The DNA-binding domain is characterized by the presence of nine highly conserved cysteine residues (see Figure 13–3) which are coordinated by zinc atoms to form the so-called two zinc fingers required for DNA binding [69]. All the other domains are located toward the carboxyl terminal and are involved not only in ligand binding and receptor dimerization but also in nuclear translocation and interaction with heat shock proteins [70]. The current concept of the retinoid signaling pathway indicates that tRA and 9-cRA, bound to either homodimers (RAR-RAR and RXR-RXR) or heterodimers of RAR and RXR (RAR-RXR), identifies and binds to specific DNA sequences called *retinoic acid responsive elements* (RAREs) in the enhancer region of the retinoid-responsive genes. In general, the specificity and affinity of RXR containing heterodimers for DNA binding is much higher than that of the homodimers; this has led to the suggestion that RXR has both transcription-activating and modulating functions [71–73]. In the transcription-activating function of RXR, 9-cRA induces the formation of RXR homodimers, which bind to a specific subset of RAREs (RXRE) found in the genes to be expressed. Homodimers of RXR have been shown to be involved in the expression of CRBP(II) and apolipoprotein A1 genes [74,75]. In the transcription-modulating function, the RXR occurs via the formation of heterodimers, with other members of the nuclear receptor superfamily, which exhibit either diminished or enhanced transcription activation functions. In the presence of 9-cRA, for example, the transcription activity of TR-RXR and VDR-RXR is diminished compared with TR-TR and VDR-VDR, respectively [76,77], whereas the transcription activities of the PPAR-RXR and RAR-RXR are higher than those of PPAR-PPAR and RAR-RAR, respectively [78].

The modulation of transcription activation is not restricted to members of the nuclear receptor superfamily, as evidenced by the ability of RAR-RXR heterodimers to inhibit the function of the AP-1 transcription factor. In the presence of both tRA and 9-cRA, the RAR-RXR dimers formed interact with the transcriptionally active c-*jun*/c-*fos* dimer, resulting in the dimers exchanging partners

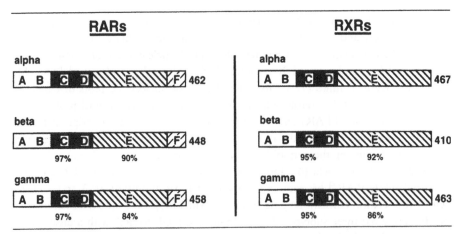

Figure 13–3. The two retinoid nuclear receptor families, RAR and RXR. Percentage indicates homology with the alpha subtype of each family.

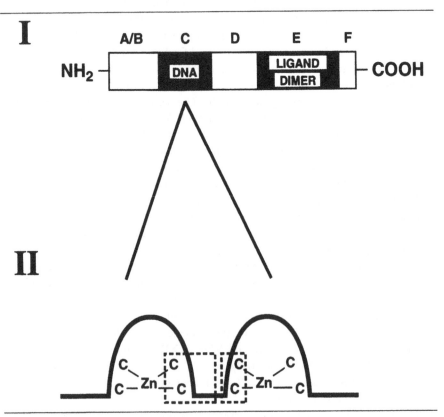

Figure 13–4. Diagramatic presentation of the functional domains of the nuclear receptor superfamily. The DNA binding domain is magnified to show clusters of cysteine amino acids forming the two zinc figures and discriminatory amino acid sequences (dotted boxes).

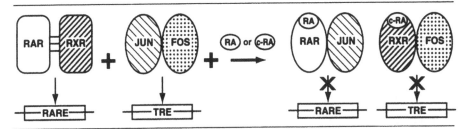

Figure 13–5. Proposed mechanism by which heterodimers of retinoid nuclear receptors disrupt the functional intergrity of transcription factor AP-1. TRE stands for TPA-responsive elements. (From Pfahl M (1994) Retinoid response pathways. In MA Livrea, G Vidali, eds. Retinoids: From Basic Science to Clinical Application, Basel: Birkhäuser Verlag, pp 115–126. With permission.)

and being unable to bind not only to the AP-1 sites on DNA but also to the RAREs [79,80] (Figure 10–5). The net effect is inhibition of AP-1 transcription activity. In this way, RXR-containing heterodimers mediate crosstalk not only with different hormones but also with different oncogenes, suppressor genes, and tumor promoters, and contribute to the wide range of biologic effects of retinoids.

Protein retinoylation

Although most of the biologic effects of retinoids can be explained by RAR- and RXR-mediated gene expression, the direct association between retinoid nuclear receptors and a response to retinoids is not always demonstrated [81]. The observation that a number of synthetic retinoids that do not bind RAR and RXR are capable of eliciting the biologic effects of retinoids further suggests that nonsignaling mechanisms may also be important. The extensive protein retinoylation routinely observed in tRA-treated cells in vitro has led to the suggestion that protein retinoylation may play a role in the biologic effects of retinoids. Not all retinoylated proteins have been fully investigated and characterized, but they include intracellular and extracellular structural proteins [82,83] and metabolic regulatory proteins, such as regulatory subunits of cAMP-dependent protein kinases of HL60 cells [84]. Since fatty acid acylation of proteins has been shown to regulate enzymatic activity [85], there is a suggestion that retinoylation of proteins may similarly modulate the enzymatic activity of proteins required for differentiation. A positive correlation between retinoylation activity and the differentiating activity of various synthetic retinoid analogues in HL60 cells has been reported [86]. This conclusion gains credibility from studies indicating that different patterns of cellular protein retinoylation in different cells result in different responses to retinoic acid [87].

BIOLOGIC BASIS OF RETINOID ANTICANCER ACTION

Scope

Retinoids are involved in numerous physiologic processes, including vision, reproduction, embryogenesis, organogenesis, morphogenesis of the nervous system and limbs, cellular differentiation, and in control of cell proliferation [88]. The biologic effects of retinoids on cell proliferation, differentiation, and programmed cell death, in addition to the immuno-stimulating, antiangiogenic, and antioxidant properties, are discussed here because they may contribute directly to the cancer chemotherapeutic and chemopreventive action of retinoids. Although these biologic effects are discussed separately, in reality they may function as a team (Figure 13–6).

Cell differentiation and growth inhibition

The majority of the current in vitro and in vivo studies of differentiating properties of retinoids have used promyelocytic hematopoietic cells and epithelial cells derived from skin, the upper aerodigestive system, and the lower genital tract systems [89–91]. This is because of the documented clinical usefulness of retinoids in the treatment of malignant and premalignant lesions arising from these sites and/or cells [92–94]. In squamous epithelial cells, the retinoid growth inhibitory effect is a prerequisite for its differentiating activity [95]. In acute promyelocytic leukemic (APL) cells, however, which have already been characterized by maturation arrest, differentiation is the main effect of retinoids. In general, growth-inhibitory concentrations are several logs higher than these required for differentiation [96,97]. Accumulating clinical data suggest that 13-cRA is most effective as a chemotherapeutic and chemopreventive agent for squamous cell malignancies [98–102], whereas tRA is excellent for remission induction of APL [92–94]. These observations support the concept that the relatively high retinoid-inhibitory concentrations required for growth inhibition are likely to be achieved with the poorly metabolized 13-cRA but not with the rapidly metabolized tRA [103].

Although the role of RARα and retinoids in myeloid cell differentiation has been appreciated for a long time [104,105], the discovery of the chromosomal translocations, t(15;17) and t(11;17), which involve the RARα gene, have led to the elucidation of the role of this nuclear receptor in the differentiation of acute promyelocytic leukemia cells both in vitro and in patients. In the t(15;17) translocation, the RARα gene on chromosome 17 is translocated to chromosome 15, where it fuses with PML, the promyelocytic leukemia gene [106–108]. The PML gene product contains a cysteine-rich region characteristic of DNA binding proteins and may represent a novel transcription factor involved in APL cell differentiation (Figure 13–7). Both in the absence and in the presence of physiologic concentrations of tRA, the PML-RARa fusion protein forms homodimers, that bind efficiently to RAREs in the genes responsible for APL differentiation and inhibit their transcription. The formation of large quantities of PML-RARa also results in nuclear sequestration and inactivation of RXR via the formation of PML-RARa-RXR heterodimers.

Other postulated nuclear interactions of PML-RARa are shown in Figure 13–8. In the presence of pharmacologic concentrations of tRA, however, the PML–RARa protein transactivates myeloid differentiation genes. The PML-RARa fusion protein is thus not only an etiologic factor in APL but also is responsible for the exquisite response of this disease to tRA [109–111]. In vitro studies using freshly

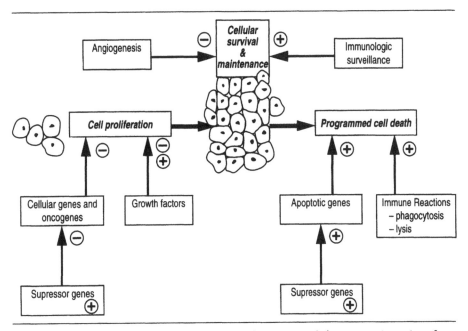

Figure 13–6. Outline of the proposed biologic sites of anticancer and chemoprevention action of retinoids: Stimulatory action (+) and inhibitory action (−).

obtained human APL cells have show that the differentiating action of tRA is superior to that of 13-cRA, in agreement with what is observed in APL patients [112]. The two isomers are, however, equipotent in cultured HL-60 and U-937 APL cell lines. This may be due to increased isomerization of 13-cRA to tRA in cultured APL cell lines compared with freshly obtained human APL cells. In the t(11;17) the RARα is translocated from chromosome 17 to a new zinc finger named PLZF (promyelocytic leukemia zinc finger) (see Figure 13–7) [113]. APL patients exhibiting t(11;17) respond poorly to tRA therapy [114].

The role of retinoids in squamous cell differentiation was first suggested by hyperkeratotic skin changes in vitamin A deficiency and hypokeratosis in vitamin A excess [115]. Vitamin A deficiency leads to increased proliferation and squamous differentiation of the skin, lower genitourinary tract, and aerodigestive tract epithelial cells. Both squamous epithelial cell proliferation and differentiation are now known to be due to impaired retinoic acid–dependent gene expression [116]. The retinoid-mediated cell growth inhibition of squamous epithelium is due to downregulation of the genes for cellular proliferation, including c-*myc*, *cdc*, and E2F-1. Down regulator of these genes is followed by cellular differentiation [95,117]. The pattern of growth inhibition and differentiation is determined not only by the type of cellular retinoic acid isomer and its concentration, but also by the profile of retinoid nuclear receptors [118]. RARα, RXRα, and RARγ are commonly expressed in epithelial cells; the expression of RARβ is variable, and RXRβ and

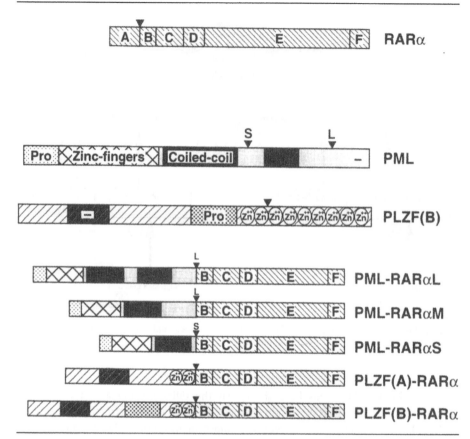

Figure 13–7. Diagrammatic presentation of the various domains of RARa, the two promyelocyte leukemia transcription factors (PML and PFZF), and the resulting fusion proteins (the long and short forms of PML-RARa, and the A and B forms of PLZF-RARa). Break and fusion sites are indicated by a solid triangle. Positive and negative signs indicate proline- and acidic amino acid–rich regions in the PML and PLZF. (Adapted with minor modifications from Zelent A (1994) Annotation. Br J Hematol 86:451–460. With permission.)

RXRγ are rarely seen [119]. The expression of RARα and RARβ is modulated by tRA, while RARγ and all the RXR subtypes are not [120]. Downregulation of the expression of RAR-β has been correlated with the progression of premaligant lesions to full-blown malignancy and is currently thought to be an important etiologic factor in aerodigestive tract neoplasia [91]. No similar correlation has been observed with either RARα, RARγ, or the RXR family of nuclear receptors.

In addition to regulating cell proliferation via cellular proto-oncogenes and suppressor genes, retinoids influence cell growth by modulating growth factors and their receptors [121]. In vitro exposure of human cancer cell lines from breast, non–small lung, and ovarian cancer cells to pharmacologic concentrations of tRA, 13-cRA, 9cRA, and 4-HPR has been shown in numerous experiments to modulate

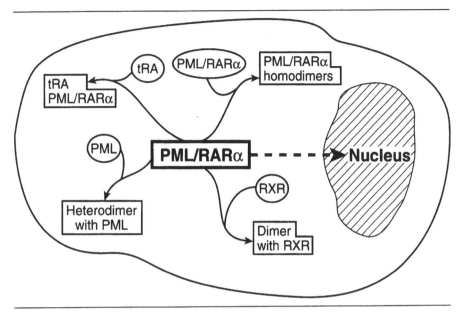

Figure 13–8. Postulated intracellular interactions of PML/RAR with retinoids. These reactions may occur in the cytoplasm or, more likely, in the nucleus.

EGF, TGF-alpha, TGF-beta, and insulin-like growth factor I (IGF1) receptor signaling pathways. In epithelial and fibroblast cell cultures, tRA increases the expression of TGF-beta receptors and TGF-beta secretion, resulting in growth inhibition and stimulation, respectively [122,123]. Similarly decreased TGF-alpha expression has been observed in leukoplakia biopsy specimens of patients treated with 13-cRA and tRA [124]. In human breast cancer cells, both tRA and the synthetic retinoid, 4-HPR, have been shown to downregulate the expression of IGF1 and to decrease plasma IGF1 levels in breast cancer patients receiving 4-HPR [125]. The mechanism by which retinoids modulate growth factors and receptors is unknown, but available experimental data suggest that nuclear retinoid and membrane growth receptor–based signaling pathways modulate each other, and that the AP-1 transcription complex is a site of convergence [79].

Induction of apoptosis

Apoptosis, or programmed cell death (PCD) is now known not to be restricted to developmental biology but to occur throughout life, and is controlled by the apoptotic genes that are transcriptionally activated by the wild-type p53 gene product [126]. Since dysregulation of apoptosis may play a role in some malignancies, selective induction of apoptosis of malignant cells is potentially a powerful weapon in the war against cancer. There is now convincing evidence that tRA, 9-cRA, and 4-HPR not only induce cell differentiation but also cause apoptosis in some human cell lines and that the two processes may occur simultaneously [127–

129]. Interestingly, 4-HPR is capable of inducing apoptosis in cells unresponsive to tRA [130]. These observations suggest the some of the cancer chemotherapeutic and chemopreventive action of retinoids may reside in their apoptotic action. Retinoic acid signaling pathways induce apoptosis either directly or indirectly via a variety proto-oncogenes and suppressor genes. The direct role of retinoic acid signaling pathways in apoptosis is clearly demonstrated in APL, a disease character-ized by a clonal expansion of hematopoietic precursors blocked at the promyelocytic stage. The PML-RAR gene product that is characteristic of APL is responsible for blockade of both differentiation and apoptosis of myeloid precursor cells; this has been confirmed by demonstrating reduced rates of PCD in cells transinfected with the PML-RARa gene compared with the control [131]. In APL cells, the block to both differentiation and apoptosis is eliminated by 9-cRA and tRA.

Retinoid signaling pathways may also influence apoptosis indirectly by modulat-ing the expression of the *bcl-2* oncogene, c-*myc*, b-*myc*, AP-1, and other transcrip-tion activators. The *bcl-2* oncogene product extends cell survival by inhibiting apoptosis [132]. Recent reports indicate that homodimers of *bcl-2* are responsible for inhibition of apoptosis, and the formation of heterodimers with *bax* (*bcl-2/bax*) abolishes this effect. The *bcl-2*–mediated anti-apoptotic action in human cell lines is not, however, reversed by retinoic acid. This is because retinoic acid upregulates the expression of the *bcl-2* oncogene product [133], which favors the formation of apoptosis inhibitory homodimers and prolongation of cell survival. HL-60 cells transinfected with *bcl-2* are similarly resistant to retinoic acid–mediated apoptosis but not differentiation [134,135]. Additional anti-apoptotic action to counteract retinoid-mediated apoptosis in myeloid cells is derived from the gene product of c-*fes*, a proto-oncogene expressed at high concentrations in the terminal stages of differentiation of granulocyte differentiation [136]. The observation that 9-cRA was 10 times more potent than tRA in inhibiting T-cell hybridoma apoptosis suggests that RXR-containing heterodimers or homodimers are more important in PCD [137]. Like *bcl-2*, a functional AP-1 is essential for repression of cell death. Disrup-tion of the structural and functional integrity of the c-*jun*/c-*fos* complex by RAR-RXR heterodimers in the presence of tRA and 9-cRA discussed previously may thus contribute to retinoid-mediated apoptosis.

The central role of the p53 in apoptosis, mentioned earlier, has led to the classification of apoptosis into p53-dependent and p53-independent pathways based on whether or not this gene is involved in the experimental model. p53-dependent apoptosis is characterized by the accumulation/stabilization of the p53 gene product in the nucleus due to reduced protein turnover [138]. High nuclear concentrations of the wild p53 gene product inhibit the activity of the cyclin/cdk complex, which results in the arrest of cell growth and subsequently death, and is commonly mechanism of cell death after DNA-damaging cancer agents. Wild-type p53 also binds to the promoter region of a number of proteins essential for cellular prolifera-tion, including c-*myc*, c-*fos*, and c-*jun*, [139–141], and modulates their transcription activity. Since the gene products of these p53-modulated promoter regions are also modulated by retinoids, c-*myc* expression is upregulated; while c-*jun* and c-*fos* interact with RAR-RXR heterodimers, indirect modulation of p53-dependent apoptosis by retinoids is obvious.

In human prostate carcinoma cells, tRA and 9-cRA induced apoptosis via a p53-independent induction of p21/waf1, which inhibits the activity of the cyclin/cdk complex [142]. The observed enhancement of cell kill and growth inhibition following pretreatment with tRA and 9-cRA may partly be due either to synergism between the p53-dependent apoptosis by DNA-damaging agents with the p53-independent and dependent retinoid-mediated apoptosis or due to retinoid-primed programmed cell death, which is accelerated by subsequent exposure to chemotherapeutic agents [143]. This may be the biologic basis for the recently reported clinical success of combining 13-cRA and tRA with DNA-damaging chemotherapeutic agents such as cisplatin and VP-16.

Antioxidant properties

In vitro studies have shown that retinoids, like their carotene precursor, are excellent scavengers of reactive oxygen species, and they protect cells from oxidative damage. Since oxidative damage and free radical damage play a central role in carcinogenesis, it is plausible that the interaction of reactive oxygen species with retinoids would reduce DNA, RNA, membrane, and protein damage to a level manageable by other cellular defense and repair mechanisms [144–147]. The hydrophobic nature of retinoids suggests that their reactive oxygen-scavenging properties will be more marked in membrane. In vitro and in vivo antioxidant properties of vitamin A and 13-cRA have been studied in microsomal preparations by measuring thiobarbituratic acid reactive substances (TBARS) and conjugated diene formation [148–150]. Published reports have shown that physiologic cellular concentrations of vitamin A can protect membrane from reactive oxygen species assault [151]. Although the relative abilities of the various retinoids to scavenge reactive oxygen species have not been evaluated in detail, one favorable characteristic for a therapeutically effective free radical scavenger would be a long biologic half-life. We therefore speculate that 13-cRA, with its long plasma half-life and longer retention in the body, would be excepted to have free radical–scavenging properties that are superior to the rapidly cleared tRA; this may explain why 13-cRA is more a efficacious chemopreventive agent for skin and head and neck cancers than tRA.

Effects on angiogenesis

An important factor in cancer pathogenesis is the development of the tumor blood circulation, which supplies the oxygen and nutrients required for growth and removes the waste products of cellular metabolism [152]. When a solid tumor outgrows its blood supply, central tumor necrosis results. The development of tumor circulation is also essential for the hematogenous spread of cancer and influences the sensitivity of the tumor cells to radiation and chemotherapy. Multiple observations correlating the degree of tumor angiogenesis, measured as microvascular density in biopsies, with tumor regression, tumor recurrence, development of loco-regional and systemic metastasis, and patient survival have been reported [153–155]. Antiangiogenic properties of the retinoic acid isomers tRA, 13-cRA, and 9-cRA have been demonstrated in tumor cell lines harboring the HPV16 and HPV18 genome using the chick embryo chorioallantois membrane test system [156–159]. Anticarcinogenesis and chemotherapeutic and chemopreventive properties of retinoids may partly be attributed to the antiangiogenic activity. Retinoids are thought to exert their antiangiogenic activity by inhibiting cellular genes, oncogenes, and suppressor genes involved in the synthesis and release of tumor-derived angiogenic factors [160].

Examples of cellular derived proteins and peptides exhibiting angiogenic properties are the basic fibroblast growth factors (bFGF) and SPARC. Tumor cells and/or infiltrating macrophage–derived bFGF is exported into the extracellular matrix in an inactive form and is subsequently activated by heparins released by mast cells or by plasminogen-mediated proteolysis [161–163]. SPARC is a transiently expressed, highly cationic extracellular matrix binding protein that, together with its proteolytic derived peptides, has potent angiogenic activity [164]. Synergism between the retinoid and interferon in laboratory experiments using HPV16- and HPV18-infected cell lines has been partly explained by their antiangiogenic actions and has now been successfully applied in the treatment of human malignancies in the clinic. Cervical cancer and recurrent respiratory papillomatosis, human diseases thought to be caused by the same viruses, are highly responsive to the 13-cRA and IFN-alpha combination [165,166]. The combination of retinoid therapy with other antiangiogenic drugs, growth factors, and cytokines is currently under intense investigation.

Immune response modulation

There is now evidence to indicate that both cellular and humoral immunity are depressed in hypovitaminosis A [167,168]. Since the functional integrity of these immunologic mechanisms is required to eliminate malignant cells, the increased incidence of cancer in vitamin A deficiency may be attributed to impaired immunologic surveillance [169–171]. Retinoid enhanced immunological surveillance and destruction of cancer cells may therefore contribute to the anticancer action of this class of drugs. The mechanism by which retinoids modulate immune responses is not known with certainty; it appears to be multifactorial. Retinol, in the form of retinyl phosphate, accepts mannose from GDP-mannose and has been shown to function as a coenzyme that carries sugar moieties for glycoprotein synthesis [172,173]. Although direct experimental evidence of the role of retinoic acid isomers in glycoprotein synthesis is lacking, because they are incapable of accepting mannose their yet identified hydroxylated metabolites can potentially do so. Glycoproteins are important structural components involved in cellular interactions, adhesion, aggregation, and recognition. A number of important membrane surface antigens, including tumor antigens and membrane surface receptors such as T-cell and antigen-presenting cell receptor complexes (lectins, thrombospondin receptors, MHC class I and class II), are gycoproteins. In the presence of optimal retinoid concentrations, the functional integrity of these important membranes components is maintained for maximal immune responses.

Retinoids may also maximize the immune responses by modulating the production of IFNg and other cytokines essential for the immune function [174]. In T-cells, retinoid deficiency results in increased expression of the IFNg gene, and these high levels of IFNg have been associated with impaired function of B-cells and the T-helper cells [175]. In contrast, retinoid deficiency results in decreased secretion of cytokines, including IL-4 and IL-5, which are essential for B-cell growth and differentiation, and IL-10, a cytokine essential for macrophage and other antigen-processing cells, is also decreased [176]. Impaired immunologic function resulting from this cytokine deficiency, together with an increased IFN level, is readily restored by retinoid therapy (4-HPR and tRA), which not only stimulates cytokine synthesis and secretion, leading to optimal macrophage function, B-cell growth, and differentiation, but also downregulates IFNg expression, resulting in an increase in the number of T-helper cells, natural killer (NK) cells, and lytic activities [177,178]. The functional integrity of the macrophage system is also essential for the recognition and phagocytic removal of cells undergoing apoptosis [179–181].

ANALYTICAL METHODS FOR RETINOIDS

Sample handling and storage

Biologic samples for quantitative determination of retinoids require protection from light in order to minimize the isomerization reaction. Samples should be collected in amber-colored vials, and extracted and analyzed under yellow light or reduced-light conditions. Clinical samples commonly assayed for retinoid contents are plasma, serum, and whole blood. Analysis of retinoids in human skin biopsies has been reported [182]. The samples are stable up to 6 months when stored at $-70°C$. Repetitive freezing and thawing of samples destroys tRA and should be avoided.

Extraction and analysis

Retinoid content of biologic samples has been assayed by reverse-phase high-pressure liquid chromatography, normal-phase adsorption chromatography, gas chromatography with mass spectrometry (GLC-MS), and by a combination of normal-phase HPLC and positive ion mass spectrometry [183–187]. The extraction of retinoids from protein-containing samples is achieved by the precipitation of proteins by organic solvents followed by liquid–liquid partition under acidic conditions. In our laboratory we have routinely used all-*trans*-9-nosityl-3,7-dimethyl-2,4,6,8 nona-tetranoic acid as an internal standard [185], but other synthetic retinoids that are stable under the extraction conditions and that do not interfere with the separation can be substituted.

Assay characteristics

Reverse-phase HPLC methods have the disadvantage of being unable to resolve the more polar metabolites because they are masked in the solvent front. The resolution of the glucuronide conjugate of retinoic acid, one of these polar metabolites in human plasma, requires 16–24 hours of incubation of the sample with beta-glucuronidase [188]. Furthermore, since the lower limit of sensitivty is approximately 10–25 ng/ml [183–185], these methods are not useful for measuring physiologic concentration retinoids in plasma. Concentration methods by evaporation of the extract or by solid-phase extraction of large samples have been used to improve the sensitivity of HPLC assay to 1–2 ng/ml and are therefore capable of measuring 2–5 ng/ml of endogenous plasma retinoid levels [189]. A more sensitive assay capable of measuring up to 0.125 ng/ml using normal-phase HPLC in combination with positive ion mass spectrometry has been developed [187].

CLINICAL PHARMACOLOGY AND PHARMACOKINETICS

Scope

This section describes the common pharmacokinetic characteristics and the general side effects of the three naturally occurring retinoic acid isomers and N-(4-hydroxyphenyl)retinamide because they are currently in clinical use. This is followed by a discussion of features characteristic of the individual retinoids.

General characteristics of all retinoids in clinical use

The pharmacokinetics of 13-cRA, tRA, and, more recently, 9-cRA have been studied in patients with advanced cancers. All the retinoids in clinical oncology are available as oral preparations, usually in the form of gelatin capsules. Formulation problems have hampered the development of suitable parental preparations for clinical use, and, as a result, there no human bioavailability studies. In experimental animals the oral route bioavailability of the 13-cRA has been estimated at 21% of the parental dose. This low bioavailability of isotretinoin following oral intestion has been attributed to a first-pass effect occurring in the gut lumen (~72%), with the gut wall and liver being responsible for the remaining 8% of the overall first-pass effect of 80% [190]. The bioavailability of retinoids is increased when taken with food rich in lipids [191].

Following oral administration, peak plasma concentrations of all retinoic acid isomers are observed within 1–3 hours [14,185,192–198]. The pharmacokinetic behavior of all isomers is characterized by tremendous intrapatient and interpatient variation in both peak plasma concentrations and area-under-the-curne (AUC) values. Results of phase I clinical studies of the three retinoic acid isomers have shown that the maximum tolerated dose for the three isomers is similar and ranges from 150 to 230 mg/m^2 for adults. The recommended phase II dose in solid tumors for all retinoic acid isomers is the same: 120–150 mg/m^2/day administered as two or three equally divided oral doses [192–195] and 200 mg/day for 4-HPR. In children the tRA maximum tolerated dose was 60 mg/m^2/day, which is significantly lower than in adults [198]. The majority of the side effects experienced by patients on retinoid therapy are mild and reversible, and are similar for all retinoids in clinical use (Table 13–1). Neither acute nor chronic oral administration of any of the three

Table 13-1. Phase II studies of all-*trans* retinoic acid as
a single agent in patients with advanced solid tumors

Study no.	Tumor type	No. pts entered	Type of response	Ref.
1	Prostate	14	None	237
2	Prostate	17	None	238
3	Head and neck	8	None	239
4	Breast	12	1 PR; soft tissue	240
5	Lung (NSCL)	11	None	241
6	Brain	25	3; objective	242

The tRA dose administered was 120–150 mg/day.
PR = partial response.

retinoic acid isomers has been associated with changes in plasma or tissue retinol concentrations.

All-*trans* retinoic acid (tretinoin)

Reports from numerous clinical studies of the day-1 pharmacokinetics of tRA have shown that the drug is cleared from plasma in a monoexponential fashion, with a half-life of 30–45 minutes, and that within 8 hours the drug concentrations are down to within the physiologic level (1–5 ng/ml) [185,187,189,192]. Until recently the only tRA metabolite detected in patient plasma was the 4-oxo-metabolite, but incubation of plasma samples has shown that 20% of the drug in circulation is conjugated to a glucuronide [185,188]. The plasma levels of the 4-oxo metabolite were less than 10% of the plasma concentration of the parent drug and were detected in a minority of patients [185]. Whereas only small quantities of 13-cRA have been detected in a minority of patients, no 9-cRA has been observed in patients on tRA therapy, suggesting no significant isomerization of tRA to either of these isomers [185].

The tremendous variation in day-1 tRA AUC values has led to the suggestion that patients may be classified into slow and rapid metabolizers of retinoic acid based on whether the AUC values were less than or greater than 300 ng.hr/ml, respectively [199,200]. This cutoff value was selected based upon the plot of 70 individual patient day-1 AUCs and because it is equivalent to the 1 μM all-*trans*-retinoic acid commonly used in vitro studies [112,201]. Nearly all patients on continuous oral tRA therapy manifest the rapid tRA metabolism phenotype within 48 hours of the start of therapy [200]. The self-induced increase in tRA metabolism has been shown to be associated with an increase in urinary 4-oxo glucuronide metabolites in a small number of APL patients, but without the corresponding increase in circulating 4-oxo tRA metabolites [185]. The increase in the CRABP content of APL cells and plasma lipid peroxides of APL and solid tumor patients, respectively, on prolonged oral retinoid therapy is thought to be responsible for the increased tRA metabolism and the observed pharmacokinetic changes [200,202].

The importance of oxidative metabolism in the pharmacokinetic behavior of tRA, and therefore therapeutic efficacy, has led to the development of a number of clinical strategies to circumvent the problem. The initial clinical studies aimed at modulating tRA pharmacokinetics by coadministration of a broad-spectrum non-specific inhibitor of the cytochrome P450 enzyme. Ketoconazole and its more water-soluble analogue, liarozole, the two most potent inhibitors of oxidative catabolism of tRA in vitro and in experimental animals [45–49], have been evaluated in the clinic. The minimum doses required to effectively improve the tRA plasma AUC value in cancer patients exhibiting the rapid tRA metabolism phenotype were 400 of ketoconazole and 300 mg of liarozole, respectively, given as a single dose 1 hour prior to oral tRA ingestion [200,203]. As expected, these inhibitors had no effect on the AUC values of normal tRA metabolizers. The long-term side effects and the impact of this combination on the differentiation and chemopreventive action of retinoids has not been investigated.

An alternative strategy for preventing self-induced tRA metabolism is to encapsulate tRA into liposomes, which has been successfully tested in vitro and in experimental animals [204]. Liposome-encapsulated tRA has a much longer elimination half-life than free tRA. Furthermore, prolonged administration of liposomal-encapsulated tRA to rats has shown no drug-induced pharmacokinetic changes, an observation supported by the lack of increased tRA catabolism by microsomes isolated from liposomal-tRA–treated animals. Microsomes from animals treated with free tRA exhibited increased rates [204]. In vitro liposomal encapsulation does not appear to affect the cytodifferentiation activity of tRA [205]. The success of liposome-encapsulated tRA may be attributed not only to its inability to induce its own catabolism but also because the first-pass effect of the gastrointestinal tract is avoided by intravenous administration. Liposome-encapsulated tRA is currently undergoing clinical evaluation. Administration of tRA on an intermittent schedule has also been advocated to prevent the self-induced tRA metabolism. Although preliminary pharmacokinetic success has been observed on a weekly schedule [206], the optimal schedule and the impact on the therapeutic efficacy of tRA remain to be investigated.

13-cis retinoic acid (isotretinoin)

The pharmacokinetic behavior of isotretinoin differs remarkably from that of tretinoin. Unlike tretinoin, isotretinoin is slowly cleared from plasma, with a terminal half-life ranging from 10 to 24 hours after a single oral dose of 80–100 mg [194,195,207]. Up to a third of the circulating 13-cRA is detected as tRA, suggesting extensive isomerization [194]. There is no evidence, however, to suggest that 13-cRA isomerizes to 9-cRA in cancer patients. The major metabolite seen in circulation is 4-oxo-13-cis retinoic acid.

The 4-oxo metabolite of 13-cRA is seen in all patients receiving the drug, and the plasma concentration may be as high as two to three times that of the parent drug [195]. Unlike tretonin, 13-cis retinoic acid does not induce its own oxidative catabolism but is associated with progressive accumulation of the 4-oxo-13-cis retinoic acid metabolites [194,207]. These pharmacokinetic differences between isotretinoin and tretinoin are currently thought to reflect differences in the oxidative metabolism of the two isomers [103].

9-*cis* retinoic acid

Preliminary results from phase I studies suggest that 9-*cis* retinoic acid has pharmacokinetic features of both of cRA and tRA [193,196,197]. 9-cRA over the 30–230 mg/m^2 dose range has a mean plasma half-life of 1.2 hours, which is close to that of tRA than 13-cRA. There is early evidence suggesting that 9-cRA may induce its own catabolism, but only when administered in doses over 100 mg/m^2/day [193,196,197]. Isomerization of 9-*cis* retinoic acid to both all-*trans* and 13-*cis* retinoic acid has been reported, but the extent of isomerization in cancer patients has not been quantitated. There is no information regarding the 4-oxo-9cRA metabolites in humans. 9,13-*dicis*-retinoic acid, the major metabolite of 9-cRA in mice and rat, has been observed in metabolic studies with microsomal preparations [5,6], but has not been identified in patients.

N-(4-hydroxyphenyl)retinamide (Fenretinide)

Fenretinide (4-HPR), a synthetic retinoid, has been developed primarily as a chemopreventive agent; comparative pharmacokinetic observations performed during the early clinical trials and after 5 years of continuous administration have been published [14,201]. comparison of 4-HPR pharmacokinetic parameters at entry into the study and at 5 years show no significant change in the peak plasma concentration (Cpmax), which remained at approximately 1 μM, indicating that 4-HPR does not induce its catabolism. The degradation of 4-HPR, like that of the naturally occurring retinoids, is primarily by oxidative catabolism, but the end products are N-(4-methoxyphenyl)-all-*trans* retinamide (4-MPR) and N-(4-ethoxyphenyl)-all-*trans* retinamide (4-EPR). As with the 4-oxo 13-cRA, the 4-MPR metabolite accumulates in the circulation. With prolonged administration, an increase in the elimination half-life of both the parent drug (from 13.7 to 27 hours) and the 4-MPR (from 23 to 54 hours) has observed [14,208]. The half-life of 4-HPR and the accumulation in circulation of its 4-methoxy metabolite are again very similar to those of 13-*cis* and its 4-oxo metabolite. The side effects of 4-HPR are similar to those of other retinoids. However, unlike both tRA and 13-cRA, 4-HPR causes visual impairment due to drug-induced plasma and tissue retinol deficiency. The mechanism by which 4-HPR reduces plasma retinol is unknown. A 3 day interruption of 4-HPR therapy at the end of every month corrects the retinol deficiency and eliminates the visual symptoms in patients receiving 200 mg/day of 4-HPR [14].

CLINICAL USE OF RETINOIDS IN ONCOLOGY

Scope

Retinoids have been and continue to be evaluated as cancer chemotherapeutic or chemopreventive agents. The majority of these clinical studies have utilized tRA and cRA, the two readily available isomers. Phase I clinical studies of 9-cRA in both hematologic and solid tumors have recently been initiated [193,196]. Published results suggest that 13-cRA and tRA may exhibit a different spectrum of antitumor and differentiation activities. tRA is now an established drug for induction of complete remission in acute promyelocytic leukemia (APL) [92–94], but its antitumor activity in solid tumors and its cancer chemopreventive activity in patients have not been fully evaluated. 13-cRA has relatively inferior remission induction activity in APL patients [112] but is used to treat advanced squamous cell cancers of the skin and cervix, and is most effective when used in combination with interferon-alpha [101,102,211]. Isotretinoin has also been used successfully to reverse preneoplastic lesions and as an effective chemopreventive agent against the development of secondary primary malignancies in patients with head and neck tumors [99,100]. Fenretinide is a highly promising chemopreventive agent for breast cancer, either alone or in combination with tamoxifen [14]. The clinical use of the individual retinoids is discussed next.

Tretinoin therapy for acute promyelocytic leukemia

The overall complete remission induction rate is over 80% for newly diagnosed APL patients treated with 45 mg/m^2/day tRA and 100% for t(15;17)-positive patients [210]. The relatively high doses used in the initial studies are probably unnecessary because similar APL complete remission induction rates have been reported with 25 mg/m^2/day, and even at 15 mg/m^2/day if tRA is given with intensive chemotherapy [211]. tRA is equally effective in inducing complete remission rates (82%) in APL patients relapsing after convectional chemotherapy [212]. Although molecular heterogeneity of the PML-RARa fusion protein has no effect on the initial response to tRA-therapy, the overall duration of remission is shorter in patients with the short form of PML-RARa fusion protein compared with those with the long form [213,214]. In clinical practice, the detection of PML-RAR mRNA is diagnostic of an APL subtype responsive to tRA, while PCR detection techniques are useful for the detection of minimal disease and for assessing the response to tRA therapy; molecular remission is characterized by the disappearance of PML-RARa mRNA. [215,216]. As previous mentioned, APL patients with t(11;17) exhibit a poor response to tRA [114].

The mechanism of tRA-induced complete remission in patients is due to progressive differentiation of APL cells, as evidenced by the change of CD33, the immature cell surface marker, to CD16, a surface marker for mature cell via cells with dual surface markers, without bone marrow suppression [92,217]. Thus, unlike the remission induction with conventional chemotherapy, which results in massive blast cell lysis, release of procoagulant and fibrinolytic substances, and bleeding diathesis, with tRA therapy there is no blast cell lysis; therefore, the duration and incidence of coagulopathies are dramatically reduced [218].

Unfortunately, the tRA-induced APL complete remissions are characteristically not durable, and the leukemic population in subsequent relapses is universally resistant to further tRA therapy [202,215]. The mechanism for clinical resistance is unknown; however, clinical evidence suggests that tRA-induced drug metabolizing enzymes (cytochrome P450 and lipoxygenase), together with the tRA-mediated increase in CRABP and lipid hydroperoxides, are responsible for increased oxidative catabolism of tRA within the tumor cell population [219–221]. This increased drug catabolism results in a failure to achieve therapeutic drug concentrations both systemically and in the target APL cells [221]. Other mechanisms of acquired retinoic acid resistance documented in cultured cells but not in patients include a C→T point mutation in the ligand binding domain of the RAR receptor in HL-60R cells and altered expression of PML/RARα in NB4.306 cells [222,223]. The mutated RARα binds tRA poorly and exhibits dominant negative transactivating activity. The altered PML-RARα in NB4.306 cells has been shown to lack immunoreactivity with antibodies to the normal PML-RARα fusion protein.

tRA therapy followed intensive consolidation chemotherapy reduces the risk of relapse and development of retinoic acid resistance in newly diagnosed APL patients [224]. Available data indicate that APL complete remissions induced by tRA therapy and consolidated by intensive chemotherapy are more durable and offer a survival advantage over conventional chemotherapy alone [210,224]. Ongoing studies are evaluating whether simultaneous administration of chemotherapy and tRA is superior to the sequential schedule and the usefulness of maintenance chemotherapy and /or tRA-therapy [225]. Because tRA therapy for APL complete remission induction can be given in the outpatient, and is not associated with bone marrow suppression, it is significantly more economical than conventional chemotherapy [226].

In additional to the usual retinoid side effects, tRA therapy for APL complete remission induction is associated with a serious and sometimes fatal complication called *retinoic acid syndrome*. This syndrome is observed in approximately 25% of APL patients receiving tRA therapy [227]. The syndrome is characterized by pyrexia, acute onset of respiratory distress, and failure pulmonary infiltrations, pleural effusions, impaired myocardial contractility, peripheral edema, episodic hypotension, and a dramatic increase in the number of circulating white cells. The etiology of this syndrome is unknown, but clogging of the pulmonary capillary bed by the increased white cells and pulmonary parenchymal damage by white cell–derived leukotrienes and cytokines may be involved [228]. This syndrome has rarely been observed in solid tumor patients on tRA therapy. There are no pre-tRA therapy features capable of predicting which patients will develop the syndrome, although white cell hyperexpression of CD13 was suggested in one study [214]. The onset of the syndrome is, however, heralded by an increased peripheral leukocyte count [226,227] and is an indication to initiate intensive chemotherapy and/or a short course of high-dose steroid therapy; both treatment regimes are highly effective. Leukophoresis or low-dose chemotherapy do not alter the morbidity or mortality from the syndrome [214].

Hypercalcaemia is another serious side effect of tRA therapy and has been observed sporadically in both hematologic and solid tumor patients [229–231]. The hypercalcaemia associated with tRA-therapy for APL is not due to ectopic PTH secretion, primary hyperparathyroidism, or increased levels of PTH related protein but is due to prostaglandin and vitamin D metabolite–independent increased osteoclastic activity [230]. In the case of multiple myeloma patients, tRA mediated downregulation of interleukin 6 receptors (IL-6R), results in increased serum IL-6 levels, leading to bone resorption and hypercalcemia [231]. Interestingly, tRA therapy is of no value in the treatment of any other hematologic malignancies, including primary and secondary myelodysplastic syndromes [232].

Tretinoin therapy in solid tumors

tRA as a single agent has shown no remarkable antitumor activity in a number of ongoing phase II clinical studies (Table 2). Unlike APL, tRA doses used are those recommended for phase II studies (120–150 mg/m^2/day). Unfortunately the clinical studies evaluating a combination of interferon (INF)-α-2a with tRA in patients with stage II or higher cervical carcinoma has been terminated prematurely because of lack of activity when compared with interferon and the 13-cRA arm of the study (M. Rothenberg, personal communication). The lack of activity is probably due the rapid elimination and changes in pharmacokinetics secondary to accelerated self-induced tRA catabolism. Topical application of 0.372% tRA, on the other hand, induces complete histologic regression in 43% of patients with cervical intraepithelial neoplasia (CIN II) compared with 27% in the placebo arm [233]. The topical use of tretinoin minimizes not only the system side effects of the therapy, but also eliminates the first-pass effects in both the gastrointestinal tract and liver, and may therefore be a useful adjunct in the treatment of early cervical neoplasia.

Clinical uses of isotretinoin

Cervical cancer

Although isotretinoin was initially used as a single agent in the treatment of cervical malignant lesions, more encouraging results have been reported when it is used in

Table 13–2. Common side effects observed in patients on retinoid therapy

Side effect	% pts with symptoms/signs of toxicity		
	13–cRA[a]	tRA	9–cRA[c]
Hypercalcemia	—	[b]	14
Skin dryness/xerostomia	90	85	55
Cheilitis	65	93	68
Conjuctivitis/epistaxis	30	18	36
Hyperlipidemia	63	86	37
Elevated transaminase/alkaline phosphatase		54	27
Headache/clogged ear sensation		69	68
Nausea/vomiting		32	14
Myalgia/arthralgia		22	23
Fatigue		37	32

[a] Incidence of side effects at 1–2 mg/kg 13-cRA dose.
[b] Data based on 52 patients entered into the phase 1 study.
[c] Seen in all six multiple myeloma patients treated at the Memorial Sloan-Kettering Cancer Center.

combination with IFN-α-2a [102]. An overall response rate of 58% was observed in previously untreated patients with stage IIB-IVA disease following 2 months of daily treatment with oral 13-cRA at a dose of 1 mg/kg and 6 million units of recombinant human IFN-α-2a administered subcutaneously. The responsiveness of cervical cancer to the 13-cRA and IFN-α-2a combination in cervical cancer is partly due the 13-cRA suppression of growth of cervical epithelial cells, together with the INF-α-2a suppression of the human papilloma transforming oncogenes E6 and E7, which are important etiologic factors in this disease [165], and the antiangiogenic effects of both drugs discussed previously. Isotretinoin is currently the recommended drug for the treatment of recurrent respiratory papillomatosis, another disease in which human papillomavirus is an etiological factor [166].

Head and neck cancers

The effectiveness of isotretinoin in the prevention of secondary malignancies in patients with head and neck cnacers was initially reported in the mid-1980s [98]. These results have been confirmed in subsequent studies in which disease-free head and neck cancer patients were randomized to receive either 13-cRA or placebo. After 1 year of follow-up, second primary tumors had developed in only 2 of the 49 patients on 13-cRA compared with 12 out of the 51 patients in the placebo group [99]. The relatively large doses of isotretinoin (50–100 mg/m²/day) in these early chemoprevention trials were associated with severe toxicity, necessitating the termination of treatment in 18% of patients, and contributed to the high noncompliance rate of 14%. Subsequent studies using high-dose isotretinoin induction therapy of 1.5 mg/kg/day for 3 months followed by lower dose maintenance isotretinoin of 0.5 mg/kg/day therapy did not compromise the cancer chemoprevention effects but was much better tolerated [100]. Further improvement in response rates has been achieved by the addition of radiotherapy to the 13-cRA and IFN-α-2a combination therapy—a complete response rate of 56% and an overall response rates of 81% [234]. The potential for further reduction of the chemopreventive isotretinoin dose when used in combination with cytokines and growth factors is real and requires clinical evaluation.

Squamous cell carcinoma of skin

Clinical use of 13-cRA as a skin cancer chemotherapeutic and chemopreventive agent is now well established [209,235,236]. High doses of 13-cRA result in an approximately 40% response rate in patients with advanced skin cancer. The doses used, however, are associated with unacceptable toxicity. In an attempt to reduce the toxicity, low doses of 13-cRA, 1 mg/kg/day given orally, have been used in combination with low-dose IFN-α, 3 million units/day administered subcutaneously. This combination has resulted in a highly effective therapy for advanced squamous cell carcinoma of the skin, with overall response rates of 93% and 67% for local disease and regional disease, respectively, but the toxicity remains severe [101].

FUTURE PROSPECTS

Retinoids have already had a major impact on the treatment and chemoprevention of cancer in humans, but their maximal clinical application has probably yet to be realized. Recent advances in the molecular basis of their anticancer and chemoprevention action has laid the foundation for their rational use in combination with chemotherapeutic agents and cytokines, the development of optimal administration schedules, and the synthesis of more potent and clinically more efficacious analogs.

To date, only interferon has been used clinically in combination with retinoids, and the results are very encouraging. In vitro and experimental animal studies suggest that combination with other cytokines is a fertile area for future clinical research. Combination of retinoids and chemotherapeutic agents, particularly DNA-damaging drugs, has already proved its clinical usefulness in APL patients undergoing remission induction therapy and needs to be extended to patients with other malignancies; studies in this area are ongoing. In vitro differentiation synergism of tRA followed by hexamethylene bisacetamide in HL-60 cells suggests that future studies will have to evaluate combinations of differentiation agents.

Our knowledge on the metabolic inter-relationship between fatty acid metabolism and retinoic acid remains very primitive. There is no good explanation for hyperlipidemia, which is commonly seen in patients on retinoid therapy, and why patients on 4-HPR therapy develop retinol deficiency. Future research will have to examine the role of bioactive lipids generated by retinoid-responsive fatty acid–metabolizing enzymes (lipoxygenase and cyclo-oxygenase, etc.) in the overall effects of retinoids.

A number of fundamental questions about retinoids remain to be answered: Although specific and selective functions of tRA and 9-cRA have now been documented, the simplistic conclusion that 13-cRA acts as a storage form needs to be re-evaluated in view of differences in the clinical efficacy of tRA and 13-cRA, and the fact that 13-cRA is not the most abundant intracellular retinoid. The function, if any, of the recently identified hydroxylated metabolites of retinoid remain elusive, but may function as carriers of sugar residues in the biosynthesis of glycoproteins.

In mammals with stable body temperature and internal organs not exposed to direct light, light- and heat-mediated isomerization probably plays no part in the isomerization reaction. Future studies should elucidate the enzymes and the physiologic conditions required for the synthesis of retinoic acid isomers and their interconversion. Knowledge of the biosynthetic pathways of the different naturally occurring retinoic isomers may led to selective induction and inhibition of the formation of these isomers in targeted cells in order to alter their biologic behavior. Research in this area has already suggested that reduced glutathione influences the synthesis of various isomers of retinoic acid. Furthermore, we know very little about transmembrane transportation of the different retinoic acid isomers and its impact on catabolism and pharmacokinetics. Theoretically the straight tetraene chain of tRA should readily intercalate into the membrane bilayer, while the kinked chain of 13-cRA may experience steric hindrances.

The ongoing identification and characterization of the physiologic functions of the various nuclear receptor subtypes and isoforms should be completed soon and will be followed by the development of their specific retinoid and nonretinoid inhibitors, which may prove to be more efficacious clinically. The currently available nonretinoid inhibitors of nuclear receptors targeted to retinoid binding domain are already undergoing clinical trials. The potential for developing inhibitors of other nuclear receptor functions (translocation to the nucleus) and domains (DNA binding, dimerization, and tranactivating) will be explored in the future. Advances in protein structure, molecular modeling, and computer graphics will accelerate research in this area.

Future research will have to establish how the retinoid signaling pathway is terminated. Accelerated termination of retinoid signaling mechanism may be important in the development of retinoid resistance. The mechanism for acquired retinoid resistance in patients remains unknown, although increased oxidative catabolism of tRA has been suggested. We do not known whether retinoids translocated to the nucleus are degraded within this organelle or in the cytosol. If tRA is degraded intranuclearly, the enzyme system involved remains a mystery. If the nuclear retinoids are subsequently degraded in the cytosol, how are they transferred back?

ACKNOWLEDGMENTS

The secretarial services of Ms. Sally White are highly appreciated. I am also very thankful for the support and encouragement I have received from Charles Young, M.D., over the years. His critical comments on this manuscript were indispensable.

REFERENCES

1. Levin AA, Sturzenbecker LJ, Kazmer S, Bosakowski T, Huselton C, Allenby G, Speck J, Kratzeisen C, Rosenberger M, Lovery A, Crippo JF (1992) 9-*Cis* retinoic acid stereoisomer binds and activates the nuclear receptor RXR. Nature 355:359–361.
2. Heyman RA, Mangelsdorf DJ, Dyck JA, Stein RB, Eichele G, Evans RM, Thaller C (1992) 9-*Cis* retinoic acid is a high affinity ligand for the retinoid X receptor. Cell 68:397–406.
3. Thaller C, Eichele G (1990) Isolation of 3,4, didehydroretinoic acid, a novel morphogenic signal in the chick wing bud. Nature 345:815–819.
4. Buck J, Derguini F, Levi E, Nakanishi K, Hammerling U (1991) Intracellular signaling by 14-hydroxy-4, 14-retro retinol. Science 254:1654–1655.
5. Tzima G, Sass JO, Wittfohl W, Elmazar MMA, Ehlers K, Nau H (1994) Identification of 9,13-*dicis*-retinoic acid as a major plasma metabolite of 9-*cis* retinoic acid and limited transfer of 9-*cis*-retinoic acid and 9,13-*dicis*-retinoic acid to the mouse and rat embryos. Drug Metab Dispos Biol Fate Chem 22:928–936.
6. Horst RL, Reinhardt TA, Goff JP, Nonnecke BJ, Gambhir VK, Fiorella PD, Napoli JL (1995) Identification of 9-*cis*,13-*cis*-retinoic acid as a major circulating retinoid in plasma. Biochemistry 34:1203–1209.
7. Stahl W, Schwarz W, Sies H (1993) Human serum concentrations of all-*trans* beta and alpha-carotene but not 9-*cis* beta carotene increase upon ingestion of natural isomer mixture obtained from *Dunaliela salina* (betatene). J Nutr 123:847–851.
8. Tsutani H, Ueda T, Uchida M, Nakamura T (1991) Pharmacological studies of retinol palmitate and its clinical effect in patients with acute non-lymphocytic leukemia. Leuk Res 15:463–471.

9. Pastorino U, Infante M, Maioli M, Chiesa G, Buyse M, Firket P, Rosmentz N, Clerici M, Soresi E, Valente Belloni PA, Ravasi G (1993) Adjuvant treatment of stage 1 lung cancer with high dose vitamin A. J Clin Oncol 11:1216–1222.

10. Omenn GS, Goodman G, Thornquist M, Grizzle J, Rosenstock L, Barnhart S, Balmes J, Cherniack MG, Cullen MR, Glass A, Keogh J, Meyskens F Jr, Valanis B, Williams J Jr (1994) The beta carotene and retinol efficacy trial (CARET) for chemoprevention of lung cancer in high risk population: Smokers and asbestos-exposed workers. Cancer Res 54:2038s–2043s.

11. Geiger JM, Ott F, Bollag W (1984) Clinical evaluation of aromatic retinoid, Ro 10–1670 in severe psoriasis. Curr Ther Res 35:735–740.

12. Moriarty M, Dunn J, Darragh A, Lambe R, Brick IH (1982) Etretinate in treatment of actinic keratosis: A double blind crossover study. Lancet 1:364.

13. Arnold A, Kowaleski B, Tozer R, Hirte H (1994) The arotinoids: Early clinical experience and discussion of future development. Leukemia 8:1817–1824.

14. Formelli F, Clerici M, Camp T, DiMauro MG, Magni A, Mascotti G, Moglia D, DePalo G, Costa A, Veronesi U (1993) Five-year administration of Fenretininide: Pharmacokinetics and effects on plasma retinol concentrations. J Clin Oncol 11:2036–2042.

15. Goodman DS, Blaner WS (1994) In MB Sporn, AB Roberts, DS Goodman, eds. The Retinoids, Vol. 2. Orlando, FL: Academic Press, pp 1–39.

16. Goodman DS, Huang HS, Shiratori T (1966) Mechanism of biosynthesis of vitamin A from beta-carotene. J Biol Chem 241:1929–1932.

17. Glover J (1960) The conversion of beta-carotene into vitamin A. In RS Harris, DJ Ingle, eds. Vitamins and Hormones, Vol. 18. New York: Academic Press, pp 371–386.

18. Wang X-D, Krinsky NI, Tang G, Russel RM (1992) Retinoic acid can be produced from eccentric cleavage of beta-carotene in human intestinal mucosa. Arch Biochem Biophys 293:298–304.

19. Goodman DS, Blomstrand R, Werner B, Huang HS, Shiratori T (1966) The intestinal absorption and metabolism of vitamin A and beta carotene in man. J Clin Invest 45:1615–1623.

20. Ong DE, Kakkad B, Macdonald PN (1987) Acyl-CoA-independent esterification of retinol bound to cellular retinol-binding protein (Type II) by microsomes from rat small intestines. J Biol Chem 262:2729–2736.

21. Helgerud P, Petersen LB, Norum KR (1983) Retinol esterification by microsomes from the mucosa of human small intestine. Evidence for acyl-coenzyme A retinol acyltransferase activity. J Clin Invest 71:747–753.

22. Blomhoff R, Green MH, Berg T, Norum KR (1990) Transport and storage of vitamin A. Science 250:399–404.

23. Chander LA, Schwartz SJ (1987) HPLC separation of cis-trans carotene isomers in fresh and processed fruits and vegetables. J Food Sci 52:669–672.

24. Stahl W, Sie H (1992) Uptake of lycopene and its geometrical isomers is greater from heat processed than from unprocessed tomato juice in human. J Nutr 122:2161–2166.

25. Stahl W, Sundquist AR, Hanusch M, Schwartz W, Sie H (1993) Separation of B-carotene and lycopene geometrical isomers in biological samples. Clin Chem 39:810–814.

26. Bernstein PS, Law WC, Rando RR (1987) Isomerization of all-trans retinoids to 11-cis retinoids in vitro. Proc Natl Acad Sci USA 84:1849–1853.

27. Deigner PS, Law WC, Canada FJ, Rando RR (1989) Membrane as the energy source in the endergonic transformation of vitamin A to 11-cis retinol. Science 244:968–971.

28. Urbach J, Rando RR (1994) Isomerization of all-trans retinoic acid to 9-cis-retinoic acid. Biochem J 299:459–465.

29. Nagao A, Olson JA (1994) Enzymatic formation of 9-cis, 13-cis and all-trans retinals from isomers of beta carotene. FASEB J 8:968–973.

30. Napoli JL, Posch KP, Fiorella PD, Boerman MHEM (1991) Physiological occurrence, biosynthesis and metabolism of retinoic acid: Evidence for roles of cellular retinol-binding protein (CRBP) and cellular retinoic acid binding protein (CRABP) in the pathway of retinoic acid homeostasis. Biomed Pharmacother 45:131–143.

31. Petkovich M, Brand NJ, Krust A, Chambon P (1987) A human retinoic acid receptor which belongs to the family of nuclear receptors. Nature 330:444–450.

32. Blomhoff R, Green MH, Berg T, Norum KR (1990) Transport and storage of vitamin A. Science 250:399–404.

33. Ottonello S, Scita G, Mantovani G, Cavazzini D, Rossi GL (1993) Retinol bound to cellular retinol-binding protein is a substrate for cytosolic retinoic acid synthesis. J Biol Chem 268:27133–27142.

34. Siegenthaler G, Saurat JH, Ponec M (1990) Retinol and retinal metabolism. Relationship to the state of differentiation of cultured human keratinocytes. Biochem J 268:371–378.
35. Posch KC, Boerman MHEM, Burns RD, Napoli JL (1991) Holocellular retinol binding protein as a substrate for microsomal retinal synthesis. Biochemistry 30:6224–6230.
36. Posch KC, Burns RD, Napoli JL (1992) Biosynthesis of all-*trans* retinoic acid from retinal. J Biol Chem 267:19676–19682.
37. Roberts AB, Frolik CA, Nichols MD, Sporn MB (1979) Retinoid-dependent induction of the in vivo and in vitro metabolism of retinoic acid in tissues of the vitamin A-deficiency hamster. J Biol Chem 254:6303–6309.
38. Leo MA, Iida S, Lieber CS (1984) Retinoic acid metabolism by a system reconstituted with cytochrome P-450. Arch Biochem Biophys 234:305–312.
39. Gubler ML, Sherman MI (1990) Metabolism of retinoic acid and retinol by intact cells and cell extracts. Methods Enzymol 189:525–536.
40. Roberts AB, Nichols MD, Newton DL, Sporn MB (1979) In vitro metabolism of retinoic acid in hamster intestines and liver. J Biol Chem 254:6296–6302.
41. Frolik CA, Roberts AB, Tavela TE, Roller PP, Newton DL, Sporn MB (1979) Isolation and identification of 4-hydroxy and 4-oxoretinoic acid in vitro metabolites of all-*trans* retinoic acid in hamster trachea and liver. Biochemistry 18:2092–2097.
42. Sato M, Lieber CS (1982) Increased metabolism of retinoic acid after chronic ethanol consumption in rat liver microsomes. Arch Biochem Biophys 213:557–564.
43. Spear PA, Garcin H, Narbonne JF (1988) Increased retinoic acid metabolism following 3,3′,4,4′,5,5′-hexabromobiphenyl injection. Can J Physiol Pharmacol 66:1181–1186.
44. Murray M, Cantrill E, Martini R, Farrell GC (1991) Increased expression of cytochrome P-450 3A2 in male rat liver after dietary vitamin A supplementation. Arch Biochem Biophys 286:618–624.
45. Williams JB, Napoli JL (1987) Inhibition of retinoic acid metabolism by imidazole antimycotics in F9 embryonal carcinoma cells. Biochem Pharmacol 36:1386–1388.
46. Van Waume JP, Coene M-C, Goossens J, Van Nijen G, Cools W, Lauwers W (1988) Ketoconazole inhibits the in vitro and in vivo metabolism of all-*trans* retinoic acid. J Pharmacol Exp Ther 245:718–722.
47. Van Waume JP, Coene M-C, Goossens J, Cools W, Monbaliu J (1990) Effect of cytochrome P-450 inhibitors on the in vivo metabolism of all-*trans* retinoic acid in rats. J Pharmacol Exp Ther 252:365–369.
48. Van Waume JP, Van Nyen G, Coene M-C, Stoppie P, Cools W, Goossens G, Borghgraef P, Janssen PAJ (1992) Liarozole, an inhibitor of retinoic acid metabolism, exerts retinoid-mimetic effects in vivo. J Pharmacol Exp Ther 261:773–779.
49. Wouters W, Van Dun J, Dillen A, Coene M-C, Cools W, DeCoster R (1992) Effects of liarozole, a new antitumor compound, on retinoic acid-induced inhibition of cell growth and on retinoic acid metabolism in MCF-7 human breast cancer cells. Cancer Res 52:2841–2846.
50. Van Waume JP, Janssen PAJ (1989) Is there a case for P-450 inhibitors in cancer treatment? J Med Chem 32:2231–2239.
51. Capdevila J, Gil L, Orellana M, Marnett LJ, Mason JI, Yadagiri P, Falck JR (1988) Inhibitors of P-450-dependent arachidonic acid metabolism. Arch Biochem Biophys 261:257–263.
52. Beetens JR, Loots W, Coenes M-C, DeClerck F (1986) Ketoconazole inhibits the biosynthesis of leukotrienes in vitro and in vivo. Biochem Pharmacol 35:883–891.
53. Steinhilber D, Jaschonek K, Knospe J, Morof O, Roth HJ (1990) Arzneim-Forch/Drug Res 40:1260–1263.
54. Muindi JF, Young CW (1993) Lipid hydroperoxides greatly increase the rate of oxidative catabolism of all-trans retinoic acid by human cell culture microsomes genetically enriched in specific cytochrome P-450 isoforms. Cancer Res 53:1226–1229.
55. Martin R, Murray M (1994) Retinal dehydrogenation and retinoic acid 4-hydroxylation in rat hepatic microsomes: Developmental studies and effect of foreign compounds on the activity. Biochem Pharmacol 47:905–909.
56. Nordblom GD, White RE, Coon MJ (1976) Studies on hydroperoxide-dependent substrate hydroxylation by purified liver microsomal cytochrome P-450. Arch Biochem Biophys 175:524–533.
57. Roberts ES, Vaz ADN, Coon MJ (1992) Role of isoenzymes of rabbit microsomal cytochrome P-450 in the metabolism of retinoic acid, retinol and retinal. Arch Biochem Biophys 41:427–433.

58. Samokyszyn VM, Marnett LJ (1987) Hydroperoxide-dependent cooxidation of 13-cis retinoic acid by prostaglandin H synthase. J Biol Chem 262:14119–14133.
59. Fiorella PD, Giguere V, Napoli JL (1993) Expression of cellular retinoic acid-binding protein (Type II) in *Escherichia coli*. J Biol Chem 268:21545–21552.
60. Fiorella PD, Napoli JL (1991) Expression of cellular retinoic acid binding protein (CRABP) in *Escherichia coli*. J Biol Chem 266:16572–16579.
61. Boyland JF, Gudas LJ (1991) Over-expression of the cellular retinoic acid binding protein-I (CRABP-I) results in a reduction in differentiation-specific gene expression in F9 teratocarcinoma cells. J Cell Biol 112:965–979.
62. Durand B, Saunders M, Leroy Leid M, Chambon P (1992) All-*trans* and 9-*cis* retinoic acid induction of CRABPII transcription is mediated by RAR-RXR heterodimers bound to DR1 and DR2 repeated motifs. Cell 71:73–85.
63. Giguere V, Lyn S, Yip P, Siu C-H, Amin S (1990) Molecular cloning of cDNA encoding a second cellular retinoic acid-binding protein. Proc Natl Acad Sci USA 87:6233–6237.
64. Evans RM (1988) The steroid and thyroid hormone receptor superfamily. Science 240:889–895.
65. Green S, Chambon P (1988) Nuclear receptors enhance our understanding of transcription regulation. Trends Genet 4:309–314.
66. Levin AA, Sturzenbecker LJ, Kazmer S, Bosakowski T, Huselton C, Allenby G, Speck J, Kratzeisen C, Rosenberger M, Lovery A, Crippo JF (1992) 9-Cis retinoic acid stereoisomer binds and activates the nuclear receptor RXR. Nature 355:359–361.
67. Ishikawa T, Umesomo K, Mangelsdorf DJ, Aburtani H, Stanger BZ, Shibasaki Y, Imaware M, Evans RM, Takaku F (1990) A functional retinoic acid receptor encoded by the gene on human chromosome 12. Mol Endocrinol 6:329–344.
68. Freedman L, Luisi B, Korzun R, Basavappa R, Singler P, Yamamoto K (1988) The function and structure of the metal coordination sites within the glucocorticoid DNA binding domain. Nature 334:543–546.
69. Beato M (1989) Gene regulation by steroid hormones. Cell 56:335–344.
70. Zhang X-K, Lehmann J, Hoffmann B, Dawson MI, Cameron J, Graupner G, Hermann T, Pfahl M (1992) Homodimer formation of retinoid X receptor induced by 9-*cis* retinoic acid. Nature 358:587–591.
71. Bugge TH, Pohl J, Lonnoy O, Stunnenberg HG (1992) RXRa, a promiscuous partner of retinoic acid and thyroid hormone receptors. EMBO J 11:1409–1418.
72. Kliewer SA, Umesono K, Mangelsdorf DJ, Evans RM (1992) Retinoid X receptor interacts with nuclear receptors in retinoic acid, thyroid hormone and vitamin D3 signaling. Nature 355:446–449.
73. Zhang X-K, Hoffmann B, Tran P, Graupner G, Pfahl M (1992) Retinoid X receptor is an auxillary protein for thyroid hormone and retinoic acid receptors. Nature 355:441–446.
74. Lehmann JM, Jong L, Fanjul A, Cameron JF, Lu XP, Haefner P, Dawson MI, Pfahl M (1992) Retinoids selective for retinoid X receptor response pathways. Science 258:1944–1946.
75. Lehmann JM, Zhang X-K, Graupner G, Hermann T, Hoffmann B, Pfahl M (1993) Formation of RXR homodimers leads to repression of T3 response: Hormonal cross talk by ligand induced squelching. Mol Cell Biol 13:7698–7707.
76. MacDonald PN, Dowd DR, Nakajima S, Galligan MA, Reeder MC, Haussler CA, Ozato K, Haussler M (1993) Retinoid X receptors stimulate and 9-*cis* retinoic acid inhibits 1,25 dihydroxyvitamin D3-activated expression of the rat osteocalcin gene. Mol Cell Biol 13:5907–5917.
77. Kliewer SA, Umesono K, Noonan DJ, Heyman RA, Evans RM (1992) Convergence of 9-*cis* retinoic acid and peroxisome proliferator signaling pathways through heterodimer formation of their receptors. Nature 358:771–774.
78. Salbert G, Fanjul A, Piedrafita J, Lu X-P, Kim S-J, Tran P, Pfahl M (1993) Retinoic acid receptors and retinoid X receptor-a down regulate the transforming growth factor-beta promoter by antagonizing AP-1 activity. Mol Endocrinol 7:1347–1356.
79. Perez P, Schonthal A, Aranda A (1993) Repression of c-fos gene expression by thyroid hormone and retinoic acid receptors. J Biol Chem 268:23538–23543.
80. Pfahl M (1993) Nuclear receptor/AP-1 interaction. Endocr Rev 14:651–658.
81. Harant H, Korschineck I, Krupitza G, Fazeny B, Dittrich C, Grunt TW (1993) Retinoic acid receptors in ovarian cancer cells. Br J Cancer 68:530–536.
82. Takahashi N, Jetten AM, Breitman TR (1991) Cytokeratins are retinoylated in normal human keratinocytes. Biochem Biophys Res Commun 180:393–400.

83. Takahashi N, Breitman TR (1994) Retinoylation of vimentin in the human myeloid leukemia cell line HL-60. J Biol Chem 269:5913–5917.
84. Takahashi N, Liapi C, Anderson WB, Breitman TR (1991) Retinoylation of the cAMP-binding regulatory subunits of type I and type II cAMP-dependent protein kinases in HL60 cells. Arch Biochem Biophys 290:293–302.
85. Berthiaume L, Deichaite I, Peseckis S, Resh MD (1994) Regulation of enzymatic activity by active site fatty acylation: A new role for long chain fatty acid acylation of proteins. J Biol Chem 269:6498–6505.
86. Takahashi N, Breitman TR (1994) Induction of differentiation and covalent binding to proteins by synthetic retinoids Ch55 and Am80. Arch Biochem Biophys 314:82–89.
87. Takahashi N, Breitman TR (1991) Retinoylation of proteins in leukemia and embryonal carcinoma, and normal kidney cell lines: Differences associated with differential responses to retinoic acid. Arch Biochem Biophys 285:105–110.
88. Leid M, Kastner P, Chambon P (1992) Multiplicity generates diversity in retinoic acid signalimrg pathway. Trends Biochem Sci 17:427–433.
89. Kizaki M, Nakajima H, Mori S, Koike T, Morikawa M, Ohta M, Saito M, Koeffler HP, Ikeda Y (1994) Novel retinoic acid, 9-cis retinoic acid, in combination with all-trans retinoic acid is an effective inducer of differentiation of retinoic acid-resistant HL-60 cells. Blood 83:3289–3297.
90. Dermime S, Grignani F, Clerici M, Nervi C, Sozzi G, Talamo GP, Marchesi E, Formelli F, Parmiani G, Pelicci PG (1993) Occurrence of resistance to retinoic acid in acute promyelocytic leukemia cell line NB4 is associated with altered expression of the pml/RaR alpha protein. Blood 82:1573–1577.
91. Lotan R (1994) Suppression of squamous cell carcinoma growth and differentiation by retinoids. Cancer Res 54:1987s–1990s.
92. Warrell RP, Frankel SR, Miller WH, Scheinberg DA, Itri IM, Hittelman WN, Vyas R, Andreeff M, Tafuri A, Jakubowski A, Gabrilove J, Gordon MS, Dimitrovsky E (1991) Differentiation therapy of acute promyelocytic leukemia with tretinoin (all-*trans* retinoic acid). N Engl J Med 324:1385–1393.
93. Castaigne S, Chomienne C, Daniel MT, Berger R, Fenaux P, Degos L (1990) All-*trans* retinoic acid as a differentiation therapy for acute promyelocytic leukemia: I Clinical results. Blood 76:1704–1709.
94. Huang M-E, Ye Y-C, Chen S-R, Chai J-R, Lu J-X, Zhoa L, Gu L-J, Wang Z-Y (1988) Use of all-*trans* retinoic acid in the treatment of acute promyelocytic leukemia. Blood 72:567–572.
95. Saunders NA, Jetten AM (1994) Control of growth regulatory and differentiation-specific genes in human epidermal keratinocytes by interferon gamma. J Biol Chem 269:2016–2022.
96. Sacks PG, Oke V, Vasey T, Lotan R (1989) Modulation of growth, differentiation and glycoprotein synthesis by beta-all-*trans* retinoic acid in a multicellular tumor spheroid model for squamous carcinoma of the head and neck. Int J Cancer 44:926–933.
97. Gallagher RE, de Cuevillas F, Chang C-S, Schwartz EL (1989) Variable regulation of sensitivity to retinoic acid-induced differentiation in wild-type and retinoic acid-resistant HL-60 cells. Cancer Commun 1:45–54.
98. Hong WK, Endicott J, Itri LM (1986) 13-*cis* retinoic acid in the treatment of oral leukoplakia. N Engl J Med 315:1501–1505.
99. Hong WK, Lippmann SM, Itri LM, Karp DD, Lee JS, Byers RM, Schantz SP, Kramer AM, Lotan R, Peters LJ, Dimery IW, Brown BW, Goepfert H (1990) Prevention of second primary tumors with isotretinoin in squamous cell carcinoma of the head and neck. N Engl J Med 323:795–801.
100. Lippmann S, Batsakis J, Toth B, Weber RS, Lee JJ, Martin JW, Hays GL, Goepfert H, Hong WK (1993) Comparison of low dose isotretinoin with beta carotene to prevent oral carcinogenesis. N Engl J Med 328:15–20.
101. Lippmann SM, Parkinson DR, Itri LM, Weber RS, Schantz SP, Ota DM, Schusterman MA, Krakoff IH, Gutterman JU, Hong WK (1992) 13-*cis* retinoic acid and interferon alpha-2a: Effective combination therapy for advanced squamous cell carcinoma of the skin. J Natl Cancer Inst 84:235–241.
102. Lippmann SM, Kavanagh JJ, Paredes-Espinoza M, Delgadillo-Madrueno F, Paredes-Casillas P, Hong WK, Holdener E, Krakoff IH (1992) 13-*cis* retinoic acid plus interferon alpha-2a: Highly active systemic therapy for squamous cell carcinoma of the cervix. J Natl Cancer Inst 84:241–245.
103. Muindi JRF, Young CW, Warrell RP Jr (1994) Clinical pharmacology of all-*trans* retinoic acid. Leukemia 8:1807–1812.

104. Bennet JM, Catovsky D, Daniel MT, Flandrin G, Galton DAG, Gralnick HR, Sultan C (1976) Proposal for the classification of acute leukemia. Br J Hematol 33:451–458.
105. Imaizumi M, Breitman TR (1987) Retinoic acid induces differentiartion of human promyeloctic leukemia cell line, HL60 and fresh human, leukemia cells in primary culture: A model for differentiation inducing therapy. Eur J Hematol 38:289–302.
106. Larson RA, Kondo K, Vardiman JW, Bulter AE, Golomb HM, Rowley JD (1984) Evidence for a 15;17 translocation in every patient with acute promyelocytic leukemia. Am J Med 76:827–841.
107. Chomienne C, Ballerini P, Balitrand N, Huang ME, Krawice I, Castaigne S, Fenaux P, Tiollai P, Dejean A, Degos L, de The H (1992) The retinoic acid receptor alpha gene is rearranged in retinoic acid-sensitive promyelocytic leukemia. Leukemia 4:802.
108. Longo L, Dionti E, Mencarelli A, Avanzi G, Pegoraro L, Alimena G, Tabilio A, Venti G, Grignani F, Pelicci PD (1990) Mapping of chromosome 17 breakpoints in acute myeloid leukemia. Oncogene 5:1557–1563.
109. Kakizuka A, Miller WH Jr, Umesono K, Warrell RP Jr, Frankel SR, Murty V, Dmitrovsky E, Evans RM (1991) Chromosomal translocation t(15:17) in human acute promyelocytic leukemia fuses RAR alpha with a novel putative transcription factor. PML. Cell 66:663–674.
110. de The H, Lavau C, Marchio A, Chomienne C, Degos L, Dejean A (1991) The PML-RAR alpha fusion mRNA generated by the t(15;17) translocation in acute promyelocytic leukemia encodes a functionally altered RAR. Cell 66:675–684.
111. Perez A, Kastner P, Sethi S, Lutz Y, Reibel C, Chambon P (1993) PML-RAR homodimers: Distinct DNA binding properties and heterodimeric interaction with RXR. EMBO J 12:3171–3182.
112. Chomienne C, Ballerini P, Balitrand N, Daniel MT, Fenaux P, Castaigne S, Degos L (1990) All-trans retinoic acid in acute promyelocytic leukemias. II. In vitro studies: Structure-function relationship. Blood 76:1710–1717.
113. Chen SJ, Zelent A, Tong JH, Yu HQ, Wang Z-Y, Derre J, Berger R, Waxman S, Chen Z (1993) Rearrangements of the retinoic acid receptor alpha and promyelocytic leukemia zinc finger genes resulting from t(11;17) (q23;q21) in a patient with acute promyelocytic leukemia. J Clin Invest 91:2260–2267.
114. Gidez F, Huang W, Tong J-H, Dubois C, Balitrand N, Waxman S, Michaux JL, Martiat P, Degos L, Chen Z (1994) Poor response to all-trans retinoic acid therapy in a t(11;17) PLZF/RAR alpha patient. Leukemia 8:312–317.
115. Kopan R, Traska G, Fuchs E (1987) Retinoids as important regulators of terminal differentiation: Examining keratin expression in individual epidermal cells at various stages of keratinization. J Cell Biol 105:427–440.
116. Darwiche N, Celli G, Sly L, Lancilotti F, DeLuca LM (1993) Retinoid status controls the appearance of reserve cells and keratin expression in mouse cervical epithelium. Cancer Res 53:2287–2299.
117. Saunders NA, Smith RJ, Jetten AM (1993) Regulation of proliferation-specific and differentiation specific genes during senescene of human epidermal keratinocyte and mammary epithelial cells. Biochem Biophys Res Commun 197:46–57.
118. Giguere V (1994) Retinoic acid receptors and cellular retinoid binding proteins: Complex interplay in retinoid signaling. Endocrinol Rev 15:61–79.
119. Nervi C, Vollberg TM, George MD, Zelent A, Chambon P, Jetten AM (1990) Expression of nuclear retinoic acid receptors in normal tracheo-bronchial epithelial cell and lung carcinoma cells. Exp Cell Res 195:163–170.
120. Roman SD, Clarke CL, Hall RE, Alexander IE, Sutherland RI (1992) Expression and regulation of retinoic acid receptors in human breast cancer cells. Cancer Res 52:2235–2242.
121. (1994) Modulation of growth factor receptors on acute myelocytic leukemia cells by all-trans retinoic acid. Jpn J Cancer Res 85:378–383.
122. Roberts AB, Sporn MB (1991) The transforming growth factor-b,. In MB Sporn, AB Roberts, eds. Peptide Growth Factors and their Receptors I. New York: Springer-Verlag, pp 419–472.
123. Derynck R (1994) The biological complexity of transforming growth factor-beta. In A Thompson, ed. The Cytokine Handbook. Boston: Academic Press, pp 319–342.
124. Tsou HC, Lee X, Si SP, Peacocke M (1994) Regulation of retinoic acid receptor expression in dermal fibroblast. Exp Cell Res 211:68–73.
125. Torrisi R, Pensa F, Orenga MA, Catsafados E, Ponzani P, Boccardo F, Costa A, Decensi A (1993) The synthetic retinoid, fenretinide, lowers plasma insulin-like growth factor I levels in breast cancer patients. Cancer Res 53:4769–4771.

126. Clarke AR, Purdie CA, Harrison DJ, Morris RG, Bird CC, Hooper ML, Wyllie AH (1993) Thymocyte apoptosis induced by p53-dependent and independent pathways. Nature 363:849–852.
127. Atencia R. Garcia-Sanz M, Unda F, Arechaga J (1994) Apoptosis during retinoic acid-induced differentiation of F9 embryonal carcinoma cells. Exp Cell Res 214:663–667.
128. Martin SJ, Bradley JG, Cotter TG (1990) HL-60 cells induced to differentiate towards neutrophils subsequently die via apoptosis. Clin Exp Immunol 79:448–453.
129. Maxwell SA, Mukhopadhyay T (1994) Transient stabilization of p53 in non-small cell lung carcinoma cultures arrested for growth by retinoic acid. Exp Cell Res 214:67–74.
130. Delia D, Aiello A, Lombardi L, Pellicci PG, Grignani F, Grignani F, Formelli F, Menard S, Costa A, Veronesi •• (1993) N-(4-hydroxyphenyl)retinamide induces apoptosis of malignant hematopoietic cell lines including those unresponsive to retinoic acid. Cancer Res 53:6036–6040.
131. Grignani F, Ferucci PF, Testa U, Talamo G, Fagioli M, Alcalay M, Mencarelli A, Grignani F, Peschle C, Nicoletti I (1993) The acute promyelocytic leukemia-specific PML-RAR alpha fusion protein inhibits differentiation and promotes survival of myeloid precursor cells. Cell 74:423–431.
132. Hockenbery D, Nunez G, Milliman C, Schreiber RD, Korsmeyer SJ (1990) Bcl-2 is an inner mitochondrial membrane protein that blocks programmed cell death. Nature 348:334–336.
133. Rodriguez-Tebar A, Rohrer H (1991) Retinoic acid induces NGF-dependent survival response and high-affinity NGF receptors in immature chick sympathetic neurons. Development 112:813–820.
134. Park JR, Robertson K, Hickstein DD, Tsai S, Hockenbery DM, Collins SJ (1994) Dysregulated bcl-2 expression inhibits apoptosis but not differentiation of retinoic acid induced HL-60 granulocytes. Blood 84:440–445.
135. Naumovski L, Cleary ML (1994) Bcl-2 inhibits apoptosis associated with terminal differentiation of HL-60 myeloid leukemia cells. Blood 83:2261–2267.
136. Manfredini R, Grande A, Tagliafico E, Barbieri D, Zucchini P, Citro G, Zupi G, Franceschi C, Torelli U, Ferrari S (1993) Inhibition of c-fes expression by antisense oligomer cause apoptosis of HL60 cells induced to granulocytic differentiation. J Exp Med 178:381–389.
137. Yang Y, Vacchio MS, Ashwell JD (1993) 9-cis retinoic acid inhibits activation-driven T-cell apoptosis: Implications for retinoid X receptor involvement in thymocyte development. Proc Natl Acad Sci USA 90:6170–6174.
138. Ryan JJ, Danish R, Gottlieb CA, Clarke MF (1993) Cell cycle analysis of p53-induced cell death in murine erthyroleukemia cells. Mol Cell Biol 13:711–719.
139. Moberg KH, Tyndall WA, Hall DJ (1992) Wild-type murine p53 represses transcription from the murine c-myc promoter in a human glial cell line. J Cell Biochem 49:208–215.
140. Ginsberg D, Mechta F, Yaniv M, Oren M (1991) Wild type p53 can downmodulate the activity of various promoters. Proc Natl Acad Sci USA 88:9979–9983.
141. Agoff SN, Hou J, Linzer DIH, Wu B (1993) Regulation of the human hsp 70 promoter by p53. Science 259:84–87.
142. Hwang MS, Thompson KL, Ahn CH (1995) p53-independent induction of p21^{WAFI} and apoptosis by all-trans retinoic acid and 9-cis retinoic acid in human prostate cancer cell lines. Proc Am Assoc Cancer Res 36:57 (abstr).
143. Guchelaar H-J, Timmer-Bosscha H, Dam-Meiring A, Uges DRA, Oosterhuis JW, DeVries EGE (1993) Enhancement of cisplatin and etoposide cytotoxicity after all-trans retinoic acid induced cellular differentiation of a murine embryonal carcinoma cell line. Int J Cancer 55:442–447.
144. Breimer LH (1990) Molecular mechanism of oxygen radical carcinogenesis and mutagenesis: The role of DNA base damage. Mol Carcinogen 3:188–197.
145. Dean RT, Hunt JV, Grant AJ, Yamamoto Y, Niki E (1991) Free radical damage to proteins: The influence of the relative localization of radical generation, antioxidants, and target proteins. Free Radic Biol Med 11:161–168.
146. Cadena E (1989) Biochemistry of oxygen toxicity. Ann Rev Biochem 58:79–110.
147. Weitzman SA, Turk PW, Milkowski DH, Kozlowski K (1994) Free radicals adducts induce alterations in DNA cytosine methylation. Proc Natl Acad Sci USA 91:1261–1264.
148. Samokyszyn VM, Marnett JL (1990) Inhibition of liver microsomal lipid peroxidation by 13-cis retinoic acid. Free Radic Biol Med 8:491–496.
149. Buege JA, Aust SD (1978) Microsomal lipid peroxidation. In S Fleischer, L Parker, eds. Methods in Enzymology, Vol. 52. New York: Academic Press, pp 302–308.
150. Gundimeda U, Hara SK, Anderson WB, Gopalakrishina R (1993) Retinoids inhibit the oxidative modification of protein kinase C induced by oxidant tumor promoters. Arch Biochem Biophys 300:526–530.
151. Tesoriere L, Ciaccio M, Valenza M, Bongiorno A, Maresi E, Albiero R, Livrea MA (1994) Effect

of vitamin A administration on resistance of rat heart against doxorubicin-induced cardiotoxicity and lethality. J Pharmacol Exp Ther 269:430–436.

152. Folkman J (1992) The role of angiogenesis in tumor growth. Semin Cancer Biol 3:65–71.

153. Weidener N, Folkman J, Pozza F, Bevilacqua P, Alfred EN, Moore DH, Meli S, Gasparini G (1992) Tumor angiogenesis: A new significant and independent prognostic indicator in early stage breast carcinoma. J Natl Cancer Inst 84:1875–1887.

154. Horak ER, Leek R, Klenk N, Lejeune S, Smith K, Stuart N, Greenall M, Stepniewska K, Harris AL (1992) Angiogenesis, assessed by platelet/endothelial cell adhesion molecule antibodies, as indicator of node metastases and survival in breast cancer. Lancet 340:1120–1124.

155. Macchiarini P, Fontanini G, Hardin MJ, Squartini F, Angeletti CA (1992) Relation of neovascularization to metastasis of non small cell lung cancer. Lancet 340:145–146.

156. Majewski S, Polakowski I, Marczal M, Jablonska S (1986) The effects of retinoids on lymphocyte and transformed cell line-induced angiogenesis. Clin Exp Dermatol 2:317–318.

157. Oikawa T, Hirotani K, Nakamura O, Shudo K, Hiragun A, Iwaguchi T (1989) A high potent antiangiogenic activity of retinoids. Cancer Lett 48:157–162.

158. Rudnicka L, Marczak M, Smurlo A, Makiela B, Skiendzielewska A, Spopinska M, Majewski S, Jablonska A (1991) Acetretin decreases tumor cell-induced angiogenesis. Skin Pharmacol 4:150–153.

159. Majewski S, Szmurlo M, Marczak M, Jablonska S, Bollag W (1994) Synergistic effect of retinoids and intereferon-alpha on tumor-induced angiogenesis: Anti-angiogenic effect on HPV-harboring tumor cell lines. Int J Cancer 57:81–85.

160. Bouck N (1990) Tumor angiogenesis: The role of oncogenes and tumor suppressor genes. Cancer Cell 2:179–185.

161. Czubayko F, Smith RV, Chung HC, Wellstein A (1994) Tumor growth and angiogenesis induced by a secreted binding protein for fibroblast growth factors. J Biol Chem 269:28243–28248.

162. Kessler D, Langer R, Pless N, Folkman F (1976) Mast cells and tumor angiogenesis. Int J Cancer 18:703–709.

163. Saksela O, Rifkin DB (1990) Release of basic fibroblast growth factor-heparan sulfate complexes from endothelial cells by plasminogen activator-mediated proteolytic activity. J Cell Biol 110:767–775.

164. Lane TF, Iruela-Arispe ML, Johnson RS, Sage EH (1994) SPARC is a source of copper-binding peptides that stimulate angiogenesis. J Cell Biol 125:929–943.

165. Agarwal C, Hembree JR, Rorker EA, Eckert RL (1994) Interferon and retinoic acid suppress the growth of human papillomavirus type 16 immortalized cervical epithelial cells, but only interferon suppresses the level of the human papillomavirus transforming oncogenes. Cancer Res 54:2108–2112.

166. Eicher SA, Taylor-Cooley LD, Donovan DT (1994) Isotretinoin therapy for recurrent respiratory papillomatosis. Arch Otolaryngol Head Neck Surg 120:405–409.

167. Ross AC (1992) Vitamin A status: Relationship to immunity and the antibody response. Proc Soc Exp Biol Med 200:303–330.

168. Ross AC, Hammerling U (1994) Retinoids and the immune system. In MB Sporn, AB Roberts, DS Goodman, eds. The Retinoids: Biology, Chemistry and Medicine. New York: Raven Press, pp 521–544.

169. Shekelle RB, Epper M, Liu S, Maliza C, Rossof AH, Raynor WJ Jr, Paul O, Shryock AM, Stamler J (1981) Dietary vitamin A and risk of cancer in the Western Electric study. Lancet 2:1186–1190.

170. Byers TE, Graham S, Haughy BP, Marshall JR, Swanson MK (1987) Diet and lung cancer risk: Findings from the western New York diet study. Am J Epidemiol 125:351–363.

171. Kark JD, Smith AH, Hames CG, Switzer BR (1981) Serum vitamin A (retinol) and cancer incidence in Evans County, Georgia. J Natl Cancer Inst 66:7–16.

172. DeLuca LM (1977) The direct involvement of vitamin A in glycosyl transfer reactions of mammalian membranes. Vitam Horm 35:1–57.

173. Lotan R (1980) Effects of vitamin A and its analogs (retinoids) on normal and neoplastic cells. Biochim Biophys Acta 605:33–91.

174. Carman JA, Hayes CE (1991) Abnormal regulation of interferon gamma secretion in vitamin A deficency. J Immunol 147:1247–1252.

175. Finkelman FD, Katona IM, Mosmann TR, Coffman RL (1988) IFN-gamma regulates the isotype of Ig secreted during in vivo humoral immune response. J Immunol 140:1022–1027.

176. Blomhoff HK, Smeland EB, Erikstein B, Rasmissen AM, Skrede B, Skjonsberg C, Blomhoff R

(1992) Vitamin A is a key regulator of cell growth, cytokine production and differentiation in normal B-cells. J Biol Chem 267:23988–23992.

177. Garbe A, Buck J, Hammerling U (1992) Retinoids are important co-factors in T cell activation. J Exp Med 176:109–117.

178. Bowman TA, Goonewardene IM, Pasatiempo AMG, Ross AC, Taylor CE (1990) Vitamin A deficiency decreases natural killer cell activity and interferon production in rats. J Nutr 120:1264–1273.

179. Savill J, Fadok V, Henson P, Haslett C (1993) Phagocyte recognition of cells undergoing apoptosis. Immunol Today 14:131–136.

180. Jarrous N, Kaempfer R (1994) Induction of human interleukin-I gene expression by retinoic acid and its regulation at processing of precursor transcripts. J Biol Chem 269:23141–23149.

181. Elias JA, Zheng T, Einarsson O, Landry M, Trow T, Rebert N, Panuska J (1994) Epithelial interleukin II. J Biol Chem 269:22261–22268.

182. Duell EA, Astrom A, Griffiths CEM, Chambon P, Voorhees J (1992) Human skin levels of retinoic acid and cytochrome P-450-derived 4-hydroxyretinoic acid after topical application of retinoic acid in vivo compared to concentrations required to stimulate retinoic acid recepor-mediated transcription in vitro. J Clin Invest 90:1269–1274.

183. Bugge CJL, Rodriguez LC, Vane FM (1985) Determination of isotretinoin or etretinate and their major metabolites in human blood by reverse-phase high-performance liquid chromatography. J Pharm Biomed Anal 3:269–277.

184. Shelley R, Price JC, Jun HW, Cadwallader DE, Capomacchia AC (1982) Improved and rapid high-performance liquid chromatographic assay for 13-cis-retinoic acid or all-trans-retinoic acid. J Pharm Sci 71:262–264.

185. Muindi JRF, Frankel SR, Huselton C, Degrazia F, Garland WA, Young CW, Warrell RP Jr (1992) Clinical pharmacology of oral all-trans retinoic acid in patients with acute promyelocytic leukemia. Cancer Res 52:2138–2142.

186. Chiang T-C (1980) Gas chromatographic-mass spectrometric assay for low levels of retinoic acid in human blood. J Chromatogr 182:335–340.

187. Huselton CA, Fayer BE, Garland WA, Liberato DJ (1990) Qantification of endogenous retinoic acid in human plasma by liquid chromatographuy/mass spectrometry. In MA Brown, ed. Liquid Chromatography/Mass Spectrometry: Applications in Agricultural, Pharmaceutical and Environmental Chemistry. Washington DC: American Chemical Society, pp 166–178.

188. Conley B, Wu S (1995) Identification of new glucuronide metabolites of all-trans retinoic acid (ATRA) in plasma of patients. Proc Am Soc Clin Oncol 359, abstr.

189. Leenheer AP, Lambert WE, Claeys I (1982) All-trans-retinoic acid: Measurement of reference values in human serum by high-performance liquid chromatography. J Lipid Res 23:1362–1367.

190. Colter S, Bugge CJL, Colburn WA (1983) Role of gut contents intestinal wall and liver on the first pass metabolism and absolute bioavailability of isotretinoin in the dog. Drug Metab Dispos Biol Fate Chem 11:458–462.

191. Colburn WA, Gibson DM, Rodriguez LC, Bugge CJL, Blumenthal HP (1985) Food increases the bioavailability of isotretinoin. J Clin Pharmacol 25:583–589.

192. Lee JS, Newman RA, Lippman SM, Huber MH, Minor T, Raber MN, Krakoff IH, Hong WK (1993) Phase I evaluation of all-trans retinoic acid in adults with solid tumors. J Clin Oncol 11:959–966.

193. Benedetti F, Miller V, Rigas J, Tong W, Ulm E, Truglia J, Gill G, Warrell RP Jr (1995) Initial clinical and pharmacokinetic study of 9-cis retinoic acid. Proc Am Assoc Cancer Res 36:1283 (abstr).

194. Goodman GE, Einspahr JG, Alberts DS, Davis TP, Leigh SA, Chen HSG, Meyskens FL (1982) Pharmacokinetics of 13-cis-retinoic acid in patients with advanced cancer. Cancer Res 42:2087–2091.

195. Kerr IG, Lippman ME, Jenkins J, Myers CE (1982) Pharmacology of 13-cis-retinoic acid in humans. Cancer Res 42:2069–2073.

196. Kurie JM, Lee JS, Griffin T, Drum P, Weber C, Massimini G, Hong WK (1995) Phase I trial of 9-cis retinoic acid in solid tumor patients. Proc Am Soc Clin Oncol 1528 (abstr).

197. Rigas JR, Miller VA, Benedetti FM, Tong WP, Gill JA, Truglia JA, Ulm E, Loewen G, Warrell RP Jr (1995) Phase I clinical and pharmacologic study of 9-cis retinoic acid (LGD1057). Proc Am Soc Clin Oncol 14:370 (abstr).

198. Smith MA, Adamson PC, Balis FM, Feusner J, Aronson L, Murphy RF, Horowitz ME, Reaman

G, Hammond GD, Fenton RM, Connaghan GD, Hittleman WN, Poplack DG (1992) Phase I and pharmacokinetic evaluation of all-trans retinoic acid in pediatric patients with cancer. J Clin Oncol 10:1666–1673.

199. Rigas JR, Francis PA, Muindi JRF, Kris MG, Huselton C, DeGrazia F, Orazem JP, Young CW, Warrell RP Jr (1993) Constitutive variability in the pharmacokinetics of the natural retinoid, all-trans retinoic acid, and its modulation by ketoconazole. J Natl Cancer Inst 85:1921–1926.

200. Muindi JF, Scher HI, Rigas JR, Warrell RP Jr, Young CW (1994) Elevated plasma lipid peroxide content correlates with rapid plasma clearance of all-*trans* retinoic acid in patients with advnaced cancer. Cancer Res 54:2125–2128.

201. Caliaro MJ, Marmouget C, Guichard S, Mazar P, Valette A, Moisand A, Bugat R, Jozan S (1994) Response of four ovarian carcinoma cell lines to all-*trans* retinoic acid: Relationship with induction of differentiation and retinoic acid receptor expression. Int J Cancer 56:743–748.

202. Cornic M, Delva L, Guidez F, Balitrand N, Degos L, Chomiene C (1992) Induction of retinoic acid-binding protein in normal and malignant human myeloid cells by retinoic acid in acute promyelocytic leukemia patients. Cancer Res 52:3329–3334.

203. Miller VA, Rigas JR, Muindi JRF, Tong WP, Venkatraman E, Kris MG, Warrell RP Jr (1994) Modulation of all-*trans* retinoic acid pharmacokinetics by liarozole. Cancer Chemother Pharmacol 34:522–526.

204. Mehta K, Sadeghi T, Mcqueen T, Lopez-Brestein G (1994) Liposome encapsulation circumvents the hepatic clearance mechanisms of all-*trans* retinoic acid. Leuk Res 18:587–596.

205. Drach J, Lopez-Berestein G, Mcqueen T, Andreeff M, Mehta K (1993) Induction of differentiation in myeloid leukemia cell lines and acute promyelocytic leukemia cells by liposomal all-*trans* retinoic acid. Cancer Res 53:2100–2104.

206. Adamson PC, Balis FM, Yarchoan R, Pluda JM, Bailey J, Murphy RF, Bauza S, Poplack DG (1994) Pharmacokinetics of all-*trans* retinoic acid administered on an intermittent schedule. Proc Am Assoc Cancer Res 34:1265 (abstr).

207. Brazzell RK, Vane FM, Ehmann CW, Colburn WA (1983) Pharmacokinetics of isotretinoin during repetitive dosing to patients. Eur J Clin Pharmacol 24:695–702.

208. Peng Y-M, Dalton WS, Alberts DS, Xu M-J, Lim H, Meyskens FL Jr (1989) Pharmacokinetics of N-(4-hydroxyphenyl)-retinamide and effect of its oral administration on plasma retinol concentrations in cancer patients. Int J Cancer 43:22–26.

209. Lippman SM, Meyskens FL (1987) Treatment of advanced squamous cell carcinoma of skin with isotretinoin. Ann Intern Med 107:499–501.

210. Warrell RP Jr, Maslak P, Eardley A, Heller G, Miller WH Jr, Frankel SR (1994) Treatment of acute promyelocytic leukemia with all-*trans* retinoic acid: An update of the New York experience. Leukemia 8:929–933.

211. Dombret H, Castaigne S, Fenaux P, Chomienne C, Degos L (1994) Induction treatment of acute promyelocytic leukemia using all-*trans* retinoic acid. Controversies about dosage, advantages and side effect management. Leukemia 8:S73–S75.

212. Cortes JE, Kantarjian H, O'Brien S, Robertson LE, Koller C, Hirsh-Ginsberg C, Stass S, Keating M, Estey •• (1994) All-*trans* retinoic acid followed by chemotherapy for salvage of refractory or relapsed acute promyelocytic leukemia. Cancer 73:2946–2952.

213. Huang W, Sun GL, Li XS, Cao Q, Lu Y, Jang GS, Zhang FQ, Chai JR, Wang ZY, Waxman S, Chen Z, Chen S-J (1993) Acute promyelocytic leukemia: Clinical relevance of two major PML-RAR alpha isoforms and detection of minimal residual disease by retro ranscriptase/polymerase chain reaction to predict relapse. Blood 82:1264–1269.

214. Vahdat L, Maslk P, Miller WH Jr, Eardley A, Heller G, Scheinberg DA, Warrell RP Jr (1994) Early mortality and the retinoic acid syndrome in acute promyelocytic leukemia: Impact of leukocytosis, low dose chemotherapy, PML/RAR-alpha isoform, and CD13 expression in patients treated with all-*trans* retinoic acid. Blood 84:3843–3849.

215. LoCoco F, Diverio D, Pandolfi PP, Biondi A, Rossi V, Avvisati G, Rambaldi A, Arcese W, Petti MC, Meloni G, Mandelli F, Grignani F, Masera G, Barbui T, Pellici PG (1992) Molecular evaluation of residual disease as a predictor of relapse in acute promyelocytic leukemia. Lancet 340:1437–1438.

216. Miller WH Jr, Kakizuka A, Frankel SR, Warrell RP Jr, Deblassio A, Levine K, Evans RM, Dmitrovsky E (1992) Reverse transcription polymerase chain reaction for the rearranged retinoic acid receptor alpha clarifies diagnosis and detects minimal residual disease in acute promyelocytic leukemia. Proc Natl Acad Sci USA 89:4840–4844.

217. Ohashi H, Ichikawa A, Takagi N, Hotta T, Naoe T, Ohnoi R, Saito H (1992) Remission

induction of acute promyelocytic leukemia by all-*trans* retinoic acid: Molecular evidence of restoration of normal hematopoiesis after differentiation and subsequent extinction of leukemic clone. Leukemia 6:859–862.

218. Kawai Y, Watanabe K, Kizaki M, Murata M, Kamata T, Uchida H, Moriki T, Yokoyama K, Tokuhira M, Nakajima H, Handa M, Ikeda Y (1994) Rapid improvement of coagulopathy by all-*trans* retinoic acid in acute promyelocytic leukemia. Am J Hematol 46:184–188.

219. Brungs M, Radmark O, Samuelsson B, Steinhilber D (1994) On the induction of 5-lipoxygenase expression and activity in HL-60 cells: Effects of vitamin D3, retinoic acid, DMSO and TGFb. Biochem Biophys Res Commun 205:1572–1580.

220. Sellmayer A, Goebl H, Obermeier H, Volk R, Reder E, Weber C, Weber PC (1994) Differential induction of eicosanoid synthesis in monocytic cells treated with retinoic acid and 1,25-dihydroxy-vitamin D3. Prostaglandins 47:203–220.

221. Muindi J, Frankel SR, Miller WH Jr, Jakubowski A, Scheinberg DA, Young CW, Dmitrovsky E, Warrell RP Jr (1992) Continuous treatment with all-*trans* retinoic acid causes a progressive decrease in plasma concentration: Implications for relapse and resistance in acute promyelocytic leukemia. Blood 79:299–303.

222. Robertson KA, Emami B, Collins SJ (1992) Retinoic acid-resistant HL-60R cells harbor a point mutation in the retinoic acid receptor ligand-binding domain that confers dominant negative activity. Blood 80:1885–1889.

223. Dermine S, Grignani F, Clerici M, Nervi C, Sozzi G, Talamo GP, Marchesi E, Formelli F, Parmiani G, Pelicci PG (1993) Occurrence of resistance to retinoic acid in acute promyelocytic leukemia cell line NB4 is associated with altered expression of the pml/RAR alpha. Blood 82:1573–1577.

224. Degos L, Dombret H, Chomuienne C, Daniel M-T, Miclea J-M, Chastang C, Castaigne S, Fenaux P (1995) All-*trans* retinoic acid as a differentiating agent in the treatment of acute promyelocytic leukemia. Blood 85:2643–2653.

225. Fenaux P (1994) Results of APL 91 European trial combining ATRA and chemotherapy: Presentation of APL 1993 trial. Leukemia 8:S70–S72.

226. Eardley AM, Heller G, Warrell RP Jr (1994) Morbidity and cost of remission induction therapy with all-*trans* retinoic acid compared with standard chemotherapy in acute promyelocytic leukemia. Leukemia 8:934–939.

227. Frankel SR, Eardley A, Lauwers G, Weiss M, Warrell RP Jr (1992) The "retinoic acid syndrome" in acute promyelocytic leukemia. Ann Intern Med 117:292–296.

228. Nakamaki T, Hino K-I, Yokoyama A, Hisatake J-I, Tomoyasu S, Honma Y, Hozumi M, Tsuruoka N (1994) Effect of cytokines on the proliferation and differentiation of acute promyelocytic leukemia cells: Possible relationship to the development of retinoic acid syndrome. Anticancer Res 14:817–823.

229. Sakakibara M, Ichikawa M, Amano Y, Matsuzawa S, Agematsu K, Mori T, Koike K, Nakahata T, Komiyama A (1993) Hypercalcaemia associated with all-*trans* retinoic acid in the treatment of acute promyelocytic leukemia. Leuk Res 17:441–443.

230. Akiyama H, Nakamura N, Sakamaki H, Onozawa Y (1992) Hypercalcaemia due to all-*trans* retinoic acid. Lancet 339:308–309.

231. Niesvizky R, Siegel DS, Busquets X, Nichols G, Muindi J, Warrell RP Jr, Michaeli J (1995) Hypercalcaemia and increased serum interleukin-6 levels induced by all-*trans* retinoic acid in patients with multiple myeloma. Br J Hematol 89:217–218.

232. Aul C, Runde V, Gattermann N (1993) All-*trans* retinoic acid in patients with myelodysplastic syndrome: Results of a pilot study. Blood 82:2967–2974.

233. Meyskens FL Jr, Surwit E, Moon TE, Childers JM, Davis JR, Dorr RT, Johnson CS, Alberts DS (1994) Enhancement of regression of cervical intra-epithelial neoplasia II (moderate dysplasia) with topically applied all-*trans*-retinoic acid: A randomized trial. J Natl Cancer Inst 86:539–543.

234. Lippman SM, Kavanagh JJ, Paredes M, Delgadillo F, Hong WK, Figuerda F, Olguin A, Freedman RS, Massiimini G, Holdener EE, Krakoff IH (1993) 13-*cis*-retinoic acid (13-cRA), interferon-alpha-2a (IFNa-2a) and radiotherapy for locally advanced cancer of the cervix. Proc Am Soc Clin Oncol 12:257.

235. Bollang W (1987) Vitamin A and retinoids: From nutrition to pharmacotherapy in dermatology and oncology. Lancet 1:860–863.

236. Kraemer KH, DiGiovanna JJ (1988) Prevention of skin cancer in xeroderma pigmentosum with the use of oral isotretinoin. N Engl J Med 318:1633–1637.

237. Kelly WK, Scher HI, Muindi J, Bajorin D, O'Moore P, Reuter V, Young CW, Curley T, Liebertz

C (1993) Phase II of all-*trans* retinoic acid in patients with adenocarcinoma of the prostate. Proc Am Assoc Cancer Res 34:1210 (abstr).

238. Trump D, Smith D, Stiff D, Adedoyin A, Bahnson R, Day R, Branch R (1994) All-*trans* retinoic acid (ATRA) in hormone refactory prostate cancer (HRPC): Ineffectiveness due to failure of drug delivery? Proc Am Soc Clin Oncol 13:752 (abstr).

239. Smith DC, Jacob HE, Branch RA, Adedoyin A, Stiff D, Trump DL, Johnson JT (1994) A phase II trial of all-*trans* retinoic acid (ATRA) in advanced squamous cell carcinoma of head and neck (SCCHN). Proc Am Soc Clin Oncol 13:930 (abstr).

240. Winer E, Sutton L, Petros W, Havlin K, King S, Iglehart J (1994) Phase II trial of all-*trans* retinoic acid (TRA) in patients (pts) with metastatic breast cancer. Proc Am Soc Clin Oncol 13:46 (abstr).

241. Friedland D, Luginbuhl W, Meehan L, Gorman G, Kaiser L, Treat J (1994) Phase II trial of all-*trans* retinoic acid in metastatic non-small cell lung cancer. Proc Am Soc Clin Oncol 13:1086 (abstr).

242. Yung WKA, Scott C, Fischbach S, Phuphanich S, Langer CJ (1994) All-*trans* retinoic acid: A phase II Radiation Therapy Oncology Group study (RTOG-9113) in patients with recurrent malignant astrocytoma. Proc Am Soc Clin Oncol 13:495 (abstr).

VIII. NOVEL MECHANISMS AND APPROACHES

14. APOPTOSIS AND CANCER CHEMOTHERAPY

STUART G. LUTZKER AND ARNOLD J. LEVINE

For many years oncologists have focused on the proliferative capacity of tumors as an indication of their aggressiveness. Mitotic index and S-phase fraction are routinely reported in some tumors and have been used to guide treatment in some instances. It is only recently than we have come to appreciate that the net growth of a tumor is directly related to both its proliferative capacity as well as the rate of programmed cell death, termed *apoptosis*. Although first described in 1972 [1] and viewed largely as a distinctive form of cell death occurring during development and normal tissue turnover [2], apoptosis occurs spontaneously in tumor cells both in vitro and in vivo, and apoptosis can be induced in cancer cells by such diverse stimuli as DNA damage and growth factor withdrawl. As is discussed in this chapter, there appears to be a heavy selection pressure for genetic changes that inhibit apoptosis in cancer cells, and inhibition of apoptosis may represent a new form of drug resistance in cancer treatment.

APOPTOSIS IS A DISTINCT FORM OF CELL DEATH

On a morphological basis, apoptosis is an ordered process that is distinct from that of necrosis [3]. Following an appropriate signal, there is condensation of chromatin at the periphery of the nuclear envelope in apoptotic cells followed by convolution of the nuclei. This is closely followed by convolution of the cytoplasm around the fragments of nuclei to form distinct morphological structures, termed *apoptotic bodies*. As opposed to necrosis, there is no swelling of mitochondria and cellular permeability is maintained until late in the apoptotic process. Apoptotic cells are rapidly phagocytized by macrophages through vitronectin receptors [4], and this process does not induce the inflammatory response often seen in necrosis.

At the biochemical level, apoptosis is energy dependent and is characterized by a number of distinct cellular processes. Concurrent with the early condensation of chromatin is the activation of a pH-neutral Ca^{2+}/Mg^{2+}-dependent endonuclease that cleaves the DNA at internucleosomal sites to generate a ladder of DNA sizes [5,6]. The formation of apoptotic bodies appears to be due to the expression of a transglutaminase [7], which crosslinks intracellular proteins to form a rigid framework. The regulation of these biochemical processes is unclear at present, but intracellular Ca^{2+} levels rise during apoptosis in some cell types [8] and apoptosis can be stimulated by calcium ionophores [9].

NONRANDOM GENETIC ALTERATIONS IN
CANCER CELLS STIMULATE APOPTOSIS

A simple view of oncogenesis is that specific growth-promoting genes are either mutated or overexpressed in tumors, which results in enhanced cellular proliferation. For example, the c-myc gene is one of the immediate early response genes that is induced in quiescent cells following mitogenic stimulation [10]. The c-myc gene is translocated and overexpressed in human Burkitt's lymphoma [11], and avian retroviruses that have transduced the c-myc gene cause leukemia [12]. Introduction of a c-myc gene under the control of the highly active tissue-specific immunoglobulin (Ig) heavy chain enhancer into the mouse germ line gives rise to lymphoid malignancies in 100% of mice, with a median time of 2 months [13], further supporting the central role of this and other transforming oncogenes in tumorgenesis.

Given the growth-promoting role of c-myc in both normal and neoplastic cells, it is perhaps surprising that c-myc also stimulates apoptosis. This observation was first made by Evan and colleagues using Rat-1 fibroblasts that were engineered to constitutively overexpress a c-myc gene [14]. These cells, unlike normal Rat-1 fibroblasts, continue to proliferate in low serum, even though there is no appreciable increase in cell number. The lack of increase in cell numbers is due to a compensatory stimulation of apoptosis by the c-myc gene. Mutations in the c-myc gene that inhibit its transformation activity also inhibit its ability to stimulate apoptosis in low serum, indicating that these two activities are tightly linked. In addition to low serum, apoptosis is induced in Rat-1 cells overexpressing c-myc following a number of stimuli that normally cause cell cycle arrest, such as thymidine excess, isoleucine deprivation, and cycloheximide. Similarly, M1 myeloid leukemia cells that overexpress a deregulated c-myc gene undergo apoptosis following exposure to DNA-damaging agents [15]. Thus c-myc is capable of inducing apoptosis in various cell types, and this apoptosis appears to be triggered when the cell receives a conflicting signal for growth arrest.

c-myc is not alone in its ability as a transforming oncogene to stimulate apoptosis. Apoptosis is also stimulated by the adenovirus E1A protein [16], as well as the human papillovirus E7 protein [17], following exposure to drugs that normally cause growth arrest. Both of these oncogenes, unlike c-*myc*, directly inactivate the retinoblatoma protein, which is crucial for growth arrest in late G1 of the cell cycle.

BCL-2 AND A NEW CLASS OF ONCOGENES

The observation that oncogenes induce both transformation and apoptosis in vitro in tissue culture cell lines could be viewed as a phenomena of the artificial conditions imposed in such systems. If oncogenes stimulate proliferation and apoptosis in vivo and net tumor growth results from proliferation in excess of apoptosis, then there would appear to be a heavy selection pressure for genetic alterations to inhibit apoptosis. Indeed, it would be predicted that these genetic alterations should be nearly as frequent as those that activate oncogenes if suppression of apoptosis is important in tumorgensis.

This hypothesis appears to be fulfilled in the case of follicular lymphomas. Approximately 90% of these tumors contain a characteristic chromosomal translocation between the long arms of chromosmes 14 and 18, t(14;18) (q32;q21). This translocation brings the *Bcl-2* gene on chromosome 18q21 under the transcriptional control of the lg heavy chain region on chromosome 14q32 and results in the deregulated expression of the *Bcl-2* protein [18,19]. Although *Bcl-2* translocation and overexpression is highly reminiscent of the c-*myc* gene described earlier in Burkitt's lymphoma, transfection experiments with *Bcl-2* do not result in enhanced cellular proliferation. In addition, the *Bcl-2* gene localizes to the outer mitochondrial membrane, nuclear membrane, and endoplasmic reticulum [20], suggesting that it plays a unique role in tumorgenesis.

The first indication that *Bcl-2* inhibits cell death came from transfection experiments demonstrating that overexpression of *Bcl-2* inhibits apoptosis induced in vitro by withdrawl of interleukin-3 (IL-3) from IL-3–dependent lymphoid and myeloid cell lines [21]. Similarly, overexpression of *Bcl-2* blocks apoptosis induced by either low serum, thymidine excess, etoposide, or heat shock in Rat-1 fibroblasts or Chinese hamster ovary cells that overexpress the c-*myc* gene [22,23]. Thus *Bcl-2* appears to function in a number of cell types and blocks apoptosis induced by a number of different external stimuli. This block is not complete, however, as cells do die over the time period assayed, albeit at a much slower rate. For example, 60 hours following a 10 Gy dose of gamma radiation, 30–80% of lymphocytes that overexpress *Bcl-2* remain viable, in contrast to unirradiated control cells, in which >95% remain viable [24].

Bcl-2 appears to function as a survival factor without inducing cellular proliferation. Transgenic mice that contain a *Bcl-2* transgene linked to the lg heavy chain enhancer accumulate a three- to fourfold expansion of small, noncycling B lymphocytes [25]. These mice develop high-grade lymphomas with a long latency (>1 year) [26], unlike c-*myc* transgenic mice, which develop lymphomas within 100 days [13]. In contrast, mice that overexpress both *Bcl-2* and c-*myc* develop lymphoid tumors at a very young age (<40 days) [27]. This synergy between *Bcl-2* and c-*myc* underscores the fact that *Bcl-2* plays a distinct role in tumorigenesis.

The mechanism by which *Bcl-2* inhibits apoptosis is unclear at present. *Bcl-2*, which exists in cells as a homodimer, is able to block apoptosis in response to stimuli as diverse as growth factor withdrawl, DNA damage, and tumor necrosis factor, suggesting that Bcl-2 functions downstream in the apoptotic process. The expression of Bcl-2 in lipid membranes such as mitochodria [20] and the observation that Bcl-2 can block apoptosis induced by H_2O_2 [28] suggests that Bcl-2 may inhibit oxidative damage of lipid membranes. Recently, however, Bcl-2 has been shown to block apoptosis induced by hypoxia, in which oxidative damage is unlikely to occur [29,30], indicating that Bcl-2 may block apoptosis through some other mechanism.

At the time that it was discovered there were no other proteins with significant homolgy to Bcl-2. Since then a number of proteins have been identified with homology clustered within two highly conserved regions of Bcl-2, termed Bcl-2 homology 1 (BH1) and homology 2 (BH2). One of the first related proteins, Bax, was isolated by virtue of the fact that it forms a heterodimer with Bcl-2 in some cell lines [31]. Unlike Bcl-2, however, the overexpression of Bax in the FL5.12 pro-B lymphocyte line hastens (rather than inhibits) apoptosis in response to IL-3 withdrawl. This appears to be due to the ability of Bax to form homodimers in cells, rather than its ability to heterodimerize with Bcl-2, since mutations in Bcl-2 that disrupt Bax–Bcl-2 heterodimerization (but do not disrupt Bcl-2 homodimerization) destroy the ability of Bcl-2 to inhibit apoptosis [32]. The level of Bax homodimers therefore appears to be critical in determining whether a cell will undergo apoptosis in response to the appropriate signal.

Bax and Bcl-2 can be viewed as positive and negative regulators, respectively, of cell death. Another gene that regulates cell death is Bcl-X, which was isolated by low stringency hybridization with a Bcl-2 probe [33]. Analysis of cDNA indicates that this gene encodes for two different proteins due to alternative mRNA splicing. The larger protein, Bcl-X_L, contains sequences homologous to the BH1 and BH2 domains discussed earlier. The smaller protein, Bcl-X_S, is identical to Bcl-X_L. except that alternate mRNA splicing results in the removal of 63 amino acids of coding sequence, including the BH1 and BH2 domains. Interestingly, these two proteins have opposite properties in that Bcl-X_S stimulates apoptosis (by binding to Bcl-2 and BCL-X_L), while Bcl-X_L inhibits apoptosis (presumably by binding to Bax). An additional protein, termed Bad [34], isolated through two-hybrid screening, contains both BH1 and BH2 sequences and shows a preference for binding to Bcl-X_L in vivo. As would be predicted, expression of Bad stimulates apoptosis by binding to Bcl-X_L and preventing its dimerization with Bax.

Bcl-2 may also function in inhibiting apoptosis independent of its ability to bind to Bax. Both Bcl-2 and E1B-19k, a gene product encoded by the adenovirus E1B region, which also inhibits apoptosis [16], interact with three cellular proteins, termed Nip-1, Nip-2, and Nip-3 [35]. The significance of this binding is unclear, but the observation that mutants of E1B-19k that fail to inhibit apoptosis also fail to bind to these cellular proteins suggests that Bcl-2 (and E1B-19k) can inhibit apoptosis through more than one pathway.

P53 GENE MUTATIONS AND APOPTOSIS

Although *Bcl-2* can block apoptosis in tumors in response to DNA damaging agents, the *Bcl-2* gene does not appear to be deregulated in most tumors outside of follicular lymphomas, which contain the t(14;18) chromosomal translocation. Most tumors, however, show some degree of resistance to DNA-damaging drugs, suggesting that other genes critical for apoptosis may be altered in tumors. One candidate gene is the p53 tumor suppressor gene, which is the most frequently detected genetic alteration found in human cancers [36].

The p53 gene is located on the short arm of chromsome 17 (17p) and encodes a protein of 393 amino acids that exists as a tetramer in cells and functions as a transcription factor. The central or core domain of p53 binds specifically to a DNA consensus sequence (A/G) (A/G) (A/G)C (A/T) (A/T)G (C/T) (C/T) (C/T) located in the promoter region or within introns of p53 regulated genes [37]. The majority of p53 gene mutations are missense mutations that occur in the central domain of the protein and are defective for DNA binding. Although mutant p53 is able to complex with and inactivate wild-type p53, most tumors exhibit loss of heterozygocity at the p53 locus and retain only mutant p53 genes through deletion or recombination. Thus there appears to be a heavy selective pressure for loss of all wild-type p53 protein in tumor cells.

p53 appears to play a critical role in maintaining the genetic integrity of a cell in response to DNA damage. This idea is supported by the observation that DNA damage with a number of agents, including gamma radiation, UV light, alkylating agents, intercalating agents, antimetabolites, and topoisomerase inhibitors, results in an increase in the steady-state level of p53 due to a marked prolongation of p53 half-life [38,39]. Exposure of excision repair–deficient xeroderma pigmentosum cells to UV light fails to induce p53 levels [39], suggesting that DNA strand breaks normally associated with the DNA repair process are the substrate that induce p53 levels.

Following DNA damage, p53 upregulates the expression of a number of genes, among them p21 [40]. p21 inhibits the kinase activity of cyclin–CDK complexes critical for progression through the G1/S check point in the cell cycle [41]. Cells that lack p53 fail to induce p21 and fail to undergo the G1 arrest required for efficient DNA repair. Cells lacking wild-type p53 function enter the S phase with damaged DNA, which leads to a high mutation rate due to errors in DNA replication. One example of this genomic instability is gene amplification, which is inhibited by wild-type p53 in most tumor cells [42]. The fact that p53-deficient fibroblasts rapidly become aneuploid upon passage in tissue culture further emphasizes the genomic instability associated with p53 gene mutation [43].

The ability of p53 to induce apoptosis was first demonstrated in a murine myeloid leukemia cell line into which was introduced a temperature-sensitive p53 gene [44]. Shifting from the nonpermisive to a permissive temperature rapidly induced apoptosis in this cell line. Introduction of an inducible p53 gene into a colon carcinoma cell line produced similar results [45]. Perhaps the most compelling experiments linking p53 and apoptosis utilized mice deficient in p53 due to homozygous deletion of their endogenous p53 genes through gene targeting [46,47]. The thymocytes from these mice are resistant to apoptosis induced by the DNA-damaging agents gamma radiation and etoposide, but not by steroids, indicating that p53 is not required for all forms of apoptosis but may function in transmitting the DNA damage signal that triggers apoptosis.

p53 is capable of inducing either G1 arrest or apoptosis following DNA damage. Mutations in p53 that inhibit its transcriptional activity affect both processes. suggesting that p53 itself does not dictate apoptosis versus G1 arrest. Rather, it appears that other gene products determine the cell's response to elevated levels of p53 following DNA damage. For example, immortalized fibroblasts undergo G1 arrest, while the same cells engineered to overexpress c-myc [14], E1A [48], or E2F [49] undergo apoptosis. Similarly, expression of v-src or activated c-Raf cause the Baf3 lymphoid cell line to undergo p53-mediated G1 arrest rather than apoptosis [50].

p53 appears to induce apoptosis in vivo in response to endogenous stimuli as well as those generated by DNA-damaging agents. Experiments by Van Dyke and colleagues [51] demonstrate that tumors of the choroid plexus appear with a latency of 26 weeks in a strain of mouse with intact p53 function but with a latency of 3–4 weeks in a p53-deficient mouse strain. Examination of preneoplastic choroid plexus in these mouse strains reveals that the longer time to tumor development correlates with increased apoptosis (6–10% in the intact p53 strain vs. <1% in the p53-deficient strain). Thus there appears to be a strong selective advantage for p53 gene mutations *in vivo* to counteract the net antiproliferative effect of p53-mediated apoptosis.

The mechanism by which p53 induces apoptosis remains unclear at present. Although mutations of p53 that inhibit its transcriptional activity also inhibit apoptosis, there are two reports that wild-type p53 can induce apoptosis in the presence of cycloheximide [52,53], suggesting that new gene expression may not be required. Others have observed that p21 and gadd45, another p53-regulated gene, are induced to different degrees in cells undergoing apoptosis versus G1 arrest [50], suggesting that p53-induced gene expression is important. p53 binding sites are present in the promoter region of the *Bax* gene [54] and in some [55–57] but not all [50] cells, elevated levels of p53 induce *Bax* gene expression. Elevated Bax levels do not by themselves induce apoptosis but rather prime the cell for apoptosis following the appropriate signal. p53 has also been shown to downregulate a number of promoters that lack p53 binding sites [58]. Expression of either *Bcl*-2 or E1B-19k (both of which inhibit p53 dependent apoptosis) reverses this downregulation, suggesting that p53 may downregulate the expression of an inhibitor of apoptosis [59]. *Bcl*-2 mRNA levels decrease in a p53-dependent manner in some cell lines [55], lending some support to this hypothesis.

It should be pointed out that apoptosis can occur following DNA damage in the absence of p53. For example, apoptosis is induced by DNA damage in Saos-2 osteosarcoma cells [60] and HL-60 myeloid leukemia cells [61], even though both cell lines lack wild-type p53. Similarly, thymic lymphoma and teratocarcinoma cell lines derived from spontaneous tumors in p53-deficient mice also undergo apoptosis following DNA damage [62,63]. In some situations higher levels of DNA-damaging drugs are needed to induce apoptosis in cells lacking p53 [63], suggesting that wild-type p53 facilitates apoptosis in some cells by sensing low levels of DNA damage.

APOPTOSIS AND CANCER CHEMOTHERAPY

As discussed earlier, the activation of oncogenes such as c-myc in tumors stimulates both proliferation and apoptosis, the latter occurring when the tumor cell receives an antiproliferative signal such as DNA damage. This is of particular interest, since the majority of chemotherapeutic drugs commonly in use, as well as gamma radiation, induce DNA damage, either directly or indirectly. There also appears to be a strong selective pressure in vivo for genetic changes that inhibit apoptosis, such as Bcl-2 translocation or p53 gene mutation. These genetic changes may contribute to the incurability of some human cancers.

The majority of experiments described earlier relate specific genetic changes to either inducing or inhibiting apoptosis in vitro. There is experimental evidence to suggest that the ability to induce apoptosis in vivo may be similarly regulated. For example, mouse embryo fibroblasts transformed with E1A plus ras (which contain endogenous wild-type p53 genes) injected subcutaneously into nude mice readily undergo apoptosis following treatment with gamma radiation or Adriamycin [64]. Resistant tumors develop in some mice after initial tumor shrinkage, and these tumors contain p53 gene mutations. Although human tumors likely have more complex genetic alterations that are not as easily discernable, this study suggests that it may be possible to predict response to treatment based upon known genetic alterations in the primary tumor.

A few retrospective studies have attempted to correlate the expression of Bcl-2 in tumors with response to chemotherapy. In 82 cases of newly diagnosed acute myclogenous leukemia (AML), high expression of Bcl-2 was associated with a low rate of complete remission after intensive chemotherapy (29% in cases with 20% or more positive cells vs. 85% in cases with less than 20%) [65]. Interestingly, in vitro survival of leukemia cells was significantly longer in cases with higher Bcl-2 expression, suggesting that Bcl-2 is functioning as a survival factor. Similar results in terms of failure to achieve a complete remission were obtained in a smaller series of patients with AML as well as acute lymphocytic leukemia (ALL), and there was a significantly higher proportion of leukemia cells expressing Bcl-2 in patients with relapsing ALL versus ALL at initial presentation [66]. None of the leukemias in this latter study contained a t(14;18) translocation, suggesting that other genetic mechanisms, either directly or indirectly, resulted in enhanced expression of Bcl-2.

Multiple studies of various tumor types have identified the p53 mutation as a poor prognostic factor that predicts shorter median survival. Relatively few studies, however, have attempted to correlate p53 gene mutations with resistance to chemotherapy. In one study of 53 patients with B-cell CLL, 27 of 29 (93%) treated patients without p53 gene mutations versus 1 of 7 (14%) treated patients with p53 gene mutations had at least a partial response to treatment (p = 0.00009) [67]. This difference was still significant, even after controlling for the fact that patients without p53 gene mutations tended to have earlier stage disease. p53 gene mutation in this study also correlated with increased resistance to chemotherapy *in vitro*, as determined by cell viability at 72 hours, suggesting that such an assay may be clinically useful.

p53 mutations tend to occur more often in poorly differentiated carcinomas and are often associated with other poor prognostic factors [68]. In some of these studies, p53 gene mutations have not correlated with response to treatment in multivariate analysis. For example, in a study of 107 patients with AML, p53 mutation was found to correlate with both older age and a complex karyotype lacking either t(8;21), inv(16), or t(15;17) rearrangements, both of which predicted response to treatment to a greater degree [69]. It is possible that the complex karyotypes associated with p53 gene mutations may reflect the role that p53 plays in maintaining genomic stability rather than inducing apoptosis.

Implicit in this discussion is the assumption that cell death in human tumors in vivo is occurring through apoptosis. Unfortunately their is only limited evidence to support this hypothesis. Following chemotherapy a higher proportion of circulating leukemic cells isolated from patients demonstrate DNA breaks consistent with apoptosis [70]. These initial studies have not been extended to other tumors, such as solid tumors, which represent the majority of human malignancies and generally do not respond as rapidly to chemotherapy. Most solid tumors are not easily biopsied during treatment, so the cause of tumor shrinkage (apoptosis vs. necrosis) cannot be readily determined. The ability to induce apoptotic cell death may be clinically significant in cancer treatment. For example, the addition of IL-3 to gamma-irradiated Baf-3 murine lymphoid cells *in vitro* inhibits p53-dependent apoptosis and stimulates p53-dependent G1 arrest. Twice the dose of gamma radiation is needed to decrease cell survival 50% for the IL-3–treated (G1-arrested) versus untreated (apoptotic) cells [50], raising the possibility that apoptotic cell death in vivo may require lower levels of DNA damage more easily obtained with standard doses of chemotherapy.

CONCLUSIONS

The appreciation that oncogenes such as c-*myc* stimulate apoptosis as well as proliferation, and that *Bcl*-2 translocations and p53 gene mutations can inhibit this process, has led to great enthusiasm for understanding further how tumor cells respond to DNA damage. Multiple genes have been identified to date that stimulate or inhibit apoptosis following DNA damage. Determining how these gene products interact will be of critical importance in predicting whether DNA damage will stimulate apoptosis. The hypothesis that tumor shrinkage following treatment may in some (or all) instances result from programmed cell death suggests that genetic changes that inhibit apoptosis may result in less efficent cell kill following the same degree of DNA damage. Failure to induce apoptosis may explain why some tumors, such as follicular lymphomas with the *Bcl*-2 translocation, are responsive to chemo-therapy but complete responses are not durable and patients ultimately relapse [71]. In contrast, testicular tumors, which never contain p53 gene mutations [72–74], are readily curable, even when widely metastatic, and these tumor cells undergo apoptosis *in vitro* in response to various DNA-damaging drugs [63] and gamma radiation [75]. More work is necessary to determine whether resistance to apoptosis represents a form of drug resistance that prevents durable remissions in human cancers.

REFERENCES

1. Kerr J, Searle J (1972) A suggested explanation for the paradoxically slow growth rate of basal-cell carcinomas that contain numerous mitotic figures. J Pathol 107:41–44.
2. Kerr J, Wyllie A, Currie A (1972) Apoptosis: A basic biological phenomenon with wide-ranging implifications in tissue kinetics. Br J Cancer 26:239–257.
3. Searle J, Kerr J, Bishop C (1982) Necrosis and apoptosis: Distinct modes of cell death with fundamentally different significance. Pathol Annu 17:229–259.
4. Savill J, Dransfield I, Hogg N, Haslett C (1990) Vitronectin receptor-mediated phagocytosis of cells undergoing apoptosis. Nature 343:170–173.
5. Cohen J, Duke R (1984) Glucocorticoid activation of a calcium-dependent endonuclease in thymocyte nuclei leads to cell death. J Immunol 132:38–42.
6. Wyllie A (1980) Glucocorticoid-induced thymocyte apoptosis is associated with endonuclease activation. Nature 284:555–556.
7. Fesus L, Davies P, Piacentini M (1991) Apoptosis: Molecular mechanisms in programmed cell death. Eur J Cell Biol 56:170–177.
8. Baffy G, Miyashita T, Williamson J, Reed J (1993) Apoptosis induced by withdrawl of iterleukin-3 (IL-3) from an IL-3-dependent hematopoietic cell line is associated with repartitioning of intracellular calcium and is blocked by Bcl-2 oncoprotein production. J Biol Chem 268:6511–6519.
9. Wesselberg S, Kabelitz D (1993) Activation-driven death of human T cell clones: Time course kinetics of the induction of cell shrinkage, DNA fragmentation and cell death. Cell Immunol 148:234–241.
10. Dean M, Levine R, Ran W, Kindy M, Sonenshein G, Campisi J (1986) Regulation of c-myc transcription and mRNA abundance by serum growth factors and cell contact. J Biol Chem 261:9161–9166.
11. Leder P, Battey J, Lenoir G, Moulding C, Murphy W, Potter H, Stewart T, Taub R (1983) Translocations among antibody genes. Science 222:765–771.
12. Potter M, Mushinski J, Mushinski E, Brust S, Wax J, Wiener F, Babonits M, Rapp U, Morse H (1987) Avian v-myc replaces chromosomal translocation in murine plasmacytomagenesis. Science 235:787–789.
13. Langdon W, Harris A, Cory S, Adams J (1986) The c-myc oncogene perturbs B lymphocyte development in E-mu-myc transgenic mice. Cell 47:11–18.
14. Evan GI, Wyllie AH, Gilbert CS, Littlewood TD, Land H, Brooks M, Waters CM, Penn LZ, Hancock DC (1992) Induction of apoptosis in fibroblasts by c-myc protein. Cell 69:119–128.
15. Lotem J, Sachs L (1993) Hematopoietic cells from mice deficient in wild-type p53 are more resistant to induction of apoptosis by some agents. Blood 82:1092–1096.
16. Rao L, Debbas M, Sabbatini P, Hockenbery D, Korsmeyer S, White E (1992) The adenovirus E1A proteins induce apoptosis, which is inhibited by the E1B 19-kDa and Bcl-2 proteins. Proc Natl Acad Sci USA 89:7742–7746.
17. White A, Livanos E, Tlsty T (1994) Differential disruption of genomic integrity and cell cycle regulation in normal human fibroblasts by the HPV oncoproteins. Genes Dev 8:666–667.
18. Bakhshi A, Jensen J, Goldman P, Wright J, McBride O, Epstein A, Korsmeyer S (1985) Cloning the chromosomal breakpoint of t(14;18) human lymphomas: Clustering around JH on chromosome 14 and near a transcriptional unit on 18. Cell 41:889–906.
19. Cleary M, Sklar J (1985) Nucleotide sequence of a t(14;18) chromosomal breakpoint in follicular lymphoma and demonstration of a breakpoint cluster region near a transcriptionally active locus on chromosome 18. Proc Natl Acad Sci USA 82:7439–7443.
20. Hockenbery D, Nunez G, Milliman C, Schreiber R, Korsmeyer S (1990) Bcl-2 is an inner mitochondrial membrane protein that blocks programmed cell death. Nature 348:334–336.
21. Vaux D, Cory S, Adams J (1988) Bcl-2 gene promotes haemopoietic cell survival and cooperates with c-myc to immortalize pre-B cells. Nature 335:440–442.

22. Bissonnette R, Echeverri F, Mahboubi A, Green D (1992) Apoptotic cell death induced by c-myc is inhibited by bcl-2. Nature 359:552–554.

23. Fanidi A, Harrington E, Evan G (1992) Cooperative interaction between c-myc and bcl-2 proto-oncogenes. Nature 359:554–556.

24. Strasser A, Harris A, Cory S (1991) Bcl-2 transgene inhibits T cell death and perturbs thymic sensorship. Cell 67:889–899.

25. McDonnell T, Deane N, Platt F, Nunez G, Jaeger U, McKearn J, Korsmeyer S (1989) Bcl-2-immunoglobulin transgenic mice demonstrate extended B cell survival and follicular lymphoproliferation. Cell 57:79–88.

26. McDonnell T, Korsmeyer S (1991) Progression from lymphoid hyperplasia to high-grade malignant lymphoma in mice transgenic for the t(14;18). Nature 349:254–256.

27. Strasser A, Harris A, Bath M, Cory S (1990) Novel primitive tumours induced in transgenic mice by cooperation between myc and bcl-2. Nature 348:331–333.

28. Hockenbery D, Oltvai Z, Yin X-M, Milliman C, Korsmeyer S (1993) Bcl-2 functions in an antioxidant pathway to prevent apoptosis. Cell 75:241–252.

29. Jacobson M, Raff M (1995) Programmed cell death and bcl-2 protection in very low oxygen. Nature 374:814–816.

30. Shimizu S, Eguchi Y, Kosaka H, Kamiike W, Matsuda H, Tsujimoto Y (1995) Prevention of hypoxia-induced cell death by bcl-2 and bcl-x$_L$. Nature 374:811–813.

31. Oltvai Z, Milliman L, Korsmeyer S (1993) Bcl-2 heterodimerizes in vivo with a conserved homologue, Bax, that accelerates programmed cell death. Cell 74:609–620.

32. Yin X-M, Oltvai Z, Korsmeyer S (1994) BH1 and BH2 domains of Bcl-2 are required for inhibition of apoptosis and heterodimerization with Bax. Nature 369:321–323.

33. Boise L, Gonzalez-Garcia M, Postema C, Ding L, Lindsten T, Turka L, Mao X, Nunez G, Thompson C (1993) bcl-x, a bcl-2-related gene that functions as a dominant regulator of apoptotic cell death. Cell 74:597–608.

34. Yang E, Zha J, Jockel J, Boise L, Thompson C, Korsmeyer S (1995) Bad, a heterodimeric partner for Bcl-X$_L$ and Bcl-2, displaces Bax and promotes cell death. Cell 80:285–291.

35. Boyd J, Malstrom S, Subramanian T, Venkatesh L, Schaeper U, Elangovan B, D'Sa-Eipper C, Chinnadurai G (1994) Adenovirus E1B 19kDa and Bcl-2 proteins interact with a common set of cellular proteins. Cell 79:341–351.

36. Levine AJ, Momand J, Finlay CA (1991) The p53 tumor suppressor gene. Nature 351:453–456.

37. Funk WD, Pak DJ, Karas RH, Wright WE, Shay JW (1992) A transcriptionally active DNA binding site for human p53 protein complexes. Mol Cell Biol 12:2866–2871.

38. Kastan MB, Onyekwere O, Sidransky D, Vogelstein B, Craig RW (1991) Participation of p53 protein in the cellular response to DNA damage. Cancer Res 51:6304–6311.

39. Nelson W, Kastan M (1994) DNA strand breaks: The DNA template alterations that trigger p53-dependent DNA damage response pathways. Mol Cell Biol 14:1815–1823.

40. El-Deiry WS, Tokino T, Velculescu VE, Levy DB, Parsons R, Trent JM, Lin D, Mercer WE, Kinzler KW, Vogelstein B (1993) WAF1, a potential mediator of p53 tumor suppression. Cell 75:817–825.

41. Xiong Y, Hannon GJ, Zhang H, Casso D, Kobayashi R, Beach D (1993) p21 is a universal inhibitor of cyclin kinases. Nature 366:701–704.

42. Livingstone LR, White A, Sprouse J, Livanos E, Jacks T, Tlsty T (1992) Altered cell cycle arrest and gene amplification potential accompany loss of wild-type p53. Cell 70:923–935.

43. Harvey M, Sands A, Weiss R, Hegi M, Wiseman R, Pantazis P, Giovanella B, Tainsky M, Bradley A, Donehower L (1993) In vitro growth characteristics of embryo fibroblasts isoalted from p53-deficient mice. Oncogene 8:2457–2567.

44. Yonish-Rouach E, Resnitzky D, Lotem J, Sachs L, Kimchi A, Oren M (1991) Wild-type p53 induces apoptosis of myeloid leukaemic cells that is inhibited by interleukin-6. Nature 352:345–347.

45. Shaw P, Bovey R, Tardy S, Sahli R, Sordat B, Costa J (1992) Induction of apoptosis by wild-type p53 in a human colon tumor-derived cell line. Proc Natl Acad Sci USA 89:4495–4499.

46. Clarke A, Purdie C, Harrison D, Morris R, Bird C, Hooper M, Wyllie A (1993) Thymocyte apoptosis induced by p53-dependent and independent pathways. Nature 362:849–852.

47. Lowe SW, Schmitt EM, Smith SW, Osborne BA, Jacks T (1993) p53 is required for radiation induced apoptosis in mouse thymocytes. Nature 362:••–••.

48. Debbas M, White E (1993) Wild-type p53 mediates apoptosis by E1A which is inhibited by E1B. Genes Dev 7:546–554.

49. Wu X, Levine AJ (1994) p53 and E2F-1 cooperate to mediate apoptosis. Proc Natl Acad Sci USA 91:3602–3606.
50. Canman C, Gilmer T, Coutts S, Kastan M (1995) Growth factor modulation of p53-mediated growth arrest versus apoptosis. Genes Dev 9:600–611.
51. Symonds H, Krall L, Remington L, Saenz-Robles M, Lowe S, Jacks T, Van Dyke T (1994) p53-dependent apoptosis suppresses tumor growth and progression in vivo. Cell 4:703–712.
52. Caelles C, Heimberg A, Karin M (1994) p53-dependent apoptosis in the absence of transcriptional activation of p53-target genes. Nature 370:220–223.
53. Wagner A, Kokontis J, Hay N (1994) Myc-mediated apoptosis requires wild-type p53 in a manner independent of cell cycle arrest and the ability of p53 tp induce p21/waf1/cip1. Genes Dev 8:2817–2830.
54. Myashita T, Reed J (1995) Tumor suppressor p53 is a direct transcriptional activator of human Bax gene. Cell 80:293–299.
55. Miyashita T, Krajewski S, Krajewska M, Wang H-K, Lieberman D, Hoffman B, Reed J (1994) Tumor suppressor p53 is a regulator of bcl-2 and bax gene expression in vitro and in vivo. Oncogene 9:1799–1805.
56. Selvakumaran M, Lin H-K, Wang H-G, Krajewski S, Reed J, Hoffman B, Lieberman D (1994) Immediate early upregulation of bax expression by p53 but not TGF-beta: A paradigm for distinct apoptotic pathways. Oncogene 9:1791–1798.
57. Zhan Q, Fan S, Bae I, Guillouf C, Liebermann D, O'Connor P, Fornace A (1994) Induction of bax by genotoxic stress in human cells correlates with normal p53 state and apoptosis. Oncogene 9:3743–3751.
58. Zambetti GP, Levine AJ (1993) A comparison of the biological activities of wild-type and mutant p53. FASEB J 7:855–865.
59. Shen Y, Shenk T (1994) Relief of p53-mediated transcriptional repression by the adenovirus E1B-19kDa protein or the cellular Bcl-2 protein. Proc Natl Acad Sci USA, in press.
60. Haas-Kogan D, Kogan S, Levi D, Dazin P, T'Ang A, Fung Y-K, Israel M (1995) Inhibition of apoptosis by the retinoblastoma gene product. EMBO J 14:461–472.
61. Gorczyca W, Gong J, Darzynkiewicz Z (1993) Detection of DNA strand breaks in individual apoptotic cells by the in situ terminal deoxynucleotidyl transferase and nick translation assays. Cancer Res 53:1945–1951.
62. Strasser A, Harris A, Jacks T, Cory S (1994) DNA damage can induce apoptosis in proliferating lymphoid cells via p53-independent mechanisms inhibitable by Bcl-2. Cell 79:329–339.
63. Lutzker S, Levine AJ (1995) Functional inactivation of p53 in testicular tumor cell lines is reversed by DNA damage and cellular differentiation. Submitted.
64. Lowe S, Bodis S, McClatchey A, Remington L, Ruley HE, Fisher D, Housman D, Jacks T (1994) p53 status and the efficiancy of cancer therapy in vivo. Science 266:807–810.
65. Maung Z, MacLean F, Reid M, Pearson A, Proctor S, Hamilton P, Hall A (1994) The relationship between bcl-2 expression and response to chemotherapy in acute leukemia. Br J Haematol 88:105–109.
66. Campos L, Rouault J-P, Sabido O, Oriol P, Roubi N, Vasselon C, Archimbaud E, Magaud J-P, Guyotat D (1993) High expression of bcl-2 protein in acute myeloid leukemia cells is associated with poor response to chemotherapy. Blood 81:3091–3096.
67. El Rouby S, Thomas A, Costin D, Rosenberg C, Potmesil M, Silber R, Newcomb E (1993) p53 gene mutation in B-cell chronic lymphocytic leukemia is associated with rug resistance and is independent of MDR1/MDR3 gene expression. Blood 82:3452–3459.
68. Rosen P, Lesser M, Arroyo C, Cranor M, Borgen P, Norton L (1995) p53 in node-negative breast carcinoma: An immunohistochemical study of epidemiologic risk factors, histologic features and prognosis. J Clin Oncol 13:821–830.
69. Wattel E, Preudhomme C, Hecquet B, Vanrumbeke M, Quesnel B, Dervite I, Morel P, Fenaux P (1994) p53 mutations are associated with resistance to chemotherapy and short survival in hematologic malignancies. Blood 84:3148–3157.
70. Gorczyca W, Bigman K, Mittelman A, Ahmed T, Gong J, Melamed M (1990) Induction of DNA strand breaks associated with apoptosis during treatment of leukemia. Leukemia 7:659–670.
71. Sander C, Yano T, Clark H, Harris C, Longo D, Jaffe E, Raffeld M (1993) p53 mutation is associated with progression in follicular lymphomas. Blood 82:1994–2004.
72. Heimdal K, Lothe RA, Lystad S, Holm R, Fossa SD, Börresen AL (1993) No germline TP3 mutations detected in familial and bilateral testicular cancers. Genes Chromosom Cancer 6:92–97.

73. Peng HQ, Hogg D, Malkin D, Bailey D, Gallie BL, Bulbul M, Jewett M, Buchanan J, Goss PE (1993) Mutations of the p53 gene do not occur in testis cancer. Cancer Res 53:3574–3578.
74. Riou G, Barrois M, Prost S, Terrier M, Theodore C, Levine AJ (1995) The p53 and mdm-2 genes in human testicular germ-cell tumors. Mol Carcinogen 12:124–131.
75. Langley R, Palayoor S, Coleman C, Bump E (1994) Radiation-induced apoptosis in F9 teratocarcinoma cells. Int J Radiat Biol 65:605–610.

15. INTERACTION OF CHEMOTHERAPY AND BIOLOGICAL RESPONSE MODIFIERS IN THE TREATMENT OF MELANOMA

CLAY M. ANDERSON, ANTONIO C. BUZAID, AND ELIZABETH A. GRIMM

Metastatic melanoma is one of the most drug-resistant human neoplasms. While single-agent cytotoxic drugs generally produce response rates of less than 20%, combination chemotherapy regimens lead to response rates of 20–40%. Durable complete remissions, however, are rare. Biologic response modifiers (biologics) have also shown modest activity when used alone. Interferon-α (IFN-α) and interleukin-2 (IL-2), the most commonly applied biologics in melanoma, produce response rates of approximately 10–20%, with only 3–5% of the patients treated exhibiting durable responses. It remains uncertain whether the combination of IFN-α plus IL-2 is superior to IL-2 alone. Although cytotoxic agents and biologics have limited activity when used alone, the combination of cisplatin-based regimens with IFN-α and IL-2 has shown promising preliminary results, with overall response rates in the 50–60% range. Approximately 10% of these patients have exhibited durable responses. The toxicity of the biochemotherapy regimens is severe, however, and their impact on survival remains to be established in ongoing controlled trials. This chapter focuses on the clinical results of the biochemotherapy regimens and addresses the possible mechanisms of enhanced activity when cytotoxic agents and biologics are combined to overcomed drug-resistant melanoma.

By the year 2000, cutaneous melanoma will be diagnosed in an estimated 1 out of 75 Americans [1]. Early primary melanoma is cured in most cases, but once the disease becomes metastatic it is nearly always resistant to standard therapies, and therefore is ultimately fatal. No definite survival benefit has been demonstrated for any therapies available today. Of all the currently employed treatment modalities, the highest clinical activity has occurred in response to cisplatin-based regimens combined with biologic agents such as IFN-α and IL-2, a modality referred to as *biochemotherapy*. The reasons for this apparent ability to abrogate, at least in part, the resistance of melanoma to therapy are unknown. It may be due to the additive effect of combining active agents, or to alteration in metabolism of the cytotoxic drugs. More likely, either the chemotherapy or biologic therapy primes the cancer cells for maximal injury and death when exposed to the other. Current research results have led to the suggestion of several possible mechanisms for this observed synergy in human melanoma therapy. Here we review the clinical studies that have used biologics and biochemotherapy to treat advanced cutaneous melanoma, and we discuss the experimental data on chemotherapy/biologic therapy interactions.

CLINICAL STUDIES

Historically, chemotherapy and biologics have been applied separately in clinical protocols with the belief that cytotoxic agents would suppress the immune system and abrogate the effectiveness of biologic therapy. More recently, however, based in part on the results of the preclinical investigations discussed later, various cytokines, including IFN-α, IL-2, IL-1, and IL-6, have been combined with cytotoxic agents known to have clinical activity against advanced melanoma. Along with an overview of biologic therapy alone, these strategies and their clinical outcomes will be described in detail.

Biologic therapy

Interferons

Initial studies of partially purified human leukocyte-derived interferon showed only minimal clinical activity against melanoma [2,3]. Since then, several groups have studied recombinant IFNs α-2a and α-2b at different dosages and schedules and have observed total response rates of 8–22% [4–6]. The greatest clinical responses to IFN-α were to long-term therapy administered daily or three times weekly, while the lowest responses were to once-weekly doses or 5-day courses every 3 weeks [5]. IFN-α has been used with equal efficacy in patients pretreated with chemotherapy in whom alternative chemotherapy is rarely effective. In less than 5% of patients the disease has been controlled for greater than 3 years [5,6]. The frequency of response to IFN-α is higher for soft tissue metastases than for disease at other distant sites; however, responses have been recorded in lung and liver metastases as well. Phase I-II studies with IFN-β and -γ are limited but suggest a lower response rate than to IFN-α [7].

Interleukin 2

The second biologic agent to show activity against metastatic melanoma was interleukin-2 (IL-2), which mediates the activation and expansion of effector lymphocytes after antigen exposure and initiates the cytokine cascade [including IL-1, tumor necrosis factor (TNF), IL-6, etc.] responsible for most of its toxicity in humans. In the original studies carried out at the National Cancer Institute (NCI), six partial responses were observed among 23 patients treated with high-dose IL-2 alone [8]. These results were subsequently confirmed by various investigators, who reported responses of 10–20% [7]. Similar response rates, but less toxicity, have been observed when IL-2 is given by continuous infusion [9]. IL-2 has also been used with lymphokine-activated killer (LAK) cells and tumor-infiltrating lymphocytes (TIL) in patients with advanced melanoma. Despite the elegant preclinical animal data and the encouraging preliminary results reported by Dr. Steven Rosenberg's group at the NCI, the results of four phase III trials show no significant advantage of IL-2 plus LAK cells compared with that of IL-2 alone in terms of response rate and survival, although Rosenberg's study suggested a trend toward improved survival in the melanoma patients treated with LAK plus IL-2 [10–13]. The combination of IL-2 with TIL, lymphocytes derived from tumor isolates cultured in the presence of IL-2, initially showed a response rate of 55% in 20 patients [14], and responses of 40% were seen in all later NCI studies up to 1991 [15]. Other investigators, however, have observed response rates between 20% and 30% using similar strategies, which is not a significant improvement over response rates reported for IL-2 alone, particularly in light of the tremendous expense and complexity of the treatment [16–19]. Another treatment being investigated by the NCI is the use of TILs, which are selected to specifically recognize specific melanoma antigens, such as the melanoma antigen gene (MAGE)-1, MAGE-2, and the melanoma antigen recognized by T-cells (MART)-1.

In summary, the activity of IL-2 in advanced melanoma is modest, although durable remissions can occur. The addition of effector cells such as LAK and TIL has not been proven to significantly enhance the antitumor effect of the IL-2s. Whether selected TIL cells that recognize specific melanoma antigens will enhance the clinical efficacy of IL-2 remains to be determined.

Interferon-α plus interleukin-2

Since IFN-α upregulates the expression of MHC class I antigens in tumor cells and activates the killing activity of mononuclear cells [2,3,20], it was hypothesized that IFN-α could enhance the antitumor activity of IL-2. This was confirmed in animal models [21]. Following this lead, various clinical studies in patients with advanced melanoma were carried out and revealed overall response rates of 10–41% in the large series [6]. Despite this promising phase II data, a randomized trial in 85 patients comparing IL-2 plus IFN to IL-2 alone showed no significant difference in response rate and survival [22]. Therefore, it remains unclear whether IL-2 plus IFN-α is indeed superior to IL-2 alone.

Most IL-2 studies have been carried out using fixed doses of IL-2. In contrast, Keilholz et al. reported the results of two phase II trials that evaluated different schedules of IFN followed by IL-2 [23]. In one of these studies, IL-2 was given at a fixed dose (referred to as the *fixed dose regimen*), while in the IL-2 was initially given in high doses followed by a rapid taper (referred to as the *decrescendo regimen*).

According to the investigators, the rationale for the decrescendo regimen was that the high doses of IL-2 up front would increase the induction of the α chain of the IL-2 receptor on lymphocytes, and the subsequent rapid taper would decrease the production of TNF and reduce toxicity. This decrescendo regimen was more active and less toxic than the fixed dose regimen, with a response rate of 41% versus 18%, respectively (p = 0.067). The results suggest that the decrescendo regimen may have a better therapeutic index than the traditionally administered fixed dose regimens and, therefore, merits further evaluation. The clinical experience with subcutaneous IL-2 plus IFN-α in melanoma is limited and does not allow definitive conclusions.

Other cytokines

Additional cytokines that have been studied in melanoma and in other solid tumors, but have shown limited antitumor activity when used alone, include TNF-α, IL-1, IL-6, and macrophage-colony stimulating factor [6,24–26]. These cytokines, however, may be more effective when combined with other biologic or cytotoxic agents, or, as is the case of the toxic cytokine, TNF-α, when used with other modalities, such as isolated limb perfusion therapy [27,28].

Biochemotherapy

Over the last 5 years the combination of cytokines, particularly IL-2 and IFN-α, with chemotherapy has been the focus of intense investigation. Such combinations are referred to as *biochemotherapy* by M.D. Anderson investigators and as *chemoimmunotherapy* by other groups. These regimens are described later by the immunotherapy used—IFN-α alone, IL-2 alone, both IFN-α and IL-2, and other biologics.

Chemotherapy in combination with interferon-α

IFN-α has been evaluated in combination with many single cytotoxic agents and with combination chemotherapy regimens. In phase II studies of IFN-α with single-agent dacarbazine (DTIC), cisplatin, *Vinca* alkaloids, and nitrosoureas, no benefit was shown when IFN-α was added [29–31]. Similarly, phase II studies of IFN-α with the combination of cisplatin, BCNU, DTIC, and tamoxifen (the Dartmouth regimen) [32–34], or with cisplatin, vinblastine, and DTIC (CVD, as used at M.D. Anderson) [35] showed response rates comparable with chemotherapy alone. In contrast, Pyrhonen et al. [36] reported impressive results with a combination of bleomycin, vincristine, lomustine, DTIC, and IFN (BOLD + IFN) in 45 patients (an overall response rate of 62% and a complete remission rate of 13%). These results await confirmation in a large number of patients. An interesting pilot study in only 12 patients, reported in abstract form, used a regimen of DTIC, 5-fluorouracil (5-FU), and IFN-α to achieve a 66% response rate and a 42% complete response rate. The same investigators had treated 31 patients with only DTIC and IFN-α, and achieved a total response rate of only 35% [37]. These results suggest a synergistic or modulatory effect of 5-FU in this combination, because 5-FU alone is not active against melanoma.

Only four phase III randomized trials comparing chemotherapy alone to chemotherapy with IFN-α have been reported, and all studies used single-agent DTIC as the cytotoxic agent. The results are summarized in Table 15–1 and show a wide range of responses [38–41]. A large randomized trial, which compares DTIC alone with dacarbazine plus IFN-α, is currently being conducted by the Eastern Cooperative Oncology Group and should better delineate the role of IFN-α in combination with DTIC.

Chemotherapy in combination with interleukin-2

The addition of IL-2 to chemotherapeutic agents has been reported by a number of investigators. The most thoroughly evaluated combination, IL-2 plus dacarbazine, has yielded response rates of 13–33% (mean, 25%) (Table 15–2); it not clearly superior to dacarbazine alone, and is definitely more toxic [42–46]. IL-2 in combination with regimens containing cisplatin has also been studied in phase II trials and has produced results that appear superior to those obtained with IL-2 plus dacarbazine, with response rates of 37–42% (Table 3) [47–49]. These encouraging results need to be confirmed in randomized studies that include assessment of survival.

Combination of chemotherapy with interferon-α plus interleukin-2

Five groups have published results of studies using cytotoxic drugs in combination with IL-2 plus IFN-α to treat patients with metastatic melanoma (Tables 4 and 5) [50–54]. The treatment strategies of the most active biochemotherapy programs are shown in Figure 1. In 1 of the 5, Richards et al. added IL-2 and IFN-α to the Dartmouth regimen (BCNU 150 mg/m^2 d1, DTIC 220 mg/m^2 d1–d3 and d22–d24, cisplatin 25 mg/m^2 d1–d3 and d22–d24, tamoxifen 10 mg po bid) [55]. IFN-α (6 mU/m^2 sc qd) and IL-2 (4.5 mIU^1/m^2 iv q8h) were given on days 4–8 and days

Table 15–1. Randomized trials of chemotherapy plus interferon-α in advanced melanoma

Study	Regimen	Number assessable	% CR	% PR	% OR	95% CI
Kirkwood et al. [38]	DTIC/IFN	21	—	19	19	5–42
	DTIC	24	—	21	21	7–42
Falkson et al. [40]	DTIC/IFN	30	40	13	53	34–72
	DTIC	34	—	18	18	7–34
Thomson et al. [41]	DTIC/IFN	87	7	14	21	13–31
	DTIC	83	2	15	17	9–27
Bajetta et al. [39]	DTIC/IFN					
	High dose	76	8	20	28	18–39
	Low dose	84	7	16	23	14–33
	DTIC	82	5	15	20	12–30

DTIC = dacarbazine; IFN = interferon-α; OR = overall response; CR = complete response; PR = partial response; CI = confidence interval.

Table 15–2. Selected trials of dacarbazine plus interleukin-2
with or without LAK cells in advanced melanoma

Study	Regimen	Number assessable	% CR	% PR	% OR	95% CI
Papadopoulos et al. [42]	DTIC/IL-2	30	13	20	33	17–53
Dillman et al. [43]	DTIC/IL-2(CI)/LAK	27	7	19	26	11–46
Stoter et al. [44]	DTIC/IL-2 (CI)	25	8	16	24	9–45
Flaherty et al. [45]	DTIC/IL-2(SQ)	32	3	19	22	9–40
Dummer et al. [46]	DTIC/IL-2 (CI)	57	2	14	16	7–28

DTIC = dacarbazine; IL-2 = interleukin-2; LAK = lymphokine activated killer; CI = continuous infusion; SQ = subcutaneously; OR = overall response; CR = complete response; PR = partial response; CI = confidence interval.

Table 15–3. Phase II trials of cisplatin-based regimens plus interleukin-2 in advanced melanoma

Study	Regimen	Number assessable	% CR	% PR	% OR	95% CI
Demchak et al. [47]	cDDP/IL-2 (bolus)	27	11	26	37	19–58
Flaherty et al. [48]	cDDP/DTIC/IL-2 (bolus)	32	15	26	41	24–60
Atkins et al. [49]	cDDP/DTIC/TAM/IL-2 (bolus)	38	8	34	42	26–59

cDDP = cisplatin; IL-2 = interleukin-2; DTIC = dacarbazine; TAM = tamoxifen; OR = overall response; CR = complete response; PR = partial response; CI = confidence interval.

Table 15–4. Trials of cisplatin-based regimens plus
interferon-α and interleukin-2 in advanced melanoma

Study	Regimen	Number assessable	% CR	% PR	% OR	95% CI
Richards et al. [50]	CBDT/IL-2/IFN	74	15	40	55	43–67
Dorval et al. [52][a]	C/IL-2/IFN	49	2	24	26	15–41
Rixe et al. [51]	C/IL-2/IFN	80	9	43	52	41–64
Ron et al. [54]	Carboplatin/DTIC IL-2(SQ)/IFN(SQ)	16	0	38	38	15–65

[a] Part of phase III study that compared C/IL-2/IFN with C/IL-2 alone (overall response rate of 17%).
IL-2 = interleukin-2; IFN = interferon-α; C = cisplatin; B = BCNU; DTIC = dacarbazine; TAM = tamoxifen; SQ = subcutaneous; OR = overall response; CR = complete response; PR = partial response; CI = confidence interval.

Table 15–5. Phase II trials of CVD chemotherapy plus interferon-
α and interleukin-2 in advanced melanoma at M.D. Anderson Cancer Center

Regimen	Number assessable	% CR	% PR	% OR	95% CI
Alternating CVD-BIO	39	5	28	33	19–50
Sequential CVD/BIO	30	30	43	73	54–88
Sequential BIO/CVD	30	17	30	47	28–66
Concurrent CVD+BIO	52	12	51	63	49–76

IL-2 = interleukin-2; IFN = interferon-α; C = cisplatin; D = dacarbazine; V = vinblastine; OR = overall response; CR = complete response; PR = partial response; CI = confidence interval.

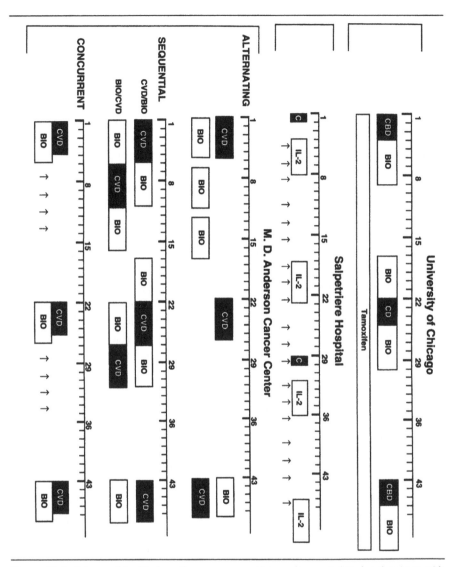

Figure 15–1. Schema of the biochemotherapy programs that combine a cisplatin-based regimen with IL-2 plus interferon-α in advanced melanoma. C = cisplatin; D = dacarbazine; B = BCNU; V = vinblastine; BIO = biotherapy consisting of IL-2 plus interferon-α.

17–21, repeated every 21 days (all IL-2 doses have been converted to IU). The overall response rate in 42 patients was 57%. In a recent update, the same overall response rate was recorded in 74 patients, while 15% of the patients achieved a complete response (median survival of more than 15 months was observed in the complete responders) [50].

Rixe et al. [51] recently reported the results of a French multicenter trial, including the Salpetriere Hospital experience, using cisplatin (100 mg/m² iv d1), IL-2 (18 mIU/m² iv by continuous infusion over 24 hours d3–d6 and d18–d22), and

IFN-α (9 mU sc 3×/wk). The overall response rate among 80 assessable patients was 52%. In contrast, a French randomized multicenter tiral comparing the Salpetriere Hospital regimen with cisplatin plus INF-α (same doses) reported a response rate of only 26% and 17%, respectively [52]. The disparity in these results may be due in part to the different level of dose intensity of IL-2 between the two study groups. A small outpatient study by Ron et al. that used carboplatin (400 mg/m^2 iv d1) and DTIC (750 mg/m^2 iv d1) with subcutaneous IL-2 (4.8 mIU/m^2 sc 5×/wk) and IFN-α (6 mIU/m^2 sc 3×/wk) reported a response rate of 38% in 16 patients but no complete responders [54]. The small number of patients in this study limits its interpretation.

To gauge the effect of schedule on the effectiveness of biochemotherapy, investigators from M.D. Anderson conducted a series of phase II trials integrating IFN-α (5 mU/m^2 sc for 5 days) and IL-2 (9 mIU/m^2 iv by continuous infusion over 24 hours for 4 days) (BIO) with cisplatin (20 mg/m^2 iv qd for 4 days), vinblastine (1.6 mg/m^2 iv qd for 4 or 5 days), and DTIC (800 mg/m^2 iv on d1) (CVD) [53,56]. The results are outlined in Table 15–5. In this "alternating biochemotherapy" study, BIO and CVD were alternated every 6 weeks to minimize toxicity and to avoid the possibility of chemotherapy interfering with the immunologic effects of biotherapy. Patients were randomly assigned to receive either CVD followed by BIO or BIO followed by CVD. The two regimens produced similar results. The combined response rate of 33% in the two groups was not superior to previous experience with CVD alone.

The unimpressive results with "alternating biochemotherapy" and Richard's encouraging preliminary results [55] led to an alteration in treatment strategy. The BIO and CVD regimens were now given one immediately after the other. This "sequential biochemotherapy" protocol was randomized so that half of the patients received CVD followed immediately by BIO (CVD/BIO; see Figure 15–1), and 6 days later, BIO followed by CVD followed by BIO (BIO/CVD/BIO). The other half of the patients received the BIO/CVD/BIO first and 6 days later, received BIO followed immediately by CVD (BIO/CVD). Compared with CVD alone, CVD/BIO produced a higher response rate (73% vs. 40%, p = 0.008), progression-free survival (8 vs. 4 months, p = 0.005), and overall survival (12 vs. 9 months, p = 0.006). CVC/BIO was also superior to BIO/CVD in response rate (73% vs. 47%, p = 0.065) and progression-free survival (8 vs. 7 months, p = 0.007) but not in overall survival (p = 0.18).

In the most recent study, biotherapy and chemotherapy were administered together ("concurrent biochemotherapy") to reduce the delivery time from 10 days to 5 days on a 21 day cycle. The doses were identical to those in the previous trials, except for vinblastine, which was given for 4 days instead of 5. In addition, the INF-α dosing was repeated during the second week of therapy on days 7, 9, 11, and 13. The overall response rate of 63% was superior to that of VCD alone (p = 0.030). However, the median duration of response was only 6 months, primarily because of recurrences in the central nervous system.

These M.D. Anderson phase II studies suggest that while alternating biochemotherapy does not produce additive clinical activity, sequential CVD/BIO biochemotherapy appears to produce better results than CVD alone or alternating BIO/CVD. Concurrent biochemotherapy also appears to be superior to CVD alone and is more convenient and less toxic than the sequential regimen. It is not yet clear, however, whether concurrent biochemotherapy is as effective as sequential biochemotherapy in terms of survival.

Toxicity has been substantial with these regimens and reflects the known side effects of both the chemotherapy and the biotherapy, including nausea, vomiting, diarrhea, fever, chills, edema, erythema, hypotension, and serious infections. Many of these toxicities are attributable to IL-2, but nausea, vomiting, cytopenias, and renal dysfunction appear to be caused by additive toxicities of the biologics and the chemotherapy agents. Reducing these toxicities without diminishing the effectiveness of the therapy will be a signficant challenge.

Because these regimens have shown encouraging phase II results with response rates consistently above 50% and possible improvement in survival, a randomized phase III trial is currently being conducted at M.D. Anderson comparing sequential biochemotherapy with CVD alone. A similar study is ongoing at the National Cancer Institute. Investigators at M.D. Anderson are also evaluating the use of neoadjuvant concurrent biochemotherapy for patients with measurable loco-regional disease.

The mechanisms underlying the apparent ability of these aggressive combined modality approaches to at least partially overcome resistance in humans with advanced melanoma are not yet clear. Nevertheless, the response rates are consistently high (>50%), especially for cisplatin-based regimens with both IL-2 and IFN, considering the poor track record (response rates of approximately 20%) for earlier systemic therapies for advanced melanoma.

Chemotherapy with other biologics

Chemotherapy combined with classic immune stimulators such as *Bacillus-Calmette-Guerin* (BCG), *Corynebacterium parvum*, and levamisole has not improved upon chemotherapy alone in melanoma patients [57–59]. Use of additional biologics has been evaluated. In one case, Lesting et al. combined IL-6 with the Dartmouth regimen in metastatic melanoma patients in hopes of improving response rates while abrogating the treatment-induced thrombocytopenia [60]. The results, however, showed no advantage for the new regimen. IL-1α in combination with carboplatin is currently being evaluated in two ongoing phase I trials [61,62]. As noted earlier, studies of TNF-α have been very limited. Two more recently discovered cytokines, IL-12 and IL-15, which are primarily produced by macrophages and are involved in the terminal differentiation and function of effector cells working in concert with IL-1 and IL-2, are showing promise in preclinical studies, including melanoma models, with a more favorable toxicity profile than the older cytokines [63–65]. Thus, these cytokines are receiving attention as possible alternatives to IL-2 alone or as additions to other cytokines or chemotherapy.

POTENTIAL MECHANISMS OF INTERACTION
BETWEEN BIOLOGICS AND CHEMOTHERAPY

The clinical rationale for most of the biochemotherapy studies so far has been based primarily on two principles: (1) the independent single activity of each component and (2) the lack of crossresistance between biologics and cytotoxic agents against melanoma. However, there is a sizable body of preclinical data that demonstrate synergism between the biologics and cytotoxic agents, mirroring their more than additive effects in clinical trials. The results of these preclinical investigations also suggest several possible mechanisms of interaction between biologics and cytotoxic agents that might account for their improved rates of response.

Direct interaction between biologics and chemotherapy

Interferons and chemotherapy

A large number of in vitro and in vivo studies have shown that IFNs can have an additive or synergistic effect with many cytotoxic agents [66]. The most extensively tested combinations have been cisplatin with IFN-α and -γ, doxorubicin with IFN-α and -γ, 5-FU with IFN-α and -β, and vinblastine with IFN-γ [66]. The extensive data, however, do not point to any combinations as being inherently more potent than others against tumor cell lines. Von Hoff used a human tumor cloning system to test multiple human tumor specimens for the activity of IFN-α combined with various cytotoxic agents [67] and found synergistic killing activity with IFN-α combined with doxorubicin, 5-FU, or etoposide. Overall, these in vitro studies support a direct interaction between IFN and cytotoxic drugs, and suggest that the host immune response is not essential for these interactions.

Despite the relative wealth of in vitro investigation on the interaction between IFN and cytotoxic drugs, the mechanism of synergism between them is not clear. In fact, the conflicting results of the clinical studies that combined IFNs with cytotoxic agents in melanoma have discouraged further study of this interaction. On the other hand, because of the relatively high clinical activity of 5-FU and IFN-α in colorectal cancer, most laboratory investigations into the mechanisms of interaction have been focused on this combination. These studies have suggested that the synergism between 5-FU and IFN-α was due to IFN's capacity to inhibit the upregulation of thymidylate synthase induced by 5-FU [68,69], an enhanced incorporation of 5-FU into tumor cell RNA or DNA [70–72], or the induction of thymidine phosphorylase, the enzyme responsible for the intracellular activation of 5-FU, thereby increasing cytotoxicity in colon and breast carcinoma cell lines [73]. Studies such as these using melanoma models may be worth re-examining now that more clinical activity has been reported with IL-2 added to IFN-α and cytotoxic agents in melanoma.

Other mechanisms of interaction between cytotoxic agents with IFNs have been reported in other in vitro systems. For instance, Jani et al. showed that IFN-α augmented cisplatin accumulation by two- to sixfold in squamous cell carcinoma cell lines [74], and Darnowski et al. reported that IFN-α in combination with AZT blocked DNA repair [75].

Most cytotoxic agent/IFN combinations studied in vitro have also been evaluated in human xenografts grown in male mice, and in native animal tumor models [66], with results similar to those obtained in the in vitro models. The greater effect of IFNs alone observed using in vivo animals with intact immune systems than was seen with in vitro studies has again suggested a role of host immune response in the mechanism of IFN antitumor activity. This does not, however, negate the synergism of cytotoxic agents in mice without intact immune systems. Together, these data suggest at least two mechanisms for this interaction: (1) a direct interaction between the IFNs and the cytotoxic agent on cancer cells, and (2) an immune-modulating effect that likely depends upon IFN-induced enhancement of effector cell function.

Interleukins and chemotherapy

IL-2 has not been demonstrated to have significant synergy with cytotoxic agents in vitro or in human xenograft models, primarily because an intact host immune system is required for the antitumor effects of IL-2. However, several studies have shown that IL-2–stimulated effector cells, such as LAK cells, are synergistic with cytotoxic agents, particularly cisplatin, against a variety of tumors in vitro and in vivo [76–79]. In addition, in animal models with implanted tumors, IL-2 and cytotoxic agents have been shown to be synergistic [80–83].

IL-1, the cytokine that initiates the immune effector and cytotoxicity cascades, has also been studied against various tumor cells in combination with cytotoxic agents. A comprehensive review by Johnson indicates that IL-1, in addition to having intrinsic antitumor activity similar to that of tumor necrosis factor (TNF), interacts synergistically with etoposide and doxorubicin in killing many human tumor cell lines [24]. The interaction with etoposide was observed against mela-noma cells but not against the breast or colon cell lines tested [24]. Very few mechanistic studies of the interaction between IL-1 and cytotoxic agents have been reported. In nude mice bearing human ovarian cancer xenografts, Wang and Sinha showed that camptothecin and IL-1α enhanced antitumor activity five- to sixfold over that of either agent alone [84]. Their in vitro studies also revealed synergy between IL-1α and camptothecin, and suggested this effect was due to upregulation of topoisomerase I, camptothecin's target enzyme [84]. Cisplatin plus IL-1α has been shown to be synergistic in other murine models [85,86]. The mechanism of interaction between cisplatin and IL-1α remains unclear. While Braunschweiger et al. failed to show a direct interaction between IL-1α and cisplatin in vitro in a head and neck cancer cell line, Benchekroun et al. demonstrated that IL-1α increased cisplatin accumulation in cells and inhibited DNA repair in human ovarian cancer cell lines [87,88]. These results have led to early clinical studies combining carboplatin with IL-1α in patients with advanced cancer, including melanoma.

Tumor necrosis factor and chemotherapy

TNF-α, produced hemorrhagic necrosis in human tumor xenograft models but is extremely toxic in humans. TNF-α has also shown synergistic interactions in vitro with various drugs, including BCNU, doxorubicin, cisplatin, etoposide, and melphalan [28,29]. In the clinical arena, however, only the combination of TNF-α and melphalan used in the isolated limb perfusion setting has shown encouraging preliminary results [27].

Chemotherapy enhancement of immune function

Cisplatin

In 1975, Dr. Barnett Rosenberg, who initially reported the antitumor activity of cisplatin, was the first to suggest that its antitumor effect could also be due to its enhancement of tumor immunogenicity [90]. Since then, a number of studies have reported the effects of cisplatin on the immune system: enhancement of monocyte-mediated cytotoxicity in vitro [91,92], possibly via the release of TNF [93]; increased production of H_2O_2, O_2 and IL-1 in murine macrophages in vitro [94]; upregulation of LAK cell killing by peripheral blood monocytes via the release of IL-1 and TNF [95]; enhancement of NK cell activity both in vitro and in vivo [92,96]; and increased activity of circulating lymphocytes that mediate tumor resistance by low-dose cisplatin [97]. Other investigators have shown that pretreatment of tumor cells with low concentrations of cisplatin increased the susceptibility of the tumor cells to killing by both NK and LAK cells [78,79,98,99]. Not surprisingly, tests in a murine model have shown that the characteristics of the tumor cells can affect the results of the interaction between cisplatin and IL-2 [100]. Bernsen et al. [100] found that two different murine tumors comparably sensitive to either IL-2 or cisplatin alone had very different sensitivities to combined therapy (sequential treatment with cisplatin and then IL-2), suggesting that cisplatin could make the tumor cells either more or less resistant to IL-2.

Clinical studies of the effects of cisplatin on the immune system in cancer patients have been limited. One of the original studies, reported by Kleinerman et al., examined spontaneous monocyte-mediated cytotoxicity in 34 patients with various malignancies treated with cisplatin-based regimens compared with that seen in 31 normal controls [101]. Compared with normal controls, cancer patients had a significantly decreased spontaneous monocyte cytotoxicity (43% vs. 7%). In seven patients, the monocyte cytotoxicity during six cycles of chemotherapy increased by at least three- to fourfold between the third and fifth cycles of therapy, suggesting that cancer patients have depressed monocyte function and that cisplatin-based chemotherapy enhanced this activity. In contrast, using non–cisplatin-based regimens, Lower and Baughman evaluated the production of hydrogen peroxide by human peripheral blood monocytes and showed that chemotherapy reversibly impaired monocyte function in breast and lung cancer patients [102]. Tsuda et al. evaluated the effects of cisplatin on the T-cell suppressor activity in 15 ovarian cancer patients and showed that cisplatin did not affect NK cell activity but selectively decreased suppressor cell activity up to 7 days after treatment [103]. Immunophenotyping revealed that the CD56+/CD16+ and CD8+/CD11+ T-cell population significantly decreased, while the CD4+/2H4+ T-cell population significantly increased after therapy. Arinaga et al. found that a single dose of cisplatin in cancer patients was able to increase the ability of peripheral blood mononuclear cells to produce LAK activity upon stimulation with IL-2 without increasing NK activity [104]. Similar results were observed by Allavena et al. [105]. Together, the preclinical and clinical data suggest that cisplatin has important direct and indirect effects on the immune system, which may be relevant to the efficacy of biochemotherapy programs.

Other cytotoxic agents

Other cytotoxic agents as well have been shown to stimulate immune function. Low-dose cyclophosphamide augments the immune response by decreasing T-cell suppressor cell activity. Maguire and Ettore were the first to demonstrate that, when given at the appropriate time, cyclophosphamide surprisingly augmented the development of allergic contact dermatitis rather than suppressing it [106]. Following this lead, Berd et al. showed a significant decrease in suppressor cell activity and a corresponding increase in delayed-type hypersensitivity in patients with advanced cancer 3–7 days after administration of standard-dose cyclophosphamide [107,108]. Kiyohara et al. showed induction of LAK-like effector cell activity after combination chemotherapy at standard doses in patients with bladder and testicular cancer [109]. In addition, Watanabe et al. showed that when human colon cancer cells were exposed to low concentrations of 5-FU, they became more susceptible to LAK killing [110]. These studies demonstrate that, like cisplatin, other cytotoxic agents may have important immunomodulatory effects.

Effect of tumor burden on immune function

Another potential mechanism by which chemotherapy drugs may enhance the effects of immunotherapy is due simply to a decrease in tumor burden, which by itself may enhance T-cell function. In murine models and in a limited number of melanoma patients, a large tumor mass has been correlated with decreased expression of the zeta chain of the T-cell receptor and downstream signal transduction proteins as well [111–113]. Papa et al. [114] evaluated the effects of cyclophosphamide, BCNU, and doxorubicin in mice with advanced lung tumors treated with IL-2 and found synergistic antitumor effects only between cyclophosphamide and IL-2. Cyclophosphamide also appeared to reduce the yield of in vivo generated LAK cells, although the LAK cells could still lyse fresh tumor targets in vitro. This study suggested that the mechanisms of synergy between cyclophosphamide and IL-2 did not involve LAK cell number and that the interaction was due in part due to reduction of tumor burden, possibly through an increase in tumor susceptibility to cellular immune lysis and/or a decrease in suppressor cell activity [114]. Formelli et al. also observed in a murine model that cisplatin, but not doxorubicin, was synergistic with immune lymphocyte infusion, apparently because cisplatin was more effective in reducing tumor burden [115]. Similarly, improved results were reported by Salup et al. using doxorubicin and LAK cells in a murine model of renal cell carcinoma after the tumor burden was reduced by nephrectomy [116]. Collectively, these studies suggest that reduction in tumor burden by cytotoxic drugs may enhance immune-mediated antitumor activity by either altering T-cell receptor function, improving effector to target cell ratios, or both.

Effect of immune system on chemotherapy drugs

Most studies reported in the literature have focused on the effects of chemotherapy on the immune system. Only a few investigators have evaluated the effects of the immune effector mechanisms on the antitumor effect of chemotherapy drugs. The original studies by Braunschweiger et al. were an important contribution to this complex area of research [86]. For instance, using a murine model of squamous cell carcinoma, they showed that cisplatin and IL-1α were synergistic in vivo. They also showed that dexamethasone, but not indomethacin, could abrogate the synergism, which suggested that prostaglandins were not involved and that the immune system, either macrophages or lymphocytes, might be playing an important a role in this interaction [86]. To study the participation of macrophages, the authors evaluated the effects of cisplatin and IL-1α using a coculture model comprised of cisplatin-pretreated tumor cells and tumor-infiltrating macrophages. In this model, pretreatment of tumor cells with cisplatin prior to exposure to IL-1α alone did not produce synergistic cell kill. However, when cisplatin-pretreated tumor cells were exposed to IL-1α in the presence of tumor-infiltrating macrophages (coculture model), marked synergistic killing was observed. In addition, this synergistic killing interaction was abrogated by catalase, suggesting that the release of hydrogen peroxide from macrophages induced by IL-1 was responsible for the synergism [88]. It was thus hypothesized that hydrogen peroxide may enhance cisplatin's antitumor effect by affecting the DNA repair process, and this theory is currently being tested. As noted earlier in this review, IL-1 has been shown to inhibit repair of cisplatin-induced DNA damage in human ovarian cancer cells in vitro [87]. This finding, however, is not likely to explain Braunschweiger's results because cisplatin and IL-1 were not synergistic in the absence of macrophages.

Immunomodulatory agents might also influence the antitumor effect of chemotherapy drugs by affecting their pharmacokinetics or pharmacodynamics. Kase et al. demonstrated an increase in fluorouridine content of tumor tissues when IFN-α was added to 5-FU in a murine tumor model [71]. In a pharmacokinetic study in melanoma patients receiving dacarbazine and IL-2 in sequence, dacarbazine and 5-aminoimidazole 4-carboxamide levels were significantly lower when intravenous dacarbazine was given 3 days after IL-2 administration than when dacarbazine was given before IL-2, suggesting that there was an increased metabolism or volume of distribution of dacarbazine after IL-2 administration [117]. In another study, Gandara et al. showed that IL-2 did not affect cisplatin pharmacokinetics when the cisplatin was administered every few days [118]. Our own preliminary results on cisplatin pharmacokinetics during concurrent and sequential biochemotherapy treatment have shown no significant difference from those when chemotherapy is given alone [Buzaid, personal communication]. In summary, biologics may enhance the effects of cytotoxic agents, directly or indirectly, possibly by inhibiting the repair of cellular damage induced by the cytotoxic drug, or by modulating the pharmacologic disposition of the drug in the cell. The effect of the biologics on the pharmacokinetics of cytotoxic agents does not appear to be critically important.

Importance of schedule in the interaction between biologics and chemotherapy

In most reports of the combination of biologics with chemotherapy, the chemotherapy preceded the biologic therapy. The dependence on schedule between biologics and chemotherapy drugs for their synergistic interaction, however, has been systematically studied by only a few investigators. Gauny et al. evaluated the combination of IL-2 with various cytotoxic agents in two murine models, Meth A sarcoma and B16 melanoma [83]. In the Meth A model, cisplatin, bleomycin, and doxorubicin had enhanced effects when administered before or concurrent with IL-2. However, no improvement was observed when IL-2 was given first. In those studies, a synergistic effect was observed only with cisplatin. In the B16 model, when cyclophosphamide was given before or concurrent with IL-2, tumors regressed completely and new tumor growth was prevented. When IL-2 was administered prior to cyclophosphadmide, it delayed but did not inhibit tumor growth. However, neither cisplatin nor 5-FU had any effect when combined with IL-2 in the B16 melanoma model [83]. Rinehart et al. showed in a mouse B16 melanoma model that IL-2 combined with cyclophosphamide, etoposide, and cisplatin chemotherapy was more effective than the chemotherapy alone only when the chemotherapy was given before the IL-2 [80]. When Formelli et al. studied the combination of immune lymphocyte infusion and cisplatin in mice bearing YC8 lymphoma cells, they observed that the antitumor effect was superior when cisplatin was administered on day 5 and the immune lymphocytes on day 7 versus when immune lymphocytes were administered on day 5 and cisplatin on day 12 (2 days after completion of the immune lymphocyte infusion) [115]. In contrast, Lumsden et al. found no schedule dependency for the effectiveness of Adriamycin and IL-2 against colonic adenocarcinoma in a rat model [81].

The importance of timing between cytotoxic drugs and IL-1α administration has also been studied. Nakamura et al. investigated the interaction of IL-1α in combination with a number of cytotoxic agents, including mitomycin-C, doxorubicin, cisplatin, cyclophosphamide, and 5-FU, in two murine models, Meth A sarcoma and colon 26 adenocarcinoma. IL-1α was administered 1 day prior to, concurrent with, or 1 day after the cytotoxic drug. Treatment was started on day 1 or 7 after intradermal transplantation of the tumor. In the sarcoma model, with drug administration starting on day 7, all drugs tested had an enhanced antitumor effect, with the greatest effect for doxorubicin and 5-FU. With doxorubicin, the timing of administration did not significantly affect the number of cures, but with 5-FU more cures were observed when the drug was administered either concurrently with or 1 day before IL-1. In the colon carcinoma model, timing was not a factor when the drugs were administered on day 1 of tumor transplantation. However, when the drugs were administered starting on day 7 of tumor transplantation, cisplatin was significantly more effective when administered concurrently with IL-1. No difference was observed when cisplatin was given 1 day before or 1 day after IL-1α. Detailed in vivo studies concerning the schedule dependency of the synergism between IL-1α and cytotoxic drugs were also performed by Braunschweiger et al. using the RIF-1 murine model. They observed that mitomycin was synergistic with IL-1 when it was administered 1 hour before IL-1, while cisplatin was synergistic when administered 6 hours prior to or up to 2 hours after IL-1 [86,119]. In contrast, Chang et al. observed opposite results with both carboplatin and cisplatin treatment with IL-1α in the same tumor model [120]. There is no obvious explanation for these differing results.

Despite some conflicting reports, most of the animal studies suggest that combination cytotoxic/biologic treatment is more effective when the cytotoxic therapy is administered either before or concurrent with the biologic agent. These findings agree with the results of the M.D. Anderson biochemotherapy studies showing that concurrent biochemotherapy is an active combination and that CVD/BIO appears to be more effective than BIO/CVD.

Mechanistic studies from biochemotherapy trials

Another form of investigation into the mechanism of biologic/cytotoxic interactions has been the laboratory study of patients undergoing biochemotherapy. A number of such investigations have been carried out, primarily using peripheral blood mononuclear cells, in cases of advanced melanoma. In one such instance, Muhonen et al. investigated phenotypic markers on peripheral lymphocytes during biochemotherapy with bleomycin, vincristine, lomustine, dacarbazine, and IFN-α (BOLD plus IFN-α) and found that all lymphocyte subsets decreased during therapy, while only changes in the CD4+/CD8+ values during therapy correlated with response and progression [121].

Eisenthal et al. reported that in patients given dacarbazine and carboplatin followed by IL-2 and IFN-α, CD16+ cells and lymphokine-activated killer cell activity decreased after chemotherapy, whereas the parameters increased after immunotherapy [122]. These patients received chemotherapy on day 1 and day 22 and immunotherapy from day 36 to day 75, and had peripheral blood cells studied on day 36 and day 76. Responding patients maintained more cytotoxic and proliferative activity in their mononuclear cells after chemotherapy and had a higher percentage of CD8+ cells after immuotherapy.

In a trial of dacarbazine and IL-2 in metastatic melanoma patients, Isacson et al. measured multiple hematologic and immunologic parameters and found only one parameter that correlated with response to therapy: a greater induction of IL-2 receptor (CD25) expression on the lymphocytes of responders [123]. A similar finding was reported by Mouawad et al. in melanoma patients treated with the Salpetriere Hospital regimen, consisting of cisplatin, IL-2, and IFN-α [124]. In Mouawad's study, those patients who had the greatest increase in the high- and intermediate-affinity IL-2 receptors on lymphocytes after IL-2 therapy were more likely to respond to therapy, and the increase in β-chain expression was limited to natural killer (NK) phenotype cells.

At M.D. Anderson, during the conduct of the concurrent biochemotherapy protocol we performed a series of laboratory studies designed to better understand the mechanism of antitumor activity in biochemotherapy. We initially hypothesized that CVD enhanced the antitumor activity of biotherapy. However, the absence of LAK and minimal NK cell cytotoxicity in our first 10 patients, including 8 responders, prompted us to reject our initial hypothesis [125]. We acknowledged however, that the immunologic effects assessed in the peripheral blood might not represent the effects observed at the site or within the tumor. Nonetheless, we next proposed that IFN-α and IL-2 could enhance the cytotoxic effect of CVD. Specifically, we attributed the synergistic interaction to biotherapy-induced activation of tumor-infiltrating macrophages. This hypothesis was based on the work of Braunschweiger et al., which suggested that the synergy between cisplatin and IL-1α is mediated by hydrogen peroxide release from tumor-infiltrating macrophages [88]. Because IL-2, like IL-1α, can also activate macrophages, we hypothesized that a similar mechanism might operate in biochemotherapy. Consequently, we evaluated macrophage activation by measuring serum neopterin levels in patients participating in the concurrent biochemotherapy study. Compared with baseline, neopterin levels increased at least sixfold in 7 of 8 responders but in only 2 of 7 nonresponders (p = 0.041). We also measured the level of DNA interstrand crosslinking in cryopreserved peripheral mononuclear cells. Based on the work of others [126], that showed cisplatin-induced DNA crosslinking of peripheral mononuclear cells correlates with response to therapy, we hypothesized that if biotherapy enhanced the cytotoxicity of cisplatin, then biochemotherapy-induced DNA damage would also correlate with response to therapy. The DNA crosslinking index, a measure of was ≥0.8 in 4 of 4 responders but in only 1 of 4 nonresponders (p = 0.14). Thus, although the number of patients studied was very small, our preliminary data supported the hypothesis that concurrent biochemotherapy exerts its antitumor effect predominantly by directly increasing cytotoxicity and that macrophages may be involved [125].

We are currently conducting a randomized trial comparing sequential biochemotherapy with CVD alone. A series of laboratory studies designed to evaluate DNA repair in peripheral mononuclear cells and tumor cells, as well as various immunologic studies, are being performed in both treatment arms to more rigorously test our working hypothesis. We anticipate that these clinical studies, although of great importance, will provide primarily circumstrantial evidence to support or refute our hypothesis and that studies in animal models will be necessary to better elucidate the mechaisms of interaction between biologics and chemotherapy drugs.

CONCLUSIONS

Biochemotherapy combining cisplatin-based chemotherapy with IL-2 and IFN-α appears quite promising as a new approach to resistant, advanced melanoma, with preliminary results from several centers showing dramatically improved response rates, complete responses, and duration of response. Hopefully these early results will foretell a significant improvement in survival over currently available therapies. Also, it will be important to reduce the toxicity of biochemotherapy with dose or schedule modifications and better supportive care. Biochemotherapy regimens were developed empirically, and the mechanism by which they produce potent antitumor effects in melanoma patients is not yet known. Only a better understanding of the antitumor mechanisms will allow us to more rationally improve upon the current results with biochemotherapy in advanced melanoma.

REFERENCES

1. Wingo P, Tong T, Bolden S (1995) Cancer Statistics, 1995. CA Cancer J Clin 45:8–30.
2. Karavodin L, Golub S (1984) Systemic administration of human leukocyte interferon to melanoma patients. III. Increased helper:suppressor ratios in melanoma patients during interferon treatment. Nat Immun Cell Growth Regul 3:193–202.
3. Hersey P, MacDonald M, Hall C, Spurling A, Edwards A, Coates A, McCarthy W (1986) Immunological effects of recombinant interferon alfa-2a in patients with disseminated melanoma. Cancer 57:1666–1674.
4. Creagan E, Ahmann D, Frytak S (1986) Phase II trials of recombinant leukocyte alpha interferon in disseminated malignant melanoma: Results in 96 patients. Cancer Treat Rep 70:619–624.
5. Legha S (1989) Current therapy for malignant melanoma. Semin Oncol 16:34–44.
6. Kirkwood J, Agarwala S (1993) Systemic cytotoxic and biologic therapy of melanoma. PPO Updates 7:1–16.
7. Creagan ET, Ahmann DL, Frytak S, Long HJ, Itri LM (1986) Recombinant leukocyte A interferon (rIFN-alphaA) in the treatment of disseminated malignant melanoma. Analysis of complete and long-term responding patients. Cancer 58:2576–2578.
8. Rosenberg S, Lotze M, Mule J (1988) New approaches to the immunotherapy of cancer using interleukin-2. Ann Intern Med 108:853–864.
9. Parkinson D, Abrams J, Wiernik P, Rayner AA, Margolin KA, Van Echo DA, Sznol M, Dutcher JP, Aronson FR, Doroshow JH, Atkins MB, Hawkins MJ (1990) Interleukin-2 therapy in patients with metastatic malignant melanoma: A phase II study. J Clin Oncol 8:1650–1656.
10. Richards J, Bajorin D, Vogelzang N, Houghton A, Seigler H, Sell K, Zeffrin J, Levitt D (1990) Treatment of metastatic melanoma with continuous infusion IL-2 +/– LAK cells: A randomized trial. Proc Am Soc Clin Oncol 9:322.
11. McCabe M, Stablein D, Hawkins M (1991) The modified group C experience—phase III randomized trials of IL-2 vs. IL-2/LAK in advanced renal cell carcinoma and advanced melanoma. Proc Am Soc Clin Oncol 10:213.
12. Koretz M, Lawson D, York R, Graham S, Murray D, Gillespie T, Levitt D, Sell K (1991) Randomized study of interleukin-2 alone vs. IL-2 plus lymphokine activated killer cells for treatment of melanoma and renal cell carcinoma. Arch Surg 126:893–903.
13. Rosenberg S, Lotze M, Yang J, Topalian SL, Chang AE, Schwartzentruber DJ, Aebersold P, Leitman S, Linehan WM, Seipp CA, White DE, Steinberg SM (1993) Prospective randomized trial of high-dose interleukin-2 alone or in conjunction with lymphokine-activated killer cells for the treatment of patients with advanced cancer. J Natl Cancer Inst 85:622–632.
14. Rosenberg S, Packard B, Aebersold P, Solomon D, Topalian S, Toy S, Simon P, Lotze M, Yang J, Seipp C (1988) Use of tumor-infiltrating lymphocytes and interleukin-2 in the immunotherapy of patients with metastatic melanoma: A preliminary report. N Engl J Med 319:1676–1680.
15. Aebersold P, Hyatt C, Johnson S (1991) Lysis of autologous melanoma cells by tumor-infiltrating lymphocytes: Association with clinical response. J Natl Cancer Inst 83:932–936.
16. Kradin R, Lazarus D, Dubinett S, Gifford J, Grove B, Kurnick J, Preffer F, Pinto C, Davidson E, Callahan R, Strauss H (1989) Tumor-infiltrating lymphocytes and interleukin-2 treatment of advanced cancer. Lancet 1:577–580.
17. Dillman RO, Oldham RK, Barth NM, Cohen RJ, Minor DR, Birch R, Yanelli JR, Maleckar JR, Sferruzza A, Arnold J, West WH (1991) Continuous infusion interleukin-2 and tumor infiltrating lymphocytes as treatment of advanced melanoma. Cancer 68:1–5.
18. Arienti F, Belli F, Rivoltini L, Gambacorti-Passerini C, Furlan L, Mascheroni L, Prada A, Rizzi M,

Marchesi E, Vaglini M, Parmiani G, Cascinelli N (1993) Adoptive immunotherapy of advanced melanoma patients with interleukin-2 and tumor-infiltrating lymphocytes selected in vitro with low doses of IL-2. Cancer Immunol Immunother 36:315–322.

19. Hanson J, Kurtz J, Rohloff C, Kabler-Babbit C, Aleem J, Rausch C, Bielinski K, Klimaszewski AD (1993) Recombinant interleukin-2 with tumor infiltrating lymphocytes for metastatic melanoma. Proc Am Soc Clin Oncol 12:396.

20. Hersey P, Hasic E, MacDonald M, Edwards A, Spurling A, Coates AS, Milton GW, McCarthy WH (1985) Effects of recombinant leukocyte interferon on tumour growth and immune response in patients with metastatic melanoma. Br J Cancer 51:815–826.

21. Brunda M, Bellantoni D, Sulich V (1987) In vivo anti-tumor activity of combinations of interferon-alpha and interleukin-2 in a murine model. Correlation of efficacy with the induction of cytotoxic cells resembling natural killer cells. Int J Cancer 40:365–371.

22. Sparano J, Fisher R, Sunderland M, Margolin K, Ernest M, Sznol M, Atkins M, Dutcher J, Micetich K, Weiss G, Doroshow J, Aronson F, Rubinstein L, Mier J (1993) Randomized phase III trial of treatment with high-dose interleukin-2 alone or in combination with interferon alpha-2a in patients with advanced melanoma. J Clin Oncol 11:1969–1977.

23. Keilholz U, Scheibenbogen C, Tilgen W, Bergmann L, Weidmann E, Seither E, Richter M, Brado B, Mitrou PS, Hunstein W (1993) Interferon-alpha and interleukin-2 in the treatment of malignant melanoma: Comparison of two phase 2 trials. Cancer 72:607–614.

24. Johnson C (1992) Modulation of chemotherapy antineoplastic agents with biologic agents: enhancement of antitumor activities by interleukin-1. Curr Opin Oncol 4:1108–1115.

25. Sznol M, Mier J, Dutcher J, Sosman J, Weiss G, Isaacs R, Margolin K (1994) A phase II trial of a daily 1-hour infusion of interleukin-6 for metastatic malignant melanoma. Proc Am Soc Clin Oncol 13:396.

26. Oppenheim J, Krakauer T, Smith J, Urba W, Longo D (1992) Therapeutic potential of interleukin-1 in neoplastic diseases. Proc Am Assoc Cancer Res 33:579.

27. Lienard D, Ewalenko P, Delmotte J, Renard N, Lejeune F (1992) High-dose recombinant tumor necrosis factor alpha in combination with interferon gamma and melphalan in isolation perfusion of the limbs for melanoma and sarcoma. J Clin Oncol 10:52–60.

28. Lejeune F, Lienard D, Eggermont A, Schraffordt-Koops H, Rosenkaimer F, Gerain J, Klaase J, Kroon B, Vanderveken J, Schmitz P (1994) Rationale for using TNF-alpha and chemotherapy in regional therapy of melanoma. J Cell Biochem 56:52–61.

29. Margolin K, Doroshow J, Akman S, Leong L, Morgan R, Odujinrin O, Raschko J, Somlo G, Blevins C, Prestifilippo J (1990) Treatment of advanced melanoma with cisdiamminedichloroplatinum (CDDP) and alpha interferon (aIFN). Proc Am Soc Clin Oncol 9:277.

30. Morton R, Creagan E, Schaid D, Kardinal C, McCormack G, McHale M, Wiesenfeld M (1991) Phase II trial of recombinant leukocyte A interferon (IFN-alpha-2a) plus 1,3-bis(2-chloroethyl)-1-nitrosourea (BCNU) and the combination cimetidine with BCNU in patients with disseminated malignant melanoma. Am J Clin Oncol 14:152–155.

31. Smith K, Green J, Eccles J (1992) Interferon alpha 2a and vindesine in the treatment of advanced malignant melanoma. Eur J Cancer 28:438–441.

32. Stark J, Schulof R, Wiemann M, Barth N, Honeycutt P, Soori G (1993) Alpha interferon and chemo-hormonal therapy in advanced melanoma: A phase I/II NBSG/MAOP study. Proc Am Soc Clin Oncol 12:392.

33. Feun L, Savaraj N, Moffat F, Robinson D, Liebmann A, Hurley J, Raub WJ, Richman S (Year) Combination of BCNU, DTIC, cisplatin, and tamoxifen with alpha-interferon in stage IV melanoma. Advances in the Biology and Clinical Management of Melanoma: 38th Annual Clinical Conference. Houston, Texas, p 101.

34. Schultz M, Buzaid A, Poo W (1996) A phase II study of interferon-alpha 2b with dacarbazine, cisplatin, carmustine, and tamoxifen in metastatic melanoma. Melanoma Res, in press.

35. Legha S, Ring S, Bedikian A, Eton O, Plager C, Papadopoulos N, Ensign L, Benjamin R (1993) Lack of benefit from tamoxifen added to a regimen of cisplatin (C), vinblastine (V), DTIC (D) and alpha interferon (IFN) in patients with metastatic melanoma. Proc Am Soc Clin Oncol 12:388.

36. Pyrhonen S, Hahka-Kemppinen M, Muhonen T (1992) A promising interferon plus four-drug chemotherapy regimen for metastatic melanoma. J Clin Oncol 10:1919–1926.

37. Mulder N, H S-K, Sleijfer D, deVries E, Willemse P (1991) Possible synergistic effect of 5-FU added to alpha-interferon and DTIC in the treatment of disseminated malignant melanoma. Proc Am Soc Clin Oncol 10:292.

38. Kirkwood J, Ernstoff M, Giuliano A, Gams R, Robinson W, Costanzi J, Pouillart P, Speyer J, Grimm M, Spiegel R (1990) Interferon alpha 2a and dacarbazine in melanoma. J Natl Cancer Inst 82:1062–1063.

39. Bajetta E, Di Leo A, Zampino M, Sertoli M, Comella G, Barduagni M, Giannotti B, Queirolo P, Tribbia G, Bernengo M, Menichetti E, Palmeri S, Russo A, Cristofolini M, Erbazzi A, Fowst C, Criscuolo D, Bufalino R, Zilembo N, Cascinelli N (1994) Multicenter randomized trial of dacarbazine alone or in combination with two different doses and schedules of interferon alpha-2a in the treatment of advanced melanoma. J Clin Oncol 12:806–811.

40. Falkson C, Falkson G, Falkson H (1991) Improved results with the addition of interferon alpha-2a to dacarbazine in the treatment of patients with metastatic malignant melanoma. J Clin Oncol 9:1403–1408.

41. Thomson D, Adena M, McLeod G, Hersey P, Gill P, Coates A, Olver I, Kefford R, Lowenthal R, Beadle G, Walpole E, Boland K, Kingston D (1993) Interferon-alpha-2a does not improve response or survival when combined with dacarbazine in metastatic malignant melanoma: results of a multi-institutional Australian randomized trial. Melanoma Res 3:133–138.

42. Papadopoulos N, Howard J, Murray J, Cunningham J, Plager C, Legha S, Reuben J, Gutterman J, Benjamin R (1990) Phase II DTIC and interleukin-2 (IL-2) trial for metastatic malignant melanoma. Proc Am Soc Clin Oncol 9:277.

43. Dillman R, Oldham R, Barth N, Birch R, Arnold J, West W (1990) Recombinant interleukin-2 and adoptive immunotherapy alternated with dacarbazine therapy in melanoma: A National Biotherapy Study Group trial. J Natl Cancer Inst 82:1345–1349.

44. Stoter G, Aamdal S, Rodenhuis S, Cleton F, Iacobelli S, Franks C, Oskam R, Shiloni E (1991) Sequential administration of recombinant human interleukin-2 and dacarbazine in metastatic melanoma: A multicenter phase II study. J Clin Oncol 9:1687–1691.

45. Flaherty L, Redman B, Chabot G, Martino S, Gualdoni S, Heilbrun L, Valdivieso M, Bradley E (1990) A phase I-II study of dacarbazine in combination with outpatient interleukin-2 in metastatic malignant melanoma. Cancer 65:2471–2477.

46. Dummer R, Gore M, Hancock B, Guillou P, Grobben H, Becker J, Oskam R, Dieleman J, Burg G (1995) A multicenter phase II clinical trial using dacarbazine and continuous infusion interleukin-2 for metastatic melanoma. Cancer 75:1038–1044.

47. Demchak P, Mier J, Robert N, O'Brien K, Gould J, Atkins M (1991) Interleukin-2 and high-dose cisplatin in patients with metastatic melanoma: A pilot study. J Clin Oncol 9:1821–1830.

48. Flaherty L, Robinson W, Redman B, Gonzales R, Martino S, Kraut M, Valdivieso M, Rudolph A (1993) A phase II study of dacarbazine and cisplatin in combination with outpatient administered interleukin-2 in metastatic melanoma. Cancer 71:3520–3525.

49. Atkins M, O'Boyle K, Sosman J, Weiss G, Margolin K, Ernest M, Kappler K, Mier J, Sparano J, Fisher R, Eckardt J, Pereira C, Aronson F (1994) Multiinstitutional phase II trial of intensive combination chemoimmunotherapy for metastatic melanoma. J Clin Oncol 12:1553–1560.

50. Richards J, Mehta N, Schroeder L, Dordal A (1992) Sequential chemotherapy/immunotherapy for metastatic melanoma. Proc Am Soc Clin Oncol 11:346.

51. Rixe O, Benhammouda A, Antoine E, Petit T, Tourani J, Borel C, Franks C, Kalif B, Mousseau M, Thomas A, Bensfia S, Nisri D, Soubrane C, Herrera A, Bizzari J, Auclerc G, Weil M, Banzet P, Khayat D (1994) Final results of a prospective multicentric study on 91 metastatic malignant melanoma patients treated by chemo-immunotherapy with cisplatin, interleukin-2, and interferon-alpha. Proc Am Soc Clin Oncol 13:399.

52. Dorval T, Negrier S, Chevreau C, Baume D, Cupissol D, Oskam R, Herrera A, Escudier B (1994) Results of a French multicentric randomized trial of chemoimmunotherapy (cisplatin, IL-2, with or without IFN) in metastatic malignant melanoma. Proc Am Soc Clin Oncol 13:395.

53. Buzaid A, Legha S (1994) Combination of chemotherapy with interleukin-2 and interferon-alpha for the treatment of advanced melanoma. Semin Oncol 21:23–28.

54. Ron I, Mordish Y, Eisenthal A, Skornick Y, Inbar M, Chaitchik S (1994) A phase II study of combined adminstration of dacarbazine and carboplatin with home therapy of recombinant interleukin-2 and interferon-alpha 2a in patients with advanced malignant melanoma. Cancer Immunol Immunother 38:379–384.

55. Richards J, Mehta N, Ramming K, Skosey P (1992) Sequential chemoimmunotherapy in the treatment of metastatic melanoma. J Clin Oncol 10:1338–1343.

56. Legha S, Buzaid A, Ring S, Bedikian A, Plager C, Eton O, Papadopoulos N, Benjamin R (1994) Improved results of treatment of metastatic melanoma with combined use of biotherapy and chemotherapy. Proc Am Soc Clin Oncol 13:394.

57. Thatcher N, Wagstaff J, Mene A, Smith D, Orton C, Craig P (1986) Corynebacterium parvum followed by chemotherapy (actinomycin D and DTIC) compared with chemotherapy alone for metastatic malignant melanoma. Eur J Cancer 22:1009–1014.

58. Verschraegen C, Legha S, Hersh E, Plager C, Papadopoulos N, Burgess M (1993) Phase II study of vindesine and dacarbazine with or without non-specific stimulation of the immune system in patients with metastatic melanoma. Eur J Cancer 29A:708–711.

59. Costanzi J, Fletcher W, Balcerzak S, Taylor S, Eyre H, O'Bryan R, Al-Sarraf M, Frank J (1984) Combination chemotherapy plus levamisole in the treatment of disseminated malignant melanoma. Cancer 53:833–836.

60. Lestingi T, Richards J, Shulman K, Gale D, Karius D, Isaacs R, Levitt D (1994) Pilot phase II study of recombinant interleukin-6 and chemotherapy in metastatic melanoma. Proc Am Soc Clin Oncol 13:395.

61. Vlock D, Johnson C, Chang M, Reyno L, Erkman K, Egorin M, Logan T, McCauley C (1993) Phase I trial of interleukin-1-alpha and carboplatin. Proc Am Assoc Cancer Res 34:296.

62. Logan T, Bishop H, Mintun M, Choi Y, Sashin D, Virji M, Billiar T, Trump D, Smith D, Kirkwood J (1994) Phase I trial of interleukin-1-alpha and carboplatin in patients with metastatic disease to the lung: Effects on tumor blood flow evaluated by positron emission tomography. Proc Am Assoc Cancer Res 35:198.

63. Brunda M, Luistro L, Warrier R, Wright R, Hubbard B, Murphy M, Wolf S, Gately M (1993) Antitumor and antimetastatic activity of interleukin-12 against murine tumors. J Exp Med 178:1223–1230.

64. Tahara H, Zeh H, Storkus W, Pappo I, Watkins S, Gubler U, Wolf S, Robbins R, Lotze M (1994) Fibroblasts genetically engineered to secrete interleukin-12 can suppress tumor growth and induce antitumor immunity to a murine melanoma in vivo. Cancer Res 54:182–189.

65. Carson W, Grabstein K, Giri J, Lindemann M, Linett M, Caligiuri M (1994) Interleukin-15 is a novel cytokine which activates human natural killer cells using components of the interleukin-2 receptor. Proc Am Soc Clin Oncol 13:296.

66. Wadler S, Schwartz E (1990) Antineoplastic activity of the combination of interferon and cytotoxic agents against experimental and human malignancies: A review. Cancer Res 50:3473–3486.

67. Von Hoff D (1991) In vitro data supporting interferon plus cytotoxic agent combinations. Sem Oncology 18 (Suppl 7):58–61.

68. Seymour M, McSheehy P, Dobson N, Rodrigues L, Clemens M, Slevin M (1992) 5-fluorouracil and interferon-alpha: Interactions in vitro and in vivo. Br J Cancer 65 (Suppl 16):17.

69. Mizunuma N, Aiba K, Shibata H, Ogawa M, Kuraish Y, Yoshida K (1992) Dual modulation with D,L leucovorin and interferon-gamma enhances cytotoxic activity of 5-fluorouracil in human colon cancer cell lines. Proc Am Assoc Cancer Res 33:426.

70. Kase S, Kubota T, Wanatabe M, Furukawa T, Tanino H, Ishibiki K, Teramoto T, Kitajima M (1993) Interferon-beta increases antitumor activity of 5-fluorouracil against human colon carcinoma cells in vitro and in vivo. Anticancer Res 13:369–374.

71. Kase S, Kubota T, Watanabe M, Teramoto T, Kitajima M, Hoffman R (1994) Recombinant human interferon-alpha 2a increases 5-fluorouracil efficacy by elevating fluorouridine concentration in tumor tissue. Cancer Res 14:1155–1160.

72. Houghton J, Adkins D, Morton C, Cheshire P, Houghton P (1992) Potentiation by interferon of 5-fluorouracil-leucovorin combinations in colon carcinoma cell lines and the interaction mechanism. Anticancer Res 12:1796–1797.

73. Schwartz E, Baptiste N, Wadler S (1994) Mechanism of induction of thymidine phosphorylase expression by interferon-alpha in vitro and in vivo. Proc Am Assoc Cancer Res 35:A1894.

74. Jani J, Xu B, Emerson E, Katoh A, Gupta V, Singh S (1995) Modulation of cisplatin (CDDP) accumulation and sensitivity by interferon-α (IFN) in human squamous carcinoma cell. Proc Am Assoc Cancer Res 36:342.

75. Darnowski J, Hankinson G, Goulette F (1995) Alpha-interferon induced inhibition of DNA repair increases the cytotoxicity of azidothymidine in HCT-8 cells. Proc Am Assoc Cancer Res 36:298.

76. Basu S, Sodhi A, Singh S, Suresh A (1991) Up-regulation of induction of lymphokine (IL-2) activated killer (LAK) cell activity by FK-565 and cisplatin. Immunol Lett 27:199–204.

77. Gazit Z, Weiss D, Shouval D, Yechezkeli M, Schirrmacher V, Notter M, Walter J, Kedar E (1992) Chemo-adoptive immunotherapy of nude mice implanted with human colorectal carcinoma and melanoma cell lines. Cancer Immunol Immunother 35:135–144.

78. Mizutani Y, Nio Y, Yoshida O (1992) Modulation by cis-diamminedichloroplatinum (II) of the susceptibilities of human T24 lined and freshly separated autologous urinary bladder transitional

carcinoma cells to peripheral blood lymphocytes and lymphokine activated killer cells. J Urol 147:505–510.

79. Mizutani Y, Bonavida B, Nio Y, Yoshida O (1993) Enhanced susceptibility of cis-diamminedichloroplatinum-treated K562 cell to lysis by peripheral blood lymphocytes and lymphokine activated killer cells. Cancer 71:1313–1321.

80. Rinehart J, Triozzi P, Lee M, Aldrich W, Young D (1992) Modulation of hematologic and immunologic effects of high dose chemotherapy by interleukin-2 in a murine tumor model. Mol Biother 4:77–82.

81. Lumsden S, Codde J, Gay B (1992) Influence of schedule on the therapeutic efficacy of chemoimmunotherapy with doxorubicin and interleukin-2. Biotherapy 5:113–118.

82. Iigo M, Tsuda H, Moriyama M (1994) Enhanced therapeutic effects of anti-tumor agents against growth and metastasis of colon carcinoma 26 when given in combination with interferon and interleukin-2. Clin Exp Metast 12:368–374.

83. Gauny S, Zimmerman R, Winkelhake J (1989) Combination therapies using interleukin-2 and chemotherapeutics in murine tumors. Proc Am Assoc Cancer Res 30:372.

84. Wang Z, Sinha B (1995) Interleukin-1-α-induced modulation of topoisomerase I and synergistic activity in vitro and in vivo. Proc Am Assoc Cancer Res 36:295.

85. Nakamura S, Kashimoto S, Kajikawa F, Nakata K (1991) Combination effect of recombinant huma interleukin-1 alpha with antitumor drugs on syngeneic tumors in mice. Cancer Res 51:215–221.

86. Braunschweiger P, Basrur V, Santos O, Markoe A, Houdek P, Schwade J (1993) Synergistic antitumor activity of cisplatin and interleukin-1 in sensitive and resistant solid tumors. Cancer Res 53:1091–1097.

87. Benchekroun M, Parker R, Reed E, Sinha B (1993) Inhibition of DNA repair and sensitization of cisplatin in human ovarian carcinoma cells by interleukin-1 alpha. Biochem Biophys Res Commun 195:294–300.

88. Braunschweiger P, Basrur V, Santos O (1993) Interleukin-1a induced oxidants increase cisplatin cytotoxicity in squamous cell carcinoma cells in vitro. Proc Am Assoc Cancer Res 34:466.

89. Parmiani G, Rivoltini L (1991) Biologic agents as modifiers of chemotherapeutic effects. Curr Opin Oncol 3:1078–1086.

90. Rosenberg B (1975) Possible mechanisms for the antitumor activity of platinum complexes. Cancer Chemother Rep 59:589–598.

91. Kleinerman E, Zwelling L, Muchmore A (1980) Enhancement of naturally occurring human spontaneous monocyte-mediated cytotoxicity by cis-diamminedichloroplatinum(II). Cancer Res 40:3099–3102.

92. Sodhi A, Pai K, Singh R, Singh S (1990) Activation of human NK cells and monocytes with cisplatin in vitro. Int J Immunopharmacol 12:893–898.

93. Gan X, Jewett A, Bonavida B (1992) Activation of human peripheral blood derived monocytes by cis-diamminedichloroplatinum: Enhanced tumoricidal activity and secretion of tumor necrosis factor-alpha. Nat Immun 11:144–155.

94. Sodhi A, Geetha B (1989) Effect of cisplatin, lipopolysaccharide, muramyl dipeptide, and recombinant interferon-gamma on murine macrophages in vitro. Nat Immun Cell Growth Regul 8:108–116.

95. Sodhi A, Basu S (1992) Up-regulation of IL-2 induced lymphokine activated killer cell activity by cisplatin and FK-565: Involvement of calcium ion. Immunol Lett 32:139–146.

96. Lichtenstein A, Pende D (1986) Enhancement of natural killer cytotoxicity by cis-diamminedichloroplatinum (II) in vivo and in vitro. Cancer Res 46:639–644.

97. Crum E (1993) Effect of cisplatin upon expression of in vivo immune tumor resistance. Cancer Immunol Immunother 36:18–24.

98. Collins J, Kao M (1989) The anticancer drug, cisplatin, increases the naturally occurring cell-mediated lysis of tumor cells. Cancer Immunol Immunother 29:17–22.

99. Mally M, Taylor C, Callewaert D (1980) Effects of platinum agents on in vitro assays of human antitumor immunity. II. Effects of cis-[Pt(NH₃)₂Cl₂] on spontaneous cell-mediated cytotoxicity. Chemotherapy 26:1–6.

100. Bernsen M, van Barlingen H, van der Velden A, Dullens H, den Otter W, Heintz P (1993) Dualistic effects of cis-diammine-dichloro-platinum on the antitumor efficacy of subsequently applied recombinant interleukin-2 therapy: A tumor-dependent phenomemon. Int J Cancer 54:513–517.

101. Kleinerman E, Howser D, Young R, Bull J, Zwelling L, Barlock A, Decker J, Muchmore A (1980)

Defective monocyte killing in patients with malignancies and restoration of function during chemotherapy. Lancet 2:1102–1105.

102. Lower E, Baughman R (1990) The effect of cancer and chemotherapy on monocyte function. J Clin Lab Immunol 31:121–125.

103. Tsuda H, Kitahashi S, Umesaki N, Kanoaka Y, Kawabata M, Ogita S (1994) Abrogation of suppressor cells activity by cis-diamminedichloroplatinum treatment using therapeutic doses in ovarian cancer patients. Gynecol Oncol 52:218–221.

104. Arinaga S, Adachi M, Karimine N, Inoue H, Asoh T, Ueo H, Akiyoshi T (1994) Enhanced induction of lymphokine-activated killer activity following a single dose of cisplatin in cancer patients. Int J Immunopharmacol 16:519–524.

105. Allavena P, Pirovano P, Bonazzi C, Colombo N, Mantovani A, D'Incalci M (1990) In vitro and in vivo effects of cisplatin on the generation of lymphokine-activated killer cells. J Natl Cancer Inst 82:139–142.

106. Maguire H, Jr, Ettore V (1967) Enhancement of dinitrochlorobenzene (DNCB) contact sensitization by cyclophosphamide in the guinea pig. J Invest Dermatol 48:39–43.

107. Berd D, Mastrangelo M, Engstrom P, Paul A, Maguire H (1982) Augmentation of the human immune response to cyclophosphamide. Cancer Res 42:4862–4866.

108. Berd D, Maguire H, Mastrangelo M (1984) Impairment of concanavalin-A-inducible suppressor activity following administration of cyclophosphamide to patients with advanced cancer. Cancer Res 44:1275–1280.

109. Kiyohara T, Taniguchi K, Kubota S, Koga S, Sakuragi T, Saitoh Y (1988) Induction of lymphokine-activated killer-like cells by cancer chemotherapy. J Exp Med 168:2355–2360.

110. Watanabe M, Kawano Y, Kubota T, Kurihara N, Nishibori H, Hoshiya Y, Teramoto T, Kitajima M (1995) Mechanism of synergistic antitumor effects of mitomycin-C, 5-fluorouracil and interleukin-2 against humon colon cancer. Proc Am Assoc Cancer Res 36:299.

111. Mizoguchi H, O'Shea J, Longo D, Loeffler C, McVicar D, Ochoa A (1992) Alterations in signal transduction molecules in T lymphocytes from tumor-bearing mice. Science 258:1795–1798.

112. Ochoa A, Mizoguchi H, Oshea J, Loeffler C, Urba W, Longo D (1993) Alterations in signal transduction molecules in T lymphocytes from tumor-bearing mice. Proc Am Assoc Cancer Res 34:451.

113. Zea A, Longo D, Mizoguchi H, Curti B, Strobl S, Creekmore S, Urba W, Ochoa A (1994) Alterations in T cell receptor and signal transduction in melanoma patients. Proc Am Assoc Cancer Res 35:A2840.

114. Papa M, Yang J, Vetto J, Shiloni E, Eisenthal A, Rosenberg S (1988) Combined effects of chemotherapy and interleukin-2 in the therapy of mice with advanced pulmonary tumors. Cancer Res 48:122–129.

115. Formelli F, Rossi C, Luisa-Sensi M, Parmiani G (1988) Potentiation of adoptive immunotherapy by cis-diamminedichloroplatinum (II), but not doxorubicin, on a disseminated mouse lymphoma and its association with reduction of tumor burden. Int J Cancer 42:952–957.

116. Salup R, Back T, Wiltrout R (1987) Successful treatment of advanced murine renal cell cancer by bicompartimental adoptive chemoimmunotherapy. J Immunol 138:641–647.

117. Chabot G, Flaherty L, Valdivieso M, Baker L (1990) Alteration of dacarbazine pharmacokinetics after interleukin-2 administration in melanoma patients. Cancer Chemother Pharmacol 27:157–160.

118. Gandara D, Perez E, Denham A, Wiebe V, DeGregorio M (1989) Pharmacokinetics of cisplatin in patients receiving interleukin-2 containing treatment regimens. Cancer Chemother Pharmacol 24:135–136.

119. Braunschweiger P, Jones S, Johnson C, Furmanki P (1991) Potentiation of mitomycin-C and porfiromycin antitumor activity in solid tumor models by recombinant human interleukin-1a. Cancer Res 51:5454–5460.

120. Chang M-J, Yu W-D, Reyno L, Modzelewski R, Egorin M, Erkmen K, Vlock D, Furmanski P, Johnson C (1994) Potentiation by interleukin-1 alpha of cisplatin and carboplatin antitumor activity: schedule-dependent and pharmacokinetic effects in RIF-1 tumor model. Cancer Res 54:5380–5386.

121. Muhonen T, Hahka-Kemppinen M, Pakkala S, Pyrhonen S (1994) Decreasing CD4/CD8 ratio during prolonged four-drug chemotherapy plus interferon treatment for metastatic melanoma. J Immunother 15:67–73.

122. Eisenthal A, Skornick Y, Ron I, Zakuth V, Chaitchik S (1993) Phenotypic and functional profile

of peripheral blood mononuclear cells isolated from melanoma patients undergoing combined immunotherapy and chemotherapy. Cancer Immunol Immunother 37:367–372.

123. Isacson R, Kedar E, Barak V, Gazit Z, Yurim O, Kalichman I, Ben-Bassat H, Biran S, Schlesinger M, Franks C (1992) Chemo-immunotherapy in patients with metastatic melanoma using sequential treatment with dacarbazine and recombinant human interleukin-2: Evaluation of hematologic and immunologic parameters and correlation with clinical response. Immunol Lett 33:127–134.

124. Mouawad R, Ichen M, Rixe O, Benhammouda A, Vuillemin E, Weil M, Khayat D (1994) Study of IL-2 receptor expression after chemoimmunotherapy in patients treated for metastatic malignant melanoma. Clin Exp Immunol 97:342–346.

125. Buzaid A, Grimm E, Ali-Osman F, Ring S, Eton O, Papadopoulos N, Bedikian A, Plager C, Legha S, Benjamin R (1994) Mechanism of the anti-tumor effect of biochemotherapy in melanoma: Preliminary results. Melanoma Res 4:327–330.

126. Reed E, Parker R, Gill I, Bicher A, Dabholkar M, Vionnet J, Bostick-Bruton F, Tarone R, Muggia F (1993) Platinum-DNA adduct in leukocyte DNA of a cohort of 49 patients with 24 different types of malignancies. Cancer Res 53:3694–3699.

16. MULTIFUNCTIONAL MODULATORS OF DRUG RESISTANCE

JOHN R. MURREN, GERMANA RAPPA, AND YUNG-CHI CHENG

A variety of specific biochemical mechanisms have been identified that allow tumors to escape the cytotoxic effect of chemotherapy. Resistance may be induced to one particular class of cytotoxins, such as the resistance to methotrexate associated with a mutational change in the target enzyme dihydrofolate reductase. Resistance may also develop to a cross section of structurally unrelated classes of chemotherapy, such as the multidrug resistance (MDR) phenotype identified in the laboratories of Tsuruo [1], Biedler [2], and Ling [3].

Since clinical experience has shown that drug resistance, once acquired, usually extends to most classes of antineoplastic agents, the identification of the MDR phenotype sparked intense interest. Several biochemical changes have been described in MDR cells, including the overexpression of P-glycoprotein and other membrane transport proteins, changes in the glutathione detoxification system, and alterations in topoisomerase enzymes. Current approaches for modulating P-glycoprotein and these other mechanisms of MDR are explored in other chapters in this volume. Since multiple phenotypic changes may be present in MDR cells, an alternative strategy would be to develop modulators that interact with multiple different targets within the cell, or that modulate a target, such as protein kinase C, that is involved in the signal transduction of multiple cellular pathways. This approach may be of additional clinical relevance since regimens that combine different classes of chemotherapy drugs are used to treat virtually every malignant disease. In this chapter, "multifunctional" modulators of resistance that may potentiate are in the early stages of clinical development are reviewed.

PROTEIN KINASE C AS A TARGET

Protein kinase C (PKC) includes a family of cytoplasmic serine/threonine kinases that are a key element in the signal transduction pathway. Of the 11 isoforms identified to date, 10 are encoded by different genes. Most cells contain more than one isoform of PKC. The pattern of isoform expression is specific to both tissue type and to the stage of cellular differentiation, implying that different isozymes perform different functions in vivo [4]. When extracellular signals, such as mitogens, lectins, hormones, and growth factors, interact with their cell surface receptors, second messengers are generated that activate PKC and induce its translocation from the cytosol to plasma membranes (Figure 18–1). Activated PKC phosphorylates a variety of proteins that trigger many different cellular responses, including cell proliferation, differentiation, membrane transport, and gene expression [reviewed in 5,6]. Activation of PKC also leads to increased sensitivity of the enzyme to proteolytic degradation. Prolonged stimulation of PKC, therefore, may lead to downregulation and loss of activity. The efficiency of downregulation is isozyme, cell, and activator dependent, and this may represent another level of control of PKC function [4,7].

Protein kinase C participates in carcinogenesis in some tumors by playing a direct role in controlling cell growth, and in others it may interact with p21^{ras} and other oncogene products to promote transformation [4,8]. Protein kinase C serves as the main receptor for phorbol esters and other tumor promoters [9]. Several lines of evidence suggest that PKC also contributes to the MDR phenotype [reviewed in 10]. The PKC family is one of the kinases that phosphorylate P-glycoprotein and thereby promote the activity of this putative drug transporter [11,12]. Increased PKC activity and altered isoform expression and subcellular distribution have been observed in several MDR cell lines [13–16]. Cotransfection of mdr1 and PKCα induces a greater degree of resistance than transfection with mdr1 alone [17]. Modulation of mdr1 may be isoform specific, since similar experiments in which PKCγ was overexpressed failed to increase resistance [18]. In some settings PKC may also regulate mdr1 gene expression [19].

Protein kinase C has also been implicated in MDR that is not mediated by the overexpression of P-glycoprotein. For example, sensitive parental cells become transiently resistant to several different classes of chemotherapy by preincubation with phorbol esters and other stimulators of PKC [20–22]. Reduced intracellular drug accumulation was identified in cells made resistant in this fashion. Decreased accumulation and subcellular redistribution of doxorubicin was also observed in a cell line without detectable P-glycoprotein selected for resistance to the growth inhibitory effects of phorbol esters [23]. Furthermore, reduced drug accumulation associated with low levels of resistance has also been accomplished by transfection and overexpression of certain isoforms of PKC [24].

Exposure to chemotherapy can produce acute changes in PKC activity, either directly or indirectly via interaction with lipids in the plasma membrane [25,26]. Both increased and decreased PKC activity has been observed [26,27]. The PKC signal pathway may be involved in the cellular response to the DNA damage

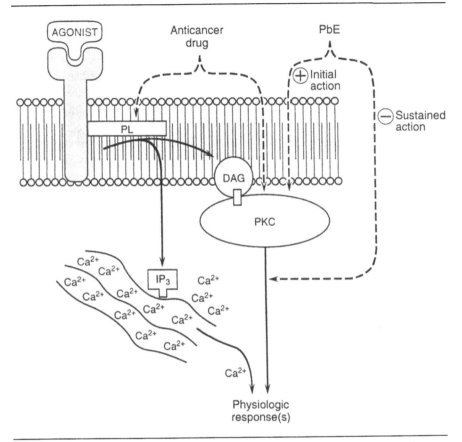

Figure 16–1. Model of protein kinase C (PKC)-mediated signal transduction. Extracellular agonists bind to specific cell membrane surface receptors and activate membrane phospholipases. These enzymes hydrolyze membrane phospholipids (PL) to inositol 1,4,5-trisphosphate (IP$_3$), 1,2-diacylglycerol (DAG), and other lipid mediators. DAG production leads to the translocation of PKC to the cell membrane, and IP$_3$ mobilizes Ca^{2+} stored in the endoplasmic reticulum. PKC catalyes the ATP-dependent phosphorylation of substrate proteins, which, together with the changes in Ca^{2+} flux, result in the physiologic response. Phorbol esters (PbE) activate PKC by direct binding and initially stimulate PKC activity. Anticancer drugs may act directly on PKC, or indirectly by inducing the production of membrane mediators. Sustained activation of PKC may lead to down regulation of enzyme activity. (Modified from Hait and Aftab [168], with permission.)

induced by chemotherapy. For example, Rubin and colleagues found that cisplatinum increased both PKC activity and c-*jun* expression in several human leukemia lines [28]. Inhibition of PKC abolished the effect of cisplatinum on c-*jun* expression. In other cell models, certain PKC isoforms have also been associated with control of c-*jun* expression [29]. Since activation of c-*jun* has been implicated in the process of apoptotic cell death, these observations suggest that modulation of PKC may enhance the activity of cytotoxic drugs.

In fact, modulators of PKC function, including both inhibitors and activators, enhance sensitivity of cells to chemotherapy under the appropriately defined conditions. Basu and coworkers have found that structurally and functionally dissimilar activators of PKC sensitize HeLa cells to cisplatinum [30–32]. They have also reported that pretreatment with epidermal growth factor (EGF) sensitized cells to cisplatin, possibly due to stimulation of PKC [33]. Mendelsohn's group has demonstrated that the combination of cisplatin and monoclonal antibodies that block the EGF receptor produce supra-additive cytotoxicity in vivo [34]. These observations may not be entirely contradictory, since PKC phosphorylates and can downregulate the EGF receptor [35].

In contrast, other groups have found that PKC inhibition potentiates cisplatinum cytotoxicity [36–38]. Inhibition of PKC has also been shown to sensitize cells to doxorubicin and to cytosine arabinoside (ara-C). For example, Grant and colleagues have reported that inhibition of PKC activity potentiates ara-C–related apoptosis, while stimulation of PKC resulted in less DNA fragmentation [39,40].

These conflicting results may be partially explained by the dose and schedule dependence of agents that modulate PKC. Within minutes of exposure to phorbol esters, for example, intracellular PKC activity is strongly activated, but if this exposure is continuously maintained for several hours, PKC enzyme activity may be completely abolished. The scheduling of PKC modulators with chemotherapy may also be important since PKC is involved in the control of cell cycle traversal. Sequencing may define whether cells undergo cycle arrest and DNA repair, or proceed toward apoptosis. Protein kinase C activity and isoform concentration varies in different cells and may contribute to the cell line specificity of modulator effect [41–44]. Furthermore, none of the modulators currently available are completely specific for PKC. Therefore, interaction with other important cellular kinases may also play a role in the divergent interactions of these modulators with cytotoxic agents. Despite the complexity of drug interaction with PKC, a broad array of PKC modulators are being actively investigated as potential anticancer agents. These include derivatives of indolocarbazole, sphingolipids, flavanoids, and lipophilic cations [reviewed in 45]. Strategies being pursued include the development of modulators that act indirectly, by enhancing tumor cell sensitivity to chemotherapy, and modulators that act directly, by inhibiting tumor cell proliferation or by inducing differentiation. Of most immediate clinical interest, the bryostatins have been shown to be potent modulators of PKC function.

BRYOSTATINS

Bryostatins are a family of over 13 compounds isolated from marine invertebrates of the phylum Bryozoa. They contain a multiringed macrolide lactone structure with varying side chains [46]. Bryostatin 1 (Figure 16–2) was identified in drug screening as having significant antineoplastic activity against a number of cancer cell lines, including melanoma, renal cell carcinoma, lymphoma, and leukemia [44,46–48]. Bryostatins were subsequently shown to bind to PKC and to modulate its activity [49–51]. Like phorbol esters, bryostatins initially enhance PKC activity but following prolonged exposure, downregulation of the enzyme may occur [32,52,53]. Perhaps through this interaction with PKC, bryostatin has been shown to induce

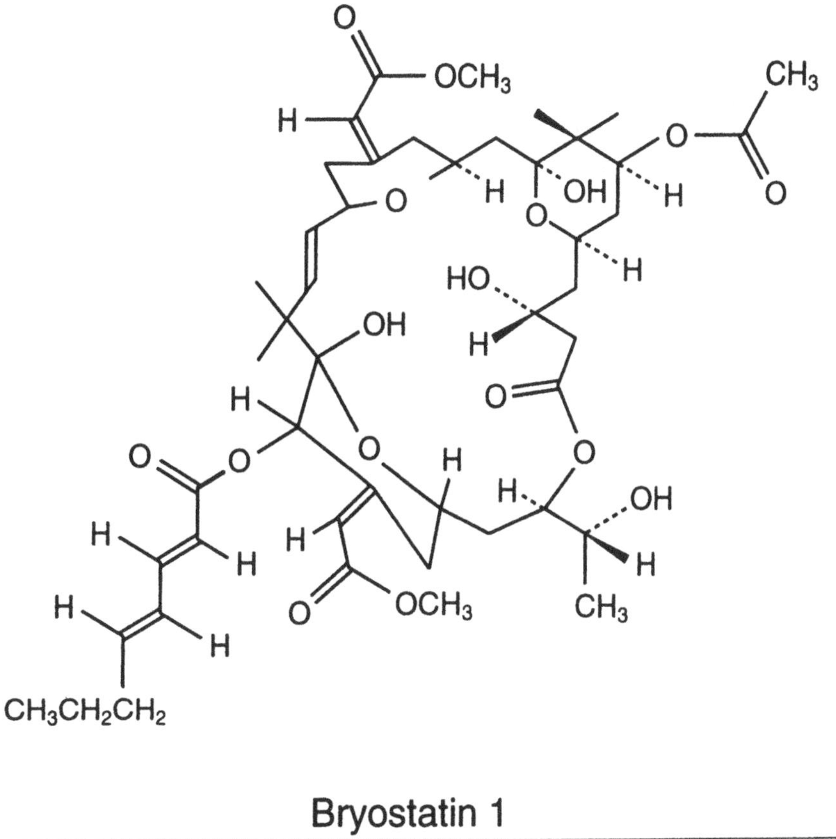

Bryostatin 1

Figure 16–2. Structure of bryostatin 1.

differentiation and to inhibit the growth of human leukemic and lymphoma cells [49,53–57]. These compounds have a number of other effects on the hematopoetic system, including induction of platelet aggregation and degranulation, stimulation of oxidative burst in neutrophils, proliferation of progenitor cells, and modulation of immune function and cytokine release [44,58,59].

Like other PKC modulators, bryostatins can sensitize cells to chemotherapy drugs, and this effect is cell line, dose, and schedule dependent. The mechanisms involved in this potentiation remain unclear and may vary depending on the cytotoxin. For example, activation of second messenger systems may enhance the intracellular accumulation of cisplatinum [30,33]. In combination with ara-C, bryostatin can increase drug phosphorylation to ara-CTP and the resultant drug-induced DNA fragmentation [39,40,60]. Since PKC has been shown to phosphorylate topoisomerases [61,62], bryostatins may also prove useful in combination with drugs directed against these enzymes [62].

To date, two dose-finding studies of bryostatin 1 have been completed in human beings [63,64]. In both studies, bryostatin was administered as a 1 hour infusion via a peripheral vein. Phlebitis related to the 60% ethanol vehicle could be partially ameliorated by aggressive concomitant saline hydration or by using a reformulated solvent. Flulike symptoms, consisting of fever, fatigue, headache, and rhinitis, occurred commonly, but the dose-limiting toxicities in both studies were myalgias and muscle tenderness. Although bryostatin induces electrical membrane instability in muscle cells in vitro [65], biochemical and electromyographic studies were generally not consistent with either ischemia or peripheral neuropathy as an etiology of this complaint. When given every 2 weeks, the recommended dose was defined as 35–50 μg/m² [64]. In another study, dose intensity could be maintained and treatment was better tolerated using a schedule of 25 μg/m²/wk for 3 of every 4 weeks [63]. Dose-related hematologic toxicity, including reductions in platelets, neutrophils, total lymphocyte counts, and hemoglobin concentration, were noted within 4 hours of drug infusion and resolved in most patients within 1 week of treatment. Despite anticipated activity predicted in preclinical studies, bryostatin did not affect coagulation or alter the proliferation of marrow progenitor cells in cloning assays. Observed effects on immunologic function included enhanced superoxide formation in primed neutrophils, a possible reduction in natural killer cell activity, induction of TNFα and IL-6 release, and in the presence of interleukin-2 (IL-2), increased production of lymphocyte activated killer cells and the expression of IL-2 receptors on lymphocytes [63,64,66]. Partial remissions were attained in two patients with previously treated malignant melanoma [63]. Additional clinical studies of bryostatin 1 evaluating alterative schedules of dosing are under way.

ALTERNATIVE APPROACHES: NOVOBIOCIN

Novobiocin (Figure 16–3) is a commercially available coumermycin antibiotic used to treat urinary tract and soft tissue infections [67,68]. Its antibacterial activity is based upon the inhibition of the enzyme DNA gyrase. Intracellular transport of novobiocin may be an important determinant of its antibacterial activity. For example, novobiocin is actively transported in *Staphylococcus aureus*, a microorganism that is very sensitive to the drug, but not in *Escherichia coli*, which is a resistant bacterium [69]. Novobiocin also inhibits the eukaryotic counterpart of the enzyme gyrase, topoisomerase II, but with an affinity that is three orders of magnitude lower than for gyrase. Rather than stabilize the covalently bound reaction intermediate between topoisomerase II and DNA, in a manner analogous to that of many other topoisomerase II inhibitors that have anticancer activity, novobiocin competitively inhibits the binding of ATP to topoisomerase II and is devoid of direct antineoplastic activity [70–72]. Other effects of novobiocin that have been reported in eukaryotes in vitro include a depletion of intracellular ATP, a change in the structure of mitochondria, the precipitation of intracellular histones, and inhibition of the transcription of RNA polymerase III. The concentrations of novobiocin required to produce these effects are generally higher than those needed to inhibit topoisomerase II [73–75]. In addition, novobiocin has also been shown to induce differentiation in leukemic and melanoma cell lines [76–79].

Eder et al. reported that novobiocin markedly increased the number of DNA interstrand crosslinks induced by alkylating agents in tumor cells in vitro, thereby

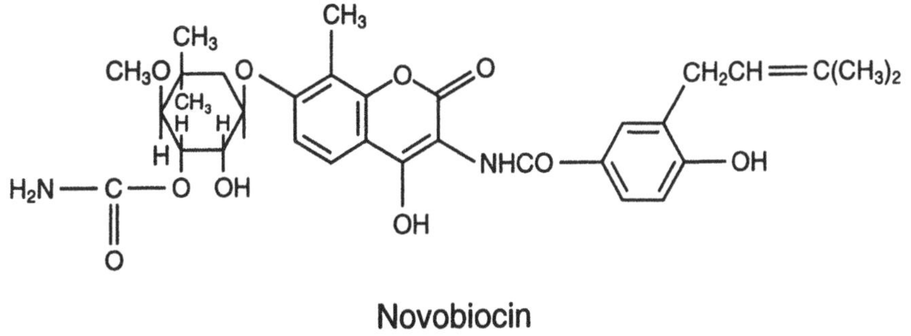

Novobiocin

Figure 16–3. Structure of novobiocin.

enhancing the cytotoxic activity of the alkylating agents [80]. It was subsequently shown that novobiocin in combination with cyclophosphamide, carmustine, or cisplatin reduced the growth of a murine fibrosarcoma in vivo, enhancing the therapeutic index [81]. Synergistic cytotoxicity was schedule dependent, in that novobiocin had to be given before, during, and after treatment with the alkylating agent. Although no clear evidence exists in the current literature that topoisomerase II is involved in the repair of alkylator-induced DNA damage, the modulatory activity of novobiocin was attributed to a delay of the repair of DNA interstrand crosslinks caused by inhibition of topoisomerase II [80,81]. Based upon these findings, clinical trials have been launched to evaluate the effects of novobiocin in combination with alkylating agents. For example, Eder and colleagues administered cyclophosphamide at a dose of 750 mg/m², with escalating doses of oral novobiocin [82]. Dose-limiting toxicity due to nausea and vomiting was seen at 6 g/day of novobiocin. Partial responses were observed in 2 of 30 evaluable patients. No correlation was observed between the dose of novobiocin and the serum blood levels that were obtained with this drug. However, at daily doses of novobiocin of 4 g or more, 18 of 19 patients achieved serum concentrations that were ≥100 µg/ ml, concentrations that are sufficient to produce synergistic cytotoxicity in combination with alkylating drugs in vitro [82].

A subsequent study confirmed that novobiocin in doses up to 4 g/day by mouth can be safely given in combination with relatively high doses of cyclophosphamide (3–6 g/m² over 4 days) or of thiotepa (up to 800 mg/m²) [83]. The most prominent and dose-limiting toxicity in this trial was gastrointestinal. All of the patients treated with the highest dose level of novobiocin (5 g/day) developed significant mucositis, nausea, and vomiting. Plasma concentrations of novobiocin equivalent to the doses that are active in laboratory systems were reached. In another study, cisplatin (100 mg/m² on days 1 and 8) was combined with novobiocin (1 g every 12 hours for 6 doses, beginning 2 days before each dose of cisplatin) [84]. The overall response and toxicity of this combination were comparable with those of other trials of high-dose cisplatin in non–small cell lung cancer. Plasma levels of novobiocin were obtained in three patients and were approximately 50% of the optimal concentration that augments the activity of cytotoxic drugs in vitro.

In all three of these clinical trials, only total levels of novobiocin were measured. Since novobiocin is highly bound to serum proteins, the concentration of free novobiocin achievable in human serum may be lower than that required for the modulatory activity observed in tissue culture. If in ongoing clinical trials this proves to be the case, potential options include testing an intravenous formulation of novobiocin, the development of more potent analogs, or administration of novobiocin in combination with other modulating agents. For example, preclinical data show that combining novobiocin with topotecan results in an even greater augmentation of cyclophosphamide cytotoxicity than when either agent is used alone with the alkylator, suggesting that the combination of novobiocin with other inhibitors of topoisomerase might be the optimal use of novobiocin and other agents that increase the activity of alkylating agents clinically [85].

Besides being a modulator of alkylating agents, novobiocin has recently been demonstrated to produce supra-additive cytotoxicity and to increase the formation of drug-stabilized topoisomerase II-DNA covalent complexes when combined with VP-16 or VM-26 [86,87]. These actions were observed after short-term exposure (1 hour) of cells to concentrations of novobiocin that do not alter topoisomerase II activity, do not initiate differentiation, and do not cause a decrease in intracellular ATP. Novobiocin did not potentiate the cytotoxic activity of other topoisomerase II inhibitors, such as doxorubicin and m-AMSA, nor did it affect the quantity of covalent complexes of topoisomerase II and DNA produced by VP-16 in isolated nuclei, suggesting that the potentiation of the activity of the epipodophyllotoxins by novobiocin was not due to its direct interaction with the nuclear topoisomerase II enzyme [86].

Lorico et al. [88] showed that the mechanism involved in producing supra-additive cytotoxicity was inhibition of VP-16 efflux by novobiocin, which in turn resulted in an increase in the formation of VP-16–stabilized topoisomerase II–DNA covalent complexes and in cytotoxicity (Figure 16–4). That the membrane transporter for VP-16 that is inhibited by novobiocin is distinct from P-glycoprotein is supported by the observation that novobiocin potentiates the cytotoxic activity of VP-16 in several cell lines that did not express P-glycoprotein [87]. Furthermore, novobiocin itself is a poor substrate for the P-glycoprotein, as demonstrated by the findings that the IC_{50} value for novobiocin is the same for both parental L1210 and resistant L1210/VMDRC0.06 cells, the latter having been transfected with the human *mdr*1 gene and overexpressing P-glycoprotein [87,89]. Furthermore, analogous preliminary data suggest that the transporter inhibited by novobiocin is distinct from the multidrug associated protein (MRP) recently described by Cole and colleagues [90]. Novobiocin has also been reported to synergistically enhance the sensitivity of two different non–P-glycoprotein–expressing MDR cell lines to VP-16 and correspondingly to increase the intracellular accumulation of VP-16 and the VP-16–induced formation of topoisomerase II–DNA covalent complexes.

These findings suggest that the synergistic antineoplastic activity that occurs between novobiocin and VP-16 is due to an effect on the steady-state intracellular concentration of VP-16, resulting in an increase in the amount of VP-16–induced

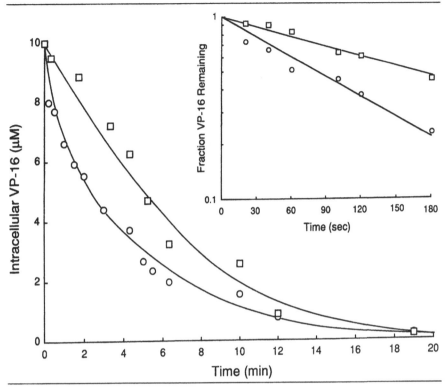

Figure 16–4. Effects of novobiocin on VP-16 efflux in WEHI-3B D⁺ cells. Cells were incubated for 60 minutes to achieve the same intracellular level of VP-16 by incubation with 10 μM ³H-VP-16 alone (○) or 4.5 μM ³H-VP-16 plus 250 μM novobiocin (□). Cells were washed free of extracellular drugs by three washings at 4°C, intracellular radioactivity was measured, and the cells were resuspended in VP-16–free medium at 37°C. Novobiocin-treated cells were again exposed to 250 μM novobiocin. Over the next 20 minutes, the intracellular radioactivity was measured. *Inset:* Log of the fraction of exchangeable VP-16 remaining in cells as a function of time after resuspension in Vp-16–free medium in the absence (○) or the presence of 250 μM novobiocin (□). Points represent the mean of two to four independent determinations. (Reprinted with permission from Lorico et al. [88].)

topoisomerase II-DNA covalent complexes. Although the effects of novobiocin on the cellular pharmacology of VP-16 are analogous to those of "classic" P-glycoprotein inhibitors, such as verapamil and cyclosporin A, these modulatory agents do not appear to function by the same mechanism [91,92]. The classic P-glycoprotein inhibitors are generally more effective in reversing multidrug resistance in cells that express high levels of the *mdr*1 gene and manifest the "classic" MDR phenotype [91–95], while novobiocin is ineffective in cells expressing high levels of P-glycoprotein [87]. Also, since novobiocin can enhance the sensitivity of a number of cell lines that are sensitive to VP-16 and have minimal or no detectable expression of the *mdr*1 gene (Table 16–1), it offers the potential of producing a much broader effect on tumor response. Furthermore, treatment with a drug regimen that includes both novobiocin and an inhibitor of P-gp may be useful against heterogenous tumors containing cell populations with both P-gp and other mechanisms of resistance.

Our recent studies evaluating tumor cell samples freshly obtained from patients with leukemia or malignant ascites due to ovarian cancer suggest that this yet unidentified novobiocin-inhibitable VP-16 transporter is of clinical relevance. In more than 50% of the tumors tested thus far, novobiocin, in a range from 150–1,000 μM, increased the intracellular accumulation of VP-16 up to 350% by inhibiting drug efflux [96]. Novobiocin was a more effective modulator of VP-16 than either verapamil or cyclosporin A, and its activity was not dependent on the expression of the *mdr*1 or MRP genes, as measured by a polymerase chain reaction method. In fact, the expression of the *mdr*1 or MRP genes was variable among both novobiocin-responsive and non-responsive tumor cell populations [96]. Recently, we initiated a dose-finding clinical trial of novobiocin and VP-16. Based on preclinical data [86], which show that the maximum potentiation of VP-16 occurred when tumor cells were exposed to the drugs simultaneously, patients are being treated with novobiocin 30 minutes before VP-16 on days 1, 3, and 5 for each cycle of chemotherapy. This intermittent exposure to novobiocin is also designed to achieve high peak plasma concentrations, in an attempt to overcome the problem of extensive protein binding of novobiocin in serum. The primary toxicity observed thus far has been myelosuppression related to the VP-16 [96]. Significant nausea has not occurred in any patient, even at the current dose of 7.0 g of novobiocin per day. Higher doses of novobiocin may be tolerated than in previous trials because of the current availability of anti-serotoninergic antiemetics.

DIPYRIDAMOLE ANALOGS

Dipyridamole is clinically available as a vasodilator and antiplatelet agent. The biochemical activities of dipyridamole include inhibition of cyclic AMP phosphodiesterase and membrane transport of nucleosides. Due to its activity in blocking nucleoside transport by facilitated diffusion, dipyridamole has been evaluated as a modulator of antimetabolites such as acivicin, N-phosphonoacetyl-L-aspartate, methotrexate, and 5-fluorouracil (5-FU) [97–100].

Dipyridamole is capable of enhancing the effects of 5-FU in vitro and in vivo in a dose- and time-dependent manner [reviewed in 101]. This modulation is achieved in several ways. By inhibiting the transport of pyrimidine nucleosides, dipyridamole prevents the efflux of the 5-FU metabolites fluorodeoxyuridine and fluorouridine from the cell. These metabolites are subsequently phosphorylated and can then be incorporated into nucleic acids. By blocking the uptake of preformed nucleosides, such as thymidine, dipyridamole also inhibits repletion of critical nucleotides from the extracellular environment. This may enhance the therapeutic index since tumor cells may rely more heavily on this nucleoside salvage pathway than does normal tissue [102]. Coupled with the inhibition of thymidylate synthetase resulting from the increased formation of fluorodeoxyuridine monophosphate [103], there results a depletion of deoxythymidine triphosphate available for the formation of DNA. Dipyridamole has no effect on the cellular uptake of 5-FU itself because this compound is a pyrimidine base.

Table 16-1. Modulation of VP-16 cytotoxicity by Novobiocin in Sensitive and Drug Resistant Cell Lines

Cell line	Relative degree of VP-16 resistance	Mechanism of VP-16 resistance	Fold increase in VP-16 cytotoxicity by 500 μM NOVO[a]	Fold increase in VP-16 accumulation by 500 μM NOVO[b]	Fold increase in VP-16 induced DPC by 500 μM NOVO[c]
WEHI-3B/S	1		3.3	4.0	3.0
WEHI-3B/NOVO	11	Non-Pgp efflux	6.2	6.5	4.0
A 549	1		7.1	4.5	3.5
A 549(VP)28	7.5	Low topo II	5.0	3.0	5.0
L 1210	1		2.0	2.5	3.2
L 1210/VMDRC0.06	21.7	Pgp efflux	1.2	0.8	0.7
HCT 116	1		2.5	2.8	2.0
HCT 116(VM)34	5	Pgp efflux	0.8	1.4	1.3

[a] Decrease in surviving fraction after simultaneous exposure for 1 hour to VP-16 and 500 μM novobiocin as compared with the effect of VP-16 alone. Concentrations of VP-16 producing approximately 50% inhibition of colony formation were used.

[b] Cells were exposed for 30 minutes to 4 μM [³H]-VP-16 (16 μM for L1210/VMDRC0.06 cells) in the absence or presence of 500 μM novobiocin and intracellular radioactivity was measured.

[c] Cells were exposed for 60 minutes to concentrations of VP-16 (ranging from 3 to 50 μM), which induced a similar number of DNA–protein crosslinks (DPC) in both parental and resistant cell lines in the presence or absence of 500 μM novobiocin. The formation of DPC was measured by the potassium-sodium dodecyl sulfate precipitation assay.

The combination of dipyridamole and fluorouracil has been evaluated in several early clinical trials [100,104–107]. A number of different schedules of both the oral and parenteral forms of dipyridamole have been investigated in these studies. When given orally in divided doses, the maximal tolerated dose was 175 mg/m² every 6 hours (700 mg/m²/day), which produced a mean peak plasma concentration of total dipyridamole of 16 µM. Overall, the mean trough concentration was 60% of the mean peak concentration, suggesting that relatively constant concentrations of dipyridamole were available during the 5 days of chemotherapy [106]. If given as a continuous intravenous infusion for 72 hours, the mean concentrations of total dipyridamole attained were slightly higher than in most studies that used an oral formulation [97,100]. The dose-limiting toxicities were stomatitis and other gastrointestinal complaints, headaches, and moderate to severe constitutional symptoms [100,105–107]. When given intravenously, a central venous catheter was necessary because of thrombophlebitis. Comparing paired courses, in which 5-FU was delivered alone for one cycle and then given at the same dose with dipyridamole, there was no significant increase in myelosuppression or stomatitis [100]. A similar absence of increased toxicity was observed in studies that evaluated 5-FU and leucovorin in combination with dipyridamole [105,106]. This lack of increased toxicity may have been related to an alteration in the pharmacokinetics of 5-FU. The total body clearance of 5-FU was increased, resulting in a significantly lower mean steady-state plasma concentration of 5-FU. Since more than 99% of dipyridamole is protein bound, the free plasma drug concentrations ranged from 25 nM to 50 nM. This approached the minimal concentration of 50 nM required in cell culture to modulate of 5-FU toxicity, but was significantly less than the optimal potentiating concentration of 500 nM [108]. As single-arm, dose-finding studies, these trials did not define the impact of dipyridamole modulation on the clinical efficacy of 5-FU.

In addition to antimetabolites such as 5-FU, dipyridamole has been shown to modulate a number of other chemotherapy drugs, including *Vinca* alkaloids, etoposide, doxorubin, and cisplatinum. Enhanced cytotoxicity has been observed in both sensitive and drug-selected resistant cell lines. The mechanism by which dipyridamole potentiates these drugs remains incompletely defined. Inhibition of nucleoside uptake does not appear to be the mechanism, since other nucleoside transport inhibitors do not potentiate these drugs [109,110]. Dipyridamole increased the steady-state intracellular concentrations of these drugs between 1.5- and 3.7-fold [111–115]. In some cases, enhanced drug accumulation could be due to modulation of MDR. Dipyridamole contains a number of the structural features characteristic of MDR modulators, including lipid solubility at physiologic pH, two planar rings, and two tertiary amines [116]. Dipyridamole concentrations of at least 10 µM, however, are required in cell culture to inhibit doxorubicin efflux in MDR cells [113,117].

Since this concentration range cannot be approached with the systemic administration of dipyridamole, two alternative strategies have been explored. Howell's group has exploited the tight protein binding of dipyridamole by administering this drug via an intraperitoneal route. They have conducted two clinical studies in which the intraperitoneal administration of dipyridamole has been explored in combination

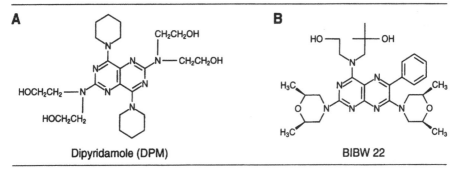

Figure 16–5. Structure of dipyridamole (*A*) and BIBW22 (*B*).

with methotrexate and with etoposide [104,118]. In both studies, mean intraperitoneal concentrations of free dipyridamole sufficient to modulate drug activity were achieved, while systemic concentrations remained insignificant. For example, when dipyridamole and etoposide were administered concurrently by 72 hour continuous infusion at doses of $24\,mg/m^2/day$ and $175\,mg/m^2/day$ respectively, the mean concentration of unbound dipyridamole in the peritoneal fluid was $20\,\mu M$, compared with a concentration of $0.2\,\mu M$ in the systemic circulation. The observed antitumor activity was modest (4 of 34 patients in the two studies), and there were no major responses.

Given the limitations of intraperitoneal therapy, an alternative approach would be to identify more effect analogs of the parent compound. Structure–activity studies by Ramu and Ramu predicted that activity of dipyridamole analogs depended on the presence of three tertiary amine groups and on the presence of a substituent with a partial electronegative charge [119]. Our screen of a group of dipyridamole derivatives has identified one such lead compound, BIBW22, a phenylpteridine analog that is a more potent modulator than dipyridamole and also fulfills these structural requirements (Figure 16–5). In the P-glycoprotein–overexpressing MDR cell line KBV20C, BIBW22 enhanced vincristine cytotoxicity at a concentration of $0.1\,\mu M$ and restored sensitivity comparable with the parental line at $0.3\,\mu M$ (Figure 16–6). The equivalent modulating concentrations of dipyridamole in this system were 10 times higher [120]. Drug-accumulation studies demonstrated that BIBW22 was 100-fold more effective than dipyridamole in blocking P-glycoprotein–mediated efflux. BIBW22, however, does not have significant activity in modulating non–P-glycoprotein–mediated multidrug resistance associated with the overexpression of the MRP protein [90,121].

Compared with dipyridamole, BIBW22 was sevenfold more effective in inhibiting nucleoside transport (Figure 16–7). Transport of ribonucleosides is more effectively blocked than are deoxyribonucleotides [122]. Photoaffinity labelling experiments have demonstrated that BIBW22 binds both to P-glycoprotein and to a 55 kDa plasma membrane protein, which may also be the receptor for other nucleoside transport inhibitors [120,123]. Although BIBW22 is less highly protein

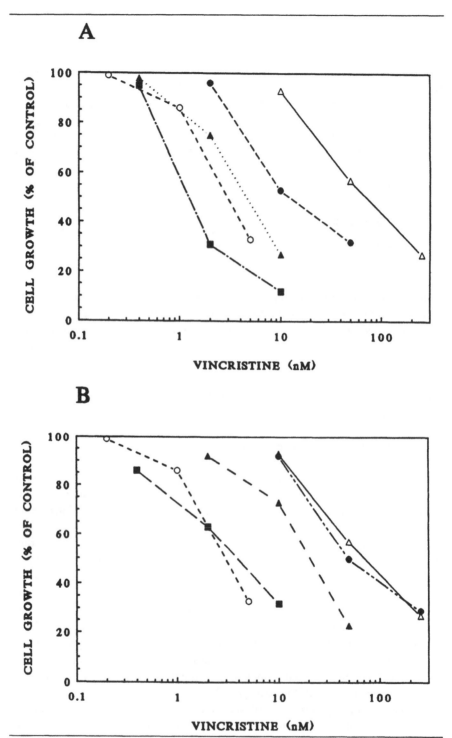

Figure 16–6. Modulating activity of dipyridamole and BIBW22 toward KB cell lines treated with vincristine. KBV20C cells were exposed to 0–250 nM vincristine for 72 hours in the absence (△) or presence (closed symbols) of modulator. Parental KB cells are shown in open symbols (o) for comparison. Dipyridamole (*A*) concentrations used were 0.3 (●), 1.0 (▲), and 3 (■) μM. BIBW22 (*B*) concentrations used were 0.1 (●), 0.3 (▲), and 1 (■) μM. (Reprinted with permission from Chen et al. [120].)

bound than dipyridamole, protein binding significantly affect the observed activity. In cell culture, the presence of 100% human serum reduces the modulation of both MDR activity and nucleoside transport by 150-fold and 5-fold, respectively [122]. However, BIBW22 has less potent cardiovascular effects than dipyridamole, suggesting that higher systemic concentrations may be tolerated. Moreover, BIBW22 has been shown to increase vincristine accumulation within MDR tumors in vivo, and in this mouse xenograft model it also significantly retarded tumor growth [124,125].

BIBW22 is as potent as dipyridamole as an antiplatelet agent, and this property may in fact be advantageous to its role in anticancer therapy. Platelet–tumor cell interactions have been implicated in the development of blood-borne metastases. Within the circulation platelets may physically shield cells within tumor emboli from the immune system, and in the capillary beds of target organs platelet-derived permeability factors and growth factors may enhance tumor cell extravasation and survival [126]. In a B16 melanoma model, in which treatment was started 24 hours after the infusion of tumor cells, the addition of a nontoxic dose of dypyridamole to

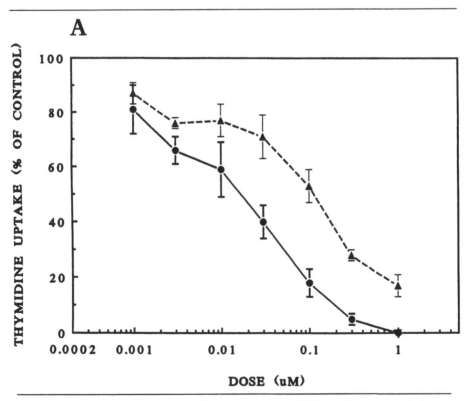

Figure 16–7. A: Modulating activity of BIBW22 on transport of [^{14}C]thymidine by KB cells. KB cells were incubated with 1 μM [^{14}C]thymidine in the absence or presence of either dipyridamole (▲) or BIBW22 (●) at the indicated concentrations for 30 seconds, and the incorporated radioactivity was determined. Points, indicate the mean of three determinations and bars the standard deviation.

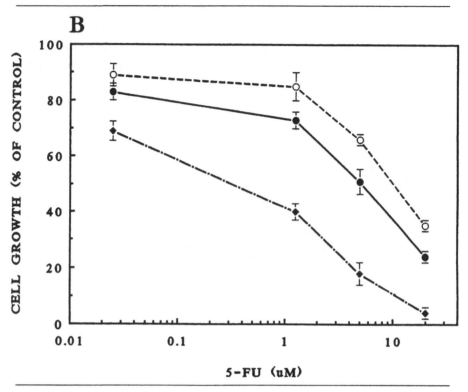

Figure 16–7. B: Modulating activity of BIBW22 on the sensitivity of KB cells to 5-fluorouracil (5-FU). KB cells were exposed to 0–20 µM 5-FU for 72 hours in the absence (O) or presence of either 1 µM dipyridamole (O) or 1 µM BIBW22 (◆). Points indicate the mean of three determinations and bars the standard deviation. (Reprinted with permission from Chen et al. [120].)

doxorubicin significantly reduced the number of lung metastases compared with doxorubicin alone at all dose levels tested [127]. Although enhanced cytotoxic activity, rather than impairment of metastatic potential, may have contributed to the result in this study, Tzanakakis and colleagues have reported that the combination of dipyridamole and the cAMP phosphodiesterase inhibitor RA-233 dramatically impaired platelet aggregation and resulted in a significant reduction ($p < 0.001$) in the development of hepatic metastases when human pancreatic carcinoma cells were injected into nude mice [128]. Neither dipyridamole nor RA-233 reduced the number of metastases when given alone. Further exploration of BIBW22 should be considered in a malignancy such as breast cancer, a disease in which resistance to both antimetabolites and to drugs transported by P-glycoprotein is clinically relevant.

LONIDAMINE

Lonidamine and related indazole-carboxylic acid derivatives were identified in early toxicology studies as possessing significant antispermatogenesis activity (Figure 16–8). Since spermatogenesis provides a model for evaluating drugs that impair cellular differentiation, Floridi and colleagues studied the biochemical activity of

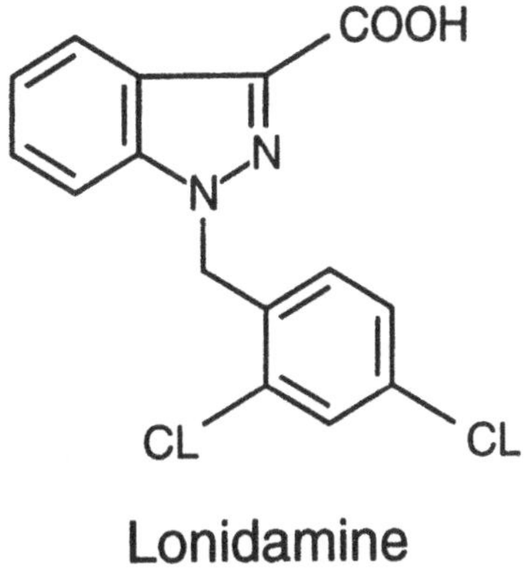

Lonidamine

Figure 16-8. Structure of lonidamine 1-[2,4-dichlorophenyl) methyl]-1H-indazole-3-carboxylic acid.

lonidamine in tumor cells [129,130]. They found that lonidamine reduced oxygen consumption and preferentially inhibited anaerobic and aerobic glycolysis in tumor cells. This selective effect on energy metabolism may be related to inhibition of mitochondrial bound hexokinase, an enzyme that is typically present on outer mitochondrial membrane of malignant but not normal differentiated cells [129,130]. Alternatively, impaired energy metabolism may be a consequence of structural damage to the mitochondrial membrane induced by lonidamine [131,132].

In cell culture systems, lonidamine has direct antiproliferative effects, but typically relatively high drug concentrations are required. In contrast, much lower concentrations ($\leq 50\,\mu g/ml$) of lonidamine are effective in potentiating a number of anticancer therapies, including hyperthermia, x-irradiation, and cytotoxins, such as alkylators, platinum agents, and anthracyclines. For example, Teicher and coworkers showed that lonidamine could enhance the cytotoxicity by up to 100-fold in a parental MCF-7 human breast cancer cell line and could reverse the 5-fold resistance in a cisplatin-selected cell line [133]. This potentiation of cytotoxicity is a function of dosage, time, and sequence of drug administration. In general, lonidamine treatment following the anticancer therapy, with or without additional lonidamine treatment before the anticancer therapy, is necessary for maximal cytotoxicity [134–137]. This schedule dependence is consistent with the hypothesis that lonidamine enhances cytotoxicity by inhibiting the energy-dependent repair of potentially lethal DNA damage. In addition, alterations in amino acid and cytotoxin uptake have been identified in alkylator-resistant cell lines, suggesting that lonidamine's effect on plasma membranes may also directly modulate drug accumulation. Animal studies confirmed the potentiating activity of lonidamine and indicated that full doses of the cytotoxin could be administered with no increase in host toxicity [85,133,137].

Drug efflux mediated by the MDR phenotype has also been shown to be energy dependent, and resistant cells have higher rates of glycolysis than sensitive cells [138]. Thus, lonidamine has been evaluated as a modulator of this form of drug resistance. In the MCF-7 ADR subline, which is 300-fold resistant to doxorubicin, Citro and colleagues showed that nontoxic concentrations of lonidamine completely reversed the MDR phenotype and increased cytotoxicity by more than two logs. Lonidamine significantly increased the intracellular doxorubicin content in the resistant cells but had no such effect on the parental cell line [139].

Lonidamine entered clinical trials over 10 years ago and has been evaluated both alone and as a modulator of other anticancer therapies. Several different dosage schedules have been tested, and it remains uncertain whether an optimal schedule has been defined. Lonidamine has a unique toxicity profile compared with traditional cytotoxins. There have been no reports of significant myelosuppression, stomatitis, or cardiopulmonary toxicities, even at the highest dosages tested. Hepatic and renal side effects are extremely rare. The dose-limiting toxicity consists of myalgias, which occurs in most patients treated at doses exceeding 300 mg daily. Treatment with corticosteroids and/or muscle relaxants has met with mixed success [140]. The cause of the myalgias is unclear but may be related to accumulation of lactate within myocytes. Other prominent toxicities unique to lonidamine are testicular pain, which occurs in about half of the males, and ototoxicity, which is frequently described as an alteration in pitch perception [141]. These toxicities are reversible with discontinuation or dose reduction of lonidamine. When given in combination with other anticancer therapies, there is no increase in the side effects associated with the chemotherapy or radiation.

As a single agent, lonidamine has very modest activity. Studies in patients with advanced breast cancer reported response rates of 16% or less, and in other solid tumors there was even less activity [140,142–145]. As a modulator, lonidamine has been most intensively studied in breast cancer. Four randomized trials have been conducted in Italy [146–151]. (Table 16–2). In the largest study, patients were randomized to FAC (5-fluorouracil, doxorubicin, and cyclophosphamide) with or without lonidamine [148,149]. After three cycles of treatment, patients were evaluated, and those responding or with stable disease were re-randomized to continue

Table 16–2. Randomized trials evaluating lonidamine in metastatic breast cancer

Treatment arms	Evaluable pts (n)	Overall resp (%)	Complete resp (%)	Median TTP (months)	Ref.
FAC	124	47	5	6	Calabresi et al. [148,149]
+LND	116	62[a]	18	9[a]	
Epi	98	40	10	NR	Dogliotti et al. [146,147]
+LND	95	59[a]	15	NR	
CNF	96	39	10	5	Lorusso et al. [150]
+LND	94	48	18	8[b]	
EM/FEC	70	61	14	9	Pacini et al. [151]
+LND	63	77	22	11	

[a] p < 0.01.
[b] p < 0.05.
pts = patients; resp = response; TTP = time to progression; FAC = 5-fluorouracil, doxorubicin, cyclophosphamide; LND = lonidamine; Epi = epirubicin; CNF = cyclophosphamide, mitoxantrone, 5-fluorouracil; EM = epirubicin, mitomycin C; FEC = 5-fluorouracil, epirubicin, cyclophosphamide.

chemotherapy until disease progression, or to continue chemotherapy until best response, defined as stability on two consecutive assessments of the extent of disease. The overall response rate and median time to progression were significantly better in the group of patients treated with lonidamine. In addition, there were more complete responders among patients treated with the regimen including this modulator (18% vs. 5%). Although there was no differences in survival between the two treatment arms, regression modeling of patient subsets identified a significant advantage from lonidamine treatment in postmenopausal women, in whom median survival was increased from 15 to 19 months (p < 0.02). Significantly higher response rates [146,147] and time to disease progression [150] in the treatment arms receiving lonidamine have been reported in some of the other randomized trials. The results of these studies are too preliminary to make any assessment regarding survival. Myalgias, epigastric pain, and fatigue were the most prominent side effects associated with chronic lonidamine administration.

In patients with metastatic breast cancer, lonidamine has also been evaluated as maintainence therapy following discontinuation of chemotherapy. Preliminary results of a randomized multi-institutional trial identified a longer median progression-free survival (10 vs. 6 months, p = 0.06) in patients treated with lonidamine compared with patients who received no further treatment [152].

Lonidamine has been evaluated as a modulator of chemotherapy in several other solid tumors, particularly cancers of the lung, ovary, and head and neck. A large randomized trial found no benefit when lonidamine was added to MACC (methotrexate, doxorubicin, cyclophosphamide, and lomustine) chemotherapy in patients with non–small cell lung cancer [153]. Results in ovarian cancer appear more promising. Ex vivo studies of primary cultures of human ovarian cancers identified synergy (in 4 tumors) or additivity (in 7 tumors) between lonidamine and cisplatinum in the 11 tumors evaluated [154]. Two small clinical trials have evaluated lonidamine modulation in patients with disease previously resistant to platinum compounds [155,156]. The response rates were 33% and 25% in combination with epirubicin and cisplatinum, respectively.

Encouraging results have also been observed in head and neck cancer. Colella and coworkers randomized 89 patients to methotrexate with or without lonidamine [157]. Despite a study design that precluded statistical comparison, the two groups appeared to be balanced. The response rate (26% vs. 18%), complete response rate (11% vs. 0%), and 1 year survival (37% vs. 18%) were better in the group of patients who received lonidamine. In a randomized trial, Magno and colleagues treated patients with locally advanced disease with hyperfractionated radiation to 60–66 Gy in combination with lonidamine or placebo. The complete remission rate was similar between the two arms, but subsequent relapse was significantly reduced in the complete responders who received lonidamine [158]. At 5 years, both overall disease-free survival (40% vs. 19%, p = 0.03) and locoregional control (43% vs. 25%, p = 0.06) were improved. Lonidamine did not increase either acute or late toxicities of the radiation, nor did it contribute to treatment delays. No survival advantage, however, was detected in this study.

Lonidamine is also being evaluated as a radiosensitizer in other diseases. A preliminary report suggested that lonidamine enhanced the activity of radiation in locally advanced non–small cell lung cancer, but this observation was not confirmed in a large multi-institutional randomized study [159,160]. Although the progression-free and overall survival in this randomized trial were similar, analysis of local control identified a possible long-term benefit for patients treated with lonidamine. The activity of lonidamine as a radiosensitizing agent is also being investigated in patients with primary and metastatic brain tumors [161,162]. The results of these investigations are thus far inconclusive.

In virtually all of the clinical trials described earlier, lonidamine was given at a dose of 300–600 mg daily in divided doses. Pharmacokinetic studies have shown that this schedule produces peak serum concentrations of 6–35 µg/ml that are typically attained within 1–4 hours after ingestion of the drug [141,163–166]. Although modulating activity is observed in experimental systems at these concentrations, most data suggest that optimal potentiation occurs when cells that have been treated with an alkylator are exposed to lonidamine for relatively brief periods of time (6–24 hours) at much higher concentrations (50–100 µg/ml). When given as a single dose of 900 mg, lonidamine was well tolerated in a small trial [167]. Future studies should define the maximum tolerated dose when lonidamine is given for a short duration with intensive supportive care following chemotherapy.

SUMMARY

The recent identification of several biochemical mechanisms contributing to multidrug resistance has led to clinical strategies designed to circumvent these specific causes. Examples include chemotherapy regimens that contain modulators that competitively inhibit drug efflux caused by P-glycoprotein, and regimens that include modulators designed to inhibit drug detoxification by depleting intracellular glutathione. In the clinical trials investigating these approaches, success in reversing established drug resistance has so far been modest and may be confined to select groups of patients. Further evaluation of these approaches awaits the completion of ongoing randomized trials in specific patient populations and the testing of new, more potent modulators directed against these mechanisms of resistance.

The available data, however, suggest that in many clinical settings MDR is due to the presence of multiple different mechanisms of drug resistance rather than to a solitary mechanism, such as the overexpression of P-glycoprotein, producing resistance to multiple different types of drugs. For patients with multiple mechanisms of resistance, alternative approaches will be necessary. One strategy is to develop modulators that enhance the activity of different classes of chemotherapy via two or more different mechanisms. Examples of this approach include analogs of novobiocin, which inhibit both drug transport and topoisomerase II, and dipyridamole derivatives, which block both nucleoside uptake and P-glycoprotein–mediated drug efflux.

Alternatively, differences between normal and neoplastic cells in signal transduction and energy metabolism could be exploited via modulators of PKC and other second messenger pathways, and by agents such as lonidamine. Optimal exploitation of these signal transduction pathways depends on a more complete understanding of these complex systems and may have implications beyond pure modulation of anticancer therapies. For example, signal transduction plays a critical role in the immune response, and modulation of PKC and similar pathways may be a means of enhancing tumor immunity. Signal transduction could potentially be manipulated to induce cells to differentiate or to proceed into apoptosis. In addition, dietary substances such as antioxidants and phorbol-like compounds can also modulate signal transduction pathways and thus may play a role both in carcinogenesis and in the modulation of established cancers. The clinical development of new classes of drugs, such as the bryostatins, that modulate PKC provides an opportunity to explore these avenues, in addition to providing a new means of modulating anticancer therapy. Bryostatins and other "multifunctional modulators," therefore, provide a promising new appoach to addressing drug resistance, the most pressing problem in cancer chemotherapy.

ACKNOWLEDGMENTS

This work was supported in part by grants from the Public Health Service, National Cancer Institute (CA 16359-20, CA 08341-26, CA-44358), and the Patrick and Catherine Weldon Donaghue Medical Research Foundation. Dr. Murren is a recipient of an American Society of Clinical Oncology Clinical Investigator Career Development Award.

REFERENCES

1. Tsuruo T (1989) Circumvention of drug resistance with calcium channel blockers and monoclonal antibodies. Cancer Treat Res 48:73–95.
2. Biedler J (1994) Drug resistance: genotype versus phenotype—Thiry-second G.H.A. Clowes memorial lecture. Cancer Res 54:666–678.
3. Childs S, Ling V (1994) The MDR superfamily of genes and its biological implications. In VT DeVita Jr, S Hellman, SA Rosenberg, eds. Important Advances in Oncology. Philadelphia: J.B. Lippincott Co:21–36.
4. Goodnight J, Mischak H, Mushinski JF (1994) Selective involvement of protein kinase C isozymes in differentiation and neoplastic transformation. Adv Cancer Res 64:159–209.
5. Nishizuka Y (1986) Studies and perspectives of protein kinase C. Science 233:305–312.
6. Nishizuka Y (1992) Intracellular signalling by hydrolysis of phospholipids and activation of protein kinase C. Science 258:607–613.
7. Nishizuka Y (1988) The molecular heterogeneity of protein kinase C and its implications for cellular regulation. Nature 334:661–665.
8. Bradshaw T, Gescher A, Pettit GR (1992) Modulation by staurosporine of phorbol-ester-induced effects on growth and protein kinase C localization in A549 human lung-carcinoma cells. Int J Cancer 51:144–148.
9. Niedel JE, Kuhn L, Vanderbark GR (1983) Phorbol diester receptor copurifies with protein kinase C. Proc Natl Acad Sci (USA) 80:36–40.
10. O'Brian CA, Ward NE, Gravitt KR, Fan D (1994) The role of protein kinase C in multidrug resistance. In LJ Goldstein, RF Ozols, eds. Anticancer drug resistance: advances in molecular and clinical research. Norwell, MA: Kluwer Academic Publishers: 41–55.
11. Chambers TC, Chalikonda I, Eilon G (1990) Correlation of protein kinase C translocation, P-glycoprotein phosphorylation and reduced drug accumulation in multidrug resistant human KB cells. Biochem Biophys Res Comm 169:253–259.
12. Ma L, Marquardt D, Takemoto L, Center M (1991) Analysis of P-glycoprotein phosphorylatoin in HL 60 cells isolated for resistance to vincristine. J Biol Chem 266:5593–5599.
13. Aquino A, Warren BS, Omichinski J, Hartman KD, Glazer RI (1990) Protein Kinase C-γ is present in adriamycin resistant HL-60 leukemia cells. Biochem Biophys Res Commun 166:723–728.

14. Lee S, Karaszkiewicz J, Anderson WB (1992) Elevated level of nuclear protein kinase C in multidrug-resistant MCF-7 human breast carcinoma cells. Cancer Res 52:3750–3759.

15. Sugawara S, Kumano N, Saijo Y, Suzuki S, Numata Y, Sato G, Motomiya M (1992) Protein kinase C activity in human leukemia cell lines with reference to sensitivity to antineoplastic agents. Tohoku J Exp Med 168:393–396.

16. Blobe GC, Sachs CW, Khan WA, Fabbro D, Stabel S, Wetsel WC, Obeid LM, Fine RL, Hannun YA (1993) Selective regulation of expression of protein kinase C (PKC) isoenzymes in multidrug-resistance MCF-7 cells. J Biol Chem 268:658–664.

17. Yu G, Ahmad S, Aquino A, Fairchild C, Trepel JB, Ohno S, Suzuki K, Tsuruo T, Cowan KH, Glazer RI (1991) Transfection with protein kinase C-α confers increased multidrug resistance to MCF-7 cells expressing P-glycoprotein. Cancer Comm 3:181–189.

18. Ahmad S, Trepel JB, Ohno S, Suzuki K, Tsuruo T, Glazer RI (1992) Role of protein kinase C in the modulation of multidrug resistance: expression of the atypical γ isoform of protein kinase C does not confer increased resistance to doxorubicin. Mol Pharmacol 42:1004–1009.

19. Chaudhary P, Roninson I (1992) Activation of *MDR1* (P-glycoprotein) gene expression in human cells by protein kinase C agonists. Oncol Res 4:281–290.

20. Ferguson PJ, Cheng Y-c (1987) Transient protection of cultured human cells against antitumor agents by 12-O-tetradecanoylphorbol-13-acetate. Cancer Res 47:433–441.

21. Fine RL, Patel J, Chabner BA (1988) Phorbol esters induce multidrug resistance in human breast cancer cells. Proc Natl Acad Sci USA 85:582–586.

22. O'Brian C, Fan D, Ward N, Dong Z, Iwamoto L, Gupta K, Earnest L, Fidler I (1991) Transient enhancement of multidrug resistance by the bile acid deoxycholate in murine fibrosarcoma cells in vitro. Biochem Pharmacol 41:797–806.

23. Takeda Y, Nishio K, Sugimoto Y, Kasahara K, Kubo S, Fujiwara Y, Niitani H, Saijo N (1991) Establishment of a human leukemia subline resistant to the growth-inhibitory effect of 12-O-tetradecanoylphorbol 13-acetate (TPA) and showing non-P-glycoprotein-mediated multi-drug resistance. Int J Cancer 48:931–937.

24. Fan D, Fidler IJ, Ward N, Seid C, Earnest LE, Housey GM, O'Brian CA (1992) Stable expression of a cDNA encoding rat brain protein kinase C-βI confers a multidrug-resistant phenotype on rat fibroblasts. Cancer Res 52:661–668.

25. Banfi P, Parolini O, Lanzi C, Gambetta A (1992) Lipid peroxidation, phosphoinositide turnover and protein kinase C activation in humor platelets treated with anthracyclines and their complexes with Fe(III). Biochem Pharmacol 43:1521–1527.

26. Lanzi C, Gambetta RA, Perego P, Banfi P, Franzi A, Guazzoni L, Zunino F (1991) Protein kinase C activation by anthracyclines in swiss 3t3 cells. Int J Cancer 47:136–142.

27. Palayoor S, Stein JM, Hait WN (1987) Inhibition of protein kinase C by antineoplastic agents implications for drug resistance. Biochem Biophys Res Comm 148:718–725.

28. Rubin E, Kharbanda S, Gunji H, Weichselbaum R, Kufe D (1992) cis-Diamminedichloroplatinum (II) induces c-jun expression in human myloid leukemia cells: potential involvement of a protein kinase c-dependent signaling pathway. Cancer Res 52:878–882.

29. Goode N, Hughes K, Woodgett JR, Parker PJ (1992) Differential regulation of glycogen synthase kinase-3β by protein kinase C isotypes. J Biol Chem 267:16878–16882.

30. Basu A, Teicher BA, Lazo JS (1990) Involvement of protein kinase C in phorbol ester-induced sensitization of HeLa cells to cis-diamminedichloroplatinum (II). J Biol Chem 265:8451–8457.

31. Basu A, Kozikowski AP, Sato K, Lazo JS (1991) Cellular sensitization to cis-diamminedichloroplatinum (II) by novel analogues of the protein kinase C activator lyngbyatoxin a. Cancer Res 51:2511–2514.

32. Basu A, Lazo JS (1992) Sensitization of human cervical carcinoma cells to cis-diamminedichloroplatinum (II) by bryostatin 1. Cancer Res 52:3119–3124.

33. Basu A, Evans RW (1994) Comparison of effects of growth factors and protein kinase C activators on cellular sensitivity to cis-diamminedichloroplatinum (II). Int J Cancer 58:587–591.

34. Fan Z, Balsega J, Masui H, Mendelsohn J (1993) Antitumor effect of anti-epidermal growth factor receptor monoclonal antibodies plus cis-diamminedichloroplatinum on well establishede A431 cell xenografts. Cancer Res 53:4673–4642.

35. Schlessinger J (1986) Allosteric regulation of the epidermal growth factor receptor kinase. J Cell Biol 103:2067–2072.

36. Hofmann J, Doppler W, Jakob A, Maly K, Posch L, Uberall F, Grunicke HH (1988) Enhancement of the antiproliferative effect of cis-diamminedichloroplatinum (ii) and nitrogen mustard by inhibitors of protein kinase c. Int J Cancer 42:382–388.

37. Hofmann J, Fiebig H, Winterhalter BR, Berger DR, Grunicke H (1990) Enhancement of the anti-proliferative activity of cis-diamminedichloroplatinum (ii) by quercetin. Int J Cancer 45:536–539.

38. Perego P, Casati G, Gambetta RA, Soranzo C, Zunino F (1993) Effect of modulation of protein kinase C activity on cisplatin cytotoxicity in cisplatin-resistant and cisplatin-sensitive human osteosarcoma cells. Cancer Lett 72:53–58.

39. Grant S, Jarvis WD, Swerlow PS, Turner AJ, Traylor RS, Wallace HJ, Lin P-s, Pettit GR, Gewirtz DA (1992) Potentiation of the activity of 1-β-D-arabinofuranosylcytosine by the protein kinase C activator bryostatin 1 in HL-60 cells: association with enhanced fragmentation of mature DNA. Cancer Res 52:6270–6278.

40. Jarvis WD, Povirk LF, Turner AJ, Traylor RS, Gewirtz DA, Pettit GR, Grant S (1994) Effects of bryostatin 1 and other pharmacological activators of protein kinase C on 1-[beta-D-arabinofuranosyl]cytosine-induced apoptosis in HL-60 human promyelocytic leukemia cells. Biochem Pharmacol 47:839–852.

41. Hocevar B, Fields A (1991) Selective translocation of βII- protein kinase c to the nucleus of human promyelocytic (HL60) leukemia cells. J Biol Chem 266:28–33.

42. Dlugosz AA, Yuspa SH (1991) Staurosporine induces protein kinase C agonist effects and maturation of normal and neoplastic mouse keratinocytes in vitro. Cancer Res 51:4677–4684.

43. Kennedy M, Prestigiacomo L, Tyler G, May W, Davidson N (1992) Differential effects of bryostatin 1 and phorbol ester on human breast cancer cell lines. Cancer Res 52:1278–1283.

44. Stanwell C, Gescher A, Bradshaw TD, Pettit GR (1994) The role of protein kinase C isoenzymes in the growth inhibition caused by bryostatin 1 in human A549 lung and MCF-7 breast carcinoma cells. Int J Cancer 56:585–592.

45. Basu A (1993) The potential of protein kinase C as a target for anticancer treatment. Pharmacol Ther 59:257–280.

46. Pettit GR, Herald CL, Doubek DL, Herald DL (1982) Isolation and structure of bryostatin. J Amer Chem Soc 104:6846–6848.

47. Hornung RL, Pearson JW, Beckwith M, Longo DL (1992) Preclinical evaluation of bryostatin as an anticancer agent against several murine tumour cell lines: in vitro versus in vivo activity. Cancer Res 52:101–107.

48. Schuchter LM, Esa AH, May WS, Laulis MK, Pettit GR, Hess AD (1991) Successful treatment of murine melanoma with bryostatin 1. Cancer Res 51:682–687.

49. Kraft AS, Smith JB, Berkow RL (1986) Bryostatin, an activator of the calcium phospholipid-dependent protein kinase, blocks phorbol ester-induced differentiation of human promyelocytic leukemia cells HL-60. Proc Nat Acad Sci USA 83:1334–1338.

50. Kazanietz MG, Lewin NE, Gao F, Pettit GR, Blumberg PM (1994) Binding of [26-³H] bryostatin 1 and analogs to calcium-dependent and calcium-independent protein kinase C isozymes. Mol Pharmacol 46:374–379.

51. Stone RM, Sariban E, Pettit GR, Kufe DW (1988) Bryostatin 1 activates protein kinase C and induces monocytic differentiation in HL-60 cells. Blood 72:208–213.

52. Dale IL, Bradshaw TD, Gescher A, Pettit GR (1989) Comparison of effects of bryostatins 1 and 2 and 12-0-tetradecanoylphorbol-13-acetate on protein kinase C activity in A549 human lung carcinoma cells. Cancer Res 49:3242–3245.

53. Isakov N, Galron D, Mustelin T, Pettit GR, Altman A (1993) Inhibition of phorbol ester-induced T cell proliferation by bryostatin is associated with rapid degradation of protein kinase C. J Immunol 150:1195–1204.

54. Li F, Grant S, Pettit GR, McCrady CW (1992) Bryostatin 1 modulates the proliferation and lineage commitment of human myeloid progenitor cells exposed to recombinant interleukin-3 and recombinant granulocyte-macrophage colony-stimulating factor. Blood 80:2495–2502.

55. Tuttle TM, Inge TH, Bethke KP, McCrady CW, Pettit GR, Bear HD (1992) Activation and growth of murine tumor-specific T-cells which have in vivo activity with bryostatin 1. Cancer Res 52:548–553.

56. Kraft AS, William F, Pettit GR, Lilly MB (1989) Varied differentiation responses of human leukemias to brryostatin 1. Cancer Res 49:1287–1293.

57. Mohammad RM, Al-Katib A, Pettit GR, Sensenbrenner LL (1993) Differential effects of bryostatin 1 on human non-Hodgkin's B-lymphoma cell lines. Leuk Res 17:1–8.

58. Patella V, Casolaro V, Ciccarelli A, Pettit GR, Culumbo M, Marone G (1995) The antineoplastic bryostatins affect human basophils and mast cells differently. Blood 85:1272–1281.

59. Berkow RL, Schlabach L, Dodson R, Benjamin Jr WH, Pettit GR, Rustagi P, Kraft AS (1993) In

vivo administration of the anticancer agent bryostatin 1 activates platelets and neutrophils and modulates protein kinase C activity. Cancer Res 53:2810–2815.

60. Grant S, Jarvis WD, Turner AJ, Wallace HJ, Pettit GR (1992) Effects of bryostatin 1 and rGM-CSF on the metabolism of 1-B-D-arabinofuranosylcytosine in human leukemic myeloblasts. Br J Haematol 82:522–528.

61. Pommier Y, Kerrrigan D, Hartman KD, Glazer RI (1990) Phosphorylation of mammalian dna topoisomerase I and activation by protein kinase C. J Biol Chem 265:9418–9422.

62. Yalowich JC, Ritke MK, Allan WP, Murray NR, Fields AP (1995) Bryostatin 1 upregulates topoisomerase II phosphorylation and potentiates VP16 activity in VP-16 resistant K562 cells. Proc Amer Assoc Cancer Res 36:342 (abstr).

63. Philip PA, Rea D, Thavasu P, Carmichael J, Stuart NSA, Rockett H, Talbot DC, Ganesan T, Pettit GR, Balkwill F, Harris AL (1993) Phase I study of bryostatin 1: assessment of interleukin 6 and tumor necrosis factor alpha induction in vivo. The Cancer Research Campaign Phase I Committee [see comments]. J Natl Cancer Inst 85:1812–1818.

64. Prendiville J, Crowther D, Thatcher N, Woll PJ, Fox BW, McGown A, Testa N, Stern P, McDermott R, Potter M, Pettit GR (1993) A phase I study of intravenous bryostatin 1 in patients with advanced cancer. Br J Cancer 68:418–425.

65. Brinkmeier H, Jockusch H (1987) Activators of protein kinase C induce myotonia by lowering chloride conductance in muscle. Biochem Biophys Res Commun 148:1283–1289.

66. Scheid C, Prendiville J, Jayson G, Crowther D, Fox B, Pettit GR, Stern PL (1994) Immunomodulation in patients receiving intravenous Bryostatin 1 in a phase I clinical study: comparison with effects of Bryostatin 1 on lymphocyte function in vitro. Cancer Immunol Immunother 39:223–30.

67. David NA, Burgner PR (1956) Antibiot. Med 2:219.

68. Hinman JW, Caron EL, Hoeksema H (1957) The structure of novobiocin. J Amer Chem Soc 79:3789–3800.

69. Barrett-Bee K, Pinder P (1994) The accumulation of novobiocin in Escherichia coli and Staphilococcus aureus. J Antimicrobial Chemother 33:1165–1171.

70. Drlica K, Franco RJ (1988) Inhibitors of DNA topoisomerases. Biochemistry 27:2253–2259.

71. Fox N, Studzinski GP (1982) DNA dependence and inhibition by novobiocin and coumermycin of the nucleolar adenosine triphosphatase (ATPase) of human fibroblasts. J Histochem Cytochem 30:364–370.

72. Gellert M (1981) DNA topoisomerases. Ann Rev Biochem 50:879–910.

73. Cotten M, Bresnahan D, Thompson S, Chalkli R (1986) Novobiocin precipitates histones at concentrations normally used to inhibit eukaryotic type II topoisomerase. Nucl Acids Res 14:3671–3686.

74. Downes CS, Ord MJ, Mulligan AM, Collins ARS (1985) Novobiocin inhibition of DNA excision repair may occur through effects on mitochondrial structure and ATP metabolism, not on repair topoisomerases. Carcinogenesis 6:1343–1352.

75. Gottesfeld JM (1986) Novobiocin inhibits RNA polymerase III transcription in vitro by a mechanism distinct from topoisomerase II. Nucl Acids Res 14:2075–2088.

76. Constantinou A, Henning-Chubb C, Huberman E (1989) Novobiocin and phorbol 12-myristate 13-acetate-induced differentiation of human leukemia cells associated with a reduction in topoisomerase II activity. Cancer Res 49:1110–1117.

77. Nordenberg J, Albukrek D, Hadar T, Fux A, Wasserman L, Novogrodsky A, Sidi Y (1992) Novobiocin-induced anti-proliferative and differentiating effects in melanoma B16. Brit J Cancer 65:183–188.

78. Rappa G, Lorico A, Sartorelli AC (1990) Induction of the differentiation of WEHI-3B D+ monomyelocytic leukemic cells by inhibitors of topoisomerase II. Cancer Res 50:6723–6730.

79. Rius C, Zorrilla AR, Cabanas C, Mata F, Bernabeu C (1991) Differentiation of human promonocytic leukemia U-937 cells with DNA topisomerase II inhibitors: induction of vimentin gene expression. Mol Pharmacol 39:442–448.

80. Eder JP, Teicher BA, Holden SA, Cathcart KNS, Schnipper LE (1987) Novobiocin enhances alkylating agent cytotoxicity and DNA interstrand crosslinks in a murine model. J Clin Invest 79:1524–1528.

81. Eder JP, Teicher BA, Holden SA, Cathcart KNS, Schnipper LE, Frei EI (1989) Effects of novobiocin on the antitumor activity and tumor cell and bone marrow survivals of three alkylating agents. Cancer Res 49:595–598.

82. Eder JP, Wheeler CA, Teicher BA, Schnipper LE (1991) A phase I clinical trial of novobiocin, a modulator of alkylating agent cytotoxicity. Cancer Res 51:510–513.

83. Kennedy MJ, Armstrong DK, Huelskamp A, Ohly K, Clarke BV, Colvin OM, Grochow B, Chen T-L, Davidson NE (1995) Phase I and pharmacologic study of the alkylating agent modulator Novobiocin in combination with high-dose chemotherapy for the treatment of metastatic breast cancer. J Clin Oncol 13:1136–1143.

84. Ellis GK, Crowley J, Livingston RB, Goodwin JW, Hutchins L, Allen A (1991) Cisplatin and novobiocin in the treatment of non-small-cell lung cancer. A Southwest Oncology Group Study. Cancer 67:2969–2973.

85. Schwartz GN, Teicher BA, Eder JP Jr, Korbut T, Holden SA, Arra G, Herman TS (1993) Modulation of antitumor alkylating agents by novobiocin, topotecan, and lonidamine. Cancer Chemother Pharmacol 32:455–462.

86. Rappa G, Lorico A, Sartorelli AC (1992) Potentiation by novobiocin of the cytotoxic activity of etoposide (VP-16) and teniposide (VM-26). Int J Cancer 51:780–787.

87. Rappa G, Lorico A, Sartorelli AC (1993) Reversal of etoposide resistance in non-P-glycoprotein expressing multidrug resistant tumor cell lines by novobiocin. Cancer Res 53:5487–5493.

88. Lorico A, Rappa G, Sartorelli AC (1992) Novobiocin-induced accumulation of etoposide (VP-16) in WEHI-3B D⁺ leukemia cells. Int J Cancer 52:903–909.

89. Yang JM, Hait WN (1991) Use of multidrug resistant L1210 cell line for in vitro and in vivo drug screenig. Proc Am Assoc Cancer Res (abstr) 32:364.

90. Cole SP, Bhardwaj G, Gerlach JH, Mackie JE, Grant CE, Almquist KC, Stewart AJ, Kurz EU, Duncan AM, Deeley RG (1992) Overexpression of a transporter gene in a multidrug resistant human lung cancer cell line. Science 258:1650–1654.

91. Yalowich JC, Ross WE (1985) Verapamil-induced augmentation of etoposide accumulation in L1210 cells in vitro. Cancer Res 47:1010–1015.

92. Ozols RF, Cunnion RE, Klecker RW Jr, Hamilton TC, Ostchega Y, Parrillo JE, Young RC (1987) Verapamil and adriamycin in the treatment of drug-resistant ovarian cancer patients. J Clin Oncol 5:641–647.

93. Akiyama SI, Fojo A, Hanover JA, Pastan I, Gottesman MM (1985) Isolation and genetic characterizaion of human KB cell lines resistant to multiple drugs. Somatic Cell Mol Genet 11:117–126.

94. Ford JM, Bruggemann EP, Pastan I, Gottesman MM, Hait WN (1990) Cellular and biochemical characterization of thioxanthenes for reversal of multidrug resistance in human and murine cell lines. Cancer Res 50:1748–1756.

95. Van der Graaf WTA, De Vries EGE, Uges DRA, Nanninga AG, Meijer C, Vellenga E, Mulder POM, Mulder NH (1991) In vitro and in vivo modulation of multi-drug resistance with amiodarone. Int J Cancer 48:616–622

96. Rappa G, Lorico A, Murren JR, Anderson S, Sartorelli AC (1995) Clinical evaluation of the modulation of the antitumor activity of VP-16 by novobiocin (Novo) in human tumors. Proc Am Assoc Cancer Res 36:291.

97. Willson JKV, Fischer PH, Tutsch K, Alberti D, Simon K, Hamilton RD, Bruggink J, Koeller JM, Tormey DC, Earhart RH, Ranhosky A, Trump DL (1988) Phase I clinical trial of a combination of dipyridamole and acivicin based upon inhibition of nucleoside salvage. Cancer Res 48:5585–5590.

98. Willson JKV, Fischer PH, Remick SC, Tutsch KD, Grem JL, Nieting L, Alberti D, Bruggink J, Trump DL (1989) Methotrexate and dipyridamole combination chemotherapy based upon inhibition of nucleoside salvage in humans. Cancer Res 49:1866–1870.

99. Chan T, Howell S (1985) Mechanism of synergy between N-phospphonacetyl-L-aspartate and dipyridamole in a human ovarian carcinoma cell line. Cancer Res 45:3598–3604

100. Remick SC, Grem JL, Fischer PH, Tutsch KD, Alberti DB, Nieting LM, Tombes MB, Bruggink J, Willson JKV, Trump DL (1990) Phase I trial of 5-fluorouracil and dipyridamole administered by seventy-two-hour concurrent continuous infusion. Cancer Res 50:2667–2672.

101. Grem JL, Fischer PH (1989) Enhancement of 5-fluorouracil's anticancer activity by dipyridamole. Pharmacol Ther 40:349–371.

102. Weber G (1983) Biochemical strategy of cancer cells and the design of chemotherapy. Cancer Res 43:3466–3492.

103. Grem J, Fischer H (1986) Alteration of fluorouracil metabolism in human colon cancer cells by dipyridamole with a selective increase in fluorodeoxyuridine monophosphate levels. Cancer Res 46:6191–6199.

104. Isonishi S, Kirmani S, Kim S, Plaxe SC, Braly PS, McClay EF, Howell SB (1991) Phase I and pharmacokinetic trial of intraperitoneal etoposide in combination with the multidrug-resistance-modulating agent dipyridamole. J Natl Cancer inst 83:621–626.

105. Bailey H, Wilding G, Tutsch KD, Arzoomanian RZ, Alberti D, Tombes MB, Grem JL, Spriggs

DR (1992) A phase I trial of 5-fluorouracil, leucovorin, and dipyridamole given by concurrent 120-h continuous infusions. Cancer Chemother Pharmacol 30:297–302.

106. Budd GT, Jayaraj A, Grabowski D, Adelstein D, Bauer L, Boyett J, Bukowski R, Murthy S, Weick J (1990) Phase I trial of dipyridamole with 5-fluorouracil and folinic acid. Cancer Res 50:7206–7211.

107. Buzaid AC, Alberts DS, Einspahr J, Mosley K, Peng Y-M, Tutsch K, Spears CP, Garewal HS (1989) Effect of dipyridamole on fluorodeoxyuridine cytocicity in vitro and in cancer patients. Cancer Chemother. Pharmacol 25:124–130.

108. Grem JL, Fischer PH (1985) Augmentation of 5-fluorouracil cytotoxicity in human colon cancer cells by dipyridamole. Cancer Res 45:2967–2972.

109. Howell SB, Hom DK, Sanga R, Vick JS, Chan TCK (1989) Dipyridamole enhancement of etoposide sensitivity. Cancer Res 49:4147–4153.

110. Kusumoto H, Maehara Y, Anai H, Kumashiro R, Sugimachi K (1991) Dipyridamole potentiates adriamycin cytotoxicity by a mechanism other than inhibiting nucleoside uptake. Anticancer Res 11:1539–1542.

111. Jekunen A, Vick J, Sanga R, Chan TCK, Howell SB (1992) Synergism between dipyridamole and cisplatin in human carcinoma cells in vitro. Cancer Res 52:3566–3571.

112. Kusumoto H, Maehara Y, Anai H, Kusumoto T, Sugimachi K (1988) Potentiation of adriamycin cytotoxicity by dippyridamole against HeLa cells in vitro and sarcoma 180 cells in vivo. Cancer Res 48:1208–1212.

113. Damle BD, Sridhar R, Desai PB (1994) Dipryridamole modulates multidrug resistance and intracellular as well as nuclear levels of doxorubicin in B16 melanoma cells. Int J Cancer 56:113–118.

114. Howell SB, Hom D, Sanga R, Vick JS, Abramson IS (1989) Comparison of the synergistic potentiation of etoposide, doxorubicin, and vinblastine cytotoxicity by dipyridamole. Cancer Res 49:3178–3183.

115. Hirose M, Takeda E, Ninomiya T, Kuroda Y, Miyao M (1987) Synergistic inhibitory effects of dipyridamole and vincristine on the growth of human leukaemia and lymphoma cells. Br J Cancer 56:413–417.

116. Ford JM, Prozialeck WC, Hait WN (1989) Structural features determining activity of phenothiazines and related drugs for inibition of cell growth and reversal of multidrug resistance. Mol Pharmacol 35:105–115.

117. Shalinsky DR, Andreeff M, Howell SB (1990) Modulation of drug sensitivity by dipyridamole in multidrug resistant cells in vitro. Cancer Res 50:7573–7543.

118. Goel R, Cleary SM, Horton C, Balis FM, Zimm S, Kirmani S, Howell SB (1989) Selective intraperitoneal biochemical modulation of methotrexate by dipyridamole. J Clin Oncol 7:262–269.

119. Ramu N, Ramu A (1989) Circumvention of adriamycin resistance by dipyridamole analogues: a structure-activity relationship study. Int J Cancer 43:487–491.

120. Chen H-x, Bamberger U, Heckel A, Guo X, Cheng Y-c (1993) BIBW 22, a dipyridamole analogue, acts as a bifunctional modulator on tumor cells by influencing both P-glycoprotein and nucleoside transport. Cancer Res 53:1974–1977.

121. Gaj CL, Anyanwutaku IO, Cole SC, Chang Y, Cheng Y-c (1995) Reversal of multidrug resistance associated protein mediated multidrug resistance in human carcinoma cell lines by the l/enatiomer of verapamil. Proc Amer Assoc Cancer Res 36:346 (abstr).

122. Chen H-x, Rhee DK, Heckel A, Bamberger U, Cheng Y-c (1994) Biochemical studies of BIBW 22, a bifunctional modulator for nucleoside transport and p-glycoprotein function. Proc Amer Assoc Cancer Res 35:361 (abstr).

123. Chen H-x, Bamberger U, Heckel A, Rhee D, Cheng Y-c (1995) Differential mechanisms of BIBW 22 in modulating multidrug-resistant phenotype and in inhibiting nucleoside transport. Proc Amer Assoc Cancer Res 36:372 (abstr).

124. Boven E, Jansen W, Van Telligen O, Beijnen J, Pinedo H (1995) Modulation of vincristine (VCR) concentrations by dexnigulpine or BIBW22S in tissues of tumor-bearing mice. Proc Amer Assoc Cancer Res 36:341 (abstr).

125. Jansen WJM, Pinedo HM, Kuiper CM, Lincke C, Bamberger U, Heckel A, Boven E (1994) Biochemical modulation of "classical" multidrug resistance by BIBW22S, a potent derivative of dipyridamole. Ann Oncol 5:733–739.

126. Karpatkin S, Pearlstein E (1981) Role of platelets in tumor cell metastases. Ann Int Med 95:636–641.

127. Sakaguchi Y, Emi Y, Maehara Y, Kohnoe S, Sugimachi K (1990) Combined treatment of

adriamycin and dipyridamole inhibits lung metastasis of B16 melanoma cells in mice. Eur Surg Res 22:213–218.

128. Tzanakakis GN, Agarwal KC, Vezeridis MP (1992) Prevention of human pancreatic cancer cell induced hepatic metastasis in nude mice by dipyridamole and its analog RA-233. Cancer 71:2466–2471.

129. Floridi A, Paggi MG, Marcante ML, Silvestrini B, Caputo A, De Martino C (1981) Lonidamine, a selective inhibitor of aerobic glycolysis of murine tumor cells. J Natl Cancer Inst 66:497–499.

130. Floridi A, Paggi MC, D'Atri S, De Martino C, Marcante ML, Silvestrini B, Caputo A (1981) Effect of lonidamine on the energy metabolism of Ehrlich ascites tumor cells. Cancer Res 41:4661–4666.

131. Arancia G, Malorni W, Crateri Trovalusci P, Isacchi G, Giannella G, De Martino C (1988) Differential effect of lonidamine on the plasma membrane of normal and leukemic human lymphocytes. Exper Mol Pathol 48:37–47.

132. De Martino C, Malorni W, Accinni L, Rosati F, Nista A, Formisano G, Silvestrini B, Arancia G (1987) Cell membrane changes induced by lonidamine in human erythrocytes and T lymphocytes, and Ehrlich ascites tumor cells. Exp Mol Pathol 46:15–30.

133. Teicher BA, Herman TS, Hoden SA, Epelbaum R, Liu S, Frei E (1991) Lonidamine as a modulator of alkylating agent activity in vitro and in vivo. Cancer Res 51:780–784.

134. Hahn GM, van Kersen I, Silverstrini B (1984) Inhibition of the recovery from potentially lethal damage by lonidamine. Br J Cancer 50:657–660.

135. Kim JH, Alfieri AA, Kim SH, Young CW (1986) Potentiation of radiation effects on two murine tumors by lonidamine. Cancer Res 46:1120–1123.

136. Raaphorst GP, Feeley MM, Heller DP, Danjoux CE, Martin L, Maroun JA, De Sanctis AJ (1990) Lonidamine can enhance the cytotoxic effect of cisplatin in human tumour cells and rodent cells. Anticancer Res 10:923–928.

137. Zupi G, Greco C, Laudonio N, Benassi M, Silvestrini B, Caputo A (1986) In vitro and in vivo potentiation by lonidamine of the antitumor effect to adriamycin. Anticancer Res 6:1245–1250.

138. Kaplan O, Navon G, Lyon RC, Faustino PJ, Straka EJ, Cohen JS (1990) Effects of 2-deoxyglucose on drug sensitive and drug resistant human breast cancer cells: toxicity and magnetic resonance spectroscopy studies of metabolism. Cancer Res 50:544–551.

139. Citro G, Cucco C, Verdina A, Zupi G (1991) Reversal of adriamycin resistance by lonidamine in a human breast cancer cell line. Br J Cancer 64:534–536.

140. Band PR, Maroun J, Pritchard K, Stewart D, Coppin CM, Wilson K, Eisenhauer EA (1986) Phase II study of lonidamine in patients with metastatic breast cancer: a National Cancer Institute of Canada Clinical Trials Group Study. Cancer Treat Rep 70:1305–1310.

141. Robustelli della Cuna G, Pedrazzoli P (1991) Toxicity and clinical tolerance of lonidamine. Semin Oncol 18 (Suppl 4):18–22.

142. Murray N, Shah A, Band P (1987) Phase II study of lonidamine in patients with small cell carcinoma of the lung. Cancer Treat Rep 71:1283–1284.

143. Pronzato P, Amoroso D, Bertelli G, Conte PF, Cusimano MP, Ciottoli GB, Gulisano M, Lionetto R, Rosso R (1989) Phase II study of lonidamine in metastatic breast cancer. Br J Cancer 59:251–253.

144. Robins HI, Neuberg DS, Benson AB, Pandya KJ, Tormey DC (1990) Phase II study of lonidamine in patients with metastatic breast cancer. Invest New Drugs 8:397–399.

145. Weinerman BH, Eisenhauer EA, Besner JG, Coppin CM, Stewart D, Band PR (1986) Phase II trial of lonidamine in patients with metastatic renal cell carcinoma. A National Cancer Institute of Canada Clinical Trial Group Study. Cancer 70:751–754.

146. Dogliotti L, Berruti A, Buniva T, Zola P, Bau MG, Farris A, Sarobba MG, Bottini A, Arquati P, Deltetto F, Gosso P, Monzeglio C, Moro G, Sussio M, Perroni D (1994) High-dose epirubicin vs high-dose epirubicin + lonidamine in advanced breast cancer. Proc Amer Soc Clin Oncol 13:58 (abstr).

147. Dogliotti L, Berruti A, Buniva T, Zola P, Bau MG, Farris A, Sarobba MG, Bottini A, Arquati P, Deltetto F, Gosso P, Monzeglio C, Moro G, Sussio M, Perroni D (1994) A randomized comparison of high dose epirubicin versus high dose epirubicin plus lonidamine in advanced breast cancer patients. First results from a cooperative group study. Int J Oncol 4:747–752.

148. Calabresi F, Marolla P, Di Lauro L, Curcio CG, Paoletti G, Lombardi A, Giannarelli D, Ballatore P, Foggi C, Di Palma M, Stolfi R, Cortesi E (1994) Lonidamine as a potentiating agent of the FAC regimen in the treatment of advanced breast cancer. Results of a multicentric clinical study. Int J Oncol 4:753–760.

149. Calabresi F (1994) Drug resistance: lonidamine. Principles & Prac. Oncol PPO Updates 8:1–15.
150. Lorusso V, Catino A, Brandi M, Piano A, Palomba G, Forcignano R, Mazzotta S, Musca F, Serravezza G, Durini E, Contillo A, Pezzella G, Pallazzo S, Chetri C, De Lena M (1994) Cyclophosphamide, mitoxantrone and fluorouracil versus Cyclophosphamide, mitoxantrone and fluorouracil plus lonidamine for the treatment of advanced breast cancer. A multicentric randomized clinical trial. Int J Oncol 4:767–772.
151. Pacini P, Algeri R, Rinaldini M, Guarnieri A, Bastiani P, Barsanti G, Neri B, Marzano S, Tucci E (1994) FEC (fluorouracil, epirubicin and cyclophosphamide) versus EM (epirubicin and mitomycin-C) with or without lonidamine as first line treatment for advanced breast cancer. A multicentric randomized study. Preliminary report. Int J Oncol 4:761–766.
152. Rosso R, Gardin G, Pronzato P, Camoriano A, Merlini L, Naso C, Rosso M, Barone C, Nascimben O, Ianniello G, Sturba F, Contu A, Baldini E, Giannessi PG, Conte PF (1993) The role of lonidamine in the treatment of breast cancer patients. Ann NY Acad Sci 698:349–356.
153. Buccheri G, Ferrigno D (1994) A randomized trial of MACC chemotherapy with or without lonidamine in advanced non-small cell lung cancer. Eur J Cancer 30A:1424–1431.
154. Orlandi L, Zaffaroni N, Gornati D, Veneroni S, Silvestrini R (1994) Potentiation of cisplatin cytotoxicity by lonidamine in primary culture of human ovarian cancer. Anticancer Res 14:1161–1164.
155. Brandi M, Lorusso V, de Mitrio A, Fioretto A, Giannuzzi A, de Lena M (1994) Cisplatin (CDDP) plus lonidamine (LND) in advanced ovarian cancer pretreated with CDDP or carboplatin (CBDCA). Anticancer Res 5 (Suppl 1):65 (abstr).
156. Gadducci A, Brunetti I, Muttini M, Fanucchi A, Dargenio F, Giannessi P, Conte P (1994) Epidoxorubicin and lonidamine in refractory of recurrent epithelial ovarian cancer. Eur J Cancer 30A:1432–1435.
157. Colella E, Merlano M, Blengio F, Angelini F, Ausili Cefaro GP, Scasso F, Lo Russo V, Cirulli S, Giannarelli D, Cognetti F (1994) Randomized phase II study of methotrexate (MTX) versus methotresxate plus lonidamine (MTX + LND) in recurrent and/or metastatic carcinoma of the head and neck. Eur J Cancer 30A:928–930.
158. Magno L, Terraneo F, Bertoni F, Tordiglione M, Bardelli D, Rosignoli MT, Ciottoli GB (1994) Double-blind randomized study of lonidamine and radiotherapy in head and neck cancer. Int J Radiat Oncol Biol Phys 29:45–55.
159. Privitera G, Ciottoli GB, Patane C, Palmucci T, Tafuri G, Marletta F, De Luca B, Magani F, De Gregorio M, Greco S (1987) Phase II double-blind randomized study of lonidamine and radiotherapy in epidermoid carcinoma of the lung. Radiother Oncol 10:285–290.
160. Scarantino CW, McCunniff AJ, Evans G, Young CW, Paggiarino DA (1994) a prospective randomized comparison of radiation therapy plus lonidamine versus radiation therapy plus placebo as initial treatment of clinically localized but nonresectable nonsmall cell lung cancer. Int J Radiat Oncol Biol Phys 29:999–1004.
161. Stewart DJ, Eapen L, Girard A, Verma S, Genest P, Evans WK (1993) Phase II study of lonidamine plus radiotherapy in the treatment of brain metastases. J Neurooncol 15:19–22.
162. Carapella CM, Paggi MG, Calvosa F, Cattani F, Floridi A, Jandolo B, Raus L, Riccio A (1991) The potential role of lonidamine in the combined treatment of malignant gliomas. A randomized stufy. Dev Oncol 66:205–207.
163. Newell DR, Mansi J, Hardy J, Button D, Jenns K, Smith IE, Picollo R, Cantanese B (1991) The pharmacokinetics of oral lonidamine in breast and lung cancer patients. Semin Oncol 18(suppl 4):11–17.
164. Young CW, Currie VE, Kim JH, O'Hehir MA, Farag FM, Kinahan JE (1984) Phase I and clinical pharmacologic evaluation of lonidamine in patients with advanced cancer. Oncology 41(suppl 1):60–65.
165. Besner J-G, Leclaire R, Band PR, Deschamps M, De Sanctis AJ, Catanese B (1984) Pharmacokinetics of lonidamine after oral administration in cancer patients. Oncology 41(Suppl 1):48–52.
166. Gatzemeier U, Toomes H, Picollo R, Christoffel V, Lucker PW, Ulmer J (1991) Single- and multiple dose pharmacokinetics of lonidamine in patients suffering from non-small-cell lung cancer. Arzneim-Forsch 41:436–439.
167. Franchi F, Seminara P, Codacci Pisanelli G, Pagani Guazzugli Bonaiuti V, Giovagnorio F, Gualdi G (1994) Elevated doses of carmustine and mitomycin C, with lonidamine enhancement and autologous bone marrow transplantation in the treatment of advanced colorectal cancer: results from a pilot study. Eur J Cancer 30A:1420–1423.
168. Hait WN, Aftab DT (1992) Rational design and pre-clinical pharmacology of drugs for reversing multidrug resistance. Biochem Pharmacol 43:103–107.

Index

Lightning Source UK Ltd.
Milton Keynes UK
UKOW06n1138040515

250837UK00008B/140/P